6th EDITION

Modules for Basic Nursing Skills

VOLUME II

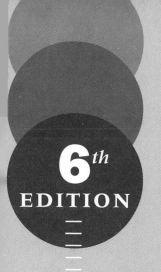

6th
EDITION

Modules for Basic Nursing Skills

VOLUME II

Janice Rider Ellis, RN, PhD

Elizabeth Ann Nowlis, RN, EdD

Patricia M. Bentz, RN, MSN

Shoreline Community College • Seattle, Washington

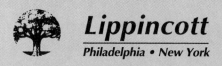

Lippincott
Philadelphia • New York

Sponsoring Editor: Mary P. Gyetvan, RN, MSN
Coordinating Editorial Assistant: Susan M. Keneally
Project Editor: Erika Kors
Design Coordinator: Melissa Olson
Production Manager: Helen Ewan
Production Coordinator: Nannette Winski
Indexer: Anne Cope

6th Edition

Library of Congress Cataloging in Publication Data

Ellis, Janice Rider.
    Modules for basic nursing skills / Janice Rider Ellis,
Elizabeth Ann Nowlis, Patricia M. Bentz. — 6th ed.
      p. cm.
    Includes bibliographical references and indexes.
    ISBN 0-397-55171-1 (v. 1 : alk. paper). — ISBN 0-397-
55170-3 (v. 2 : alk. paper)
    1. Nursing—Outlines, syllabi, etc. 2. Nursing—
Problems, exercises, etc. I. Nowlis, Elizabeth Ann.
II. Bentz, Patricia M. III. Title.
    [DNLM: 1. Nursing—programmed instruction.
WY 18.2 E47m 1996]
RT52.E44 1996
610.73'076—dc20
DNLM/DLC
for Library of Congress   95-37176
                      CIP

9 8 7 6 5 4 3 2 1

CONTENTS

☰ LIST OF SKILLS

The following skills are included in this volume. For easy reference, a module number and a page number are provided for each skill.

TO THE INSTRUCTOR

The sixth edition of *Modules for Basic Nursing Skills* continues to provide a resource for students to learn basic skills and procedures. We have used the same nursing-process-oriented, self-instructional approach that has proven valuable in previous editions, while improving visual appeal through the use of two colors.

In preparing this edition, we have tried to look at our instructions and directions from a student's standpoint. We have tried to clarify the new language of healthcare that students are learning at the same time they are mastering skills. We recognize that the formal, official terms used for equipment and skills are not always the same as the "shorthand" that students will hear in a clinical setting. Therefore, we have provided both sets of terms in many instances.

As more students enter the college setting with varied educational backgrounds, language and reading levels become ever more important. In a skills text, perhaps more than anywhere else, the focus must be on clear, straightforward language. We are grateful for the responses of our students in helping us with this task.

COMPREHENSIVE SKILLS COVERAGE

There are now 58 modules in two volumes. Volume 1 contains the most basic skills and is appropriate by itself for some courses enrolling nursing assistants. Volumes 1 and 2 together are most useful in programs for LPN/LVN and RN students although the LPN/LVN will not use all of them. Because programs vary considerably from state to state and from institution to institution, we have tried to make the two volumes as adaptable as possible to many different programs by offering comprehensive coverage of nursing skills.

ORGANIZATION

The modules are organized into units that reflect broad concepts of nursing care. This structured presentation will help the student understand how individual skills relate to particular human needs and to the nursing process. The first unit focuses on skills that students must master in order to deal safely and effectively with patients. As in the previous edition, throughout the two volumes skills are arranged in a progression from simple to complex, but each module is self-contained so that skills can be omitted or reordered according to the needs of particular programs.

SELF-INSTRUCTIONAL FORMAT

By consistently emphasizing the nursing process and appropriately highlighting rationale, the format of the modules focuses on the student's practice and mastery of skills and procedures. The elaborate program of features is designed to encourage understanding, independent learning, and self-instruction.

Module Contents

An outline of the module contents helps the student identify the information and specific skills that are included in the module.

Prerequisites

The list of prerequisites lets the student know what other modules and significant material are essential to successful completion of the particular module. This information is especially helpful when the order of modules is adjusted to meet the needs of individual nursing programs. It can also be used advantageously by the student who wishes to prepare for a particular patient-care situation.

Overall Objective

A general statement of the overall objective concisely describes what the student can expect to learn in the module.

Specific Learning Objectives

Arranged in tabular form, the outline of learning objectives previews the important steps in the skill and indicates what basic knowledge and application of knowledge are required in addition to psychomotor skills.

Learning Activities

The learning activities provide additional guidance to the student about what steps to take in order to accomplish the desired objectives. Note that each module directs the student to prepare as if planning to *teach* the skill to others. Because teaching is so integral to the nursing role, we believed students should consider that from the start.

Vocabulary

A list of key terms for each skill is provided. These terms are defined in the glossary at the back of each volume.

MODULE CORE

The discussion of each procedure includes necessary background information and step-by-step instructions, with carefully chosen photographs and technically precise illustrations.

Instructions are presented in a nursing process format when the skill is one that is used with patients and when the nursing process is appropriate to the skill. The steps in the process—Assessment, Planning, Implementation, and Evaluation—are clearly delineated by headings. This emphasis reinforces for students the fact that nursing process is relevant to practice. Nursing diagnoses are not included in the procedure itself. Where appropriate, the nursing diagnoses for which the particular skill might be used are presented in a separate display.

Documentation is included with every skill. The increasing emphasis on documentation for both evaluative and legal reasons makes the learning of correct documentation essential. Our premise is that although systems differ in *how* documentation is done, *what* needs to be documented is fairly standard. We have included specific examples of flow sheets and progress notes (in narrative, SOAP, and focus formats) to help students make the transition to the record system they will be asked to use.

Rationale for the use of each skill is explained at the beginning of every module. Rationale for the specific actions that are part of the procedure is emphasized throughout the discussion by the use of italic type.

Because the approach to many skills is the same, whenever possible a general procedure for a group of specific procedures has been identified. The purpose of this is to facilitate the student's ability to transfer basic principles from one situation to another. We have tried to do this in a way that does not create confusion and that can be followed when practicing the skill.

Illustrations were carefully chosen to help the students as they work through the module independently. We have expanded the examples of charting and have placed the examples of nursing progress notes on chart facsimiles to help the student transfer knowledge to the actual clinical setting.

A glove icon, new in the sixth edition, reminds the nursing student to wear gloves for procedures requiring Standard Precautions. To provide consistency and easy readability, we use this icon for the appropriate procedures that are formatted according to the nursing process. This does not imply that gloves are not required in other situations mentioned in the book.

Critical Thinking Exercises

Skill development for the nurse must constantly be framed within the context of the individual patient. In order to focus on this important concept, we have added critical thinking exercises to each module. These exercises assist the student in placing the skills into the context of providing nursing care for each unique patient. Students are asked to consider a patient situation that has problematic aspects and to determine needs, priorities, or approaches that would be appropriate for the particular patient. There are no "right" answers to these situations. They might form the basis for a discussion, for a written paper, or for personal thoughtful study.

References

The references given are to research data regarding the skill or the recommendations of an authoritative agency such as the Centers For Disease Control and Prevention (CDC). The most recent research is cited. In the case of skills, this research may be older than expected. For example, the many excellent studies on the procedure and timing used for taking temperatures were done 10 years ago, but remain the basis for current recommendations. The CDC change their recommendations only when their decision-making bodies determine that the data warrant a change.

Unfortunately, there is little research data to support many of the nursing techniques used. Therefore, you will also note an emphasis within the modules on consulting policy and procedure manuals in institutions. These are generally established by groups of nurses working together with legal as well as healthcare goals in mind. Learning to use the official policy and procedure manual will be an asset both to the student and to the practicing nurse.

Performance Checklist

The performance checklist follows the nursing process approach and can be used for quick review and for evaluation of the student's performance in terms of psychomotor skills. To facilitate review and evaluation, all steps of each procedure, including those that are first presented as part of a general procedure, are outlined in the performance checklist. In the sixth edition, the format of the performance checklist has been modified to allow more space for feedback.

Quiz

A self-test is provided at the end of each module to allow students to test their mastery of the material in the module. The quizzes may also be used by instructors for evaluation purposes.

Glossary

The terms in the vocabulary lists are defined in the glossary at the back of each volume. The glossaries are a convenient reference source for students.

The glossary defines terms within the context in which they are used in nursing and healthcare. This is particularly useful for the beginning student who often finds that words have special connotations in nursing and healthcare that are not included in the traditional dictionary definition.

Answers to Quizzes

Answers to the quizzes are given at the end of each volume.

Index

An index is provided at the back of each volume.

CONVENIENT PACKAGING

The pages of both volumes are three-hole punched and perforated, so students can either tear them out and hand them in or keep them in notebooks.

TESTING SUPPLEMENT

A test bank accompanying Volumes 1 and 2 includes multiple-choice questions for all the skills that are covered.

Modules for Basic Nursing Skills, Volumes 1 and 2, Sixth Edition, can be used in conjunction with the text by Ellis and Nowlis, *Nursing: A Human Needs Approach*, Fifth Edition, which treats the theory behind nursing practice. However, the two volumes of modules are designed to stand alone and can be used by themselves in a course addressing nursing skills. *Modules for Basic Nursing Skills* can also be used in conjunction with any other text covering nursing theory or fundamentals.

ACKNOWLEDGMENTS

We would like to thank the following individuals for their reviews of the manuscript at various stages and for their many useful suggestions:

Suzanna Johnson, MSN, ARNP
Skills Laboratory Coordinator
Shoreline Community College
Seattle, WA

Janet T. Barrett, PhD, RN
Director, BSN Program
Deaconess College of Nursing
St. Louis, MO

Marty Carlson, RN, MSN, MEd
Instructor
Life Sciences Division
Parkland College
Champaign, IL

Vicki Christenson, RNC, MN
Pediatric Nursing Faculty
Intercollegiate Nursing Center
Spokane, WA

Judy Davy, RN, BSN, FNP
Professor of Nursing
Department of Nursing
Humboldt State University
Arcata, CA

Marilyn Deig, RN, MSN
Instructor
Indiana Vocational Technical College—Evansville
Evansville, IN

Latrell Fowler, RN, PhD
Instructor
Medical University of South Carolina Satellite
at Francis Marion University
Florence, SC

Gay Greaves, RN, BNSc, MEd, EdD
Assistant Professor
Queens University School of Nursing
Kingston, Ontario

Karen Halbasch, RN, EdD
Associate Professor
Department of Nursing
Community College of Philadelphia
Philadelphia, PA

Joyce Ann Harney, RNC, CNA, MSN
Director of Health & Human Services
Ivy Tech State College
Columbus, IN

Genevieve A. Harris, RN, MSN
Assistant Professor of Nursing
Richard J. Daley College
Chicago, IL

Elizabeth Krekorian, PhD, RN
President/CEO
Deaconess College of Nursing
St. Louis, MO

Mary C. Shoemaker, PhD, RN
Associate Professor, Level I Coordinator
Saint Francis Medical Center
College of Nursing
Peoria, IL

Barbara Taylor, RN, MSN
ADN Instructor
Chipola Junior College
Marianna, FL

Bonnie Young, RN, BSN
Lead Instructor
Sharon Regional Health System
School of Nursing
Sharon, PA

We are especially grateful to all our students and colleagues who used the modules as they were originally written, worked through the changes made for the first five editions, and assisted in the planning of this revision. Their constant feedback has been essential to us.

J.R.E.
E.A.N.
P.M.B.

TO THE STUDENT

The modules in these two volumes are designed to enable you to learn the procedures that are basic to your role as a healthcare provider. Each module contains the following parts, unless they are not applicable to a particular skill:

Module Contents

The outline of the module contents provides you with an overview of all the information and specific skills contained in the module. Often a module contains several skills, and these will all be listed in the contents.

Prerequisites

The list of prerequisites describes the specific skills or abilities needed to master the new skill and indicates other modules that contain information necessary to an understanding of the skill.

Overall Objective

A general statement of the overall objective describes the basic skill that is taught in the module.

Specific Learning Objectives

A table of specific learning objectives breaks down the basic skill you are studying into specific subskills on which you can test yourself after completing the module.

Learning Activities

The learning activities are designed to help you progress safely and gradually into performing the new skill. Practice, in whatever setting is available, is essential to skillful performance. The amount of practice needed by each student will differ, depending on manual dexterity and previous experience. If your school provides audiovisual aids to use with the module, view them after reading the module but before actually practicing the skill. Do not hesitate to contact your instructor if you encounter difficul-

ties. Note that you are asked to study as if planning to *teach* the skill. Teaching others to provide care for self, family, and others is an integral part of the nursing role.

Vocabulary

The vocabulary list gives key terms used in the module. A glossary at the back of each volume gives the definitions of these terms, though some are best understood in the context of the module itself.

Module Core

The discussion of each procedure includes necessary background information and step-by-step instructions, with carefully chosen photographs and technically precise illustrations.

Instructions are presented in a nursing process format when the skill is one that is used with patients and when the nursing process is appropriate to the skill. The steps in the process—Assessment, Planning, Implementation, and Evaluation—are clearly delineated by headings. This emphasis reinforces for students the fact that nursing process is relevant to practice. Nursing diagnoses are not included in the procedure itself. Where appropriate, the nursing diagnoses for which the particular skill might be used are presented in a separate display.

Documentation is included with every skill. The increasing emphasis on documentation for both evaluative and legal reasons makes the learning of correct documentation essential. Our premise is that although systems differ in *how* documentation is done, *what* needs to be documented is fairly standard. We have included specific examples of flow sheets and progress notes (in narrative, SOAP, and focus formats) to help students make the transition to the record system they will be asked to use.

Rationale for the use of each skill is explained at the beginning of every module. Rationale for the specific actions that are part of the procedure is emphasized throughout the discussion by the use of italic type.

Because the approach to many skills is the same,

xiii

whenever possible a general procedure for a group of specific procedures has been identified. The purpose of this is to facilitate the student's ability to transfer basic principles from one situation to another. We have tried to do this in a way that does not create confusion and that can be followed when practicing the skill.

A glove icon, new in the sixth edition, reminds the nursing student to wear gloves for procedures requiring Standard Precautions. To provide consistency and easy readability, we use this icon for the appropriate procedures that are formatted according to the nursing process. This does not imply that gloves are not required in other situations mentioned in the book.

An increasing number of people are being cared for at home who were previously cared for in the acute care hospital. Therefore, in the sixth edition, we have expanded our discussion of how you would integrate the information on a particular skill into your planning for home care. Another area of increasing importance in healthcare is long-term care. In long-term care, adaptations of procedures and techniques may also be needed. We have added references to these changes and adaptations where appropriate. Unique icons make Home Care and Long-Term Care instantly recognizable.

Critical Thinking Exercises

Skill development for the nurse must constantly be framed within the context of the individual patient. In order to focus on this important concept, we have added critical thinking exercises to each module. These exercises will assist you in placing the skills into the context of providing nursing care for each unique patient. In the critical thinking exercises, you are asked to consider a patient situation that has problematic aspects and to determine needs, priorities, or approaches that would be appropriate for the particular patient. There are no "right" answers to these situations. They might form the basis for a discussion, for a written paper, or for personal thoughtful study.

References

The references given are to research data regarding the skill or the recommendations of an authoritative agency such as the Centers For Disease Control and Prevention (CDC). The most recent research is cited. In the case of skills, this research may be older than expected. For example, the many excellent studies on the procedures and timing used for taking temperatures were done 10 years ago, but remain the basis for current recommendations. The CDC change their recommendations only when their decision-making bodies determine that the data warrant a change.

Unfortunately, there is little research data to support many of the nursing techniques used. Therefore, you will also note an emphasis within the modules on consulting policy and procedure manuals in institutions. These are generally established by groups of nurses working together with legal as well as healthcare goals in mind. Learning to use the official policy and procedure manual will be an asset both to the student and to the practicing nurse.

Performance Checklist

The performance checklist is used as a guide for practicing the skill and judging your performance of it.

Quiz

The quiz is a brief review for self-testing.

Glossary

The glossary at the back of each volume provides definitions for the key vocabulary terms.

Answers to Quizzes

The answer key at the end of each volume allows you to score yourself on the quizzes.

Index

An index is provided at the back of each volume.

We hope you will find gaining these essential skills to be a satisfying endeavor, and we wish you our best as you begin your studies.

J.R.E.
E.A.N.
P.M.B.

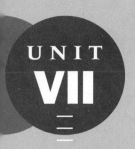

UNIT
VII

Complex Infection Control

MODULE

32

ISOLATION TECHNIQUE

MODULE CONTENTS

PREREQUISITES

Successful completion of the following modules:

OVERALL OBJECTIVE

To carry out correct isolation technique, placing emphasis on safety from infectious agents for patients, visitors, staff, and self while maintaining high-quality patient care.

SPECIFIC LEARNING OBJECTIVES

Know Facts and Principles	Apply Facts and Principles	Demonstrate Ability	Evaluate Performance

1. Purpose
  a. *To protect patient*
  b. *To protect environment*
Know two major purposes of isolation.
	Given a patient situation, identify which of two major purposes of isolation should be used.	In the clinical setting, identify purposes for isolation in use.	Evaluate with instructor.

2. Types
  a. *Rationale*
  b. *Transmission-based*
    (1) *Airborne*
    (2) *Droplet*
    (3) *Contact*
  c. *Disease-specific*
  d. *Category-specific*
    (1) *Strict*
    (2) *Respiratory*
    (3) *Wound and skin*
    (4) *Enteric*
    (5) *Protective*
    (6) *Compromised host*
Discuss various types of isolation and rationale for use of each.
	Given a patient situation, identify type of isolation procedure appropriate.	In the clinical setting, choose appropriate type of isolation for patient.	Evaluate own performance with instructor.

3. Procedures
  a. *Preparing the room*
  b. *Entering the room (gown, mask, gloves)*
  c. *Double-bagging*
  d. *Caring for linen*
  e. *Caring for dishes and food trays*
  f. *Leaving the room*
  g. *Transporting the patient in isolation*
  h. *General procedure*
Describe various procedures necessary for patient isolation.
	Given a patient situation, state which procedure would be appropriate to carry out.	Carry out various types of isolation procedures correctly.	Evaluate own performance with instructor using Performance Checklist.

(continued)

SPECIFIC LEARNING OBJECTIVES (continued)

Know Facts and Principles	Apply Facts and Principles	Demonstrate Ability	Evaluate Performance
4. Teaching List important facts to teach patient, family, and auxiliary staff.	Given a patient situation, plan teaching appropriate for type of isolation.	Instruct patient, family, and auxiliary staff on isolation procedure.	Evaluate own performance with patient, family, staff, and instructor.
5. Sensory deprivation State causes and effects of sensory deprivation. List techniques that can be used to prevent or decrease effects of sensory deprivation.	Given a patient situation, identify possible effects of sensory deprivation and list nursing techniques that could be used to decrease them.	Recognize potential and real effects of sensory deprivation and use nursing techniques to intervene.	Evaluate own performance by sharing experience with instructor and classmate.

LEARNING ACTIVITIES

1. Review the Specific Learning Objectives.
2. Read the section on isolation in the chapter on infection in Ellis and Nowlis, *Nursing: A Human Needs Approach,* or comparable material in another textbook.
3. Look up the module vocabulary terms in the glossary.
4. Read through the module as though you were preparing to teach these concepts to another person. Read about all three systems for planning isolation to be sure you understand the underlying principles and then focus your study on the system in use where you currently have clinical practice. Mentally practice the techniques.
5. In the practice setting:
   a. With a partner, practice preparing to enter and leave the various types of isolation rooms based on the technique needed. Evaluate each other's performance using the Performance Checklist.
   b. With a partner, practice double-bagging, alternating so that each of you has a turn being inside the room and outside the room. After you have done the procedure the first time, evaluate yourselves, using the Performance Checklist. Then switch roles and repeat the procedure. Again, evaluate yourselves and repeat the procedure as necessary.
   c. When you are satisfied that you can carry out the procedure, have your instructor evaluate your performances.
6. In the clinical setting:
   a. Consult your clinical instructor for an opportunity to carry out isolation procedures.

VOCABULARY

AIDS
category-specific
   precautions

compromised host
disease-specific
   precautions

isolation
microorganisms
sensory deprivation

transmission-based
   precautions

Isolation Technique

Rationale for the Use of This Skill

The isolation of an institutionalized patient may become necessary when "a person is known or suspected to be infected or colonized with epidemiologically important pathogens that can be transmitted by airborne or droplet transmission or by contact with dry skin and contaminated surfaces" (Centers for Disease Control and Prevention, 1994). The nurse must understand the rationale and be able to carry out the procedure correctly. This is true not only to maintain safety for the patient and others, but also to provide explanations regarding the procedures to the patient, the patient's family, and the auxiliary staff.

Since 1983 two main systems have been used for placing the patient in isolation: disease-specific isolation precautions and category-specific isolation precautions. Both approaches are accepted by the Centers for Disease Control and Prevention (CDC), and facilities chose to implement either type. In November of 1994, the Centers for Disease Control and Prevention published draft guidelines for a new approach to isolation (Centers for Disease Control and Prevention, 1994). This new approach is called transmission-based precautions. Final guidelines are anticipated as this text goes to press. You should be familiar with the basic principles of all three approaches. Then you will want to focus your study on the system in use where you will be practicing.

In this module, we will discuss the three types of isolation and the guidelines for their use. Specific techniques that can be used for any system including the preparation of the room for isolation and the correct method for entering and leaving the room will be outlined. We also consider sensory deprivation as a potential problem for the isolated patient.[1]

▼ NURSING DIAGNOSES

The following nursing diagnoses are problems commonly experienced by patients in isolation. Assessment for these problems is an important part of caring for the patient in isolation.

Social Isolation: Related to confinement imposed by isolation regimen. This occurs when individuals become cut off from their support systems, causing them to feel alone and in distress. A patient may experience this either as a result of the effects of the isolation procedures or as a result of concerns about safety for family and friends.

Knowledge Deficit: Related to lack of experience with infection control measures. Isolation procedures are better tolerated when the individual understands them.

Diversional Activity Deficit: Related to confinement imposed by isolation. This is a particular concern when an individual has a chronic infectious condition. As the individual reaches a convalescent state, the lack of diversional activities may be very distressing.

Sensory/Perceptual Alterations: Related to lack of stimuli in environment. Certain conditions restrict stimuli. For instance, persons entering an isolation room may be unrecognizable, and the room may have been stripped of amenities to prevent contamination. However, when an individual is acutely ill, it is possible for sensory/perceptual overload related to multiple procedures and caregivers to occur.

Risk for Infection: Related to suppressed immune system or to the overgrowth of resistant organisms. The individual whose original infection is related to a suppressed immune system may lack the body resources to fight off additional infections. When severe infections are treated, microorganisms not susceptible to the anti-infective drug may have a chance to proliferate, creating secondary infections.

RESOURCES FOR ISOLATION PROCEDURES

To meet the healthcare agency accreditation standards, each facility must have an infection control officer. This officer is commonly a nurse with specific expertise in infection control or someone on the laboratory staff. In large medical centers, the infection control officer is sometimes a physician epidemiologist. The infection control officer monitors infections and helps establish policy regarding all infection control procedures and training within the facility.

A facility's procedure manual outlines the specific isolation methods staff members are required to use. Review this resource *for clarification* regarding isolation if you are unsure how to proceed in an individual situation. If written materials do not pro-

---

[1]Rationale for action is emphasized throughout the module by the use of italics.

vide the information you need, contact the infection control officer for direction.

CREATING BARRIERS TO MICROORGANISMS

The principle behind isolation technique is to create a physical barrier that prevents the transfer of infectious agents. To do this you have to know how the organisms are transmitted and take measures to prevent that transmission. For example, if an organism is airborne, it is reasonable to start wearing masks and keep the door of the patient's room closed. If, however, the organisms are only transferred by contact with drainage or secretions on linen and items used in care, masks are unnecessary, and only direct contact with the patient is hazardous.

The barriers created for effective isolation should be appropriate to the goal—preventing the spread of select microorganisms from the patient to the environment or from the environment to the patient.

For many years, the CDC supported techniques called Category-Specific Isolation Precautions. Then in 1983 the CDC introduced a new system, Disease-Specific Isolation Precautions, which set up appropriate isolation measures for specific infectious diseases. However, many facilities continue to use the Category-Specific Isolation Precautions. Because each system has its advantages and disadvantages, both systems may be combined and used in some healthcare agencies.

With the widespread use of Standard Precautions, many facilities use a specific isolation designation only rarely because all patients are being treated as if they have infections that can be transferred by blood, body fluids, or any other body substance (see Module 2, Basic Infection Control). A specific isolation designation may be used only for those whose infections are not contained by these measures.

The transmission precautions disseminated in the 1994 Draft Guidelines from the CDC recognize this fact and are based on the use of Standard Precautions for all individuals. Thus, the only situations requiring any additional isolation precautions are those whose transmission occurs in ways other than through contact with moist body substances.

TRANSMISSION-BASED PRECAUTIONS

There are three methods of transmission covered by transmission-based precautions: airborne, by droplet, or by contact with dry skin or contaminated objects.

Airborne transmission occurs when the infectious agent is found on small particles (5 microns or less in diameter) that move about on air currents and enter the nose or mouth and land on the mucous membranes. These particles may be dried droplets or droplet nuclei. Airborne transmission occurs in such diseases as measles, chicken pox, and tuberculosis.

Droplet transmission involves large droplets of moisture that contain the infectious agent. These are dispersed through talking, coughing, or sneezing, and travel only short distances (approximately three feet or less). These droplets are deposited in the nose and mouth of another person. Droplet transmission occurs in such diseases as mumps, pertussis, and influenza.

Contact transmission involves the transfer of an infectious agent from dry skin through direct contact (skin to skin) or through indirect contact (skin to object to skin). Contact transmission occurs with some wound infections, impetigo, scabies, or herpes zoster in the immune competent person.

Some diseases, such as chicken pox, are transmitted by a combination of airborne and contact methods. In these instances both sets of precautions are used. The Draft Guidelines provide a list of diseases and infectious agents and the precautions recommended for each (Table 32–1). Remember that these precautions are always in addition to Standard Precautions.

Airborne Precautions

The patient should be in a private room with a negative air pressure and appropriate ventilation safeguards so that air from the room is not recirculated to other areas. The room door should be kept closed. All persons entering the room of a patient with tuberculosis should wear respiratory protection that provides a barrier to small particles. This is called a HEPA filter and is described below under disease-specific precautions. Individuals who are not immune to measles or chicken pox should not enter the rooms of those with these diseases. Patients should be transported as little as possible. They are asked to wear a surgical mask during transport.

Droplet Precautions

For droplet precautions the patient should be in a private room if at all possible. Those working within 3 feet of the patient must wear a mask. The Guidelines note that some facilities may prefer to have individuals wear a mask upon entry into the room. This can be a standard surgical mask. Patient transport should be minimized and the patient should wear a mask during transport.

Table 32–1. Transmission-Based Isolation Precautions for Selected Conditions (Centers for Disease Control and Prevention, 1994)

Disease	Precautions
Chickenpox (varicella)	Airborne, Contact, Standard
Decubitus ulcer, infected	
(1) Major	Contact, Standard
(2) Minor or limited	Standard
Diarrhea:	
(1) Acute diarrhea with a likely infectious cause in an incontinent or diapered patient. (Likely cause an enteric pathogen.)	Contact, Standard
(2) Diarrhea in an adult with a history of broad spectrum or long-term antibiotics. (Likely cause clostridium difficile)	Contact, Standard
Epiglottis, due to Haemophilus influenzae	Droplet, Standard
Epstein-Barr virus infection, including infectious monnucleosis	Standard
Hepatitis, viral;	
Type A in diapered or incontinent patient	Contact, Standard
Type B-HbsAg positive	Standard
Type A, C, unspecified non-A, non-B, E	Standard
Herpes simplex	
Encephalitis	Standard
Neonatal	Contact, Standard
Mucocutaneous, disseminated or primary, severe	Contact, Standard
Herpes zoster (varicella zoster)	
Localized in immunocompromised patient, or disseminated.	Airborne, Contact, Standard
Localized in normal patient	
Human Immunodeficiency Virus	Standard
Measles (Rubeola)	Airborne, Standard
Mumps	Droplet, Standard
Pertussis (whooping cough)	Droplet, Standard
Respiratory Infections especially bronchiolitis and croup in infants and young children. (Likely cause respiratory syncytial virus or parainfluenza virus.)	Contact, Standard
Rubella (German Measles)	Droplet, Standard
Tuberculosis	
Extrapulmonary, draining lesion	Standard
Extrapulmonary, meningitis	Standard
Pulmonary, confirmed or suspected, or laryngeal disease	Airborne, Standard
Skin test positive with no evidence of current pulmonary disease	Standard
Wound infection or abscess that is draining and cannot be contained. (Causative organism staphlococcus aureus, Group A streptococcus)	Contact, Standard
Wound infection that is minor or contained.	Standard

Contact Precautions

The patient should be in a private room if possible. In addition to wearing gloves when required by Standard Precautions, gloves are worn while providing direct care to the patient or touching any surface in the room. Gloves are removed before exiting from the room, hands are washed thoroughly, and nothing is touched before exiting the room. In addition to wearing a gown when required by Standard Precautions, a gown is worn when entering the room if there will be contact with the patient, environmental surfaces (such as sheets), or objects used in care. Remove the gown cautiously before leaving the room. Be sure that your clothing does not touch any surface as you leave. When possible, all patient care items should be restricted to the single patient or else adequately cleaned and disinfected after use.

DISEASE-SPECIFIC ISOLATION PRECAUTIONS

Under Disease-Specific Isolation Precautions, each infectious disease is considered separately, and guidelines that use only those procedures considered necessary to attain the goal are then set up (Table 32–2). An advantage of this system is that it is adaptable to individualized care plans. This approach has also been termed more cost-effective *because it minimizes unnecessary precautions and equipment use.* Staff and visitors are more likely to comply with all procedures because there is a logical rationale for the use of each precautionary measure based on the way the individual disease is transmitted. A disadvantage is that every patient situation may differ and this may cause confusion, especially when care providers lack knowledge.

After consulting a list of diseases with recommendations for isolation, nurses can fill out a single door card that lists the appropriate precautions to take for a specific disease (Fig. 32–1). This information may also be placed in a care plan or separate kardex.

Tuberculosis Isolation

Those individuals with documented or suggested tuberculosis are now cared for with disease-specific isolation precautions because of the occurrence of drug-resistant tuberculosis and the greater danger that this disease poses. Therefore, even if category-specific isolation is used for other conditions, you will see disease-specific procedures used for tuberculosis. This has been recommended by the CDC (1994) and further mandated in regulations developed by the Occupational Safety and Health Administration (OSHA, 1993) to protect healthcare workers from tuberculosis. In some agencies, this isolation is listed as AFB (acid-fast bacillus) Isolation to provide patient confidentiality. (See Fig. 32–2 for an example of an AFB isolation sign for a patient's door.)

You will need to learn about tuberculosis and its prevention, diagnosis, treatment, and management from your medical-surgical nursing text. Of particular importance is decision-making regarding when to initiate isolation and when to discontinue it. Tuberculosis isolation is instituted both for those diagnosed with tuberculosis and for those in whom tuberculosis is suggested until a firm diagnosis of the condition is made. The focus here is on the specific isolation procedures that may be used.

The following precautions are included in AFB or tuberculosis isolation:

1. Place the individual in an isolation room that has negative air pressure (ensuring that air from the room does not exit to the rest of the institution when the door is opened).
2. Ensure that the isolation room has six or more exchanges of air per hour and that air be exhausted to the outside or be recirculated through HEPA (high-efficiency particulate air) filters. This type of filter can remove very small microbes from air.
3. Be aware that all healthcare workers caring for the patient should be protected by wearing a special type of isolation mask, the HEPA filter respirator, which is capable of providing a barrier to all microorganisms. These masks must be individually fitted to ensure that all air moves only through the mask itself. The fit test must be redone annually. The masks are hot and somewhat uncomfortable to wear. They also muffle voices, making oral communication more difficult.

   The masks cannot be properly fitted over beards, long sideburns, or mustaches. These must be shaved for proper fit. Most agencies have adopted personnel policies requiring individuals to meet these standards if they work where they might care for patients with tuberculosis. Some agencies allow an individual to wait until the situation arises before requiring shaving.

   Some individuals have facial features, skin scarring, or other factors that make it impossible to obtain a tight fit on these masks. Medical conditions such as sensitivity to latex, certain skin conditions, and cardiopulmonary conditions may also pose a problem for those wearing these masks. Those who cannot wear a HEPA filter respirator for these reasons are usually not required to care for patients needing AFB isolation.
4. Wear a gown when needed to prevent gross contamination of clothing (Standard Precautions).
5. Wear gloves for contact with moist body substances and nonintact skin (Standard Precautions).
6. Wash hands after touching the patient or potentially contaminated articles (tissues used for covering coughs are of special concern) and after removing gloves (Standard Precautions).
7. Discard, clean, or bag and send for processing any articles used by the patient on removal from the room.
8. Keep the door to the room closed at all times.
9. Have the patient wear a mask when being transported outside of the room. If the patient cannot wear a mask, the healthcare worker transporting the patient should wear a HEPA respirator.

(text continues on page 13)

Table 32-2. Disease-Specific Isolation Precautions

Disease	Precautions Indicated					Infective Material	Apply Precautions How Long?	Comments
	Private Room?	Masks?	Gowns?	Gloves?				
Decubitus ulcer, infected								
Draining, major	Yes	No	Yes, if soiling is likely	Yes, for touching infective material		Pus	Duration of illness	Major = draining and not covered by dressing or dressing does not adequately contain the pus.
Draining, minor	No	No	Yes, if soiling is likely	Yes, for touching infective material		Pus	Duration of illness	Minor or limited = dressing covers and adequately contains the pus, or infected area is very small.
Diarrhea, acute—infective etiology suspected (see gastroenteritis)	Yes, if patient hygiene is poor	No	Yes, if soiling is likely	Yes, for touching infective material		Feces	Duration of illness	
Diphtheria, Cutaneous	Yes	No	Yes, if soiling is likely	Yes, for touching infective material		Lesion secretions	Until 2 cultures from skin lesions, taken at least 24 hrs apart after cessation of antimicrobial therapy, are negative for *Corynebacterium diphtheriae*	
Pharyngeal	Yes	Yes	Yes, if soiling is likely	Yes, for touching infective material		Respiratory secretions	Until 2 cultures from both nose and throat taken at least 24 hrs apart after cessation of antimicrobial therapy	
Meningococcemia (meningococcal sepsis)	Yes	Yes, for those close to patient	No	No		Respiratory secretions	For 24 hrs after start of effective therapy	See CDC Guideline for Infection Control in Hospital Personnel for recommendations for prophylaxis after exposure.

(*continued*)

Table 32-2. Continued

Disease	Precautions Indicated				Infective Material	Apply Precautions How Long?	Comments
	Private Room?	Masks?	Gowns?	Gloves?			
Gastrointestinal	Yes	No	Yes, if soiling is likely	Yes, for touching infective material	Feces	Until off antimicrobials and culture-negative	In outbreaks, cohorting of infected and colonized patients may be indicated if private rooms are not available.
Respiratory General	Yes	Yes, for those close to patient	Yes, if soiling is likely	Yes, for touching infective material	Respiratory secretions and possibly feces	Until off antimicrobials and culture-negative	In outbreaks, cohorting of infected and colonized patients may be indicated if private rooms are not available.
Tuberculosis (new, active case)	Yes	Yes, if patient coughing	Yes, if soiling with respiratory secretions likely	Yes, for touching infective material, such as tissues used for cough	Respiratory secretions	For 2 weeks after antituberculosis therapy initiated	Use of ultraviolet lights or filtered air systems recommended.
Skin, wound or burn	Yes	No	Yes, if soiling is likely	Yes, for touching infective material	Pus and possibly feces	Until off antimicrobials and culture-negative	In outbreaks, cohorting of infected and colonized patients may be indicated if private rooms are not available.
Urinary	Yes	No	No	Yes, for touching infective material	Urine and possibly feces	Until off antimicrobials and culture-negative	Urine and urine-measuring devices are sources of infections, especially if the patient (or any nearby patients) has indwelling urinary catheter. In outbreaks, cohorting of infected and colonized patients may be indicated if private rooms are not available.

(Front of Card)

Visitors—Report to Nurses' Station Before Entering Room

1. Private room indicated?
   - _____ No
   - _____ Yes
2. Masks indicated?
   - _____ No
   - _____ Yes for those close to patient
   - _____ Yes for all persons entering room
3. Gowns indicated?
   - _____ No
   - _____ Yes if soiling is likely
   - _____ Yes for all persons entering room
4. Gloves indicated?
   - _____ No
   - _____ Yes for touching infective material
   - _____ Yes for all persons entering room
5. Special precautions indicated for handling blood?
   - _____ No
   - _____ Yes
6. Hands must be washed after touching the patient or potentially contaminated articles and before taking care of another patient.
7. Articles contaminated with _____ should be

infective material(s)

discarded or bagged and labeled before being sent for decontamination and reprocessing.

(Back of Card)

Instructions

1. On Table B, Disease-Specific Precautions, locate the disease for which isolation precautions are indicated.
2. Write disease in blank space here: _____
3. Determine if a private room is indicated. In general, patients infected with the same organism may share a room. For some diseases or conditions, a private room is indicated if patient hygiene is poor. A patient with poor hygiene does not wash hands after touching infective material (feces, purulent drainage, or secretions), contaminates the environment with infective material, or shares contaminated articles with other patients.
4. Place a check mark beside the indicated precautions on front of card.
5. Cross through precautions that are *not* indicated.
6. Write infective material in blank space in item 7 on front of card.

Figure 32–1. Sample instruction card for disease-specific isolation precautions.

Although HEPA respirators are effective barriers, many healthcare workers believe that the research data do not clearly establish that they significantly change infection rates among healthcare workers and that the costs will be millions of dollars per year to acute care facilities (Adal et al., 1994).

A major factor in tuberculosis transmission lies in droplet nuclei deposited in tissues and the hands of the infected individual. Handwashing by patients and all others in the environment is most effective against this transmission. Coughing into the air by patients is responsible for most airborne transmission of tuberculosis. Patients can be taught to cover coughs with a disposable tissue, dispose of tissues correctly, and wash their hands. Healthcare workers can also maintain distance from patients with tuberculosis as much as possible even while wearing masks. The greatest danger of tuberculosis transmis-

AFB Isolation

Visitors—Report to Nurses' Station Before Entering Room

1. Masks are to be worn in the patient's room.

2. Gowns are indicated if needed to prevent gross contamination of clothing.

3. Gloves are indicated for body fluids and non-intact skin.

4. HANDS MUST BE WASHED AFTER TOUCHING THE PATIENT OR POTENTIALLY CONTAMINATED ARTICLES AND AFTER REMOVING GLOVES.

5. Articles should be discarded, cleaned, or sent for decontamination and reprocessing.

6. The door to the room is to remain closed.

7. The patient is to wear a mask for transportation outside the room.

Figure 32–2. Isolation precautions used for tuberculosis.

sion is often during the period before the tuberculosis is suggested or diagnosed.

In the light of these factors, some workers do not want to adopt a mask that interferes with effective patient communication and is uncomfortable. For the facility itself, the cost of fitting large numbers of healthcare workers with these special masks is a concern in light of cost–benefit ratios. As always, we recommend that you follow the current regulations and the policy of your facility and that you continue to read the literature for the latest recommendations and requirements.

CATEGORY-SPECIFIC ISOLATION PRECAUTIONS

Many hospitals continue to use the system known as category-specific isolation *to protect people from pathogens infecting a given patient*. This approach divides infectious diseases into a few broad categories, which are determined by how the organisms are transmitted. The five categories of isolation generally used in this system are strict isolation, respiratory isolation, wound and skin precautions (sometimes referred to as "contact isolation"), enteric precautions, and blood/body fluid (universal) precautions. The rationale for this approach is that it is easier for staff to remember the procedures for these broad

categories than to remember what to do for individual infectious diseases.

In view of the current concern about diseases transmitted by blood and body fluids, blood/body fluid precautions are now used for all individuals in all healthcare situations. In facilities in which body substance precautions are used, enteric precautions, which are limited to vomitus and feces, are omitted because the precautions necessary for this category as well as those for the blood/body fluid category are included in body substance precautions. Both universal precautions and body substance precautions were described in Module 2, Basic Infection Control.

Additional categories of isolation are used in both systems to protect patients who have a suppressed immune system and are therefore highly susceptible to contracting an infection. One category is called *compromised host precautions,* and the other is termed *protective isolation.* Although it has been proved that the most effective measure for infection control is handwashing, additional precautions are added to provide these individuals with increased safety.

Strict Isolation

Strict isolation is used if the identified pathogens are transmitted both through the air and by contact. Strict isolation is also used when the organism is particularly virulent and resistant to the major antibiotics. Precautions to be taken include placing the patient in a private room with the door closed; wearing a gown, mask, and gloves when entering the room; washing hands on entering and leaving the room; and double-bagging (for decontamination) linens and other articles used in the care of the patient (Fig. 32–3).

Respiratory Isolation

If the pathogens involved are airborne, respiratory isolation is carried out. It is desirable to place the patient in a private room with the door closed. Masks must be worn, but gowns and gloves are not necessary *unless there is direct contact with linens or secretions.* Hands should be washed on entering and leaving the room. Any article contaminated with secretions from the patient must be disinfected or double-bagged for disposal or decontamination (Fig. 32–4).

Wound and Skin Precautions

For the patient with a wound infected with microorganisms that can be spread by contact, wound and skin precautions are observed. Isolation of the patient is not required, but a private room is desirable. Gowns must be worn when in direct contact with the patient, the linen, or the dressings to protect your uniform from possible contamination.

Gloves should be used when in direct contact with the infected area or when handling dressings or anything contaminated with drainage. Masks are necessary only during dressing changes. Hands are washed on entering and leaving the room. Instruments, dressings, and linens must be placed in moisture-impervious bags or double-bagged for decontamination or disposal (Fig. 32–5).

Enteric Precautions

Enteric precautions are used when the pathogens involved are transmitted by direct contact with gastrointestinal secretions, vomitus, or feces. A private room is necessary for the pediatric patient *because children cannot be trusted to remain only on their own beds.* Gowns must be worn when in direct contact with the patient or contaminated linens. Gloves are worn when in direct contact with the patient's perineal area, feces, vomitus, or contaminated materials. Masks are not necessary. Hands are washed on entering and leaving the room. Linen should be double-bagged or placed in moisture-impervious bags. Urine, feces, and vomitus should be discarded in an adjoining private bathroom, and any articles contaminated with them must be discarded or disinfected. (Urine is included *because of the proximity of the urinary and intestinal tracts.*)(Fig. 32–6).

Strict Isolation
Visitors-Report to Nurses' Station Before Entering Room

1. **Private Room**—necessary; door must be kept closed.
2. **Gowns**—must be worn by all persons entering room.
3. **Masks**—must be worn by all persons entering room.
4. **Hands**—must be washed on entering and leaving room.
5. **Gloves**—must be worn by all persons entering room.
6. **Articles**—must be discarded, or wrapped before being sent to Central Supply for disinfection or sterilization.

Figure 32–3. Strict isolation sign. (Courtesy Shamrock, Inc., Bellwood, Illinois)

Respiratory Isolation
Visitors-Report to Nurses' Station Before Entering Room

1. **Private Room**—necessary; door must be kept closed.

2. **Gowns**—not necessary.

3. **Masks**—must be worn by all persons entering room if susceptible to disease.

4. **Hands**—must be washed on entering and leaving room.

5. **Gloves**—not necessary.

6. **Articles**—those contaminated with secretions must be disinfected.

7. **Caution**—all persons susceptible to the specific disease should be excluded from patient area; if contact is necessary, susceptibles must wear masks.

Figure 32–4. Respiratory isolation sign. (Courtesy Shamrock, Inc., Bellwood, Illinois)

Protective Isolation

The patient who is particularly susceptible to infection may be placed in protective (also called reverse) isolation *to provide protection from environmental pathogens.* A private room with the door closed is required. Gowns and masks must be worn by all who enter the room. Gloves must be worn by those having direct contact with the patient. Hands are washed on entering and leaving the room. All items taken into the room should be individually evaluated for their potential to carry pathogens and harm

Wound & Skin Precautions
Visitors—Report to Nurses' Station Before Entering Room

1. **Private Room**—desirable.

2. **Gowns**—must be worn by all persons having direct contact with patient.

3. **Masks**—not necessary except during dressing changes.

4. **Hands**—must be washed on entering and leaving room.

5. **Gloves**—must be worn by all persons having direct contact with infected area.

6. **Articles**—special precautions necessary for instruments, dressings, and linen.

NOTE: See Manual for Special Dressing Techniques to be used when changing dressings.

Figure 32–5. Wound and skin precautions sign. (Courtesy Shamrock, Inc., Bellwood, Illinois)

Enteric Precautions
Visitors-Report to Nurses' Station
Before Entering Room

1. **Private Room**—necessary for children only.
2. **Gowns**—must be worn by all persons having direct contact with patient.
3. **Masks**—not necessary.
4. **Hands**—must be washed on entering and leaving room.
5. **Gloves**—must be worn by all persons having direct contact with patient or with articles contaminated with fecal material.
6. **Articles**—special precautions necessary for articles contaminated with urine and feces. Articles must be disinfected or discarded.

Figure 32–6. Enteric precautions sign. (Courtesy Shamrock, Inc., Bellwood, Illinois)

the patient. Usually plants are removed because of the microorganisms in the soil. Flowers are not permitted because the standing water becomes a reservoir for microbial growth. *Because the room and its contents are considered clean,* no special measures are taken when removing articles and linens (Fig. 32–7). The most strict use of protective isolation occurs when the profoundly compromised patient is placed in a laminar airflow room and care providers wear sterile garb and all visitors are restricted. Each facility having this type of protective isolation provides careful instruction for all personnel.

Protective Isolation
Visitors—Report to Nurses' Station
Before Entering Room

1. **Private Room**—necessary; door must be kept closed.
2. **Gowns**—must be worn by all persons entering room.
3. **Masks**—must be worn by all persons entering room.
4. **Hands**—must be washed on entering and leaving room.
5. **Gloves**—must be worn by all persons having direct contact with patient.
6. **Articles**—see manual text.

Figure 32–7. Protective isolation sign. (Courtesy Shamrock, Inc., Bellwood, Illinois)

Compromised Host

The designation *compromised host* usually means that the patient has a suppressed immune system and is therefore *less capable of self-protection against pathogens.* Many facilities are now using the procedure for compromised host more often than that for protective isolation, *because it appears to be as effective and is less restrictive to the person involved.* The procedure is less stringent and usually does not require use of mask and gown; *this is why it is more acceptable to patients.* It includes meticulous handwashing by both staff and visitors and the requirement that persons who have a cold or other infection not enter the room or come close to the patient. Patients are also instructed in careful handwashing to protect them from what others may bring in and the microorganisms they carry in their own intestinal tract. Some facilities prohibit live plants and flowers in the environment just as in protective isolation. Commonly, visitors are limited to immediate family and special friends, and an attempt is made to have the same caregivers to decrease the number of different organisms to which the person is exposed.

SPECIFIC ISOLATION PROCEDURES

The following discussion provides information about a variety of specific procedures that you will use as part of isolation technique. For instance, you must know how to prepare the isolation room, enter it correctly, and care for equipment and supplies in it. You also must know how to leave the room correctly. Occasionally, the patient in the isolation room must be transported to another department for a procedure or a test; you must know how to accomplish this correctly. A General Procedure for approaching all isolation situations, in which you choose the specific procedures you need to care for the individual patient, is provided at the end.

Preparing the Room

Preparation of a room for isolation procedure varies, depending on the type of isolation required. In some instances, such as strict isolation, it is appropriate to remove unnecessary furniture and equipment from the room. In other cases, the room does not need to be changed in any way. If good handwashing technique is followed, patients under wound and skin precautions and blood and body fluid precautions can share a room with another patient, according to CDC guidelines. We recommend that you review the policy at your facility, but generally you will need to

1. Be sure the patient is in a private room with running water.
2. Post sign on the outside of the door indicating what preparation is needed before entering the room and which type of isolation is being carried out (see Figs. 32–2 through 32–7).
3. Place a stand of some sort (often a bedside stand is used) just outside the door to hold isolation laundry bags, gowns, masks, gloves, and other items specific to the care of an individual patient. In some hospitals these stands are prepared and kept in the central supply department and requisitioned when needed.
4. Obtain a laundry hamper for inside the room.
5. Be sure the room contains a wastebasket (preferably large) lined with a plastic bag.
6. Ensure that a thermometer and blood pressure equipment, including stethoscope, are left in the room.
7. Make certain a special container for used needles, syringes, and instruments is available.

In facilities that have areas especially designed for use with isolation patients, necessary items are stored in the anteroom outside the patient's room. Such special areas are also equipped with sinks with knee controls.

Entering the Room

One component of care that will prove helpful as you prepare to enter an isolation room is *organization.* Make sure you have all the equipment you need before you are gowned and in the room. *To stand helpless in the room, waiting for someone to bring you forgotten items, is frustrating and time-consuming for you and other staff members, not to mention the patient.*

You may need to wear a gown, a mask, and gloves, depending on the specific situation. Determine which items you need to wear. Specific directions for those items follow.

1. Obtain needed equipment.
2. Wash hands for infection control. Take off any rings *because the regular handwashing procedure may not remove microorganisms lodged beneath them.*
3. If the room does not have a wall clock and you need a watch to perform some aspect of care, remove your watch and place it in a plastic bag so that it is protected but visible.
4. Put on gown if needed:

a. Put on gown, making sure that all parts of your uniform are covered.

b. Fasten the ties securely.

An isolation gown is used to protect the care provider's clothing from microorganisms that can be spread on clothing. Gowns are usually worn for strict and respiratory isolation and when providing direct care to patients who have drainage or secretions that may contain infectious organisms. Isolation gowns may be made of washable cotton cloth or disposable paper.

5. Put on mask if needed.

a. Place clean mask over nose and mouth.

b. Fasten both sets of ties securely.

c. Tuck bottom edge under chin and fit the top edge snugly across the bridge of nose. If you wear glasses, tuck the mask under the lower edge of your glasses *to prevent your glasses from steaming up from your breath.* Some masks have a metal strip that can be molded to fit snugly over the bridge of your nose and under your eyes.

Masks are made of disposable material. *They protect against airborne microorganisms and the droplet nuclei on which they are carried.* To do this effectively, all inhaled air must pass through the mask material before reaching the mouth and nose. *As masks are worn, they become moist from the wearer's breath and can therefore wick microorganisms through from the surface to the wearer.* Because of this, masks should be changed as soon as moisture is detected on the surface. In addition, *masks collect microorganisms on the outside surface, concentrating them in that location.* For this reason, do not hang a mask around your neck and reuse it. *This increases the chance of contaminating your hands with organisms from the mask and of transferring organisms from your hands to the mask that will be over your mouth and nose.*

6. Put on clean gloves if needed:

a. Put on both gloves.

b. Tuck the sleeves of the gown securely inside the cuffs of the gloves.

Gloves are always used in isolation in the same way as they are used for other patients. Gloves should be kept inside of the room *so that they can be put on and changed as needed when providing care.* In addition, clean gloves may be worn for all care in a strict isolation situation. In these situations, gloves must be kept outside of the room and put on before entering. When a particularly virulent organism is being treated, you may wish to double-glove (that is, put one pair over the other) *to provide protection from torn gloves and to keep your hands covered when you are changing gloves.*

Procedures Used During Care

Double-Bagging

You may use a double-bagging technique for contaminated items removed from an isolation room (except a protective isolation room). One nurse inside of the room and one nurse outside carry out this procedure, which may be used for wet linen or for items that are being sent to another department.

Double-bagging of items sent for decontamination is not required by the CDC if the bag is sturdy so that it will not break and the outside of the bag is kept clean when contaminated items are placed inside of it. However, many facilities routinely double-bag all items as an extra precaution.

1. If you are the inside nurse, place used items in appropriate containers: linen in the linen hamper, glass bottles and jars in a brown paper bag, paper garbage in a plastic-lined wastebasket. Take care not to fill the bags too full, *because full bags are difficult to double-bag without breaking technique.* Carefully close and secure the bag.

2. If you are the outside nurse, form a cuff on another bag, spreading it to receive the bag from the nurse on the inside. *The cuff protects your hands from contact with the contaminated items inside the bag.*

3. If you are the inside nurse, place the bag holding contaminated items directly into the bag being held by the outside nurse. Be careful to touch only the inside of the bag (Fig. 32–8).

4. If you are the outside nurse, fold over and carefully secure the top of the outside bag.

5. Mark the bag in the manner prescribed by the facility. Most isolation linen bags are red (as opposed to another color for regular linen) or have a red stripe sewn on them. Brightly colored plastic tape can be used to mark paper or plastic bags. A felt-tipped marking pen is often used to indicate the contents of the bag, so that proper sterilization or destruction processes can be carried out.

6. Dispose of the bag in the proper place. Check the procedure book at your facility for any special procedures related to the care of nondisposable equipment.

As an alternative to having two nurses, an open laundry hamper may be set up outside of the isolation room. The inside nurse can then place the soiled laundry bag into the clean bag. Other items are more difficult to double-bag without a second nurse. Paper bags set on a stand outside of the isolation room tend to fall over or close, making it difficult to put an item in the bag.

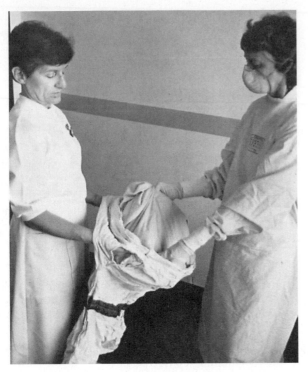

Figure 32–8. Double-bagging wet linens from a strict isolation room. (Courtesy Ivan Ellis)

Note: Do not put lids or caps on glass jars or bottles being sent to be sterilized or incinerated. *A jar or bottle with a lid or cap in place will explode in an autoclave or incinerator, possibly causing injury to hospital staff.*

Caring for Linen

1. Handle soiled linen with gloved hands.
2. Touch only the inside of the laundry bag with the soiled linen or contaminated hands. *This maintains the outside as clean as is possible.* The clean, dry bag of soiled linen may be handled just as any soiled linen bag is handled *because all are considered contaminated.*
3. Use the double-bagging technique, which is recommended by the CDC whenever linen is contaminated with moisture that might leak through to those handling the bag at any point. This provides extra protection to hospital workers. In some facilities all soiled linen from isolation rooms is handled by double-bagging as an extra precaution. Other facilities use moisture-impervious linen bags.

Caring for Dishes and Food Trays

Whether food trays are cleaned or disposed of depends on whether the disease can be transmitted by oral secretions such as saliva.

1. For patients with organisms that can be transmitted on eating utensils (eg, for patients with hepatitis A), place the trays in marked plastic bags before putting them on the unit's cart for used diet trays. The standard institutional dishwashing procedure disinfects dishes. Disposable dishes are rarely used because they add expense and are distasteful to patients. They are never required; however, they do prevent transmission of infectious agents.
2. For patients with organisms that are not transmitted on eating utensils, treat the trays as you would any others. For example, the trays from patients with infected wounds can be removed from the room and placed on the unit's cart for used diet trays, because the organism is not communicated through saliva.

Leaving the Room

This procedure assumes you are wearing a gown, mask, and gloves. You can modify it if you are not using all three.

1. Complete your work in the room.
2. Remove your gloves and dispose of them as follows:
   a. Peel first glove off, turning it inside out and touching only the outside with other gloved hand.
   b. Hold first glove in second gloved hand.
   c. Slide ungloved fingers inside of second glove and turn glove inside out over first glove while removing it.
   When removing soiled gloves, it is wise to turn them inside out as you pull them off. *This encloses the contaminated surface inside of the glove.* Small items to be disposed of may be encased in a soiled glove by turning the glove inside out over the item. This provides a compact, moisture-proof cover *to decrease the number of microorganisms being released into the room and to prevent contamination of your hands.*
3. Untie waist ties of your gown.
4. Wash your hands.
5. Untie neckline ties, dropping the gown over your shoulders. Do not touch the outside of the gown.
6. Pull off the gown, touching the inside only and turning the gown inside out as you take it off. Fold it with all outside surfaces toward the center and place it in the laundry hamper (Fig. 32–9) or waste container if disposable gowns are used.
7. Touching the ties only, untie your mask and discard it in a wastebasket.

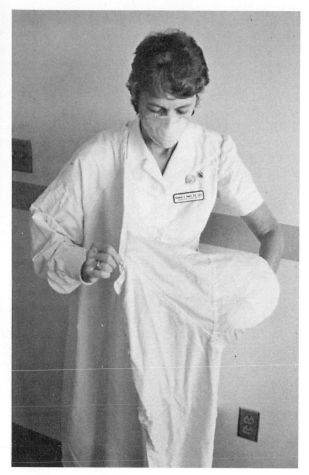

a mask during transport, and all who care for the patient in another department must wear gowns and masks. During transport, a patient in respiratory, airborne, or droplet isolation must wear a mask to protect others. A patient in wound or contact isolation should wear a gown but a mask would not be necessary. A patient in strict isolation must wear a gown and mask and should be covered by a sheet or bath blanket. All items that are touched by the patient must be disinfected. Consult your facility procedure book for specific instructions.

GENERAL PROCEDURE FOR ISOLATION

Assessment

1. Check the type of isolation ordered for the patient *to plan for care.*
2. Identify the type of infection or the reason for protective precautions.
3. Check the equipment on the stand outside the door or in the anteroom and inside the room *to be sure you have everything you need* for the procedure you intend to perform.

Planning

4. Wash your hands *for infection control.*
5. Gather any equipment you need that is not outside the door or inside the room.

Implementation

6. Identify the patient from the door *to be sure you are performing the procedure for the correct patient.* Explain to the patient what you are doing. This may be unnecessary if the patient has been in isolation for an extended period. This also lets the patient see your face before you put on a mask (if one is required) and facilitates developing a relationship with the patient.
7. When entering the room, carry out the aspects of isolation technique necessary for this patient according to the type of isolation being used.
8. Give care as planned, using appropriate techniques.
9. When leaving the room, carry out the aspects of isolation technique necessary for this patient according to the type of isolation being used.

Evaluation

10. Evaluate, using the following criteria:
    a. All necessary equipment readily available
    b. All aspects of the particular isolation procedure correctly carried out
    c. Patient cared for safely and made comfortable
    d. No nosocomial infections originate with this patient.

Figure 32–9. Removing an isolation gown by touching only the neck and inside surfaces. (Courtesy Ivan Ellis)

8. Wash your hands.
9. Using a paper towel as a barrier on the door handle, open the door. Discard the paper towel inside the room.
10. Wash your hands outside the room.

Note: The reuse technique for gowns is seldom used, except perhaps in protective isolation situations. If it is used in your facility, check the procedure book *to be certain you are following the exact procedure.*

Transporting the Patient in Isolation

Sometimes a patient in isolation must be transported to another area. This should be done only when absolutely necessary. Precautions vary according to the type of isolation in use. Generally, it is essential to keep in mind *whom* you are protecting and from what type of infection you are protecting. *A patient in protective isolation must be protected from all those with whom he or she comes in contact.* This patient may wear

DATE/TIME	
3/12/99 1620	*Pt placed in respiratory isolation per order after report on sputum specimen. Weak but comfortable. States, "I just want to rest."* ————————————— *S. Danton, RN*

Example of Nursing Progress Notes Using Narrative Format.

DATE/TIME	
3/14/99 1800	*Psychosocial status:* ——————————— *S "I feel so bored. I wish more of my friends would visit me."* *O Appears sad and restless. Pacing room for long periods of time this PM.* *A Diversional deficit.* *P Consult with family regarding visits from friends and possible diversional activities.* ———————— *S. Danton, RN*

Example of Nursing Progress Notes Using SOAP Format.

Documentation

11. Document care given appropriately. There may be a place to check (√) that isolation procedure was carried out.

PATIENT, FAMILY, AND STAFF COOPERATION

A responsibility inherent in carrying out isolation procedure is making sure the patient and the patient's family understand the reasons for the isolation procedures being carried out and that they respond to this knowledge with appropriate actions. This responsibility extends to the hospital staff and the physician as well. Remember that the chain will only be as strong as its weakest link.

No one likes isolation procedures, perhaps the patient least of all. For this reason, emphasize the do's rather than the don'ts. *A positive approach may yield more in terms of observable results.*

COMBATING SENSORY DEPRIVATION

Closely related to the idea that isolation procedure is extra work that no one really likes to do is the idea that patients in isolation feel that the staff is reluctant to take care of them. This feeling may be prompted by the fact that they are always the last to be cared for, by careless remarks made outside doors but within hearing of the patient, and by countless nonverbal exchanges. In addition, those who do come to visit isolated patients (family, friends, staff) are often covered from head to toe, making normal communication impossible. Isolation rooms are usually stripped of pictures, plants, and other decorative items, making the total setting rather dismal. The variety of stimulation isolated patients receive is less, and it can be less meaningful too. Usually these patients have limited interaction with others. As a result, patients in isolation can develop decreased alertness and motivation, increased complaints, loneliness, depression, and anger.

You can intervene positively by giving care to an isolated patient first, by answering the call light promptly, and by stopping in the doorway to wave. Provide the patient with puzzles, paperback books, and other paper items that can be disposed of when no longer needed. Typically, the family can provide such items.

LONG-TERM CARE

Most long-term care facilities use category-specific isolation procedures. That system is often easier in a setting where isolation is a rare occurrence.

Isolation requirements for tuberculosis include engineering standards regarding air circulation and exchange. Long-term care facilities do not usually meet these standards. Furthermore, tuberculosis would be a rare occurrence in these settings. As a result, these facilities usually elect to transfer any patient thought to have tuberculosis to an acute care hospital that has these structural elements in place.

HOME CARE

When individuals with infectious diseases are being cared for at home, the client, the family, and caregivers are taught how to protect themselves from infection. Isolation techniques are not used because they are unwieldy in that environment. The general instructions for basic infection control given in Module 2 are given to the family. It is critical to teach the client how to avoid spreading infection. Especially in the case of respiratory illness, the client plays a crucial role in protecting others, through careful attention to covering coughs, disposing of tissues in a paper bag, and washing hands. In addition, when a respiratory illness is present, those not needed for care are instructed to avoid entering the client's room. This is especially true for children, the elderly, and those with chronic illnesses, who are often more susceptible to infection.

When the client has tuberculosis, you should be sure that your teaching conforms to the latest information on the transmission of that disease. When a child has a communicable disease such as chickenpox, the family may be concerned about when the child may return to school or day care. Consult your local health department for the most current recommendations regarding these communicable diseases.

CRITICAL THINKING EXERCISES

• Martin Jameson was admitted to the hospital with an infected, draining ulcer on his leg. Based on the policies at your facility, what type of isolation, if any, would you establish? Determine what isolation procedures need to be carried out. Identify what teaching regarding infection control needs to be provided for the patient, the family, and other staff members.

• Marjorie Willis was admitted to the hospital with a severe respiratory infection and was just diagnosed with tuberculosis. Identify your concerns regarding initiating infection control procedures. What procedures does your facility prescribe? Summarize the concerns you have for staff members, and develop a patient teaching program.

References

Adal, K. A., Anglim, A. M., Palumbo, C. L., Titus, M. G., Coyner, B. J., & Farr, B. M. (1994). The use of high-efficiency particulate air-filter respirators to protect hospital workers from tuberculosis: A cost-effectiveness analysis. *New England Journal of Medicine, 331*(3), 169–173.

Centers for Disease Control. (1983). *Guidelines for isolation precautions in hospitals.* U.S. Department of Health and Human Services.

Centers for Disease Control. (1985). *Guidelines for handwashing and hospital environmental control.* U.S. Department of Health and Human Services.

Centers for Disease Control. (1994). *Guidelines for preventing the transmission of tuberculosis in health-care facilities, MMWR, 43*(RR–13), 1–132.

Centers for Disease Control. (1987). Recommendations for prevention of HIV transmission in health-care settings. *MMWR, 36*(25), 1–16.

Centers for Disease Control. (1988). Update: Universal precautions for prevention of transmission of human immunodeficiency virus, hepatitis B virus, and other blood borne pathogens in health-care settings. *MMWR, 37*(24), 377–382, 387–388.

Centers for Disease Control and Prevention. (1994, November 7). Draft Guideline for Isolation Precautions in Hospitals: Part I. "Evolution of Isolation Practices" and Part II. "Recommendations for Isolation Precautions in Hospitals". *Federal Register, 59,(214), 55552–55570.*

OSHA enforcement policy and procedures for occupational exposure to tuberculosis. (1993). *Infection Control and Hospital Epidemiology, 14*(12), 694–699.

PERFORMANCE CHECKLIST

Preparing the Room	Needs More Practice	Satisfactory	Comments
1. Be sure patient will be in a private room with running water.			
2. Post sign outside indicating type of isolation.			
3. Be sure a stand is outside with appropriate supplies (disposal bags, gowns, masks, gloves as needed).			
4. Have laundry hamper for inside room.			
5. Be sure a wastebasket with plastic liner is inside of room.			
6. Be sure a thermometer, blood pressure cuff, and stethoscope are inside of room.			
7. Make certain a special container for used needles and instruments is readily available.			
Entering the Room			
1. Obtain all needed equipment.			
2. Wash hands for infection control.			
3. Put watch in plastic bag.			
4. Put on gown, if needed. a. Put on gown, making sure uniform is covered.			
b. Fasten ties securely.			
5. Put on mask, if needed. a. Place mask over nose and mouth.			
b. Fasten both sets of ties securely.			
c. Tuck bottom edge under chin and fit the top edge snugly across the bridge of nose.			
6. Put on clean gloves, if needed. a. Put on both gloves.			
b. Tuck sleeves of gown securely inside of gloves.			
Double Bagging			
1. Inside nurse: Place used items in appropriate containers or bags. Carefully close and secure each bag.			

(continued)

	Needs More Practice	Satisfactory	Comments
Double Bagging *(Continued)*			
2. Outside nurse: Form a cuff on outer bag and hold with hands underneath for protection.			
3. Inside nurse: Place the bag holding contaminated items directly into the bag being held by the outside nurse, being careful to touch only the inside of that bag.			
4. Outside nurse: Fold over and carefully secure top of bag.			
5. Mark bag in manner prescribed by facility.			
6. Dispose of bag in proper place			
Caring for Linen			
1. Handle soiled linen with gloved hands.			
2. Touch only inside of laundry bag when placing soiled linen into bag.			
3. Double-bag wet linen.			
Caring for Dishes and Food Trays			
1. Place tray in plastic bag or use disposables if organisms transmitted on eating utensils.			
2. Treat as other trays if organisms not transmitted on eating utensils.			
Leaving the Room			
1. Complete your work in the room.			
2. Remove soiled gloves by turning inside out as you pull gloves off. a. Peel first glove off, touching only the outside with other gloved hand.			
b. Hold first glove in second hand.			
c. Slide ungloved fingers inside of second glove and turn glove inside out over first glove while removing it.			
3. Untie waist ties.			
4. Wash your hands.			
5. Untie neck ties, dropping gown over shoulders.			
6. Pull off gown, touching only inside, and place in laundry hamper or waste basket.			

(continued)

Leaving the Room *(Continued)*	Needs More Practice	Satisfactory	Comments
7. Untie mask ties and discard mask carefully, touching ties only.			
8. Wash your hands.			
9. Open door, using paper towel as barrier.			
10. Wash your hands outside room.			
General Procedure for Isolation Technique			
Assessment			
1. Check type of isolation ordered.			
2. Identify reason for isolation.			
3. Check equipment outside and inside the patient's room to make sure you have everything you need.			
Planning			
4. Wash your hands.			
5. Gather necessary equipment not outside or inside the patient's room.			
Implementation			
6. Identify the patient. Explain what you are doing.			
7. Carry out techniques necessary to enter room.			
8. Give care as planned.			
9. Carry out techniques necessary to leave room.			
Evaluation			
10. Evaluate, using the following criteria: **a.** Necessary equipment readily available.			
b. Isolation procedure correctly carried out.			
c. Patient left comfortable and safe.			
d. No nosomial infections originate from this patient.			
Documentation			
11. Document appropriately.			

?   Q U I Z

Short-Answer Questions

1. What are the two major purposes of isolation?

   a. _____

   b. _____

2. The organism that is causing Mr. Paulson's illness can be transmitted either by air or by contact. What type of isolation would be appropriate for him? Consider each system of isolation. _____

   _____

3. Mrs. Raymond is a postoperative patient whose care has been complicated by the presence of a pathogen transmitted by direct contact, the mode of transmission being the gastrointestinal system. What type of isolation would be appropriate for her? Consider each system of isolation.

   _____

4. List three items required in the preparation of a room for isolation procedure when the organism is airborne.

   a. _____

   b. _____

   c. _____

5. How are items removed from a protective isolation room? _____

   _____

6. If you are the outside nurse double-bagging an isolation room and the inside bag touches your hand, what should you do? _____

   _____

7. A patient with severe leukemia has been ordered placed in protective isolation. What is the purpose of isolation for this patient? _____

   _____

   Situation: Mrs. Rogers has been in isolation for 10 days. She seems irritable and shows no interest in eating or in the activities ordered by the physician.

8. What could be the source of her problem? _____

9. List at least three nursing actions that might help Mrs. Rogers.

   a. _____

   b. _____

   c. _____

MODULE

33

STERILE TECHNIQUE

MODULE CONTENTS

PREREQUISITES

Successful completion of the following modules:

VOLUME 1

OVERALL OBJECTIVES

To identify situations in which sterile technique is needed and to recognize breaks in technique when they occur. To open a sterile pack, set up a sterile field, add sterile items or fluid to a sterile area, and put on sterile gloves.

SPECIFIC LEARNING OBJECTIVES

Know Facts and Principles	Apply Facts and Principles	Demonstrate Ability	Evaluate Performance
1. Situations requiring sterile technique			
List common situations in which sterile technique is indicated.	Given a patient situation, identify which procedures require sterile technique.	In the clinical setting, decide correctly when to use sterile technique.	Evaluate decision with instructor.
2. Methods of sterilization			
Define *sterile*. List eight methods of sterilization and give an example of when each is used. State common ways to identify sterility.	Given a situation in which sterilization is needed, identify the appropriate process.	Identify whether a package is sterile.	Evaluate own performance using Performance Checklist.
3. Movement of microorganisms			
State six ways microorganisms move from one area to another. Identify methods used to maintain sterile field.	Given a situation in which a sterile field is used, identify any actions that would potentially contaminate it.	Open sterile pack correctly. Add sterile objects to sterile field without contaminating them. Pour liquid into sterile container. Put on sterile gloves.	Evaluate own performance using Performance Checklist.
4. Rationale for disinfection			
List common situations in which disinfection is used.	Given a patient situation, identify if disinfection is appropriate.	In a clinical setting, use disinfection appropriately.	Evaluate with instructor.
5. Methods of disinfection			
List two types of disinfectants, give an example of when each would be used, and state appropriate safety measures.	Given a situation in which disinfection is needed, identify the appropriate method.	In a clinical setting, use disinfection appropriately.	Evaluate with instructor.

LEARNING ACTIVITIES

1. Review the Specific Learning Objectives.
2. Read the chapter related to performing nursing procedures and the chapter on infection control in Ellis and Nowlis, *Nursing: A Human Needs Approach,* or comparable chapters in another textbook.
3. Look up the module vocabulary terms in the glossary.
4. Read through the module as though you were preparing to teach this information to another person. Mentally practice specific procedures.
5. Review the Performance Checklist.
6. In the practice setting:
   a. Open sterile packs.
   b. Add items to a sterile field.
   c. Pour liquids into sterile containers.
   d. Put on sterile gloves. Use the Performance Checklist as a guide.
7. When you can perform these tasks correctly, select a partner.
   a. Have your partner observe your performance and evaluate you, using the Performance Checklist.
   b. Observe and evaluate your partner, using the Checklist.
   Repeat this exercise until you have mastered the skill. Arrange with your instructor for a time to have your technique checked.
8. In the clinical setting:
   a. Arrange a visit to the department responsible for sterilizing equipment and supplies for your clinical group. Observe the methods of sterilization used in your facility.
   b. Identify situations in which sterile technique is needed.
   c. With other students, discuss situations that require sterile technique and how to proceed when technique is broken.

VOCABULARY

antiseptic	microorganism	sterilant	surgical asepsis
contaminated	pathogen	sterile technique	transfer forceps
disinfect	spore	sterilize	
disinfectant	sterile	sterilizer	

Sterile Technique

Rationale for the Use of This Skill

Strict sterile technique, or surgical asepsis, is frequently necessary in nursing. It is used most extensively in operating and delivery rooms, but it is also essential when performing such nursing procedures as injections, catheterizations, dressing changes, and intravenous therapy.

The purpose of sterilization is to eliminate all microorganisms as well as vegetative states such as spores from objects that come into contact with the tissues of the body that are normally sterile. Sterile technique is also used to protect patients from possible infection when normal body defenses are not intact. Nurses are responsible for identifying situations in which sterile technique is needed and for carrying out sterile procedures precisely.[1]

▼ NURSING DIAGNOSES

The most common nursing diagnoses relating to the need for sterile technique are:

Risk for Infection related to interruption of skin integrity by presence of surgical incision

Risk for Infection related to diminished immune response

Risk for Infection: Urinary, related to indwelling urinary catheter

PROCEDURES REQUIRING STERILE TECHNIQUE

Healthy, intact skin and mucous membranes provide an effective barrier to microorganisms, but underlying tissues provide an excellent medium for their growth. Therefore, when underlying tissues are exposed because of a wound or surgical incision, they must be protected against the entry of microorganisms by sterile technique.

Some internal body areas, such as the urinary bladder and the lungs, are normally sterile. To maintain this status, sterile technique is used whenever such an area must be entered. Although the eyes are not normally sterile, sterile technique is used in all procedures relating to them, *because the eyes are susceptible to infection, and the consequences of even a minor infection in the eye can be serious.*

Common situations in which sterile technique is used are inserting urinary catheters, changing sur-

[1]Rationale for action is emphasized throughout the module by the use of italics.

gical dressings, and preparing and administering injections.

STERILIZATION

The ideal method of sterilization not only should render an item free of all microorganisms (including spores and vegetative forms) but also should not damage the item being sterilized and should be relatively simple to use, inexpensive, and safe to those in the workplace. Unfortunately, no single method of sterilization meets all these criteria for all items that must be sterilized.

Many items used in modern healthcare facilities arrive from manufacturers in presterilized packages. However, sterilization of many items may still be done in a central department of the facility.

As a general staff nurse, you will be involved in using sterile materials in patient care activities and in sending items to the appropriate processing department for sterilization. Familiarity with sterilization and disinfection methods available in your setting, as well as with the care and handling of sterile materials, is important to the safe care of patients and equipment. If you are employed at a facility where you are required to carry out sterilization procedures, you will need more extensive education.

Any items to be sterilized must first be completely clean, no matter which method of sterilization is used. Among other reasons, *protein,* which is a part of all body secretions and excrement, *often coagulates, providing a protective barrier for microorganisms that helps them survive even the most careful sterilization procedure.*

Thermal

Moist Heat—Steam Under Pressure

Steam under pressure is the most reliable and commonly used sterilization procedure in healthcare facilities today. It is also the fastest, safest, and least expensive method available (Atkinson, 1992). *The high-pressure system enables the steam to reach a much higher temperature than is otherwise possible, and it is the temperature—not the pressure—that destroys microorganisms.*

Some items are not appropriate for steam sterilization. Rubber and plastics *may soften or melt, and delicate electronic devices may be damaged by moisture and high temperatures.* These items can be sterilized using other methods.

Every surface of items that are sterilized using steam under pressure must be reached by the steam during the processing time. For this to happen, the steam must be able to penetrate the packaging material. At the same time, the packaging material must be able to maintain the sterility of the item after the sterilization process. Items should be left in the steam sterilizer, also referred to as an autoclave, until they are cool and dry, *so that the exterior of a wrapped package can be handled, maintaining the sterility of the contents. Remember, moisture enhances the movement of microorganisms.*

Hot Air—Dry Heat

Hot air can penetrate substances that cannot be sterilized using other methods. It is used primarily to sterilize anhydrous oils, petroleum products, and bulk powders that steam under pressure and ethylene oxide cannot penetrate. When there is no moisture present, higher temperatures are required to destroy microorganisms.

Microwaves

Microwave sterilization uses low-pressure steam along with the nonionizing radiation of microwaves to produce temperatures sufficiently high to destroy microorganisms. The temperature required is lower than that of steam, and the time necessary is less.

Chemical

Ethylene Oxide Gas

Items that are sensitive to heat or moisture, such as equipment with plastic and electronic components, cannot be sterilized using steam under pressure but can be sterilized in an ethylene oxide (EO) gas sterilizer. The process must be carefully monitored *because EO is highly flammable and explosive in air*. It is reliable and safe when used properly, but *toxic emissions and residues of ethylene oxide can be hazardous to personnel and patients alike.* Because of this, Occupational Safety and Health Administration (OSHA) standards have been established governing the length of time an employee can be exposed to ethylene oxide. In addition, all absorbent materials that will come in contact with body tissues must be adequately aerated before being used. Manufacturers' recommendations for processing of specific products suitable for EO gas sterilization must be followed. An item that can be safely steam sterilized should never be gas sterilized (AORN Recommended Practices Committee, 1994).

Hydrogen Peroxide Plasma/Vapor

Hydrogen peroxide plasma is created by activating hydrogen peroxide to produce a reactive plasma or vapor. *Sterilization is achieved at low temperatures,* making it safe for some heat-sensitive items. *The process is nontoxic,* making aeration unnecessary. *Hydrogen peroxide plasma sterilization can be used for both moisture-stable and moisture-sensitive items,* and so may be substituted for EO and steam sterilization in healthcare facilities.

Ozone Gas

Ozone is generated from oxygen, and the ozone sterilizer is inexpensive and easy to operate. Ozone sterilization is appropriate for many heat- and moisture-sensitive items and *has the added benefit of leaving no residue,* therefore requiring no aeration period. *Ozone can be corrosive,* and so should not be used for items made of steel, brass, and aluminum. Also, it will destroy items made of natural gum rubber, such as latex (Atkinson, 1992).

Liquid Chemical Sterilant—Peracetic Acid

Peracetic acid is an example of a liquid sterilant and is suitable for sterilizing heat-sensitive items that are not harmed by moisture. It provides an alternative to gas or plasma sterilization if the item to be sterilized can be immersed. Although no aeration period is required, rinsing in sterile distilled water is required before items can be used. Instruments to be used immediately in a sterile procedure must also be dried with a sterile towel before being placed on a sterile field.

Ionizing Radiation

A less common method of sterilization is exposure to irradiation. Irradiation can be used to sterilize most heat- and moisture-sensitive items and generates no residual radiation. It is capable of penetrating large bulky items. Irradiation sterilization is currently limited to commercial use because of its cost. Cobalt 60 is the most commonly used source for irradiation sterilization.

DISINFECTION

Disinfection is used when items cannot be sterilized or in situations where no method of sterilization is available. Disinfection is done to eliminate as many microorganisms from an item or from the environment as possible, but does not eliminate spores. *Low-level disinfectants* are used for housekeeping purposes and for noncritical items that either do not touch the patient or only contact intact skin. *Intermediate-level disinfectants* are used for semicritical items that come in contact with intact skin or mucous membranes but do not enter body tissues. *High-level disinfectants* are used for critical items that *will* come in contact with body tissues below the skin or mucous membranes but will not be introduced into the intravascular system (Atkinson, 1992). When possible, critical items should be sterilized.

Chemical Disinfectants

A disinfectant is defined by the Environmental Protection Agency (EPA) as an agent that kills growing or vegetative forms of bacteria. Agents are labeled "virucidal" if effective against viruses, "fungicidal" if effective against fungi, and "sporicidal" if effective against spores. Only agents labeled as "tuberculocidal" are effective against the tubercle bacillus. Disinfectants labeled "tuberculocidal" are also effective against the human immunodeficiency virus (HIV). The hepatitis B virus is able to survive exposure to many disinfectants (Atkinson, 1992).

Items should be disinfected immediately before and after use. The nature of the contamination, the composition of the items to be disinfected, and the chemical agent to be used will all affect the method of application chosen. Read the label on the container and follow the policies in your setting. Wear gloves *to protect your hands* when handling disinfectants, because most are harsh to skin. Alcohol, chlorine compounds (such as household bleach in water), and iodophors (such as Betadine) are examples of chemical disinfectants.

For use in the home, a simple household bleach solution, considered a low-level disinfectant, can be used. This solution can kill weak viruses, such as the HIV virus, and bacteria but not all microorganisms. It must be made clear that this agent merely disinfects and *does not sterilize* items the solution contacts.

Physical Disinfectants

Boiling water is an old method of disinfection, but is still valuable in some situations, such as in the home and in circumstances where other methods of disinfection or sterilization are not available. This method is no longer used in contemporary healthcare facilities.

To use boiling water for disinfection, completely cover the items so that all surface areas are exposed to the water. Start timing only after a rolling boil has begun. Boil for a minimum of 30 minutes. If sodium carbonate is added to the water to make a 2 percent solution, the recommended boiling time is 15 minutes. This method is most often used for items that need disinfection between uses, such as bedpans and emesis basins. Some spore forms are not destroyed by boiling water.

Ultraviolet (UV) rays can kill vegetative bacteria, fungi, and lipoprotein viruses. *Because the rays must make direct contact with the organisms*, the use of UV irradiation is limited. Some operating rooms use ultraviolet lights to decrease airborne microorganism levels, but lights are turned on only when rooms are unoccupied, *because UV rays can cause skin burns and conjunctivitis of the eyes*. If you are required to work under exposure to UV irradiation, you must wear protective skin covering and goggles or a visor over your eyes.

You may also encounter UV lights in hospital isolation rooms designed especially for patients with infectious tuberculosis. In these situations, the lights are shielded, so that the persons in the rooms are not required to wear special protective clothing. Ultraviolet irradiation does not kill spores or the hepatitis B virus.

INDICATORS OF STERILITY

Indicators that react to steam under pressure or gas when exposed to it for a prolonged period are used to demonstrate an item's sterility. These indicators are commonly seen on packs in the form of special tape. Dark lines appear on the tape after a package has been exposed to a temperature for sufficient time to sterilize the item. Small glass-tubing indicators that contain a substance sensitive to heat are sometimes placed inside large packs to indicate sterility. The sterility of bottles of liquids is usually identified by the presence of a vacuum seal.

Every commercial product has some indicator of sterility. It is your responsibility to check the manufacturer's literature for this information, so you can confirm the sterility of an item before using it.

Wrapped packages retain their sterility for various lengths of time, depending on the type of wrapping material, the conditions of storage, and the integrity of the package. An expiration date should appear on the sterile package. Do not use the contents after that date until the item or items inside have been resterilized.

GENERAL PRINCIPLES

Microorganisms move through space on air currents. Thus, items that are exposed to the air for a prolonged period are considered contaminated. For this reason, it is important to minimize air movement or to control its direction through special ventilation to limit the movement of microorganisms. When a sterile field is open, keep doors closed, and do not shake drapes and gowns, even if they are sterile.

Microorganisms are transferred from one surface to another whenever a nonsterile object touches another object. Keep sterile objects at a distance from nonsterile ones to prevent the transfer of microorganisms. *Any contact, no matter how brief, renders sterile items nonsterile.* To preserve sterility, pick up sterile items with sterile gloves or with transfer forceps. When in doubt about the sterility of any item, consider it unsterile.

Microorganisms move from one object to another as a result of gravity when a nonsterile item is held above another item. For this reason, it is important to keep nonsterile objects, among them your own arm, from being over the sterile field.

Microorganisms travel rapidly along any moisture through a wicking action. If moisture connects a nonsterile surface to a sterile one, the sterile surface is considered contaminated.

Microorganisms move slowly along a dry surface. If one side of a dry object is touched, that side is contaminated, but the opposite side is still considered to be sterile. When someone picks up sterile forceps, the handle is immediately contaminated but the tips, which have not been touched, are sterile. Maintain a safety margin of at least 1 inch around a contaminated portion.

Microorganisms are released into the air on droplet nuclei whenever a person breathes or speaks. In a situation where sterility is critical (for example, the operating room), personnel wear masks to stop this source of contamination. In the general setting a mask may be omitted, but avoid talking across a sterile field, turn your head away when speaking, and speak only when necessary in a sterile environment.

Because microorganisms are in constant motion in a variety of ways, sterile areas must be protected by providing wide margins for safety. *Because you cannot guarantee what you cannot see,* it is common practice to consider anything that is out of sight to be nonsterile. *A person's back is considered nonsterile, even when clothed in an originally sterile gown.* Therefore, two persons in sterile gowns should always pass face to face or back to back, *so there is no danger of the sterile front touching the nonsterile back.* Keep gloved hands in front of you, in your line of vision. Remember that all items below your waist or below table level are considered nonsterile *because they are out of full view.*

The edge of any sterile field is potentially contaminated by microorganisms moving in from the outside. Therefore, keep sterile objects away from the edge of the field. Again, 1 inch is considered a minimum safety margin.

If you must set up a sterile field ahead of time or leave it during use, cover it with a sterile drape of some type *to prevent contamination.* Use a single thickness of paper drape or a double thickness of cloth drapes.

STERILE PROCEDURES

Arranging a Sterile Field

1. Wash your hands.
2. Choose a flat, hard, dry surface on which to prepare a sterile field. Clear a sufficient area, *so you have plenty of room to work.* As a beginner, you will find you need at least a 12-inch-square field.
3. Before sterilization, objects are wrapped *so that they can be opened without contaminating the contents.* The wrapper, when opened, provides a sterile field.
4. As you add additional sterile items, place them well within the edge of the sterile field.

Opening a Sterile Pack

1. Wash your hands.
2. When you open a sterile package, do not reach over a sterile object or area.
3. Grasp only the outside edge of the wrapper. To accomplish this, open the far flap first, then the side flaps, and finally the flap closest to you. The item can also be turned, or you can walk around it. In some instances you may reach around the object, but it is difficult to do this without contaminating the item. Figure 33–1 shows the proper sequence for opening a sterile package.
4. Do not allow anything nonsterile to touch the contents of the package.

Adding Items to a Sterile Field

When you add additional sterile items to a sterile field, you must take care that contamination does not occur.

1. Wash your hands.
2. Unwrap the item as for any sterile package. Pick it up by sliding your hand underneath the sterile

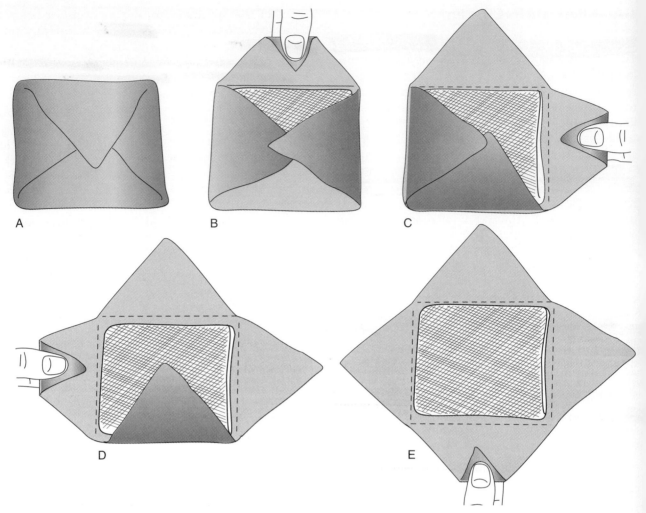

Figure 33–1. Opening a sterile package. Remember not to reach over a sterile object. **(A)** Unopened package. **(B)** First flap opened. **(C)** Second flap opened. **(D)** Third flap opened. **(E)** Fourth flap opened, sterile object in center of sterile field.

covering. Gather the ends of the covering back around your wrist, forming a sterile cover for your hand, and keep the ends from dragging.

Commercially packaged sterile dressings usually come in packages that peel open. Remember that *the ends you have grasped to peel back are contaminated* and should not touch the dressing, nor should they be held over the sterile field. If one peeled-back side is folded under, it is possible to slide the dressing off over the sterile folded edge.

3. Place items well within the sterile field, keeping your hands as far away from the field as possible. Small items, such as gauze dressings, may be dropped from 6–8 inches above the sterile field (Fig. 33–2); large items should be put down carefully. You can use sterile forceps to remove an item from a package and place it in the sterile field.

4. Avoid reaching over the sterile field with your arm as much as possible.

Adding Liquids to a Sterile Field

1. Wash your hands.
2. Pour a small amount of a nonsterile solution (e.g., Betadine) into a waste receptacle (*to clean the lip of the container*) before you pour the contents into the sterile receptacle.
3. To pour a liquid into a container in the sterile field, pour it from 6 to 8 inches above the receiving container, *to avoid the possibility of the two containers touching* (Fig. 33–3).
4. Pour slowly *to prevent splashing.*

If liquid is spilled onto the sterile field, the spot is considered contaminated if the moisture can soak through to the nonsterile surface beneath.

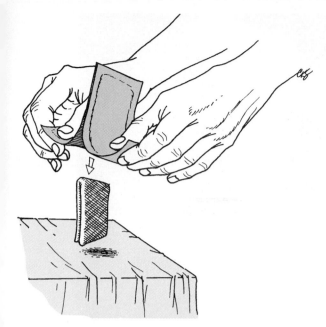

Figure 33–2. The nurse holds the package by touching only the outside and drops the sterile contents onto the sterile field.

Remember that *microorganisms move rapidly through moisture.* If the drape is waterproof (many disposable drapes have a plastic layer) and the sterile liquid pools up on the surface, the area is still sterile. Usually, however, this area is covered with a dry drape *because moisture may attract microorganisms in the air.*

5. Keep your arm as far as possible from the sterile field. Avoid reaching over the sterile field if possible.

Putting on Sterile Gloves

1. Remove all rings and wash your hands before putting on sterile gloves. *Gloves may have small imperfections or may tear, and bacteria can multiply rapidly on the skin of gloved hands. A ring can also tear the glove and can harbor microorganisms.* Module 2, Basic Infection Control, outlines general handwashing procedure. Module 34, Surgical Asepsis: Scrubbing, Gowning, and Gloving, gives the procedure for a surgical scrub, required in operating and delivery rooms and before some invasive procedures. For sterile procedures such as urinary catheterizations and dressing changes, carrying out the 2-minute handwashing procedure described in Module 2, Basic Infection Control, is generally considered adequate preparation for putting on gloves.

    Put on sterile gloves without touching the outside of the gloves, *so contamination does not occur.*

Gloves are packaged uniformly *to facilitate this procedure.*

2. Sterile gloves are sealed in a sterile package. Open the package in the same way you would open any other sterile package, unless it is a commercially prepared paper package. In that instance, instructions for opening are printed on the outside of the package.

    Inside the sterile package is a folder containing the gloves. A small, folded-back margin is provided over each glove, *so you can open the folder without touching the gloves.* The gloves in the package are arranged palm upward, with the left glove on the left side and the right glove on the right side. A cuff of 2 to 4 inches is folded down over each glove. Figure 33–4 shows the correct sequence for opening and putting on sterile gloves.

3. Open one side of the folder, either left or right, touching only the center lower corner. Pick up the exposed glove with your opposite hand (the left glove with the right hand or the right glove with the left hand). Be careful to touch only the folded cuff.

4. Insert your free hand into the glove without touching skin to the outside of the glove. (The rhyme "sk*in* side to *in*side" may help you re-

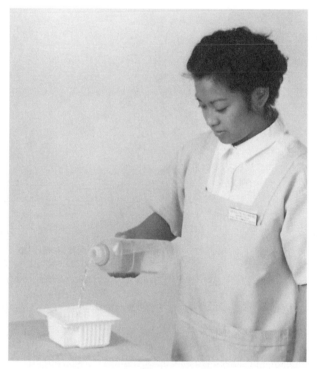

Figure 33–3. The nurse pours into a container on the sterile field by not reaching over the field and not pouring from a height that could cause splashing.

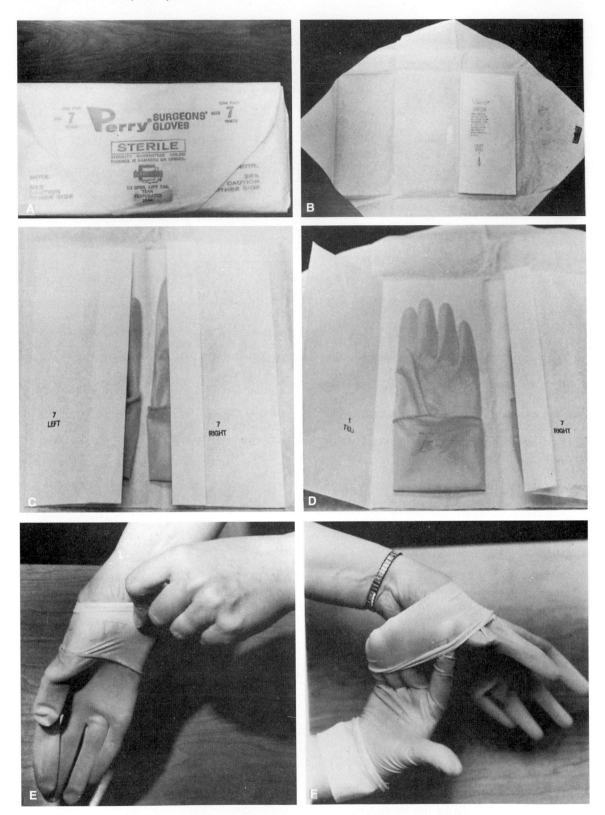

Figure 33–4. Putting on sterile gloves. **(A)** Obtain a sealed package of gloves. **(B)** Open the outer wrapper, following the directions on the package. **(C and D)** Open the inner folder at the corner without touching the gloves. **(E)** Pick up the right glove with your left hand, touching only the folded cuff, and put it on. **(F)** Grasp the left glove under the cuff and put it on. (Courtesy Ivan Ellis)

member this.) Be sure you hold the glove well away from your body and from the table or package as you work. A common error is to brush the tips of the glove fingers against a nonsterile surface while maneuvering, thus contaminating the gloves.

5. Open the second side of the folder with your ungloved hand, exposing the second glove. Pick up the glove with your gloved hand from under the cuff, which is the outside surface. Be sure to keep the thumb of the gloved hand rigidly extended outward or folded against the palm, *so you are not tempted to use it to grasp the other glove.* Hold the glove under its cuff by your four gloved fingers. *The cuff on the second glove protects the gloved hand from contamination by touching and also from microorganisms moving by gravity.*

6. Carefully maneuver the second hand into the glove.

7. When both gloves are on, turn the cuffs up by flipping them, taking care not to roll the outside of the gloves onto your skin. You may then make any necessary adjustments so the gloves fit smoothly.

HOME CARE

Patients needing sterile dressing changes are often discharged home. Some of these adult and pediatric patients have central lines in place that may require regular sterile dressing changes. The materials and equipment are available from commercial companies.

As a nurse in the hospital or as a nurse in home healthcare, you may be involved in performing the procedure yourself or teaching sterile technique to the care provider. Demonstrating the principles outlined in this module and having the designated care provider return the demonstration under your supervision are helpful in teaching a technique that will prevent infection. You should also teach the patient and caregiver(s) that pets should not be in the room while a sterile procedure is being done.

Some procedures carried out using sterile technique in the hospital or nursing home are commonly done using clean technique in the home setting.

CRITICAL THINKING EXERCISES

You are changing a surgical dressing when you inadvertently contaminate your left glove (you are right-handed). There is no other staff member in the room who can get another pair of gloves for you. Propose several ways you could handle this situation.

References

AORN Recommended Practices Committee. (1994). Proposed recommended practices for sterilization in the practice setting. *AORN Journal, 60*(1), 109–119.

Atkinson, L. (1992). *Berry & Kohn's operating room technique* (7th ed.). St. Louis: Mosby.

✔ **PERFORMANCE CHECKLIST**

	Needs More Practice	Satisfactory	Comments
Arranging a Sterile Field			
1. Wash your hands.			
2. Choose a flat, hard, dry surface.			
3. Open sterile pack, using wrapper for sterile field.			
4. Add additional sterile items, placing them well within edge of sterile field.			
Opening a Sterile Pack or Set			
1. Wash your hands.			
2. Do not cross your hand or arm over sterile area.			
3. Touch wrapper on outside only.			
4. Do not allow anything nonsterile to touch contents of pack.			
Adding Items to Sterile Field			
1. Wash your hands.			
2. Open package away from sterile field.			
3. Drop sterile item onto sterile field, keeping hands as far from field as possible.			
4. Avoid reaching over field with arm as much as possible.			
Adding Liquid to Sterile Field			
1. Wash your hands.			
2. If the liquid is nonsterile, pour small amount over lip of bottle first, into waste receptacle.			
3. Pour from 6–8 inches above sterile container; do not touch lip of bottle to container.			
4. Pour slowly.			
5. Keep arm as far as possible from sterile field. Avoid reaching over field if possible.			
Putting on Sterile Gloves			
1. Remove rings and wash your hands.			
2. Open wrapper so that areas touched do not touch gloves.			

(continued)

Putting on Sterile Gloves *(Continued)*	Needs More Practice	Satisfactory	Comments
3. Pick up first glove, touching only inside surface (cuff).			
4. Put on first glove without allowing outside to touch anything.			
5. Pick up second glove from under cuff with fingers (only) of gloved hand.			
6. Put on second glove, touching only inside of second glove with bare hand.			
7. Turn up cuffs, touching gloved hand only to outside of other glove. Do not let outside of glove touch your skin.			

MODULE

34

SURGICAL ASEPSIS: SCRUBBING, GOWNING, AND GLOVING

MODULE CONTENTS

PREREQUISITES

Successful completion of the following modules:

OVERALL OBJECTIVES

To scrub the hands and arms in a thorough manner to decrease the bacterial count preparatory to participating in procedures that require surgical technique. To put on and function appropriately in sterile attire, identifying breaks in technique if they occur and taking corrective action.

SPECIFIC LEARNING OBJECTIVES

Know Facts and Principles	Apply Facts and Principles	Demonstrate Ability	Evaluate Performance
1. Purposes State three purposes of surgical scrub.	Identify which persons in a specific situation must perform surgical scrubs.		
2. Scrubbing *a. Equipment* List equipment needed for surgical scrub and rationale for use.		Obtain and set up needed equipment for surgical scrub.	Check module to be sure all equipment is ready.
b. Types of scrub State two major bases for planning scrub procedure.	Given a specific scrub procedure, identify major basis for planning procedure.		
c. Procedure List steps in scrubbing procedure.	Explain rationale for each step in scrubbing procedure.	Scrub, using procedure outlined in module.	Evaluate own performance using Performance Checklist. Verify procedure with observer.
3. Gowning and gloving List steps for putting on sterile gown. List steps of closed-glove technique. Identify part of gown considered sterile.	Identify situations in which gowning and gloving are necessary. Explain rationale for wearing gowns. Explain rationale for closed-glove technique.	Put on gown correctly. Put on sterile gloves correctly, using closed-glove technique.	Evaluate own performance using Performance Checklist. Verify with observer that contamination did not occur.
4. Guidelines for functioning in sterile attire List six guidelines for functioning in sterile attire.	Identify reasons for guidelines.	Preserve sterility of own attire. Identify contamination if it occurs and take immediate corrective action.	Evaluate own performance. Validate with observer.

LEARNING ACTIVITIES

1. Review the Specific Learning Objectives.
2. Look up the module vocabulary terms in the glossary.
3. Read through the module as though you were preparing to teach the concepts and skills to another person. Mentally practice the procedure.
4. Read the scrub procedures of the facility where you are assigned, if available.
5. With a partner, in the practice setting:
   a. Look at the scrub equipment available.
   b. Compare it with what is described in the module.
   c. Adapt the equipment as needed. For example, if sink foot controls are not available, arrange for someone else to turn off the water.
   d. Prepare the equipment, including a gown and gloves.
   e. Scrub your hands and arms, using the Performance Checklist (or your facility's procedure) as a guide.
   f. Have your partner observe and evaluate your performance.
   g. Put on the sterile gown and gloves, using the Performance Checklist as a guide.
   h. Have your partner observe and evaluate your performance.
   i. Reverse roles and repeat steps d through h.
   j. Repeat practice until you have mastered these skills.
   k. Ask your instructor to evaluate your performance.
6. Ask your instructor for an opportunity to observe in an area where scrubbing, gowning, and gloving are carried out.
7. In class or clinical postconference, discuss with your classmates the similarities and differences between the procedure you learned and the one(s) you observed. Be prepared to present rationale for recommended practices.
8. Ask your instructor for an opportunity to scrub in an area where you are prepared to function appropriately in the nursing role, for example, as an assistant to the nurse in the delivery room or operating room.

VOCABULARY

antimicrobial	culture	medial	sterile
antiseptic	disinfectant	microorganism	subungual
axilla	lateral	normal flora	surgical asepsis

Surgical Asepsis: Scrubbing, Gowning, and Gloving

Rationale for the Use of This Skill

Handwashing alone does not eliminate normal flora on the hands. This normal flora can produce infection when introduced into an open wound. During surgical procedures, deliveries, and invasive diagnostic procedures, sterile gloves are worn. However, gloves can tear in the course of a procedure, so it is important that the hands be rendered as nearly free of microorganisms as possible. *A gown, too, can become moist, allowing microorganisms to move from the arms to the surface of the gown.*

Surgical scrubbing *lowers the total count of microorganisms on the hands and arms. It also removes dirt and oil from the skin, decreasing the ability of remaining microorganisms to multiply. After scrubbing, a residue of antimicrobial cleansing agent remains on the skin, which further reduces the growth of microorganisms.*

Gowns and gloves worn for sterile procedures must be put on in a way that ensures that nothing nonsterile touches their outer surfaces. To maintain the highest standard of sterility, proper scrubbing, gowning, and gloving technique is essential.[1]

SCRUBBING

Every facility has its own routine for performing a surgical scrub. *The use of a specific routine ensures that all individuals maintain the same high standard.* Always follow the procedure established by your facility or, if none exists, work to establish an appropriate procedure.

It is recommended that consultation with the infection control committee should take place in each practice setting regarding scrub policies and procedures (AORN, 1990). Presented here are the general principles related to the surgical scrub as well as an example of a scrub procedure.

Equipment

A nail-cleaning device such as a metal nail file or plastic nail cleaner is necessary *to remove debris from the subungual area under the nail of each finger.* Wooden cleaning sticks (orange sticks) are not recommended, *because the wood can splinter and harbor microorganisms.*

The scrubbing device may be a sterilized reusable scrub brush or a disposable sponge. Disposable products are individually packaged and are often impregnated with one of a variety of antiseptic detergent agents.

Liquid antibacterial soap or detergent, preferably in a container that can be operated by a foot pedal, is necessary *to reduce the number of microorganisms on the skin.* Many facilities provide a choice of cleansing agents, *so if you are sensitive to one type, you can use another type.*

The scrub sink should be deep and wide enough *so you can hold both arms over it and water cannot splash out onto your scrub attire. Moisture can contaminate the sterile gown put on over scrub attire.* Foot- or knee-operated faucets (rather than hand-operated ones) are preferred *to prevent contamination of the hands after you have scrubbed them.*

Before you begin to scrub, adjust your cap and mask *because you may not touch them during or after scrubbing.* Open a pack that contains a sterile gown and a sterile towel for drying the hands and arms after scrubbing. Place these in a convenient location along with gloves of the correct size.

Types of Scrubs

Counted Brush-Stroke Method

This method dictates a specified number of strokes for each surface of the fingers, hands, and arms. *It ensures complete and thorough coverage of all areas, no matter how rapidly you scrub.*

Timed Method

With this method you scrub each surface of the fingers, hands, and arms for a specified time, using a prescribed anatomic pattern *to ensure that no area is missed. Timed scrubs ensure optimum contact with the cleansing agent.*

Policies and procedures for the surgical scrub should be standardized and reviewed annually in individual facilities. The approved procedure should be posted in each scrub room.

The specific procedure for scrubbing may differ from one facility to another, but certain principles of aseptic technique are common to both the counted brush-stroke scrub and the timed scrub. Either method, if properly done, is effective and ensures sufficient exposure of all skin surfaces to friction and the antibacterial soap or detergent.

Atkinson (1992) recommends thinking of the fingers, hands, and arms as having four sides or surfaces. She further recommends following an anatomic pattern of scrub: "four surfaces of each fin-

---

[1]Rationale for action is emphasized throughout the module by the use of italics.

ger, beginning with the thumb and moving from one finger to the next, down the outer edge of the fifth finger, over the dorsal (back) surface of the hand, the palmar (palm) surface of the hand, or vice versa, from small finger to thumb, over the wrists and up the arm, in thirds, ending 2 inches (5 cm) above the elbow." *Because the hands are in the most direct contact with the sterile field,* begin the steps of any scrub procedure with the hands and finish with the elbows. Also, keep the hands higher than the elbows during the scrub procedure, *to allow water to flow from the cleanest area (the hands) to the less clean area (the elbows)* (AORN, 1990).

Properly done, a surgical scrub usually takes about 5 minutes. Facilities are encouraged to use the scrub agent manufacturer's recommendations when instituting policies and procedures for scrub times. All scrubs should follow the same procedure as the initial scrub of the day (Rehork & Ruden, 1991). Follow the policies and procedure established in your facility.

PROCEDURE FOR SCRUBBING

1. Prepare yourself for the scrub.
   a. Put on the proper surgical attire used in your facility. These are called "scrub" garments. *Wearing surgical attire prevents bringing outside organisms into the area.* All personnel should wear scrub attire consisting of a two-piece pantsuit. The scrub shirt should be tucked into the scrub pants or fit close to the body *so that loose garments do not come into contact with scrubbed hands and arms or with the sterile drying towel.*
   b. Put on a cap or hood, shoe covers, a mask, and, if necessary, protective eye gear *to cover common sources of contamination* (Fig. 34–1).
      (1) Cap or hood–All facial and head hair must be completely covered. If pierced-ear studs are worn, they must be completely covered by the cap or hood.
      (2) Shoe covers–Shoe covers are worn *to protect personnel from exposure to blood and body fluids that might contain infectious agents when spills or splashes are anticipated.*
      (3) Mask–The mask should cover both nose and mouth. Although there is some doubt as to the value of masks in preventing infection in patients, they may have value as protection to the surgical team (Mathias, 1993). Handle only the ties of a used mask when discarding a mask after use *to prevent contamination of the hands by a soiled*

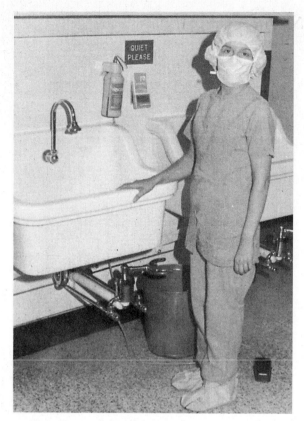

Figure 34–1. Before scrubbing, the nurse puts on surgical attire (scrub garments). Note foot pedal for liquid soap and knee-operated faucet. (Courtesy Ivan Ellis)

mask. It is generally accepted policy for masks to be worn in sterile settings and for individuals to remask with a fresh mask between procedures (Atkinson, 1992).
      (4) Eye wear–Protective eye gear must be worn *when personnel are at risk for a splash or spray to the eyes or face.* Attachments that provide protection from side splash are available for eye glasses. Individuals who wear glasses should clean them before scrubbing. A new mask is available with an added splash guard (Fig. 34–2).
   Each facility should have clear policies and procedures established for proper scrub attire to be worn in that setting. All personnel must conform to the established policy.
   c. Examine your hands and forearms for cuts or blemishes. Do not scrub if there are any open lesions or breaks in skin integrity *because they can contaminate surgical wounds.*
   d. Remove all watches, rings, and bracelets *because they harbor microorganisms beneath them* (Atkinson, 1992).
   e. Ensure that fingernails are in good condition and no longer than the tips of the fingers *to*

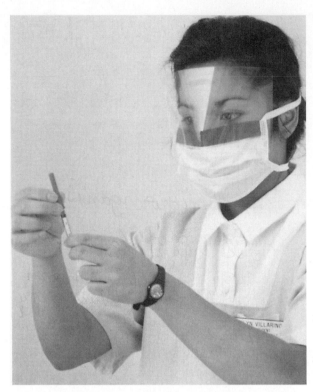

Figure 34–2. A splash guard mask protects the eyes and mucous membranes from accidental blood splashes.

prevent puncturing the gloves. Nail polish that is obviously chipped has a tendency to harbor microorganisms. If policy in your facility allows the wearing of nail polish, you should change the nail polish every 4 days *so that your nails remain well manicured.* Artificial fingernails should not be worn *because studies have shown that a higher number of microorganisms have been cultured from the fingertips of nurses wearing artificial nails than from the fingertips of nurses with natural nails.* Additionally, *because of moisture being trapped between the natural and artificial nails,* fungal growth often occurs under artificial nails (Meeker & Rothrock, 1991).

2. Perform the prescrub.
    a. Turn on the water and adjust the temperature so that it is comfortably warm. *Warm water emulsifies fats more effectively than cold water does, and hot water is harsh to the skin.*
    b. Moisten your hands and arms, keeping your hands higher than your elbows *so that water will drain off your elbows, flowing from the cleanest area to the less clean area.*
    c. Using one of the surgical hand scrub agents provided, lather your hands and arms for 1 minute.
    d. Remove a reusable brush or prepackaged, disposable brush or sponge from the dispenser

and clean under each fingernail and around each cuticle with the nail cleaner included. Rinse the nail cleaner after cleaning each fingernail.
    e. Rinse hands and arms thoroughly, passing them through the water *in one direction only,* from fingertips to elbow. Do not move your arms back and forth through the water.
3. Scrub.
    a. Counted brush-stroke method
        (1) Select a sterile brush or sponge. Apply a liquid cleanser if the brush or sponge is not impregnated with one.
        (2) Scrub the nails of the left hand 30 strokes and all skin surfaces 20 strokes, using the anatomic pattern of scrub previously outlined (Atkinson, 1992) (Fig. 34–3).
            (a) Four surfaces of each finger, thumb to fifth finger
            (b) Over dorsal surface of hand, small finger to thumb
            (c) Over palmar surface of hand, small finger to thumb
            (d) Over the wrist
            (e) Up the arm in thirds, ending 2 inches above the elbow
        (3) Repeat step (2) for the right hand and arm.
    b. Timed method
        (1) Select a sterile brush or sponge and apply liquid cleanser if the brush or sponge is not impregnated with one.
        (2) Scrub the nails, fingers, hand, and wrist of your left arm for 1½ minutes, using the anatomic pattern of scrub described above.

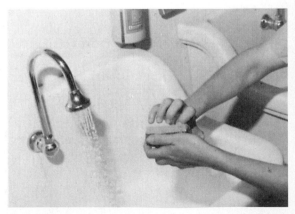

Figure 34–3. The nurse scrubs the nails briskly with a small sterile brush after the prescrub has been completed. (Courtesy Ivan Ellis)

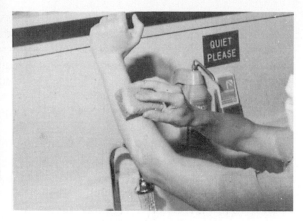

Figure 34–4. The hands and forearms are scrubbed with a sterile brush or sponge after the nails are cleaned and brushed. (Courtesy Ivan Ellis)

(3) Repeat for the right nails, fingers, hand, and wrist.

(4) Scrub from the wrist to 2 inches above the elbow, spending 1 minute on each arm (Fig. 34–4).

4. Rinse.

   a. Rinse hands and arms as previously described, passing through the water in one direction from fingertips to elbow (Fig. 34–5).

   b. Keep hands extended in front of you and above the height of your waist *to avoid contamination.* If a sterile towel is not available near the scrub sink, walk to the table where the towels are kept. If you must go through closed doors, back through. Allow water to drip from your elbows (Fig. 34–6).

5. Dry your hands and arms.

   a. Pick up the sterile towel by one end.

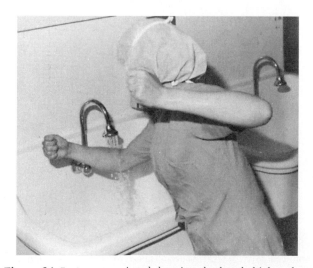

Figure 34–5. Arms are rinsed, keeping the hands higher than the elbows. (Courtesy Ivan Ellis)

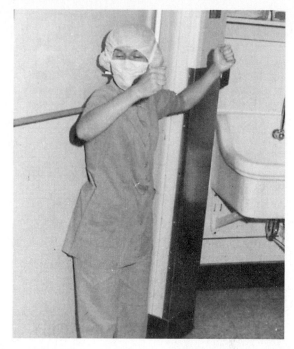

Figure 34–6. The nurse backs through a closed door with arms raised to prevent contamination. (Courtesy Ivan Ellis)

   b. Allow the towel to unfold.

   c. Place one hand under half of the towel. Use that half to blot the opposite hand dry (Fig. 34–7). Start at the fingers and move gradually up the arm.

   d. Use the other half of the towel to blot the second arm dry. Again, start at the fingers and move up the arm.

   e. Push the cuticles of your fingernails back with the towel as you dry your hands. *This helps to prevent ragged cuticle edges, decreasing the possibility of harboring bacteria. You are now ready to put on a sterile gown and gloves.*

GOWNING AND GLOVING

After you have scrubbed and dried your hands, you are ready to put on a sterile gown. Remember to keep your hands above your waist and higher than your elbows at all times *to make sure they do not touch anything nonsterile.*

Gowning is a two-person procedure. You will need an assistant to put on a sterile gown safely, and your assistant will need sterile forceps.

The closed-glove technique, which is described in step 7 below, is in widespread use because *it provides a way to put on gloves without the possibility that they will be touched on the outside by the bare hand.* You will put on the right glove first, and then the left glove.

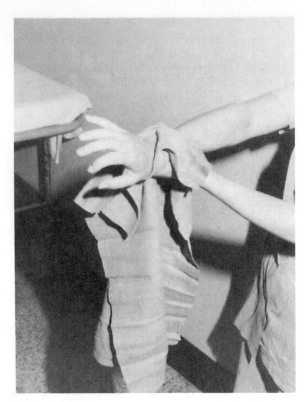

Figure 34–7. Hands and arms are dried with a sterile towel. (Courtesy Ivan Ellis)

(Open-glove technique is described in Module 33, Sterile Technique.)

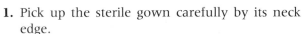

PROCEDURE FOR GOWNING AND GLOVING

1. Pick up the sterile gown carefully by its neck edge.
2. Facing the sterile field, hold the gown by the inside, top neckline in front of you and allow it to unfold (Fig. 34–8).
3. Position it so that you are facing the back opening.
4. Work your hands and arms carefully into the gown and into the sleeves, as far as the seam between the sleeve and the cuff. Take your time and proceed slowly. Do not push your hands out through the ends of the sleeves.
5. Turn your back to your assistant, who will now grasp the inside of the back, pull it securely onto your shoulders, and tie the neck and back waistline ties.
6. Leave the front waistline tie tied in front of you.
7. Using the closed-glove technique, put on the sterile gloves.
   a. Use your left hand still inside the gown to pick up the folded edge of the right glove.

b. Hold your right hand out, with the palm up, still inside the sleeve.
c. Lay the right glove on the right palm (which is still inside the sleeve). Position it with the glove fingers pointing toward the elbow and the cuff end pointing toward the fingertips. The thumb of the glove should be over the thumb of your right hand (Fig. 34–9).
d. Use your right hand (which is still inside the gown sleeve) to grasp the bottom fold of the cuff end of the right glove. You are touching sterile gown to sterile glove.
e. With your left hand (which is still inside the gown sleeve), grasp the right glove cuff by the top fold of the cuff end, and pull the right glove cuff up and over the right gown cuff (Fig. 34–10).
f. Adjust the right glove cuff over the right gown cuff as necessary, keeping the left hand inside the gown.
g. Work your right hand down into the glove. If the fingers are not in place, do not be concerned. *You can correct them when both gloves are on.*

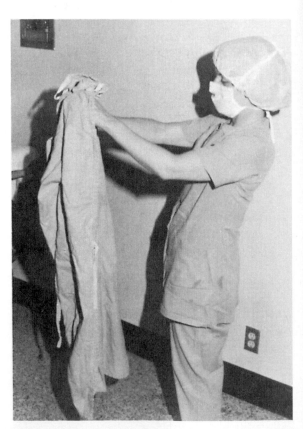

Figure 34–8. To put on a sterile gown, face the sterile field and hold the gown by the inside neckline. Allow it to fall open and work your hands and arms carefully into the gown. (Courtesy Ivan Ellis)

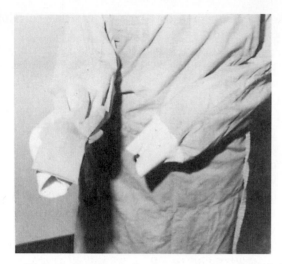

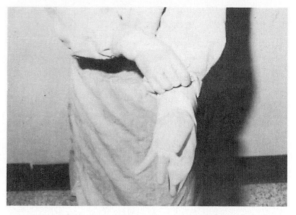

Figure 34–11. The second glove can be pulled up by the hand wearing the sterile glove. (Courtesy Ivan Ellis)

Figure 34–9. Position the sterile glove by reaching through the gown with your opposite hand. (Courtesy Ivan Ellis)

h. Pick up the left glove with the gloved right hand.

i. Hold your left hand, palm up, inside the gown sleeve.

j. Place the left glove on the left palm (which is still inside the gown), with the glove fingers pointing toward the elbow and the cuff end pointing toward your fingertips. Position the glove thumb over the left thumb of your hand.

k. Use your left hand (which is still inside the sleeve) to grasp the bottom fold of the cuff end of the left glove.

l. Grasp the top fold of the cuff edge with the gloved right hand, and pull the glove cuff up and over the gown cuff (Fig. 34–11).

m. Work your left hand down into the left glove.

n. Turn up and adjust the cuffs of both gloves (Fig 34–12).

o. Pull the glove fingers out at the ends to reposition your fingers if necessary.

8. With your gloved hands, untie the front waist tie of your gown.

9. Hold the ends carefully, keeping them above your waist.

10. Hold the shorter tie in one hand.

11. With the other hand, hold the longer tie out for your assistant to grasp with sterile forceps.

12. While your assistant is holding the tie, turn around carefully, wrapping the gown around you as you turn. This completely covers your back with the sterile gown. Be sure you are well away from all equipment when you turn.

13. Retrieve the tie from your assistant, and tie the two ties together in the front. You are now prepared to handle sterile equipment and to assist

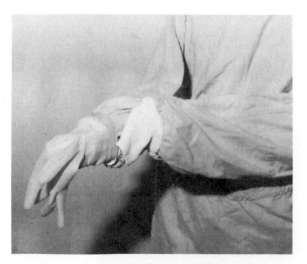

Figure 34–10. Pull up the first glove with your opposite hand still inside the gown. (Courtesy Ivan Ellis)

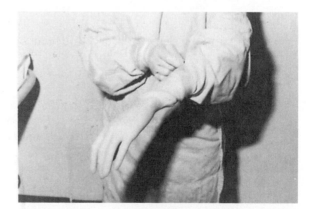

Figure 34–12. When sterile gloves are on both hands, the cuffs can be safely adjusted. (Courtesy Ivan Ellis)

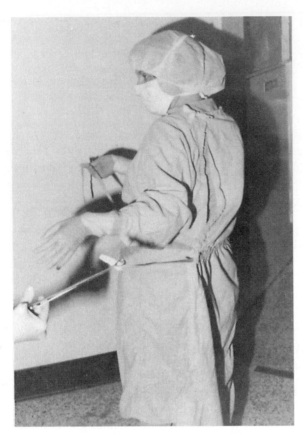

Figure 34–13. Take the tie from the forceps held by your assistant and tie the sterile gown. (Courtesy Ivan Ellis)

the physician performing a surgical procedure (Fig. 34–13).

You are now in scrub attire (Fig. 34–14).

GUIDELINES FOR WORKING IN STERILE ATTIRE

1. *Everything below the waist or table height is considered nonsterile.* Therefore, keep your hands above your waist and keep sterile equipment on top of the tables. When you are waiting, it is often convenient to clasp your gloved hands together in front of you *to protect them.*
2. *Your back is considered potentially contaminated because you cannot see if it touches anything unsterile.* Do not turn your back on any sterile area. Always pass with your face toward the sterile area.
3. For the same reason, when passing another person in sterile attire, pass either face to face or back to back. If you must stand behind someone, fasten a sterile towel over that person's back.
4. *Sterility is a matter of certainty, not conjecture.* If you even suspect that a part of your attire has been contaminated, notify the appropriate person (circulating nurse, perhaps) for assistance in changing.
5. *Moisture allows microorganisms to wick quickly and easily from one area to another.* If your attire becomes wet, consider it contaminated and change, or cover the wet area with a sterile towel.
6. *Contamination commonly occurs accidentally.* To prevent this, whenever you move close to anyone, warn them verbally. Do not assume that you will be seen.

CRITICAL THINKING EXERCISES

Imagine that you have been asked to participate in a procedure for which you must scrub, gown, and glove. Imagine further that you are dressed in exactly the same clothing as you have on right now as you read this. Identify the preparations you will need to make and the scrub attire you will need to put on, including rationale for the attire. Compare your work with that of another student. Critique one another's work, discussing similarities and differences.

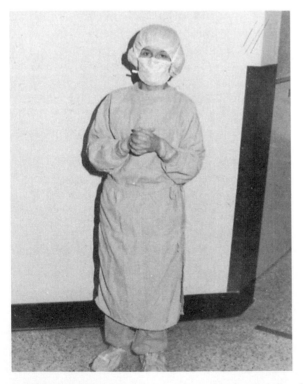

Figure 34–14. The nurse is now properly scrubbed, gowned, and gloved. (Courtesy Ivan Ellis)

References

Atkinson, L. (1992). *Berry and Kohn's introduction to operating room technique* (7th ed.). New York: Mc-Graw Hill.

Mathias, J. (1993). Experts discuss merits of surgical masks. *OR Manager, 9*(1), 8–10.

Meeker, M., & Rothrock, J. (1991). *Alexander's care of the patient in surgery* (9th ed.). St. Louis: C. V. Mosby.

Rehork, B., & Ruden, H. (1991). Investigations into the efficacy of different procedures for surgical hand disinfection between consecutive operations. *Journal of Hospital Infection, 19*, 124.

Standards and recommended practices for perioperative nursing. (1990). The Association for Operating Room Nurses, Inc. (AORN).

Procedure for Scrubbing	Needs More Practice	Satisfactory	Comments
1. Prepare yourself. **a.** Put on surgical attire ("scrub" garments).			
b. Put on cap or hood, shoe covers, and mask.			
c. Examine hands and forearms for cuts or blemishes.			
d. Remove watches, rings, and bracelets.			
e. Remove nail polish or artificial nails if worn, and clip nails so they are no longer in length than the fingertips.			
2. Perform the prescrub. **a.** Turn on water and adjust temperature.			
b. Moisten hands and arms.			
c. Lather hands and arms for 1 minute.			
d. Remove brush from dispenser and clean nails, rinsing after each nail.			
e. Rinse hands and arms, keeping hands higher than elbows.			
3. Scrub. **a.** Counted brush-stroke method (1) Select sterile brush or sponge, adding liquid cleanser if necessary.			
(2) Scrub nails of left hand 30 strokes and all skin surfaces 20 strokes, using anatomic pattern outlined. (a) Four surfaces of each finger, thumb to fifth finger			
(b) Over dorsal surface of hand, small finger to thumb			
(c) Over palmar surface of hand, small finger to thumb			
(d) Over the wrist			
(e) Up the arm in thirds, ending 2 inches above the elbow			
(3) Repeat step (2) for the right hand and arm.			

(continued)

Procedure for Scrubbing *(Continued)*	Needs More Practice	Satisfactory	Comments
b. Timed method (1) Select sterile brush or sponge, adding liquid cleanser if necessary.			
(2) Scrub nails, fingers, hand, and wrist of left arm for 1½ minutes, using anatomic pattern outlined above.			
(3) Repeat for right nails, fingers, hand, and wrist.			
(4) Scrub from wrist to 2 inches above elbow, spending 1 minute on each arm.			
4. Rinse. **a.** Rinse hands and arms, keeping hands above elbows.			
b. Keep your hands in front of you, above the waist and not higher than the axilla, and move to location of sterile towels.			
5. Dry hands and arms. **a.** Pick up sterile towel.			
b. Allow towel to unfold.			
c. Use half to dry first hand and arm.			
d. Use second half to dry second hand and arm.			
e. Push cuticles back as you dry.			
Procedure for Gowning and Closed Gloving			
1. Pick up gown by neck edge.			
2. Facing the sterile field, hold gown by the inside top neckline and allow it to unfold.			
3. Position gown so that you are facing the back opening.			
4. Work hands and arms into gown to seam between gown and cuff.			
5. Turn your back to assistant for securing gown at neck and back.			
6. Leave front tie tied.			

(continued)

Procedure for Gowning and Closed Gloving *(Continued)*	Needs More Practice	Satisfactory	Comments
7. Using closed-glove technique, put on sterile gloves. 　**a.** Use left hand inside gown to pick up folded edge of right glove.			
b. Hold right hand, palm up, inside gown.			
c. Position right glove on right palm.			
d. Use right hand inside gown to grasp bottom fold of cuff.			
e. Use left hand inside gown to pull right glove cuff over right gown cuff.			
f. Adjust right glove over right gown cuff.			
g. Work right hand into glove.			
h. Using gloved right hand, pick up left glove.			
i. Hold left hand, palm up, inside gown.			
j. Position left glove over left palm.			
k. Use left hand inside gown to grasp fold of glove cuff.			
l. Use gloved right hand to grasp top of fold and pull glove cuff over gown cuff.			
m. Work left hand into glove.			
n. Turn up and adjust cuffs.			
o. Reposition fingers as needed.			
8. Untie front waist tie.			
9. Hold ends above waist.			
10. Hold shorter tie in one hand.			
11. Hold longer tie out for assistant to grasp with sterile forceps.			
12. Turn around carefully, wrapping gown around you.			
13. Retrieve tie from assistant and tie two ties in front.			

(continued)

Working in Sterile Attire	Needs More Practice	Satisfactory	Comments
1. Keep your hands in front of you and above waist level, below axilla.			
2. Do not turn your back on sterile field.			
3. Pass front to front or back to back with others in sterile attire.			
4. Change attire when contaminated.			
5. Change or cover attire if wet.			
6. Warn others of your movements.			

MODULE

35

WOUND CARE

MODULE CONTENTS

PREREQUISITES

Successful completion of the following modules:

VOLUME 1

VOLUME 2

[1]For stump dressings, see Module 26, Applying Bandages and Binders. For colostomy dressings, see Module 36, Ostomy Care. For tracheostomy dressings, see Module 41, Tracheostomy Care and Suctioning. For central line dressings, see Module 54, Caring for Central Intravenous Catheters.

OVERALL OBJECTIVE

To care for wounds by changing dressings and removing sutures or staples, maintaining safety for both patient and nurse.

SPECIFIC LEARNING OBJECTIVES

Know Facts and Principles	Apply Facts and Principles	Demonstrate Ability	Evaluate Performance
1. Function of dressings State three functions of dressings.	Given a patient situation, identify function of particular dressing.	In the clinical setting, identify function of all dressings observed.	Evaluate effectiveness of dressing in performing identified function.
2. Drains State two reasons for use of wound drains. List three types of surgery in which drains are often used.	Given a patient situation, identify purpose of wound drain in use.	Shorten Penrose drain correctly under supervision.	Evaluate performance with instructor.
3. Observations State observations to be made during dressing change.	Given a patient situation, describe observations accurately, using correct terminology.	Make pertinent observations during dressing change.	Evaluate own performance with instructor, using Performance Checklist.
4. Dressing materials List and describe common dressing materials.	Identify various dressing materials by name. Give rationale for use of different dressing materials in various situations.	Use various types of dressing materials appropriately.	Evaluate use of dressing materials with instructor.
5. Procedure for dressing change Explain how to change dressing. Explain rationale for using sterile technique.	Given a patient situation, identify correct ways to perform procedure. Give rationale for correct performance of procedure. Give rationale for using wet-to-dry dressing.	Change dressing correctly under supervision. Apply wet-to-dry dressing correctly under supervision.	Evaluate own performance with instructor. Evaluate own performance with instructor.
6. Removing sutures or staples Describe the procedure for removing sutures or staples.		In the clinical setting, under supervision, remove sutures or staples.	Evaluate with your instructor.

(continued)

SPECIFIC LEARNING OBJECTIVES (continued)

Know Facts and Principles	Apply Facts and Principles	Demonstrate Ability	Evaluate Performance
7. *Emptying and restarting a wound suction device*			
Describe the procedure for emptying and restarting a wound suction device.	Given a patient situation, determine whether wound suction device should be emptied and restarted.	In the clinical setting, under supervision, empty and restart a wound suction device.	Evaluate own performance with instructor.
8. *Documentation*			
State items to be included on progress note regarding dressing change, removing staples or sutures, or a wound suction device.	Given a patient situation, write progress note descriptive of dressing change and wound. Give rationale for items to be included in progress note regarding dressing change and wound.	In the clinical setting, write complete and accurate progress note regarding dressing change and wound.	Evaluate own documentation with instructor.

LEARNING ACTIVITIES

1. Review the Specific Learning Objectives.
2. Read the chapters on procedures and infection in Ellis and Nowlis, *Nursing: A Human Needs Approach*, or comparable chapters in another textbook.
3. Look up the module vocabulary terms in the glossary.
4. Read through the module and mentally practice the skills. Study as though you will be teaching these skills to another person.
5. In the practice setting:
   a. Identify the various types of dressing materials available by name. In what kind of situation is each appropriate?
   b. Using a manikin or wound model, practice doing a dressing change on an abdomen, with the Performance Checklist as a guide. What adaptation would you make if a drain were present? If a drain were to be shortened?
   c. When you are satisfied with your performance, have another student evaluate you.
   d. Have your instructor evaluate your performance.
   e. Repeat steps b through d for a wet-to-dry dressing.
6. Examine a suture removal kit. Practice using the forceps to pick up a small thread and clip it with the scissors.
7. Examine a staple remover. Note how it operates.
8. Examine a wound suction device. Practice opening, draining, and reestablishing the suction.
9. In the clinical setting:
   a. Change a sterile dressing under the supervision of your instructor or a staff nurse.
   b. Remove staples under the supervision of your instructor or a staff nurse.
   c. Seek opportunities to manage wound suction devices.

VOCABULARY

approximated	epithelialization	purulent	serosanguineous
aseptic	excoriation	sanguineous	serous
contaminated	first-intention healing	second-intention	sterile
debride	Penrose drain	healing	

Wound Care

Rationale for the Use of This Skill

Open wounds such as surgical wounds, decubitus ulcers, and burns require care that will promote healing and prevent further injury or deterioration of the wound. An essential nursing responsibility is to observe and describe the wound carefully to determine its progress in healing. Another responsibility is to choose the most appropriate dressing materials available and to apply them in the most secure and comfortable way possible.

Dressings over open wounds must be sterile; therefore sterile technique is essential when changing these dressings. Any wound where subcutaneous tissue is visible or that is draining is still open. A wound with a drain in place is being kept open artificially to facilitate drainage. Clean, approximated surgical wounds seal before healing is completed, usually within 24 to 48 hours after surgery. These wounds are often left open to the air after this period. If a dressing is used, the aim is to maintain cleanliness, but sterile technique is not essential.[2]

▼ NURSING DIAGNOSES

The individual with the nursing diagnosis "Impaired Skin Integrity" specifically related to an open surgical wound, decubitus ulcer, or burn is in need of appropriate wound care.

Individuals with open wounds may have "Pain" related to the wound. This is often exacerbated by movement and by dressing changes. The nursing diagnosis of "Fear" related to painful wound care procedures" may be present in an individual with an extensive wound.

OBSERVING AND DESCRIBING THE WOUND

Careful observation and accurate description of the wound are integral parts of changing a dressing. Observe the following:

1. *Healing status*. Are the edges approximated? Does the wound have a smooth contour? Are inflammation and edema (swelling) present? If so, to what degree? A wound that has approximated edges, a smooth contour, displays minimal inflammation and swelling, and is healing across all layers is said to be healing by *primary (first) intention*. Scarring is minimal with this type of healing. If the wound opens or if the edges never were closely approximated, the wound heals from the inside out, and the gap fills with granulation tissue. This type of healing is called healing by *secondary intention*. It takes longer and leaves a larger scar.

2. *Drainage*. Is there drainage from the surface of the wound? Drainage may be primarily *serous* (composed of serum from the body), *serosanguineous* (composed of blood and serum), or *purulent* (containing pus). You must identify and document the color, amount, and odor of the drainage. Note the amount by stating the number of dressings saturated or stained by the drainage. Odors are best described by comparing them with a familiar smell such as feces or ammonia, if that is possible. A flow sheet is commonly used to document wound assessment and treatment.

All types of wound drainage support the growth of microorganisms. Therefore, many measures are used to keep the wound surface clean and to move the drainage away from it. *Drainage can also irritate the skin around the wound*, so heavily draining wounds may need special dressing techniques to protect the skin.

[handwritten: Why dressings   1. Protection   2. Absorption   3. Pressure   4. Keep moist]

DRAINS

Drains are sometimes placed during surgery *to enhance the flow of drainage from the wound, thus promoting wound healing*. A drain may also be used *to help keep the operated area dry*.

The Penrose drain is an example of such a drain (Fig. 35–1). The Penrose is a soft latex rubber tubing material. One end is placed in the bottom of the wound and the other opens to the outside of the body, either through the wound itself or through a small surgical "stab" wound (a small puncture wound made by the surgeon) beside a larger wound. A sterile safety pin is attached to the Penrose drain to prevent it from sliding down into the wound.

If a considerable amount of drainage is expected postoperatively, a closed wound suction device is placed at surgery. This portable system consists of a drainage tube with multiple openings that is attached to a vacuum unit that gently suctions fluid from the wound. The Hemovac is an example of this type of setup (Fig. 35–2).

Other brands have a different shape, such as a small plastic bottle, but operate on the same principle of low suction. These closed wound suction de-

---

[2]Rationale for action is emphasized throughout the module by the use of italics.

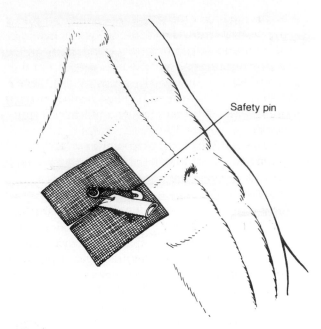

Figure 35–1. Split gauze surrounding a Penrose drain.

vices are commonly used after breast, hip, or perineal surgery, help keep the wound dry, and are easily moved when the patient moves.

Rarely, a large, rigid plastic drainage tube is placed into a wound and attached to a connection tube that is connected to the wall suction device. This is done when a very large volume of drainage is expected.

DRESSING MATERIALS

The type of dressing materials used varies from facility to facility. Here are some of the most common types, although they may be called by different names:

1. *4 × 4s:* These are folded gauze pads, 4 inches by 4 inches in size. They are available in both sterile and nonsterile forms. In most facilities, 2 × 2s and 3 × 3s are also available.
2. *Fluffs:* These are large pieces of sterile or nonsterile gauze that are loosely folded *to absorb drainage.* They are also used to pack wounds.
3. *ABDs (combines, combination pads):* These are large, sterile or nonsterile, absorbent pads (usually a coarse gauze covered by a finer gauze). Normally they are used over smaller dressing materials, and most are moisture resistant on one side.
4. *Nonadherents:* These are special sterile dressings that have a surface that will not stick to wound surfaces. Impregnated nonadherent dressings

have petrolatum, antimicrobials, or other agents on the woven material *to prevent adherence.* Other nonadherent dressings, such as Telfa, have a synthetic material attached to one side of the gauze dressing. Nonadherent dressings are used directly on incisions or open wound surfaces *to prevent injury to tissues when the dressing is removed.* They may be cut to appropriate size.

5. *Moisture-vapor-permeable (MVP) transparent film:* These dressings look like a thin sheet of plastic and are often called by their brand names, such as Bioclusive, Opsite, and Tegaderm. One surface has an adhesive that adheres to dry, intact skin but not to a moist wound surface. The dressings are semipermeable and allow gases, such as moisture vapor and oxygen, to move through them. Larger molecules, such as those found in the drainage or in bacteria, do not pass through the material. Bacteria can move from the skin surrounding the dressing to the area under it through very small crevices in the skin that are not sealed off by the dressing. MVP dressings provide a moist surface that encour-

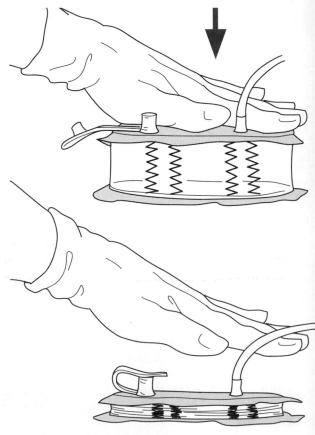

Figure 35–2. Hemovac wound suction. Open the valve and push down to reestablish suction. (Courtesy Zimmer, Inc., Warsaw, Indiana)

ages epithelialization of the wound surface. These are used primarily over small wounds and sometimes for intravenous dressings. However, they are also very effective when placed over wounds with black eschar or necrotic debris because they help to liquefy the material (Barnes, 1993.)

6. *Hydrocolloid dressings:* A common brand of this type of dressing is Duoderm, a soft wafer that can be cut to the desired shape and size and placed over an open wound. The colloidal substance absorbs drainage at the wound surface, providing a moist environment for epithelialization and healing. The hydrocolloidal dressing is impermeable to both small and large molecules, but bacteria can move under it, as they do with MVP dressings. Hydrocolloid dressings are used over decubitus ulcers and other open skin lesions and may be left in place for up to 1 week.

7. *Polyurethane foam:* These dressings may be used around tubes or drains *to hold them away from skin and prevent abrasion.* Although they will absorb small amounts of drainage, they are best used with other materials if drainage is profuse. They will stick to the surface of wounds that do not have drainage.

8. *Skin barriers:* Materials developed to protect the skin from stool or urine after an ostomy are also valuable for protecting the skin around heavily draining wounds. They can also be used to protect skin from tape irritation—if they are placed over intact skin where tape must be removed frequently, the tape can be affixed to the skin barrier instead of the skin. One of these products, karaya, is available as a pliable wafer that can be cut to any shape and adheres to the skin. It also comes in a powder form, to be used on skin irregularities, such as those caused by a scar or the umbilicus, that are near the wound. Another type, Stomadhesive, comes as a wafer or paste. A lesser degree of protection is offered by clear liquids, such as tincture of benzoin, which dry to form a thin protective covering on the skin.

9. *Roller gauze:* This is sterile gauze that comes in various widths. It is used for packing and wrapping wounds as well as to secure dressings.

10. *Tape:* Tape comes in a variety of materials (adhesive, plastic, paper, and other) and in widths from ¼ inch to 6 inches. Paper tape is generally considered hypoallergenic.

11. *Montgomery straps or ties:* These straps are used to tie across large or bulky dressings that need frequent changing (Fig. 35–3). This avoids the skin irritation caused by repeated tape removal.

Commercially available tapes may be cut to the desired width. Each tape would include one or more eyelets. Generally, twill tape, roller gauze, or rubber bands attached with safety pins are used to secure these straps or ties. Straps may remain on the dressing until soiled, but ties are usually changed more frequently. Montgomery straps can be made from wide tape folded back, with holes cut for eyelets.

12. *Drainage bags:* Disposable plastic drainage bags are sometimes used over profusely draining wounds. These bags attach to the skin with a variety of adhesives. Most have a ring that is attached to the skin and a bag that can be removed and replaced. The bags allow staff to measure drainage precisely and observe the wound. They control odor and moisture, making the patient more comfortable (Fig. 35–4).

PROCEDURE FOR CHANGING DRESSINGS

Assessment

1. Check the orders for the dressing change. Sometimes the physician will want to do the first dressing change after surgery and then will write an order: "Change dressing prn." Or, you may be responsible for all dressing changes. In any case, a dressing may always be reinforced, meaning that you can apply additional dressings on top of dressings already in place *to absorb drainage.* Sterile dressings are used over a previous dressing *to avoid introducing organisms.* However, because they are placed on the contaminated exterior surface of the old dressing, they do not prevent the possibility of wound contamination. Keep in mind that *once drainage has penetrated to the outside of a dressing, organisms may be carried to the wound through moisture.*

2. Check the current dressing *to determine the general size of the wound and the type and amount of dressing materials necessary.* This information may be on the Nursing Care Plan.

3. Check the patient's unit for supplies and equipment that may already be in the room. Remember that dressing materials in packages that have previously been opened are no longer sterile *because they have been exposed to the microbes in the air.*

Planning

4. Wash your hands *for infection control.*

5. Gather the equipment. Some facilities use commercially prepared packages that include all the instruments needed. Your facility may use a partially prepared dressing tray, in which case you

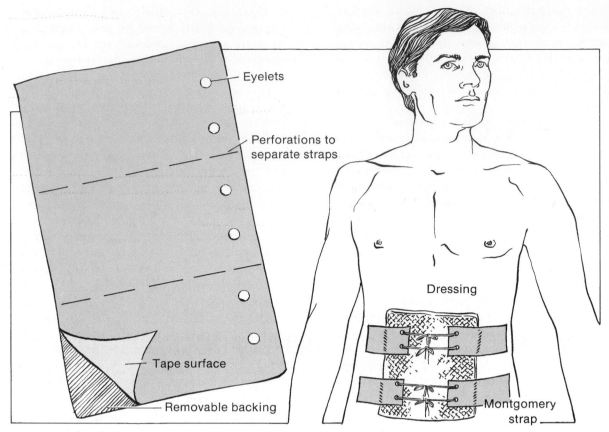

Figure 35–3. Montgomery straps allow multiple dressing changes without removing and reapplying tape each time.

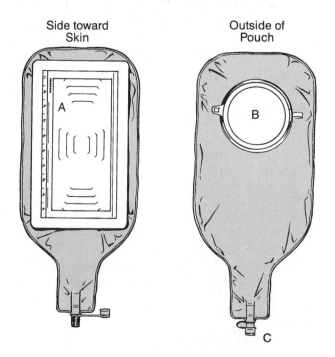

Figure 35–4. Wound or drainage collection pouch. **(A)** Adhesive area, cut to fit shape of wound. **(B)** Access opening for wound observation and care. **(C)** Drainage port for emptying drainage.

must add the additional sterile supplies needed. Or you may have to assemble all the sterile supplies, using a sterile towel or the individual sterile packages as a sterile field. Items you may need include scissors, thumb forceps (pickups), 4 × 4s and ABDs or other dressing materials, tape, antiseptic solution, cotton-tipped applicators, and sterile gloves. Some facilities have special bags or paper *for the disposal of soiled dressings.* In others, the bedside waste bag is used. If you follow this latter procedure, the bag should be discarded in the appropriate disposal container and replaced immediately after the dressing change.

Implementation

6. Identify the patient *to be sure you are performing the procedure for the correct patient.*
7. Explain what you intend to do. Allow the patient to ask questions *to help ensure his or her cooperation.* In the case of a very complex wound when pain is expected, arrange for pain medications before beginning. Ask the patient to keep his or her hands away from the dressing area and to avoid talking during the procedure *to limit the number of microorganisms moving in the air.*

Limit your own conversation to essential information while the open wound is exposed. In some situations it may be necessary for both patient and nurse to wear masks during a dressing change *to decrease microbes in the air.*

8. Prepare the environment. Close windows and doors *to eliminate drafts that might chill the patient or carry microorganisms into the open wound.* Pull the drapes and draw the curtains around the bed *to provide privacy.* The patient should be lying flat or in low Fowler's position. Clear a working space—the overbed table serves this purpose well. Make sure your work surface is clean and dry *to prevent contamination of supplies.* Place a bag or paper *for soiled dressings* within easy reach. The bag edges can be taped to the mattress edge *for convenience.*

9. Expose the area to be dressed and drape the patient, if necessary, *for modesty.* You can use a bath blanket or top sheet for this purpose.

10. Prepare to remove the current dressing. Loosen tapes, starting from the outside and working toward the dressing *to minimize disruption of wound healing. If body hair makes this activity uncomfortable for the patient,* you may want to shave the area before applying more tape. Some dressings are covered with an elastic or cloth binder, in which case you must unhook or unpin the binder before beginning.

11. Put on clean gloves and remove the dressings. This can be done in many ways. Your facility may have a preferred procedure, so be sure to consult its procedure book. Take the outer dressings off by grasping them at the center (without applying pressure) and removing them to the side. Avoid passing dressings over any sterile area. Wear clean gloves to remove all dressings; *doing so protects you from wound drainage.* Rarely, you may find that you must touch and move drains, retention sutures, and other devices in the wound to remove a soiled dressing. In such cases, put on sterile gloves *to avoid introducing microorganisms to this area.*

Notice how many of which type of dressings are soiled *to indicate the amount of drainage when you chart.* Place the soiled dressings in the bag or on the paper designated for that use. Discard gloves into the container with the dressings.

12. Wash your hands.

13. Observe the wound, noting the approximation of the wound's edges, the presence of inflammation and edema, and the presence, appearance, and odor of drainage, if any.

14. Set up equipment and supplies.
    a. Open all packages and arrange the sterile equipment conveniently.

b. Tear strips of tape in correct lengths and place them on the edge of an easily reached surface. Determine whether the patient has an allergy to adhesive tape, in which case you should use paper or plastic tape. If Montgomery straps or a binder are used, you will not need tape. You may need a clean binder if the one being worn is soiled. If you are changing Montgomery straps, set them up at this time.

c. Set up cleansing materials, if needed. Use the antiseptic solution of the physician's choice or the one currently used at your facility. In some facilities, the solution is available in small bottles for individual use and does not have to be poured. In any case, if you need a container for the solution, it must be sterile. Be careful not to drip solution around the basin, especially on the cloth drapes. Also available for use in this situation are antiseptic-soaked swabsticks and small foil packages of antiseptic solution.

The most common agents used for cleansing are the iodophor compounds (Betadine, Acudyne, povidone), which provide long-lasting antimicrobial protection. However, *they also cause skin reactions in some individuals,* so you should assess the skin carefully for early signs of redness and edema when you are using them. Hibiclens is another commonly used antibacterial agent. Hydrogen peroxide is less effective as an antimicrobial, but it does clean and is less likely to provoke skin reactions. Sterile normal saline may be all that is needed to cleanse the surface of most wounds. *Antimicrobials applied directly to a wound surface inhibit epithelialization and blood flow and therefore retard healing. When applied repeatedly to extensive open wounds, povidone-iodine compounds may be absorbed and cause iodine toxicity.*

d. Prepare solution for wet-to-dry dressings as needed. Obtain a sterile basin, open the dressings into the basin, and pour the solution over the dressings in the basin. Another method is to open the solution container and plan to hold the dressings in a sterile gloved hand as you pour solution over them.

15. Change the dressing as appropriate.
    a. *Sealed (Closed) Wound Dressings.* When the wound has sealed, place a simple dry dressing over the surface *to protect it from abrasion.* Inspect the wound after the dressing has been removed. If it appears still sealed:
    (1) Handle the dressing by the outside of the

corners only *to maintain sterility of the surface in contact with the wound.*

(2) Place it over the wound.

(3) Tape dressing in place.

b. *Open Wound Dressings*

(1) Put on sterile gloves (see Module 33, Sterile Technique).

(2) Clean the skin around the wound with antiseptic solution if indicated or ordered by the physician. Using cotton balls or prepared swabs, clean around the wound.

If the wound is small or is a surgical "stab" wound (a small puncture wound made by the surgeon), clean in ever-widening circles away from it, moving from the area it is most necessary to keep clean to the more contaminated (dirty) area (Fig. 35–5) to move microbes away from the open wound.

For a longer wound, you may need to use consecutive long strokes, starting each stroke at the top of the wound and moving to the bottom. Each successive stroke is farther from the wound on that side. Use another swab to clean the other side of the wound, starting at the wound edge and gradually moving out (Fig. 35–6). Use each swab only once. These actions move microbes away from the open wound. Clean two or three times as indicated.

If there are multiple wounds, such as a

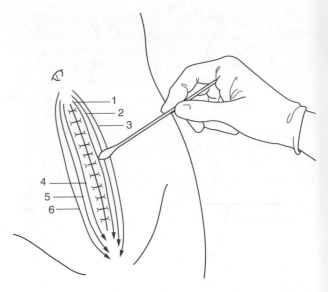

Figure 35–6. Cleaning along a large wound. Use one swab for strokes 1, 2, and 3. Use a second swab for strokes 4, 5, and 6.

central incision with several drains, clean each wound separately, using fresh swabs *to avoid moving microbes from one site to another.*

(3) Redress the wound, placing dressing materials securely *so that they remain in place.* Use materials in the order they were in when the old dressing was removed, if that seemed effective. If not, redress *for greater effectiveness.*

If the wound is deep and is to be packed, place the dressings so that they contact all surfaces of the wound. Fill the wound firmly but not so tightly that pressure is placed on its surface.

If a drain is in place, the bulk of the dressing should cover the drain area, usually in a dependent position *to absorb drainage most effectively. To prevent excoriation of the skin around the drain site,* partially split a 4 × 4 with sterile scissors and place it snugly around the drain (see Fig. 35–1). A drain site may also be dressed with two 4 × 4s. Open the 4 × 4s and fold them in half lengthwise. By folding each at right angles, each can serve as two sides of the dressing (Fig. 35–7). Prenotched gauze squares are also available.

(4) Remove your gloves and place them in the bag of soiled dressing materials.

(5) Secure the dressing with tape, Montgomery straps, or a binder as indicated. Use enough tape to hold the dressing in

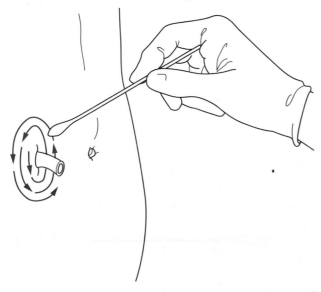

Figure 35–5. Clean around a drain by using a widening spiral starting at the drain and moving outward.

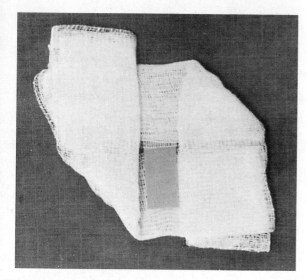

Figure 35–7. Two 4 × 4s surrounding a Penrose drain. (Courtesy Ivan Ellis)

place, but do not use more than necessary. Avoid putting tension on the tape because *this can create skin irritation and tape burns* (Fig. 35–8).

c. *Wet-to-Dry Dressings.* Wet-to-dry dressings may be used to *debride* (clean away adherent material from) the wound surface. Moist gauze, which is placed in the wound, absorbs drainage from the wound readily. As it begins to dry, it adheres to debris on the surface of the wound. When the dressing is removed, the surface debris is removed along with it. This may be uncomfortable for the patient, but moistening the dressing to prevent pulling on the surface negates the purpose of the wet-to-dry dressing. *Dressings removed in*

this way may also disturb fresh granulation tissue, so it may be appropriate to use saline to carefully remoisten areas of the dressing that have adhered to granulating tissue rather than to debris.

Some facilities refer to any dressing that is moist at the wound surface and covered with a dry dressing as a wet-to-dry dressing. Some moist dressings are designed to provide a moist healing environment, not to debride the wound. Be sure that you clearly understand the purpose of the dressing before proceeding.

(1) Put on sterile gloves.
(2) Remove wet dressings from solution or pour the fluid from a container over the gauze, which is held in the sterile gloved hand or with sterile forceps. The hand that holds the fluid container is contaminated and cannot then be used for placing the sterile dressings (Fig. 35–9).
(3) Place the gauze that has been moistened with saline in contact with the wound surface.
(4) Cover moist dressings with dry dressings.
(5) Remove gloves and place with soiled dressings.
(6) Tape the dressing in place.
16. Assist the patient to a comfortable position.
17. Put on gloves and care for the equipment. Remove the bag used for soiled dressings and other materials and dispose of it the appropriate

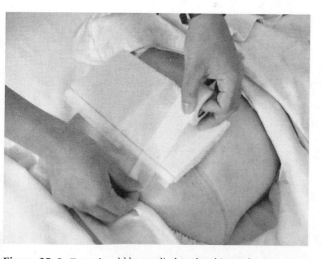

Figure 35–8. Tape should be applied to the skin without tension to prevent tape burns and skin irritation.

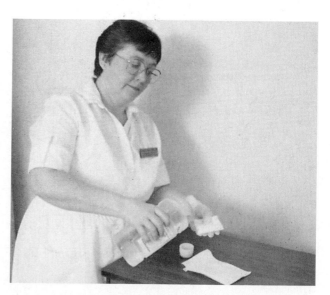

Figure 35–9. A sterile dressing can be moistened by pouring solution. The hand that holds the sterile dressing wears a sterile glove and the hand that holds the container is contaminated and cannot touch the dressing or wound.

place, commonly a special garbage receptacle in the soiled utility room. Rinse any glass or metal materials used *to remove protein substances* before sending them to the central processing department. Dispose of gloves.

18. Wash your hands.

Evaluation

19. Evaluate using the following criteria:
    a. Appropriate technique maintained
    b. Dressing applied securely
    c. Patient made comfortable after procedure

Documentation

20. Document the procedure on the patient's chart, including the time the procedure was performed, observations made, dressing materials and antiseptic solution used, and any of the pa-

tient's reactions. This information is sometimes entered on a flow sheet (Fig. 35–10).

SHORTENING A PENROSE DRAIN

The physician may order that a Penrose drain (described above) be shortened by a specific amount, usually *to encourage the closure of the wound from the inside out.* The drain is pulled out of the wound the specified distance, and its length inside of the wound is thus shortened. A sterile safety pin is commonly used to prevent the drain from slipping back inside the wound. If a drain is stapled or sutured to the skin, remove the staple or suture before you shorten or remove the drain. The drain is shortened dur-

STAGE I	Skin is pink, red or mottled; blanches on touch—lasting up to 15 min after pressure is released. Skin feels firm & warm.
STAGE II	Skin appears cracked, blistered, & broken. Surrounding area red.
STAGE III	Full thickness skin loss. May include subcutaneous tissue and produce serosanguineous drainage.
STAGE IV	Full thickness skin loss with deep tissue, muscle, or bone involved.
ESCHAR	If present, should be measured and documented.
POSTOP	Debridement, flap, rotation closure (sutures, staples, drains).

☒ Present on admission?　　From: *Home*

THERAPEUTIC MEASURES/PHYSICIAN'S ORDERS FOR:

Present Surface:
Alternating Pressure
☒ Elbow Protectors
☒ Heel Protectors
☒ Turn Sched Q *2 hr*

☐ PT ☐ Range of Motion Exercise
☐ Whirlpool Therapy
☐ Catheter
☐ Hydration

☐ Dietary Assessment
☐ G Tube ☐ NG Tube
☐ Protein Supplement
☐ Multi Vits/Zinc/Iron
☐ Current HGB/HCT

Height *53"*　Weight *50 Kg*　Ideal Body Wt ☐

Other *Clean and apply Duoderm as needed.*

Illustrate Position of Affected Area in Red
Utilize One Sheet Per Affected Area

CULTURES DONE: Date: *1-29-95*　　Date:_____　　Date:_____　　Date:_____

Date	#	Site	Stage	Length/Width (CM)	Drainage/Type	Treatment	MD Notified
1-29-99	*1*	*Coccyx*	*III*	*2 X 2.5*	*Yellow purulent*	*Cleaned with H₂O₂ Duoderm applied*	
Depth	**Undermining/Tunneling**			**Odor**	**Color**	**Response**	**RN Signature**
2 mm	*None*			*Musty*	*Red under drainage*	*States pain when cleansed*	*K. Lang*
Comments							

Date	#	Site	Stage	Length/Width (CM)	Drainage/Type	Treatment	MD Notified
Depth	**Undermining/Tunneling**			**Odor**	**Color**	**Response**	**RN Signature**
Comments							

Figure 35–10. Example of a wound care flow sheet. A full page would contain spaces for five entries and patient identification.

DATE/TIME	
4/4/99 0930	Abd dressing changed, 3 fluffs and 1 ABD saturated with serosanguineous drainage. Edges of wound approximated with no puffiness noted and only slight redness at drain site. Patient unwilling to look at wound but offered no complaints. Resting comfortably at present. —————— H. Gray, RN

Example of Nursing Progress Notes Using Narrative Format.

DATE/TIME	
4/4/99 0930	Impaired skin integrity: surgical wound —————— S Reports minimal pain in wound area. States does not want to observe wound. O Abd drsg: 3 fluffs and 1 ABD saturated with serosanguineous drainage. Wound surface appears clean. Sterile drsg applied. A Healing progressing. P Change drsg q shift. —————— H. Gray, RN

Example of Nursing Progress Notes Using SOAP Format.

DATE/TIME	
5/22/99	D: Abd. wound is reddened and edematous with moderate amount of yellow drainage on drsg. A: Wound cleansed with sterile saline and redressed. R: Pt. resting comfortably. —————— G. Williams, NS

Example of Nursing Progress Notes Using Focus Format.

ing the dressing change, which is an open wound dressing change.

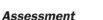

PROCEDURE FOR SHORTENING A PENROSE DRAIN

Assessment

1.–3. Follow the steps of the Procedure for Changing Dressings.

Planning

4.–5. Follow the steps of the Procedure for Changing Dressings.

Implementation

6.–14. Follow the steps of the Procedure for Changing Dressings.

15. Shorten the Penrose drain and redress the wound.

   a. Put on sterile gloves.

   b. Clean the skin around the wound as indicated (see step 15.b.(2) of the Procedure for Changing Dressings).

   c. Grasp the Penrose drain with a pair of sterile forceps.

   d. Gently but firmly pull the drain out the specified distance.

   e. If a sterile safety pin is to be placed on the drain, handle it with sterile gloved hands. Remove and replace it at wound surface.

   f. Using sterile scissors, clip off the excess drain, making sure that 2 inches of drain remain visible outside the wound. *Doing so prevents the drain from sliding back into the wound, where a surgical incision would be needed to remove it.*

   g. Complete dressing the wound.

   h. Remove gloves and place with soiled dressings.

   i. Secure the dressing.

16.–18. Follow the steps of the Procedure for Changing Dressings.

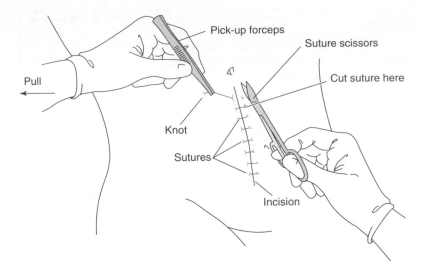

Figure 35–11. Removing sutures. Clip the suture close to the skin. Remove it by pulling in line with the stitch. Do not pull a knot into tissue.

Pick-up forceps

Suture scissors

Pull

Cut suture here

Knot

Sutures

Incision

Evaluation
19. Follow the Procedure for Changing Dressings.

Documentation
20. Follow the Procedure for Changing Dressings.

PROCEDURE FOR REMOVING SUTURES OR SKIN STAPLES

Assessment
1. Check for an order to remove sutures or skin staples or clips.

Planning
2. Wash your hands *for infection control.*
3. Gather the equipment you will need. The suture removal kits and staple removers used in your facility may be either disposable or nondisposable. The latter type is sterilized and packaged in the central processing department.

Implementation
4. Identify the patient *to be sure you are performing the procedure for the correct patient.*
5. Explain to the patient what you are going to do. Removal of sutures or staples may produce a pinching or pulling sensation but does not usually cause pain. If pain is present or anticipated based on the condition of the wound, give the patient the ordered pain relief medication about 30 minutes before the procedure is to be performed.
6. If a dressing is in place, remove it as described in step 11 of the Procedure for Changing Dressings.
7. If the patient's wound has been closed with sutures, put on gloves and gently lift each suture away from the skin with the pickup forceps. Then snip the suture close to the skin. Pull it out by pulling in line with the suture that is still inside

the tissue, *so as not to traumatize tissue at the suture exit site* (Fig. 35–11). *Clipping close to the skin ensures that suture material that was outside the tissue is not pulled inside, which could contaminate the wound.*

To remove skin staples or clips, use a special instrument that is placed under the staple and pinched down to exert pressure on its center. This motion raises the ends, allowing you to remove the staple easily (Fig. 35–12). Remove every other suture or staple first *to determine whether the wound will hold.* Then remove remaining staples.
8. Apply tape, if ordered or if included in the procedure at your facility, *to help keep the wound edges together.* Commercially available sterile tapes (Steri-strips) are usually used to approximate skin edges after suture or staple removal.

Evaluation
9. Evaluate using the following criteria:
   a. Patient comfort
   b. Appearance of wound: approximation of wound's edges; presence of inflammation and

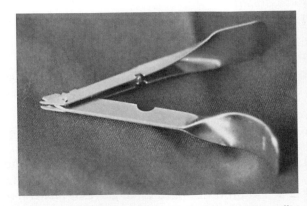

Figure 35–12. A wound staple remover. (Courtesy Ivan Ellis)

DATE/TIME	
1/23/99 0830	*Impaired skin integrity: surgical wound* S *"Feels good to get those stitches out."* O *Skin sutures removed. Skin edges approximated without redness or puffiness.* A *Wound healing without obvious problems* P *Continue to observe.* *M. Wong, SN*

Example of Nursing Progress Notes Using SOAP Format.

DATE/TIME	
1/23/99 0830	*Skin sutures removed per order of Dr. Mark. Skin edges approximated. No puffiness noted. Small, reddened area at left end of incision. Patient resting comfortably. N. Sturtevant, RN*

Example of Nursing Progress Notes Using Narrative Format.

edema; presence, appearance, and odor of drainage, if any.

Documentation

10. Document the procedure on the patient's record, including the time the procedure was performed, observations of the wound, and any reactions of the patient. Update the Nursing Care Plan as needed.

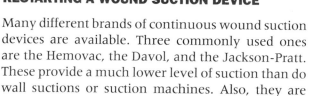

PROCEDURE FOR EMPTYING AND RESTARTING A WOUND SUCTION DEVICE

Many different brands of continuous wound suction devices are available. Three commonly used ones are the Hemovac, the Davol, and the Jackson-Pratt. These provide a much lower level of suction than do wall suctions or suction machines. Also, they are lightweight and allow the patient freedom of movement.

Assessment

1. Identify the type of suction device and its location.
2. Check the device *to determine whether the drainage chamber contains fluid and the suction container has reexpanded.*

Planning

3. Wash your hands *for infection control.*
4. Obtain a clean towel or absorbent pad *to protect the bed* and a container *in which to measure the drainage.* You will need clean gloves *to protect you from contact with the drainage.*

Implementation

5. Identify the patient *to be sure you are performing the procedure for the correct patient.*
6. Explain what you plan to do and allow the patient to ask questions.
7. Put on gloves.
8. Open the drainage port, avoiding contamination, and empty the contents into the container for measurement.
9. Clean the port with an alcohol or iodine swab.
10. Compress the suction chamber. For the Hemovac, you do this by pressing firmly down on the top of the chamber (see Fig. 35–2). In the type with a bulb syringe, squeeze the bulb firmly to fill the balloon inside the suction chamber. While pressing down or squeezing firmly, reseal the drainage port. *This reestablishes the vacuum and the suction.*
11. Measure and empty the drainage and discard or clean the container.
12. Remove the gloves and wash your hands.

Evaluation

13. Evaluate using the following criteria:
    a. Container is properly closed to prevent leaks
    b. Suction is working in the device

Documentation

14. Document the amount and describe the drainage on a flow sheet if one is available. If not, you can add this information to the narrative progress notes. Also note the amount on the intake and output record, under "drainage."

LONG-TERM CARE

In the long-term care setting, the most common types of wounds are skin ulcers created by circulatory problems or by pressure. These wounds often take a long time to heal because of underlying physiologic deficits in circulation, nutrition, and oxygenation. The slow healing rate makes progress difficult to assess. The Nursing Care Plan may specify the care techniques to be used, and documentation of wound status may be done on a weekly basis rather than daily. The nurse and the physician must work collaboratively on these difficult problems. Sometimes you may need to take a trial-and-error approach to finding the most successful care techniques.

In addition to care of the wound itself, the nurse must be highly aware of the multiple factors involved in healing and strive to support the resident through nutrition, stress reduction, positioning, activity, and oxygenation. Your nursing theory text provides more detailed information on the factors that affect wound healing.

HOME CARE

The patient who returns home with a surgical wound may need little more than instruction to keep the area clean and dry as healing is completed. Occasionally, the patient may return home with an extensive wound that requires complex management. Before discharge, plan how this is to be done at home while there is still time to teach the patient. Modifications of technique may be necessary when hospital equipment and supplies are not available at home.

For some long-term chronic wounds, such as leg ulcers arising from poor circulation, clients may be instructed to use clean rather than sterile technique for home care. Sterile supplies are expensive and may be unaffordable for a person on a limited income. The body's own defenses may be adequate to prevent infection if the individual is in the home without contact with new and more virulent organisms such as those that might be in a care setting. Careful handwashing and the use of meticulously clean supplies may be adequate protection in this setting.

The home care nurse can teach the client and any caregiver to assess the progress of the wound. Some of the same concerns regarding healing in the long-term care setting may also apply to the home-bound person. Other physiologic problems may interfere with healing, making attention to the whole person essential.

CRITICAL THINKING EXERCISES

As you listen to report, the off-going nurse states that she has changed a patient's dressing every hour because of the volume of drainage. Based on this information, what are your concerns for the patient? Considering what you know about dressing materials, recommend some options for effectively dressing this wound.

In addition to planning specific actions for wound care, what other nursing interventions will you undertake? Determine how you will evaluate the effectiveness of your interventions. If your plan is successful, explain how you will communicate it to other nurses.

Reference
Barnes, H. R. (1993). Wound care: Fact and fictions about hydrocolloid dressings. *Journal of Gerontological Nursing, 19*(6), 23–26.

Procedure for Changing Dressings	Needs More Practice	Satisfactory	Comments
Assessment			
1. Check orders.			
2. Check the present dressing.			
3. Check the patient's unit for supplies.			
Planning			
4. Wash your hands.			
5. Gather necessary equipment.			
Implementation			
6. Identify patient.			
7. Explain procedure.			
8. Prepare environment.			
9. Expose dressing, draping patient as necessary.			
10. Loosen tapes.			
11. Put on gloves, remove dressing, and dispose of dressing and gloves in bag.			
12. Wash your hands.			
13. Observe the wound.			
14. Set up equipment. a. Open sterile packages.			
b. Tear strips of tape.			
c. Set up cleansing materials, if needed.			
d. Prepare solution as needed. Pour solution over dressings in container or set up solution to be poured over dressings in gloved hand, if using wet dressings.			
15. Change dressing as appropriate. a. Sealed (closed) wound dressing (1) Handle dressing by corners.			
(2) Place dressing over wound.			
(3) Tape in place.			

(continued)

Procedure for Changing Dressings *(Continued)*	Needs More Practice	Satisfactory	Comments
b. Open wound dressing (1) Put on sterile gloves.			
(2) Clean skin around wound as indicated.			
(3) Place dressings over the wound.			
(4) Remove gloves and place with soiled dressings.			
(5) Secure dressing with tape.			
c. Wet-to-dry dressing (1) Put on sterile gloves.			
(2) Remove wet dressings one at a time from solution, or use one hand to hold dressing while pouring solution with the other hand.			
(3) Place dressings in contact with wound surface, maintaining sterility.			
(4) Cover wet dressings with dry dressings.			
(5) Remove gloves and place with soiled dressings.			
(6) Tape dressings in place.			
16. Assist patient to comfortable position.			
17. Put on gloves and care for equipment.			
18. Wash your hands.			
Evaluation			
19. Evaluate, using the following criteria: **a.** Appropriate technique maintained.			
b. Dressing secure.			
c. Patient comfortable.			
Documentation			
20. Document time, observations of wound, dressing materials and antiseptic solution used, and patient reaction.			

(continued

© 1996 by Lippincott-Raven Publishers

Procedure for Shortening a Penrose Drain	Needs More Practice	Satisfactory	Comments
Assessment			
1.–3. Follow Checklist steps 1–3 of the Procedure for Changing Dressings (check orders, the current dressing, and the patient's unit).			
Planning			
4.–5. Follow Checklist steps 4 and 5 of the Procedure for Changing Dressings (wash hands and gather necessary equipment, including sterile scissors, sterile forceps, and sterile safety pin).			
Implementation			
6.–14. Follow Checklist steps 6–14 of the Procedure for Changing Dressings (identify patient, explain procedure, prepare environment, expose dressing, loosen tapes, put on gloves and remove soiled dressing, remove gloves and wash your hands, observe the wound, and set up equipment).			
15. Shorten Penrose drain and redress wound. **a.** Put on sterile gloves.			
b. Clean skin around wound as indicated.			
c. Grasp Penrose drain with forceps.			
d. Pull drain out the specified distance.			
e. Place sterile safety pin at level of wound surface.			
f. Clip off excess drain, leaving 2 inches.			
g. Redress wound.			
h. Remove gloves and place with soiled dressings.			
i. Secure dressing.			
16.–18. Follow Checklist steps 16–18 of the Procedure for Changing Dressings (assist patient to comfortable position, put on gloves and care for equipment, and wash your hands).			

(continued)

Procedure for Shortening a Penrose Drain *(Continued)*	Needs More Practice	Satisfactory	Comments
Evaluation			
19. Evaluate as in Checklist step 19 of the Procedure for Changing Dressings (appropriate technique maintained, dressing secure, patient comfortable).			
Documentation			
20. Document as in Checklist step 19 of the Procedure for Changing Dressings (time, observations of wound, dressing materials and antiseptic solution used, shortening of Penrose drain, and patient reaction).			
Procedure for Removing Sutures or Staples			
Assessment			
1. Check orders			
Planning			
2. Wash your hands.			
3. Gather necessary equipment.			
Implementation			
4. Identify the patient.			
5. Explain the procedure.			
6. Remove dressing, if necessary.			
7. Remove sutures or skin staples or clips.			
8. Apply tape as ordered or appropriate.			
Evaluation			
9. Evaluate using the following criteria: **a.** Patient comfort			
b. Appearance of wound: approximation of wound's edges; presence of inflammation and edema; presence, appearance, and odor of drainage, if any.			
Documentation			
10. Document the time, observations made, and patient reaction.			

(continued

Procedure for Emptying and Restarting a Wound Suction Device	Needs More Practice	Satisfactory	Comments
Assessment			
1. Identify type and location of suction device.			
2. Check device for drainage and suction area reexpansion.			
Planning			
3. Wash your hands.			
4. Obtain clean towel or absorbent pad, measuring container, and clean gloves.			
Implementation			
5. Identify patient.			
6. Explain what you plan to do.			
7. Put on gloves.			
8. Open drainage port and empty contents into container.			
9. Clean the drainage port.			
10. Compress suction chamber as appropriate and reclose drainage port while compressing.			
11. Measure and empty drainage and care for container.			
12. Remove gloves and wash your hands.			
Evaluation			
13. Evaluate using the following criteria: a. Container is properly closed to prevent leaks.			
b. Suction is working in device.			
Documentation			
14. Document amount and description of drainage on flow sheet or narrative and on intake and output record.			

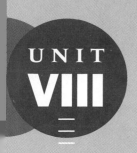

UNIT VIII

Complex Procedures Related to Elimination

36

OSTOMY CARE

MODULE CONTENTS

PREREQUISITES

Successful completion of the following modules:

OVERALL OBJECTIVE

To care for patients with an "ostomy," using safe and appropriate technique while maintaining cleanliness and an environment conducive to the patient's dignity and self-respect.

SPECIFIC LEARNING OBJECTIVES

Know Facts and Principles	Apply Facts and Principles	Demonstrate Ability	Evaluate Performance
1. Types of ostomies Differentiate between various types of ostomies.	Explain why skin care is different for different ostomies, based on effect of urine and feces on skin.	Correctly identify type of drainage to expect when assigned patient with ostomy.	Verify identification with instructor.
2. Appliances Describe various appliances available.		In the clinical setting, choose an appropriate appliance.	Evaluate with your instructor.
3. Changing a colostomy or ileostomy pouch List steps in procedure for changing colostomy pouch.	Given a patient situation, decide whether pouch should be changed.	Change colostomy or ileostomy pouch correctly.	Check pouch for security, leaks, and cleanliness. Evaluate own performance using Performance Checklist.
4. Observations List observations to make before, during, and after procedure.	Given a patient situation, identify observations that are significant.	Identify which observations are significant. Institute corrective action if necessary.	Evaluate own performance with clinical instructor.
5. Documentation State information and observations that need to be documented.	Given a patient situation, record data as though on chart.	Document procedure and observations correctly.	Evaluate with instructor.

LEARNING ACTIVITIES

1. Review the Specific Learning Objectives.
2. Look up the module vocabulary terms in the glossary.
3. Read through the module as though you were preparing to teach the contents to another person. Mentally practice the procedures.
4. In the practice setting:
   a. Examine the various types of appliances available.
   b. Read the instructions on any appliances and adhesives available.
   c. Examine colostomy irrigation equipment.
   d. Using a simulated ostomy on a manikin:
      (1) Change the ostomy pouch using the Performance Checklist as a guide.
      (2) Set up a colostomy irrigation using the equipment available. Do a mock irrigation if possible, using the Performance Checklist as a guide.
      (3) When you have mastered these skills, ask your instructor to check your performance.
5. In the clinical setting:
   a. Arrange with your instructor to perform any of the following procedures for a patient with a colostomy:
      (1) Changing an ostomy pouch.
      (2) Teaching the procedure for changing an ostomy pouch.
      (3) Performing a colostomy irrigation.
      (4) Teaching the irrigation of a colostomy.
   b. Ask your instructor to evaluate your performance.

VOCABULARY

adhesive
asepto syringe
anastomose
appliance
asymmetry
cauterize
cecostomy

colostomy
descending
transverse
double-barrel
continent urinary
   reservoir (CUR)

enterostomal therapist
  (ET)
excoriate
ileoconduit
ileobladder
ileoloop

ileostomy
ostomate
ostomy
skin barrier
stoma
ureterostomy

Ostomy Care

Rationale for the Use of This Skill

Advanced surgical techniques have led to increasing numbers of patients with surgical diversions of fecal and urinary elimination pathways. Comprehensive care requires that the nurse understand the different types of diversions and the reasons for them. Cleanliness, skin care, and odor control are other concerns. Because a surgical diversion is a profound change in body structure and function, the nurse must also provide supportive care, helping patients to make the necessary psychosocial adjustments.

Ostomies drain either fecal material or urine through a surgically altered passage. Rarely does the same ostomy drain both. Bowel diversion ostomies and urinary diversion ostomies, although similar in appearance and in appliances used, differ in one important element: urine drains from the sterile ureters, and any opening into the urinary system offers a pathway for infection directly to the kidneys.

The nurse must also constantly assess the condition of the skin surrounding the ostomy for problems that can be caused by constant moisture on the skin as well as by urine or fecal material.[1]

▼ NURSING DIAGNOSES

Examples of some nursing diagnoses that may be appropriate for the patient with an ostomy include:

Risk for Impaired Skin Integrity: Related to skin around stoma being exposed to urine or fecal material.

Body Image Disturbance: Actual related to presence of stoma and surgical alteration of elimination.

Knowledge Deficit: Management of the ostomy and performance of procedures for care.

BOWEL DIVERSION OSTOMIES

Bowel diversion ostomies may be temporary or permanent. Persons with a chronic disease of the bowel may have an ostomy *so that the diseased bowel can rest for a time to heal.* Others who have severe bowel injury that requires reconstructive surgery may also have a temporary diversion *so that healing can take place.* More commonly, a permanent bowel diversion is performed for the person who has a malignancy of the rectum or lower bowel.

All bowel diversion ostomies drain fecal material. The consistency of the material depends on the portion of the bowel that remains, the length of time the ostomy has been in place, and the location chosen for the placement of the ostomy.

An ileostomy empties from the end of the small intestine. *Because a large part of the water in the stool in the ileum is normally absorbed in the intestinal tract, the fecal material may be very liquid.* After the ileostomy has been in place for a time, the ileum often assumes a degree of this water-absorbing function, which results in a less liquid stool, although not one that is truly formed. The discharge from the stoma also *contains digestive enzymes, which increase the risk for impaired skin integrity.* Odor is not usually a major problem.

A cecostomy empties from the first part of the large intestine. Some digestive enzymes are usually present, and the stool may be liquid. Neither the cecostomy nor the ileostomy should need to be irrigated, *because the stool is not formed and moves through the intestinal tract without stimulation.*

A person with an ileostomy or a cecostomy wears a drainage pouch, formerly referred to as a bag. A new surgical ileostomy technique, called the continent ileostomy or Kock pouch, has been devised. During this procedure, a pouch of small intestine is formed to serve as a reservoir for feces for the person whose entire large bowel has been removed.

A "nipple" valve is formed where the pouch is attached to the skin. A catheter is introduced at regular intervals to drain the liquid fecal material. When not accessed, the valve closes *so that stool does not drain, and therefore the patient does not need to wear an appliance.* Sometimes a small amount of leakage occurs. In that case, the person wears a light dressing for absorption.

A colostomy can be located anywhere along the entire length of the large intestine. The further along the bowel it is located, the more solid the stool, *because the large intestine reabsorbs water, and the colon is less active than more proximal portions of the intestine.* The larger the portion of intestine that remains, the less frequent the bowel movements, *because there is more space for fecal material to accumulate.*

There are several types of colostomies. When a descending or sigmoid colostomy is done, the diseased portion of the colon is removed, and a permanent colostomy is formed. A transverse colostomy is done by removing a portion of the diseased transverse colon and forming a loop of bowel, which is either cauterized in the operating room (a current

---

[1]Rationale for action is emphasized throughout the module by the use of italics.

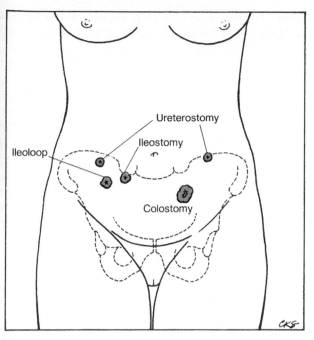

Figure 36–1. Common ostomy sites.

procedure) or brought through the abdominal wall with a glass rod beneath the loop, to be cauterized later (an older procedure). After the diseased portions of the colon are surgically removed, both ends of the intestine are brought to the surface, forming a double-barrel colostomy. Two stomas are formed: the proximal delivers stool, and the distal, which connects to the rectum, produces mucus. The latter is sometimes referred to as a *mucus fistula*. Both loop and double-barrel colostomies may be temporary in cases in which the distal bowel primarily needs a period in which to heal from severe infection or surgery. The ends of the severed bowel are reanastomosed later.

As with the ileostomy and cecostomy, the longer a colostomy has been in place, the more normal the consistency of the stool, *because remaining portions of the intestine increase water reabsorption to compensate for the excised bowel*. The general location of a planned ostomy, which depends on the underlying pathology, is determined by the surgeon. However, in many large medical centers the *enterostomal therapist* (ET), usually a nurse, is consulted. Several factors regarding the placement of the stoma are taken into consideration. Patients should be able to see the stoma easily, *so that if they are caring for themselves, they can see what they are doing*. The stoma should never be placed in areas such as a body crease, near scar tissue, or by bony prominences, *because any of these could interfere with the appliance's secure fit* (Fig. 36–1).

URINARY DIVERSION OSTOMIES

All urinary diversions provide drainage of urine that bypasses the bladder. *A ureterostomy is an opening of a ureter directly onto the abdominal surface.* Ureterostomies can be right, left, or bilateral. In the bilateral ureterostomy, each opening is covered by a separate appliance. Another variation is to anastomose (suture) one ureter into the other and bring that ureter to the skin, forming only one stoma. The opening is small—about as large in diameter as a pencil—and drains urine continuously so that an appliance must be worn.

To produce the urinary diversion, the physician may perform a more elaborate surgical procedure called *ileoloop, ileobladder, or ileoconduit*. (The prefix *ileal* is also used.) In this procedure a section of the ileum (small intestine) or some other part of the intestine, such as the cecum, is dissected from the rest of the intestine, and the intestinal ends are reattached. (Although some surgeons use sections other than the ileum, the term *ileo* is still used.) Both ureters are attached to this separate segment of intestine and drain into it. One end of the intestinal segment is closed, forming a substitute bladder and the other passage opens onto the abdomen as a stoma (Fig. 36–2). The stoma is the size of an ileostomy (about 1½ inches in diameter) and drains urine continuously. *The advantage of this type of urinary diversion is having one stoma that is larger and more easily fitted with an appliance. This procedure reduces the risk of ascending kidney infection because the mucous membrane of the intestinal segment serves as a barrier to microorganisms.*

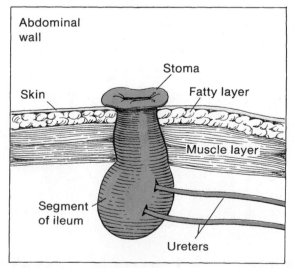

Figure 36–2. To form an ileoloop, a portion of the ileum is formed into a pouch for storing urine.

A technique being done with increasing frequency is the continent urinary reservoir (CUR). The advantage for the patient of having this procedure is that no appliance needs to be worn. It is similar to the bowel diversion technique known as the continent ileostomy or Kock pouch. A portion of the ileum is dissected and folded back on itself to form a structure for urine storage. A "nipple" valve is constructed onto the skin so that a stoma is formed and a catheter can be introduced at intervals to drain the urine (Fig. 36–3). Module 37, Catheterization, describes the procedure for draining the continent urinary reservoir.

OSTOMY APPLIANCES

Ostomy appliances are manufactured by a number of companies, and no one type of appliance is best for all patients. An enterostomal therapist is the best resource person to consult when making a selection. If no therapist is available, a representative from the surgical supply store may be able to explain the various types of appliances. For convenience, many facilities carry only one brand of appliance, but the patient should be made aware of all available options *so he or she can make a personal choice for ongoing care.* Ostomy appliances and accessories can also be ordered at most pharmacies (Table 36–1).

While in the hospital, the patient can use a temporary, disposable pouch with a peel-off adhesive square (Fig. 36–4A). An opening measuring the size of the stoma is cut in the square. Only the mucous membrane of the stoma is permitted to project through the hole. (*The mucus protects the membrane from irritation.*) *The skin surrounding the stoma can be irritated easily if there is contact with urine or stool.* After the opening is cut, the covering is peeled from the adhesive and the pouch is applied to the skin.

It is important to use a "see-through" appliance while the patient is in the hospital with a new stoma, *so that staff can see the stoma and assess its condition.* If the pouch is partially full, it can be opened and drained from the bottom. It can then be rinsed with an asepto syringe and warm water while in place. *Removing and reapplying adhesive pouches can irritate the skin.*

Most patients use a disposable pouch, but patients who have had a colostomy for some time may be more familiar and comfortable with a reusable (permanent) pouch. Generally, some patients who have had an ostomy for a long time did not have the option of using a disposable pouch and have continued the procedures that relate to a reusable pouch.

Reusable pouches have a solid plastic faceplate that fits around the stoma (Fig. 36–4B). Faceplates come in various sizes, and the size needed by an individual patient may change over time as the tissue shrinks. The pouch is fastened to the faceplate, which is held in place by a skin barrier: a karaya gum ring, a solid-pectin adhesive (such as Stomahesive), or a liquid adhesive. A belt is usually attached to the faceplate and worn around the patient's waist (Fig 36–4C). *The belt is designed to support the weight of the pouch as it fills, preventing it from pulling the adhesive loose and causing leakage.* Most pouches have a closure at the bottom, so they can be drained. The closure clip may be reused even if the pouch is disposable.

Colostomy dressings are uncommon except in the case of a newly created colostomy that is nonfunctioning. Because most colostomies are functioning the patient returns from the operating room with an appliance in place. If a colostomy dressing is used, a sterile 4 × 4 held in place with paper tape is usually sufficient. After healing, a person who has established good colostomy control may wear only a flat dressing over the stoma except when irrigating the colostomy.

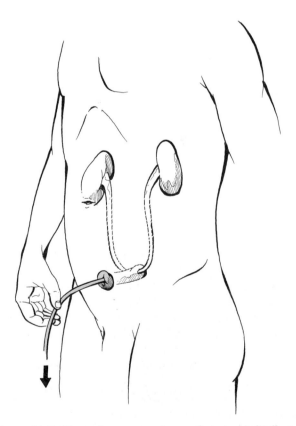

Figure 36–3. The patient uses a clean catheter periodically to drain a continent ileoconduit.

Table 36–1. Commonly Used Ostomy Products

Product	Manufacturer	Uses
Moisturizing cream	Hollister Cream (Hollister) Special Care Cream (Bard) Sween Cream (Sween)	Applied to lubricate dry skin around stoma. Applied sparingly so that the skin barrier used will adhere.
Powders	Stomahesive (ConvaTec) Karaya (many manufacturers) Baby powder (many manufacturers) Corn starch (many manufacturers)	Powders applied to irritated or moist skin enable barriers to adhere more tightly to the skin.
Skin sealers	Skin Gel (Hollister) Bard Protective Barrier (Bard) Skin Prep (United)	Can be used over powder to protect the skin from adhesive barriers.
Skin barriers	Premium Skin Barrier (Hollister) ReliaSeal (Bard) Stomahesive Barrier (ConvaTec) Comfeel (Coloplast) Various sheets, rings, and wafers (many manufacturers)	Skin barriers help protect the skin from irritation caused by the discharge from the ostomy. Most skin barriers can be applied to moist or irritated skin.
Sealing pastes	Premium paste (Hollister) Karaya Paste (Hollister) Stomahesive Paste (ConvaTec) Comfeel Paste (Coloplast)	These pastes fill in skin cracks and crevices to ensure a tight seal.
Deodorants	UltraFresh (Mentor) Ostozyme (Shelton) Banish (United) White vinegar (household 1:3 water)	Deodorants are used in the pouch to decrease odor.

Appliances used for urinary drainage ostomies that are not CURs are similar to those already described. Special adhesives that cannot be broken down by urine are used. Urinary pouches are drained from the bottom. They are replaced every 2 to 3 days to prevent urinary infection.

APPEARANCE OF A NORMAL STOMA

It is important that patients with an ostomy as well as nurses recognize the appearance of a normal stoma *so that changes can be identified, problems prevented, and interventions planned if necessary.* The normal stoma is highly vascular, appears red and smooth, and resembles other mucous membranes of the body. *Because there are no nerve endings in this tissue,* the stoma can be irritated and even necrotic without causing the patient pain. This fact mandates careful and continual assessment. Although the stoma is edematous (swollen) at first, this subsides in 5 to 10 days. Any of the following conditions indicates a peristomal skin problem and should be promptly reported. The skin may have a chemical burn producing redness from contact with urine or feces. Hair follicles can develop bacterial infections, and fungal infections of the skin cause what appears to be "pimples" surrounding the stoma. Some patients develop a contact dermatitis from the products being used (Van Niel, 1991). Any abnormal physical sign such as a rash, bluish color, excoriation, or asymmetry should be reported and documented.

To avoid early complications, assess the appearance of the stoma every 2 hours for the first 24 hours and then every 4 hours for the next 48 to 72 hours.

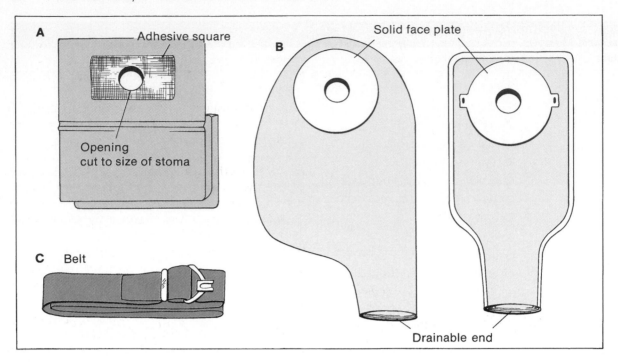

Figure 36–4. Examples of equipment used for colostomy. **(A)** Temporary pouch held on skin by an adhesive square. Adhesive squares are also called "wafers." **(B)** Reusable pouches. **(C)** Belt with hooks support pouch, length adjustable.

HEALTH TEACHING TOWARD SELF-CARE

Unless the patient is very debilitated or seriously ill, an important nursing goal is to teach the patient to perform ostomy self-care. The nurse must be both totally accepting of the appearance of the stoma and competent and knowledgeable in the care of ostomies. After the nurse has mastered the various procedures, a teaching plan should be set up and shared with the healthcare team.

Some hospitals have a health teaching outline for teaching the patient with a new ostomy. If the facility has an enterostomal therapist on the staff, this person may give instructions to the patient or be a useful resource to you so that you can teach the patient. At first, the patient may be reluctant to actively enter a teaching program *because of both fear and depression related to the realization that such a basic function as elimination has been surgically altered.* This may be particularly true if the surgery has been done as an emergency and the patient had little time to prepare. One study showed that many patients with ostomies do not have sufficient proficiency in self-care at the time of discharge and need to continue to improve their performance after leaving the hospital. Community resources may need to be contacted. Your approach in the healthcare setting is one that is straightforward and supportive of the patient who will quickly understand the goal as one of regaining independence.

OBTAINING SPECIMENS FROM OSTOMIES

At times, a stool or urine specimen is needed from the patient with a fecal or urinary diversion *to identify the presence of blood, glucose, bacteria, or parasites.* Even if the pouch has just been changed, it is preferable to secure the specimen directly from the stoma, *because it will not have had time to deteriorate in the pouch or to become contaminated if the pouch is not new.* Use a tongue blade to gently collect a specimen of stool from an intestinal stoma and a syringe without a needle to aspirate a small amount of urine from a urinary diversion. Review these procedures in Module 11, Collecting Specimens and Performing Common Laboratory Tests.

GENERAL PROCEDURE FOR CHANGING AN OSTOMY POUCH

Assessment
1. Identify the type of ostomy the patient has and its location.
2. Assess skin integrity around the stoma and its general appearance.

3. Note the amount and characteristics of any fecal material or urine in the pouch or on the dressing.
4. Determine whether the patient is being taught self-care at this time.

Planning

5. Wash your hands *for infection control.*
6. Gather the following equipment needed to change a pouch or dressing:
   a. Cleansing supplies, including tissues, warm water, mild soap, a washcloth, and a towel. In some facilities, clean disposable cloths are used for cleaning colostomies.
   b. Clean pouch of the type currently being used.
   c. Seal or use tape *to prevent leakage.* (This may be attached to the pouch.)
   d. Clean belt. The patient usually has two: one to be worn while the other is washed and dried. The belt being worn can be used again if it is clean. Temporary appliances may not have a belt.
   e. Dressing materials.
   f. Receptacle for the soiled pouch or dressing. A bedpan can be used initially. *For both aseptic and aesthetic reasons,* place the soiled pouch or dressing in a paper bag or wrap it in newspaper or paper towels for disposal. *This keeps the linen clean and helps contain odor.*
   g. Protective spray. The skin around the stoma may be protected by spraying with a liquid skin protector.
   h. Clean gloves.
7. Determine whether the patient is to participate actively.
8. Choose the appropriate location for performing the procedure. *The bathroom offers the patient more privacy and is more like the setting the patient will use at home.* The bedside can also be used and is usually more convenient for the nurse *because the stoma can be clearly seen and there is a place to put needed equipment.* Always plan based on the patient's needs.

Implementation

9. Identify the patient *to be sure you are performing the procedure for the correct patient.*
10. Explain what you are planning to do. If the patient is to participate, explain each step, including the rationale.
11. Put on clean gloves *for infection control.* Wear gloves when *handling any soiled material.*
12. Assist the patient to the bathroom or provide privacy.
13. Remove the soiled dressing or appliance (see specific instructions below). At home, instruct the patient to wear clean gloves if desirable when performing self-care *for aesthetic reasons.* Nurses and care providers wear clean gloves *for infection control.*
14. Using warm water and a mild soap, cleanse the skin around the stoma thoroughly *to remove feces or urine.* Inspect the skin for redness or irritation.
15. Cover the stoma with a tissue *to prevent feces or urine from contacting the clean skin.* Change tissues as necessary during the procedure.
16. Dry the skin around the stoma carefully, patting gently. Do not rub, *to avoid irritating the skin.*
17. Apply a skin protective if needed. Use sparingly *because a thin coating is sufficient for protection and will not interfere with pouch attachment.*
18. Allow the skin to dry thoroughly *so the pouch will adhere firmly.* Some patients use a hair dryer on a low setting at least eighteen inches from the skin for this purpose.
19. Remove the tissue from the stoma and apply the clean pouch or dressing as outlined below.
20. Remove your gloves and wash your hands thoroughly *for infection control.*

Evaluation

21. Evaluate using the following criteria:
   a. Pouch or dressing secure
   b. Area clean
   c. Odor-free
   d. Patient comfortable
   If the patient is being taught the procedure, add these criteria:
   e. Patient is able to change pouch using correct technique.
   f. Patient verbalizes understanding of key points in care.

Documentation

22. Record the following information:
   a. The amount, color, and consistency of the fecal material or urine in the pouch
   b. The application of the clean pouch and dressing change
   c. The knowledge and ability of the patient to participate in the procedure or ability to change the pouch independently

IRRIGATING A COLOSTOMY

The physician determines whether a colostomy should be irrigated. Not all colostomies need to be irrigated for effective functioning, although irrigation may be done *if constipation develops.* For some people, a colostomy does not function well without irrigation. When irrigation is performed daily, a reg-

DATE/TIME	
8/18/99	S *"I'm really worried about how red the intestine looks."*
1020	O *Stoma appears to be of normal color; no evidence of excoriation or infection.*
	A *Knowledge deficit regarding normal tissue appearance.*
	P *Teach patient about expected characteristics of stoma.*
	— M. Shaw, RN

Example of Nursing Progress Notes Using SOAP Format.

ular routine should be established *to facilitate cleanliness and odor control and to prevent embarrassing emptying of the bowel at inconvenient times and places.* To this end, set up a regular time for irrigation, accommodating to the patient's personal schedule. Select a time when the patient will be relaxed and be able to pay careful attention to detail. The patient's privacy is also important. Often you will have to teach the procedure to the patient or caregiver. The more the irrigation in the hospital can be made to resemble the way it will be done at home, the easier the patient's transition will be.

The physician may decide which one of two general types of irrigation will be used, or your facility may have a policy regarding the type to be used.

The large-volume, enema-type irrigation stimulates the bowel to evacuate. Some patients using this method may have to irrigate only every 2 or 3 days. Its disadvantages may include the retention of fluid and, later, dribbling; excessive distention of the colon; electrolyte depletion; and the prolonged amount of time required for the procedure. Also, some patients increase the volume of the irrigation beyond what is ordered or insert the tubing a longer distance than recommended into the colon, both of which can damage the colon.

The small-volume, bulb-syringe method is used to stimulate the bowel to do its own emptying. Because the tip on the syringe is short, it is impossible for the patient to insert it too far *and cause bowel damage. A disadvantage of the method is that it may not empty the bowel adequately, so that stool might be excreted later.* Also, the *hard bulb may be too stiff for weak or arthritic elderly persons to squeeze.* In this case, the enema-type equipment is used for a smaller-volume irrigation. Usually the small-volume irrigation must be done daily.

Both methods are described below. Review the general procedure for enema administration outlined in Module 28, Administering Enemas, as a guide, with the following directions for the specific irrigation:

PROCEDURE FOR IRRIGATING A COLOSTOMY

Assessment
1. Verify the type of irrigation to be done.
2. Find out if the patient is being taught self-care.

Planning
3. Wash your hands *for infection control.*
4. Obtain the necessary equipment.
   a. For either large-volume method or bulb-syringe method:
      (1) Bath blanket or large towel
      (2) Water-soluble lubricant
      (3) Clean gloves
      (4) Container for soiled pouch or dressings
      (5) Clean colostomy pouch or dressings
      (6) Irrigation sleeve or pouch
      (7) Bedpan and two disposable protective pads (if the patient must remain in bed)
   b. For large-volume method (Figure 36–5):

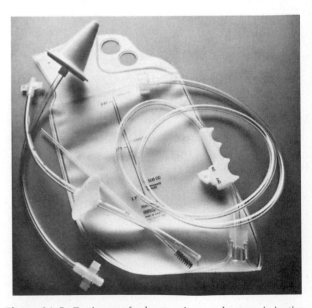

Figure 36–5. Equipment for large-volume colostomy irrigation.

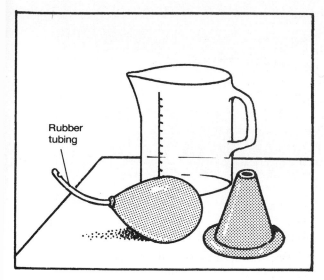

Figure 36–6. Cone catheter and bulb-syringe colostomy irrigating equipment.

   (1) Irrigation bag containing 1,000 mL warm tap water or other solution as ordered. This bag is usually equipped with a flow regulator and a number 28 cone-tipped catheter. A cone may be substituted for the catheter. An advantage of the cone is that it cannot be inserted too far.
   (2) Intravenous (IV) pole or other hook
   (3) Rubber nipple *to prevent back flow.* (This fits over the catheter. It is not necessary if a cone tip is on the tubing.)
  c. For bulb-syringe method (Fig. 36–6):
   (1) 8-oz bulb syringe with a number 28 cone-tipped catheter attached. A large ear syringe without a catheter may be substituted.
   (2) Container filled with 750 mL warm tap water.
5. Choose an appropriate location for the procedure. *The bathroom simulates the setting in which the patient will perform an irrigation at home. If the patient is weak or debilitated, the bedside is more appropriate.*

Implementation

6. Identify the patient *to be sure you are performing the procedure for the correct patient.*
7. Explain what you are planning to do. If the patient is to participate, explain each step, including rationale.
8. Provide privacy.
9. Put on clean gloves.
10. Remove the soiled pouch.
11. Wash around the stoma with warm water and mild soap. Dry well.

12. Place the irrigation bag or sleeve over the colostomy.
13. Position and drape the patient.
  a. In the bathroom, the patient sits on the toilet or commode. Place the end of the irrigation bag between the legs, *so the bag can drain directly into the toilet.* You may drape a towel or bath blanket over the patient's lap *for warmth and modesty* (Fig. 36–7).
  b. In bed, position the patient on the side. Place the bedpan on a disposable protective pad on the bed. Then place the end of the irrigation sleeve in the bedpan (Fig. 36–8). Use the other disposable pad to cover the bedpan as the colostomy empties, *to help contain odor.* Sometimes a patient who cannot sit on a commode but can sit in bed is placed in high Fowler's position. The bedpan is then placed beside the patient's hips.
14. Irrigate the colostomy.
  a. Large-volume method:
   (1) Hang the irrigation container on the IV pole, with the fluid level approximately 12 to 18 inches above the stoma. This positions the bottom of the container at the patient's shoulder *for appropriate pressure.*

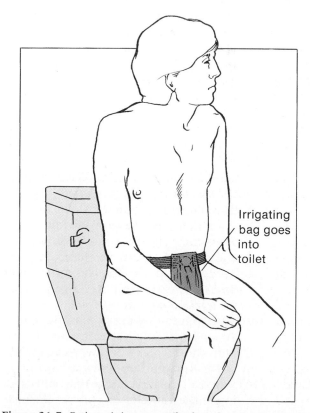

Irrigating bag goes into toilet

Figure 36–7. Patient sitting on a toilet for colostomy irrigation.

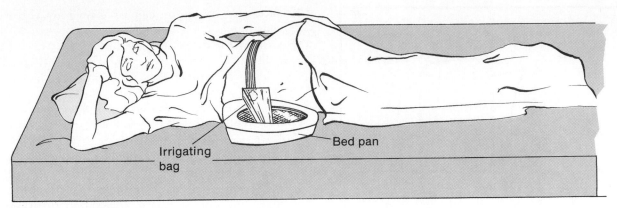

Figure 36–8. Patient lying on side for colostomy irrigation.

(2) Expel all air from the tubing.

(3) Place the nipple over the end of the catheter, and insert it down to ~~3 to 5~~ inches from the end, or attach the cone to the tubing.

(4) Lubricate the tip of the catheter or the cone.

(5) Lubricate your gloved little finger.

(6) Gently dilate the stoma by putting your lubricated finger through the open top of the irrigation sleeve (or the hole provided in the bag) into the opening. Check the direction of the lumen. If the colostomy is double-barreled (has two stomas), you will be irrigating the proximal loop.

(7) Gently thread the catheter through the opening in the irrigation bag into the stoma. Insert the catheter only 3 to 5 inches. If you detect any obstruction, do not force the catheter. Rotate it gently, allowing a small amount of fluid to flow in. *This measure often opens the lumen.* If you still cannot insert the catheter, seek help. Although a remote occurrence, *it is possible to perforate a bowel or to traumatize the mucosa severely by forceful pushing.* The cone tip fits into the stoma only far enough to dam the flow of water.

(8) Press the nipple or cone firmly against the stoma *to occlude the opening around the catheter.* If a nipple or cone is not available, press with the fingers *to close the stoma around the catheter.*

(9) Unclamp the tubing *to allow the fluid to flow into the bowel.* If cramping occurs, stop the flow and wait, as you would with a conventional enema.

(10) When all the fluid has been instilled, remove the catheter or cone *to allow the bowel to empty.*

b. Bulb-syringe (small-volume) method:

(1) Fill the syringe with water. Be sure to hold up the opening and expel all air.

(2) Dilate the stoma with your gloved and lubricated little finger.

(3) Gently insert the catheter of the syringe 3 to 5 inches into the stoma.

(4) Gently squeeze the bulb, instilling all the water, as you press around the stoma *to prevent backflow.* Do not allow the bulb to reinflate while in the stoma *to prevent damage to tissues.* There may be some return after the catheter is withdrawn.

(5) Remove and refill the syringe two more times, for a total of three syringes full (750 mL) of fluid. Do not instill more than this amount, even if some fluid is returned between instillations.

15. Instruct the patient to sit for approximately 15 minutes *to allow the bowel to empty. You or the patient can encourage emptying* by gently massaging the abdomen.

16. Clean off the bottom of the irrigation sleeve, fold it up, and fasten it closed.

17. Wait an additional 30 minutes *to allow the colostomy to complete emptying.* During this time the patient can move around, shave, bathe, and so on.

18. Drain the irrigation sleeve again, then rinse and remove it.

19. Apply a clean pouch, using the General Procedure for Changing an Ostomy Pouch (above).

20. Clean all the equipment, dry it, and put it away for future use.

21. Remove gloves and wash your hands.

Evaluation

22. Evaluate using the following criteria:

a. The amount and consistency of stool returned

b. If patient participated, understanding and ability to carry out the procedure.

DATE/TIME	
4/12/99 1100	D: *Patient is to be discharged in 3 days with colostomy. Has refused to look at or care for stoma.*
	A: *Used pictures and diagrams to explain stoma. Supported patient and family emotionally.*
	R: *Patient stated, "I really appreciate all your help and information. I know I have to learn to take care of myself and now I think I can do it." Agreed to look at stoma in AM.*
	R. Lash, RN

Example of Nursing Progress Notes Using Focus Format.

Documentation

23. Record the irrigation, including the amount of fluid instilled and returned, a description of return, and the patient's reaction.

24. Document the patient's level of knowledge and ability to carry out the procedure by having the patient demonstrate the procedure.

Colostomy Irrigation Problems

1. *The fluid does not return.* First, try to siphon fluid back. *Do not* instill additional fluid. Watch the patient carefully for later fluid return.

2. *No stool returns.* If the bulb-syringe method is used, you may either repeat the procedure immediately, wait a few hours and repeat, or wait 24 hours and repeat, depending on the physician's decision and your facility's procedure. *Repeating the procedure immediately may excessively fatigue the patient.* A large-volume irrigation is not usually repeated without specific consultation with the physician *because of electrolyte depletion.*

3. *The fluid flows out as fast as you put it in.* This action will not promote adequate emptying of the bowel. Stop the irrigation and devise a better way to occlude the stoma opening before you begin again.

4. *A patient with an old colostomy tells you he or she uses a lot more fluid than you are planning to use.* Some patients increase the amount of fluid instilled on their own at home and have been known to instill 4,000 to 5,000 mL and to take 2 hours for an irrigation. Explain to the patient the rationale for the procedure as you are going to do it. Then consult with your team leader or head nurse. You may have to increase the amount of fluid *to obtain any results.* Also, inform the physician of the patient's current practice.

5. *The patient states that he or she always inserts the catheter 8 or 10 inches.* Explain the rationale for the short distance and do not insert the catheter any further. One of the advantages of the bulb syringe

(or cone) is that the patient cannot insert the device too far *because it is so short.*

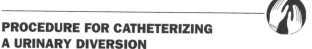

PROCEDURE FOR CATHETERIZING A URINARY DIVERSION

To obtain a sterile urine specimen or drain a continent urinary reservoir, it is necessary to catheterize the patient through the stoma. Before doing this procedure you should complete Module 33, Sterile Technique, and Module 37, Catheterization.

Assessment

1. Identify the type of urinary diversion the patient has.

2. Check the order for the catheterized specimen.

Planning

3. Wash your hands *for infection control.*

4. Obtain the equipment listed below. Some of these items may be included in a straight catheterization set. Sterile equipment is used *to avoid introducing pathogenic organisms into the urinary tract.*

   a. Sterile straight catheter
   b. Sterile gloves
   c. Sterile water-soluble lubricant
   d. Sterile container for the urine specimen
   e. Materials for applying a new appliance.

Implementation

5. Identify the patient *to make sure you are performing the procedure on the correct patient.*

6. Explain what you are going to do.

7. Remove the existing drainage pouch from the stoma, following the steps of the General Procedure for Changing an Ostomy Pouch (above).

8. Open the sterile equipment packages.

9. Put on sterile gloves.

10. Prepare the sterile field and lubricate the catheter as described in Module 37, Catheterization.

DATE/TIME	
5/22/99 0930	Colostomy irrigated with 750 ml, tap water, 50 ml, returned. Stoma siphoned with bulb syringe. Remainder of water returned containing small amount of liquid medium brown feces. Patient comfortable after procedure. ⎯⎯⎯⎯⎯⎯⎯⎯⎯ I, Sumi, RN

Example of Nursing Progress Notes Using Narrative Format.

11. Hold the sterile catheter approximately 3 inches from the catheter tip *to provide good control while preserving sterility.*

12. Insert the catheter into the stoma until urine begins to flow, but never insert it further than 2 inches. *This prevents trauma to the lining of the urinary diversion.* If you meet resistance, do not force the catheter but gently rotate its tip *to see if it will slide in with ease.*

13. After the specimen has been obtained, remove the catheter.

14. Replace the appliance according to the above procedure.

15. Measure the amount of urine for later documentation; if a specimen is ordered, place a portion of the urine into a specimen container and label accurately. Place in a plastic bag before sending it to the laboratory.

16. Remove your gloves and wash your hands.

Evaluation

17. Evaluate using the following criteria:
    a. Clarity and color of urine
    b. Patient's comfort during procedure

Documentation

18. Document the catheterization of the stoma, the collection of the specimen, and the drainage pouch change in the manner prescribed by your facility. This information may be placed on a flow sheet or on the nurses' progress notes.

19. Document any significant response of the patient to the procedure.

LONG-TERM CARE

The nurse in the long-term care setting has an added responsibility when caring for the older resident who has had an ostomy for some time and may be living in the facility because of impairments other than elimination. Some of these people have been performing their own ostomy care for years but find they have gradually lost the ability to continue giving themselves ostomy care. It is important for you to understand the type of ostomy and the procedure needed for a specific resident *so that you can offer what has been usual and satisfactory to the resident.* It also becomes vital to maintain proper exercise and diet *to maintain adequate fecal elimination through an ostomy. To ensure adequate urinary elimination and decrease the risk of urinary tract infection,* it is essential to provide enough oral fluids for the resident in your care who has a urinary diversion. With adaptations for the individual resident, you can modify certain procedures in this module for use within the long-term care setting.

HOME CARE

After the person with an ostomy (these persons are referred to as "ostomates") is discharged from the hospital, visits from the home health nurse *make the transition much easier*. The nurse can promote self-care as the client faces what may be a new and frightening experience.

Researchers have noted that the pouch that worked well for the patient in the hospital may be unsatisfactory when used at home because of the resumption of normal activity. If this is the case, the home health nurse can consult with the enterostomal therapist to identify a pouch that may be more effective. Again, it is important to emphasize exercise and adequate diet and fluid intake *so that elimination, both bowel and urinary, is facilitated. To avoid excessive intestinal gas formation,* teach clients to avoid gas-producing foods.

The home health nurse can also act as a resource. Self-help groups within most communities meet regularly to talk about the physical and psychological impacts of living with an ostomy. These groups offer ways of overcoming any disruptions in life *caused by having an ostomy* and have proven invaluable for many people with temporary or permanent elimination diversion.

CRITICAL THINKING EXERCISES

You are to teach two patients to irrigate their own colostomies. The first patient is a 72-year-old male gas station owner who had his colon and rectum removed because of cancer. The second patient is a 23-year-old female college student who had a portion of her colon resected because of a chronic inflammation of the bowel. Analyze how and why your teaching methods might be similar or different for these two patients. Contrast both physical and psychosocial concerns.

References

Van Niel, J. (1991). What's wrong with this peristomal skin? *American Journal of Nursing, 91*(12), 44–45.

Procedure for Changing an Ostomy Pouch	Needs More Practice	Satisfactory	Comments
Assessment			
1. Identify type and location of ostomy.			
2. Assess skin integrity around the stoma.			
3. Note the amount and appearance of any fecal material or urine.			
4. Determine whether patient is being taught self-care.			
Planning			
5. Wash your hands.			
6. Gather the following equipment to change a pouch or dressing: a. Cleansing supplies			
b. Clean pouch of correct type			
c. Seal or adhesive			
d. Clean belt			
e. Dressing materials			
f. Receptacle for soiled pouch or dressing			
g. Protective spray			
h. Clean gloves.			
7. Determine whether patient is to participate actively.			
8. Choose appropriate location for procedure.			
Implementation			
9. Identify the patient.			
10. Explain the procedure.			
11. Put on clean gloves.			
12. Assist the patient to the bathroom or provide privacy.			
13. Remove soiled dressing or appliance.			
14. Using warm water and mild soap, cleanse around the stoma.			
15. Cover the stoma with a tissue.			

(*continued*)

Procedure for Changing an Ostomy Pouch *(Continued)*	Needs More Practice	Satisfactory	Comments
16. Dry the skin around the stoma.			
17. Apply skin protective.			
18. Allow skin to dry thoroughly.			
19. Remove the tissue and apply the clean pouch or dressing. (See specific instructions below.)			
20. Remove gloves and wash your hands.			
Evaluation			
21. Evaluate using the following criteria: a. Pouch or dressing secure			
b. Area clean			
c. Odor free			
d. Patient comfort			
22. If the patient is being taught procedure, add: e. Able to change pouch, using correct technique.			
f. Verbalizes understanding.			
Documentation			
23. Record the following information: a. Amount, color, and consistency of fecal material or urine.			
b. Application of pouch and dressing change.			
c. Knowledge, understanding, and ability of patient's participation.			
Procedure for Irrigating a Colostomy			
Assessment			
1. Verify type of irrigation.			
2. Find out if patient is being taught self-care.			
Planning			
3. Wash your hands.			
4. Obtain necessary equipment. a. For either large-volume method or bulb-syringe method: (1) Bath blanket or large towel			

(continued

Procedure for Irrigating a Colostomy *(Continued)*	Needs More Practice	Satisfactory	Comments
(2) Lubricant			
(3) Clean gloves			
(4) Container for soiled pouch or dressing			
(5) Clean colostomy pouch or dressings			
(6) Irrigation sleeve or pouch			
(7) Bedpan and two disposable pads (for bed patient).			
b. For large-volume method: (1) Irrigation bag containing 1,000 mL warm tap water			
(2) IV pole or hook			
(3) Rubber nipple if irrigation bag does not have a cone tip.			
c. For bulb-syringe method: (1) 8-oz bulb syringe with number 28 separate catheter			
(2) Container filled with 750 mL warm tap water.			
5. Choose an appropriate place for irrigation.			
Implementation			
6. Identify the patient.			
7. Explain the procedure.			
8. Provide for patient's privacy.			
9. Put on clean gloves.			
10. Remove the soiled pouch.			
11. Wash around stoma with soap and warm water, then dry well.			
12. Place irrigation bag or sleeve over colostomy.			
13. Position and drape the patient, with end of bag in bedpan or toilet or commode.			
14. Irrigate the colostomy. **a.** Large-volume method: (1) Hang container on IV pole, with fluid 12–18 inches above the stoma.			
(2) Expel air from tubing.			

(continued)

Procedure for Irrigating a Colostomy *(Continued)*	Needs More Practice	Satisfactory	Comments
(3) Place nipple over end of catheter, approximately 3–5 inches from end, or attach cone.			
(4) Lubricate tip.			
(5) Lubricate gloved little finger.			
(6) Gently dilate stoma and check direction of the lumen with lubricated finger.			
(7) Thread catheter into stoma 3–5 inches.			
(8) Press nipple or cone firmly against stoma.			
(9) Unclamp tubing and allow fluid to flow.			
(10) When all fluid has been instilled, remove catheter and allow bowel to empty.			
b. Bulb-syringe method: (1) Fill syringe with water after expelling all air.			
(2) Dilate the stoma with gloved and lubricated little finger.			
(3) Insert catheter 3–5 inches.			
(4) Gently squeeze bulb, instilling all the water. (During this step, press around the stoma to prevent backflow.)			
(5) Remove and refill the syringe two more times until 750 mL has been instilled.			
15. Instruct patient to sit for 15 minutes to allow the bowel to empty.			
16. Clean off bottom of irrigation bag, fold it up, and fasten it closed.			
17. Wait an additional 30 minutes to allow complete emptying.			
18. Drain the irrigation sleeve again and remove it.			
19. Apply clean pouch.			

(continued)

Procedure for Irrigating a Colostomy *(Continued)*	Needs More Practice	Satisfactory	Comments
20. Clean all equipment, dry it, and put it away.			
21. Remove gloves and wash your hands.			
Evaluation			
22. Evaluate using the following criteria: **a.** Amount and consistency of stool returned.			
b. Patient's understanding and ability to carry out procedure.			
Documentation			
23. Record the irrigation, including amount of fluid instilled and returned, description of return, and patient's reaction.			
24. Document patient's level of knowledge and ability to carry out procedure.			
Procedure for Catheterizing a Urinary Diversion			
Assessment			
1. Identify type of urinary diversion.			
2. Check order for catheterization specimen.			
Planning			
3. Wash your hands.			
4. Obtain the needed equipment. **a.** Sterile straight catheter			
b. Sterile gloves			
c. Sterile water-soluble lubricant			
d. Sterile container for urine			
e. Materials for applying new appliance.			
Implementation			
5. Identify the patient.			
6. Explain the procedure.			
7. Remove existing appliance.			
8. Open sterile equipment packages.			
9. Put on sterile gloves.			
10. Prepare sterile field and lubricate catheter as described in Module 37, Catheterization.			

(continued)

Procedure for Catheterizing a Urinary Diversion (Continued)	Needs More Practice	Satisfactory	Comments
11. Hold sterile catheter 3 inches from tip.			
12. Insert catheter until urine begins to flow, but not further than 2 inches.			
13. After specimen has been obtained, remove catheter.			
14. Replace the appliance according to above procedure.			
15. Measure amount of urine; obtain specimen if ordered.			
16. Remove your gloves and wash your hands.			
Evaluation			
17. Evaluate using the following criteria: a. Clarity and color of urine			
b. Patient's comfort during procedure			
Documentation			
18. Document the procedure, collection of a specimen, and drainage pouch change.			
19. Document any significant response of the patient.			

MODULE

37

CATHETERIZATION

MODULE CONTENTS

PREREQUISITES

Successful completion of the following modules:

VOLUME 1
Module 1 An Approach to Nursing Skills
Module 2 Basic Infection Control
Module 3 Safety
Module 5 Documentation
Module 6 Introduction to Assessment Skills

VOLUME 2
Module 33 Sterile Technique

Review of the anatomy of the urinary system

OVERALL OBJECTIVE

To insert a urinary catheter using correct sterile technique. To establish, maintain, and discontinue continuous urinary drainage when appropriate.

SPECIFIC LEARNING OBJECTIVES

Know Facts and Principles	Apply Facts and Principles	Demonstrate Ability	Evaluate Performance
1. Patient concerns State usual concerns of patient regarding catheterization.	Given a patient situation, identify what concerns have and have not been met.	In the clinical setting: a. Prepare patient by teaching. b. Provide privacy and drape. c. Allow time for patient's questions. d. Leave patient comfortable.	Evaluate own performance using Performance Checklist.
2. Catheterization procedure List common ways contamination occurs in catheterization. Identify all items needed for catheterization of the bladder, urinary diversion, or self-catheterization and their purpose. State usual length of urethra in male and female. State rationale for sterile technique. Identify and explain principles of sterile technique used in catheterization.	Describe proper way to clean external meatus. Given a patient situation, state how to expose urinary meatus. Given a patient situation, state how far to insert catheter.	In the practice setting: a. Correctly set up equipment and arrange sterile field for catheterization. b. Carry out catheterization without contamination. c. Correctly identify meatus. d. Insert catheter correct distance.	Evaluate own performance using Performance Checklist and consulting with instructor.
3. Maintaining continuous drainage List major concerns related to continuous drainage.	Given a patient situation, identify errors in continuous drainage setup.	In the clinical setting: a. Assess patient with continuous drainage to identify problems. b. Correct errors in continuous drainage setup.	Evaluate own performance using Performance Checklist.

(continued)

Know Facts and Principles	Apply Facts and Principles	Demonstrate Ability	Evaluate Performance
4. Removing a Foley catheter			
Describe procedure for removing Foley catheter.	Plan teaching regarding Foley catheter removal.	In the clinical setting: a. Teach patient regarding removal of Foley catheter. b. Remove Foley catheter correctly.	Evaluate own performance using Performance Checklist.
5. Documentation			
List observations to be recorded.	Given a patient situation, identify information that should be recorded. Write nurses' progress note that would be appropriate for situation.	In the clinical setting, record catheterization in appropriate places on patient chart.	Evaluate with instructor.

LEARNING ACTIVITIES

1. Review the Specific Learning Objectives.
2. Read the section on the urinary system in the chapter on elimination in Ellis and Nowlis, *Nursing: A Human Needs Approach,* or comparable material in another textbook.
3. Look up the module vocabulary terms in the Glossary.
4. Review the anatomy of the urinary system.
5. Read through the module as though you are preparing to teach the concepts and skills to another person. Mentally practice the specific procedures.
6. In the practice setting:
   a. Obtain a catheterization set.
   b. Open the set properly, noting the arrangement of all equipment. If more than one type or brand of equipment is available, compare the different sets.
   c. Repack the set as it was originally.
   d. Using the Performance Checklist as a guide, go through the entire procedure, preferably using a manikin, or improvise an area to represent a patient (pillows will work for this). Repeat the procedure until you feel comfortable with the equipment and you remember the steps.
   e. With a partner, arrange for a time to use a manikin.
   f. Take turns going through the procedure and evaluate each other's performance using the Performance Checklist.
   g. With a partner as the "patient," assume that an indwelling catheter is to be removed and do health teaching in the four appropriate areas.
   h. Have your instructor evaluate your performance.
7. In the clinical setting:
   a. Consult with your clinical instructor regarding an opportunity to perform catheterization under supervision.
   b. Evaluate your own performance using the Performance Checklist.
   c. Consult your instructor regarding your performance.
8. If the opportunity arises, observe the teaching of a patient who is learning self-catheterization or learning to perform catheterization of a urinary diversion.

VOCABULARY

catheter	foreskin	penis	straight catheter
catheterization	homeostasis	perineum	urethra
Foley catheter	meatus	stoma	void

Catheterization

Rationale for the Use of This Skill

A catheter is used to drain urine from the bladder or to instill solution into the bladder. Patients' bladders are catheterized for various diagnostic and therapeutic reasons. It is the nurse's responsibility to carry out this task or delegate it to a skilled staff person. Because the inside of the bladder is sterile and provides direct access to the kidneys, the primary concern must be preventing contamination of the bladder. Urinary tract infections are common in those who have indwelling catheters in place. Even a single catheterization carries with it the danger of contaminating the urethra, the bladder, or both. Although bladder infections can be serious in themselves, they can also lead to kidney infections, which may be life-threatening.

It is also the nurse's responsibility to know the anatomy of the urinary system to avoid damage to the urethra during catheterization. Once the catheter is in place, the nurse must establish correct drainage.

The patient with neuromuscular disease or obstruction that temporarily or permanently interferes with voluntary bladder emptying may be taught to perform self-catheterization. Patients who have had a surgical urinary diversion are taught to use the procedure of periodic stomal catheterization to empty the continent ileal pouch that has been surgically formed.

The nurse is responsible not only to perform catheterization procedures effectively and safely but also to provide patient teaching and relieve anxiety.[1]

▼ NURSING DIAGNOSES

The following are common nursing diagnoses for the patient who is to be catheterized or the patient with an indwelling catheter:

Altered Urinary Elimination. This may be related to a variety of urinary problems, such as incontinence, urgency, or bladder distention.

Urinary Retention. This may arise after surgery and be caused by exposure to anesthesia.

Risk for Infection related to presence of indwelling catheter.

Dependence on Urinary Catheter related to incontinence. Although this is not a NANDA-approved nursing diagnosis, it may be applicable.

Rationale for action is emphasized throughout the module by the use of italics.

PREPARING THE PATIENT

Many patients are anxious about catheterization, fearing pain and discomfort. They react emotionally to any procedure related to the genitourinary system—one that involves penetration of the body. Some facilities *protect privacy by* establishing a policy for male patients to be catheterized by male nurses and female patients to be catheterized by female nurses, unless the catheterization is an emergency. If an emergency occurs, and because there are relatively few male nurses, some facilities have specially trained male technicians or nursing assistants who can catheterize male patients. Other institutions permit both male and female nurses to perform catheterizations on a patient of either sex, but permission is often asked. Always assess the patient's feelings about the procedure and review the policy of your facility *to cause the patient as little embarrassment as possible.* In preparing the patient, use a calm, straightforward, professional manner *to relieve the patient's anxiety.* Explain the procedure completely, and tell the patient what to expect. Give the patient an opportunity to ask questions and express concerns. Pay careful attention to privacy by closing doors, draping the patient, and exposing only the area involved in the procedure. *These actions show your concern for the patient's privacy and should alleviate some distress.*

EQUIPMENT

A catheterization set contains the basic equipment needed for the procedure (Fig. 37–1). Some variation from one brand to another may exist, but usually the following items are included:

1. **Sterile catheter.** Either a plain (straight) catheter or an indwelling catheter can be used. Indwelling catheters are often referred to as "Foley" catheters, named after their originator. *The indwelling catheter has a balloon at the end that is inflated to hold the catheter in the bladder.*

   Balloons are available in several sizes. Nurses most commonly insert catheters with balloons that hold 5 or 6 mL sterile water, depending on the manufacturer. Catheters with larger balloons are available and can be used for patients who have difficulty retaining the indwelling catheter. The larger balloon is needed to secure it within the bladder. During surgery, physicians sometimes insert catheters with balloons as large as 30 mL, which they secure with traction to provide hemostasis at a urologic surgical site

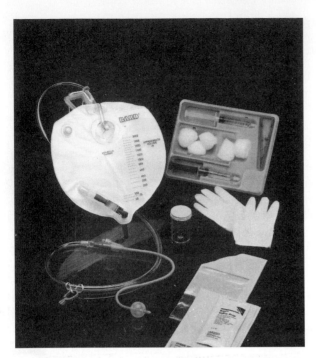

Figure 37–1. Indwelling catheterization set.

(Fig. 37–2). This type of catheter is used when continuous drainage is required.

Catheters are available in sizes 8 to 20 French. (French is a method of sizing.) Size 8 French is used for infants and young children. Size 16 French is the size commonly used for adults. For patients who drain urine around an indwelling catheter, size 18 or 20 French is used.

A sterile prefilled syringe (in the set) to fill the balloon is attached to indwelling catheters. The syringe contains an additional amount of sterile water *to fill the catheter chamber as well as the inflated balloon.*

It has been found that the selection of the smallest size of the catheter that will be effective *decreases the likelihood of infection. Larger catheters irritate the wall of the urethra, causing it to be prone to invasion by microorganisms.* This is very important when an indwelling catheter is to be inserted *because it remains in contact with the urethra for a longer time.* The substance of the catheter to be used also makes a difference in infection rates. Researchers have recommended the use of silicone catheters. *Silicone catheters are softer, cause less irritation than latex catheters, and therefore can be left in place longer with less possibility of infection.*

The balloon on an indwelling catheter usually holds either 5 mL or 30 mL sterile water. A size 8 French catheter, used for the pediatric patient, has a 3-mL balloon. The 5-mL balloon

catheter is used routinely for urinary drainage of adult patients. The 30-mL balloon catheter is often ordered for a confused patient *who has pulled out a catheter with a smaller balloon.* Patients undergoing surgery of the prostate may have a 30-mL balloon catheter inserted before or during surgery and taped to the leg with traction *to provide hemostasis* (retard the tendency to bleed).

2. **Sterile wrapper.** When opened, the inside of the wrapper provides a sterile field. The outside is usually impervious to moisture.
3. **Sterile gloves.** These are usually on top, so all other items can be set up using sterile technique. As a beginner, you may want to have an extra pair of gloves in the room.
4. **Sterile drapes.** Two drapes are usually provided. One is a plain drape to slide under the female patient or to spread out under the penis. The other drape is often fenestrated (has a hole in it). The fenestrated drape is placed over the perineum,

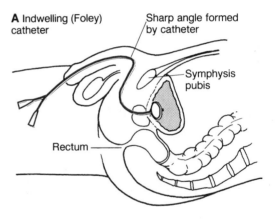
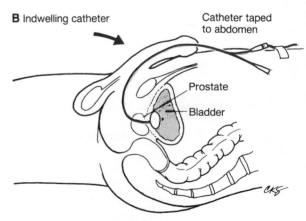

Figure 37–2. The inflated balloon holds the catheter in the bladder. **(A)** Note the sharp angle formed at the penile-scrotal junction when the penis is directed toward the thigh. **(B)** Note how correct taping of the catheter in the male patient eliminates the potential for abrasion and erosion of the penile-scrotal angle.

with the opening over the meatus for a female patient or around the penis of a male patient.

5. **Sterile cleansing swabs.** These may be cotton balls or swabs with a short handle attached.

6. **Thumb forceps, or pickups.** You will need these to handle the cotton balls without contaminating your gloves.

Cleansing solution. These may vary, according to the manufacturer. Most sets contain a water-soluble iodine solution, which is an excellent antibacterial agent.

8. **Syringe prefilled with sterile water.** This is used to fill the retention balloon of an indwelling catheter.

9. **Water-soluble lubricant** for lubricating the catheter.

10. **Specimen container and label.**

11. **Safety pin and rubber band or plastic clamp** (in some sets). These are used to secure the catheter tubing to the bed if the catheter is indwelling. If they are not in the set, you will have to obtain them separately. If it is policy to use tape, you will have to obtain this.

12. **Drainage tubing and collection bag.** These are often packaged with the set. If not, obtain them separately.

13. **Tape.** Tape for securing the catheter to the patient is not included in the set. A disposable cloth peel-off patch with Velcro (Cath-Secure) or a leg strap can be used in place of tape.

PROCEDURE FOR CATHETERIZATION

Assessment

1. Assess the patient and check the order *to be sure that catheterization has been ordered for the patient.*

2. Determine whether the procedure is to be a straight or indwelling catheterization.

3. Find out whether a urine specimen is needed. When in doubt, always obtain a specimen. It can be discarded later if it is not needed.

Planning

4. Wash your hands *for infection control.*

5. Select the specific type and size of catheter to be used.

6. Collect the appropriate equipment, including the correct catheterization set, additional lighting if the room does not have adequate lighting (a portable gooseneck lamp or a flashlight may be used to improve existing lighting), and a bath blanket or sheet *to drape the patient.* You may wish to have extra equipment available *in case an item is contaminated.*

Implementation

7. Identify the patient *to be sure you are performing the procedure on the correct patient.*

8. Explain the procedure to the patient and answer any questions.

9. Close the door of the room or draw the bed curtains *for privacy.* Raise the bed to a comfortable working height and drape the patient.

   a. *For a pediatric patient or one who is disoriented or confused,* you may need another person (sometimes two others) *to assist the patient to maintain the proper position.*

   b. Place a female patient in the dorsal recumbent position, with knees flexed and legs spread, *because it provides good visualization* and is *usually most convenient* (Fig. 37–3). Sometimes it is more comfortable for the patient to have her knees supported with pillows. Drape the bath blanket so that both legs are covered and only the perineum is exposed, *to protect privacy. If the patient cannot assume the dorsal recumbent position,* the Sims' position can be used.

   c. Place the male patient in the supine position. Expose only the penis and a small surrounding area (see Module 17, Assisting with Elimination and Perineal Care).

10. Set up the equipment.

    a. Arrange the lighting *so that you can see the perineum easily.* If the perineal area is soiled, provide perineal care, wearing clean gloves, with soap and water before you begin catheterization. You may be able to identify the meatus while providing perineal care.

    b. Open the catheterization set and arrange the sterile field in a convenient location (on an overbed table at the foot of the bed or on the bed between the patient's legs).

    c. Set up a receptacle for soiled cleansing swabs. The plastic bag that contained the set, a bedside bag, or several paper towels stacked together can be used for this purpose. The set itself may have a "well" for this purpose.

    d. If the drainage bag is in a separate package, open it and attach it to the bed.

    e. If a sterile drape is on top of the set, grasp it by one corner and open it with care, touching only the underside and edges to keep the top sterile. Ask the female patient to lift her hips and carefully slide the drape under the buttocks. The soft side should be up against the patient, and the shiny waterproof side should be down (Fig. 37–4).

       Even though the drape is placed carefully, this area should be considered clean and not sterile throughout the procedure *because it is*

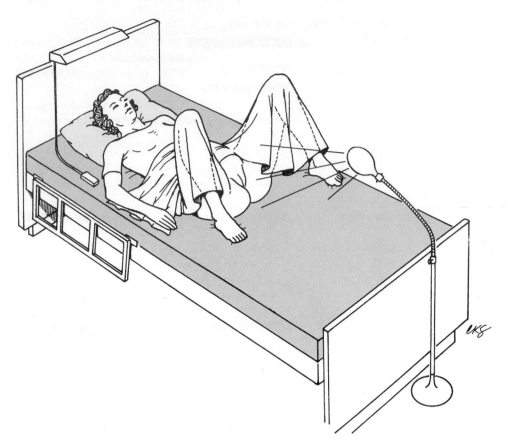

Figure 37–3. Female in dorsal recumbent position.

difficult to maintain sterility here. For the male patient, slide the drape under the penis, across the groin. This area can be considered sterile. Put on sterile gloves.

f. If sterile gloves (not drape) are on top, put

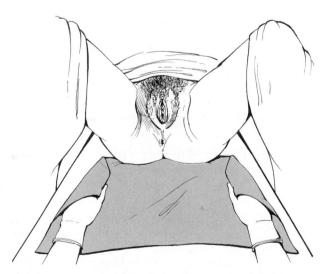

Figure 37–4. Placing a sterile drape under the female patient without contaminating sterile gloves.

them on first, *so nothing is contaminated as you work*. Then, carefully take the first drape and unfold it, keeping your gloved hands at the top of the drape. Grasp two adjacent corners of the drape and turn your hands, so that the drape covers the gloves *to protect them from contamination*. Next, place the drape as described above to provide a sterile field, keeping the top sterile and not touching anything but the top side of the drape with your gloved hands.

g. Place the second drape *to secure and enlarge the sterile field*. If it is fenestrated, place the opening over the penis of the male patient. The drape can be placed over the meatus of the female patient, but many nurses find that it tends to fall forward, obscuring their vision and potentially contaminating the catheter. An alternative is to fold the drape in half and place it over the pubic area.

h. Open the cleansing solution and pour it over the swabs.

i. Open the lubricant and place it along the end of the catheter. *Lubricant minimizes trauma and discomfort to the urethra when the catheter is inserted*.

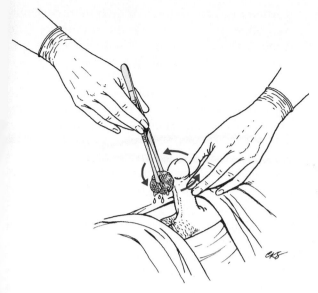

Figure 37–5. The nurse cleaning the male patient for catheterization. Clean the penis with circular strokes.

j. If an indwelling catheter is being inserted, attach the prefilled syringe to the balloon port. Test the balloon by instilling all of the sterile water and then deflating it by withdrawing the water. Leave the syringe attached. (This can simplify later work because you will want to hold the catheter in place with one hand, which leaves you only one hand to manipulate the syringe.) If the catheter is defective, ask someone to get another catheter or remove your gloves and get both another catheter and another pair of gloves *to proceed.*

k. Set the specimen container and its cap upside down *so that it is convenient and remains sterile.*

l. If the drainage bag is in the set, connect the distal end of the catheter to the drainage tube. *This prevents urine spilling from a collecting container while you are performing the procedure.* If a specimen is needed, you can either not connect the catheter to the drainage tube at this time and use the specimen container as a collection device or obtain a specimen from the drainage bag after you have finished.

11. Catheterize the patient.

a. Use your nondominant hand to expose the meatus. Remember that this hand is now contaminated and cannot be used to handle equipment again.

For a man or boy, raise the penis at a 45° angle from the scrotum and retract the foreskin. For a woman or girl, separate both the labia majora and the labia minora. Retract the labia in an outward direction. A common

error is to place the fingers too high to expose the meatus. If the meatus is not identifiable, move your hand for better exposure. Always identify the meatus before any other equipment is contaminated. Cleansing, the next step, will help you positively identify it. You may ask the patient to cough *because coughing usually causes the meatus to open slightly and aids identification.*

b. After the meatus is exposed and identified, begin cleaning.

Use forceps to handle the cleansing swabs *to maintain sterility of your dominant gloved hand for handling the catheter.* Use each swab only once, and then discard in the prepared location, *where it will not contaminate your field. To prevent bacteria from falling onto the sterile field,* do not pass the used cleaning swabs over the sterile field. For a man or boy, clean in a circular motion, starting at the meatus, without retracing any area *to move bacteria away from the meatus* (Fig. 37–5).

For a female, use each swab from front to back, starting with the outside labia and moving toward the center (Fig. 37–6). Clean one side first and then the other. The final stroke should be vertical to clean the meatus itself. The principle behind this pattern is to *move from the area of lesser accumulation of secretions and organisms (labia) to the area of greater concentration (meatus).* The last stroke, if done slowly, may open the meatus slightly, thereby assuring identification.

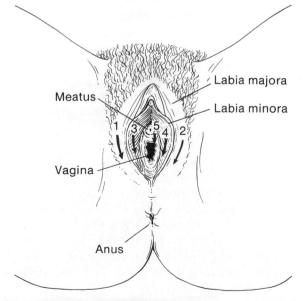

Figure 37–6. Cleaning the female for catheterization. Clean the genitalia from anterior to posterior.

Some persons recommend that the first cleansing strokes be down the center, across the meatus, and that subsequent strokes move outward. The principle for this pattern is *to move from the area you want to be the cleanest area (meatus) to the area that is less critical (labia).*

Research has not identified which of these procedures is better. The most critical point seems to be that each swab be used only once and that the path of the swab be from anterior to posterior *to avoid moving microorganisms from the rectal area to the meatus.* For this step, follow your facility's policy or procedure.

c. Use the sterile-gloved dominant hand to move the tray containing the catheter close to the patient (between the legs of the female patient and beside the male patient). Touch only the inside of the tray. Pick up the catheter several inches back from the tip *to keep the tip sterile.* If a collecting bag is not attached, be sure to keep the end of the catheter in the tray.

d. Insert the lubricated catheter smoothly, approximately 2 to 3 inches into the female and 6 to 9 inches into the male, beyond the urethra into the bladder. Do not use force. If you encounter resistance, ask the patient to breathe deeply (*to relax the muscles*) and gently rotate the catheter to see if it will penetrate. If it still will not enter, consult a physician before trying again. *It is possible to damage the urethra and the urinary sphincters by pushing against resistant tissue.*

The return of urine indicates that the catheter is in the bladder. To inflate the balloon, insert the catheter 1 inch further after urine is returned *to make sure that the balloon does not inflate in the urethra.*

12. If you are using a straight catheter, hold the catheter in place while you fill the specimen container. Drain the bladder, pinch the catheter closed to prevent further draining, and remove the catheter. Recent research indicates that whichever type of catheter you use, it is not harmful to drain the bladder completely, regardless of the quantity. It was once thought that draining more than 1,000 mL at one time could lead to a shocklike reaction, but researchers have found that this does not appear to be true. Although there may be small changes in blood pressure and pulse, these are not usually clinically significant.

13. If you are inserting an indwelling catheter, hold it in place while you fill the balloon. The catheter can continue to drain into the receptacle while this is done. Use the amount of fluid indicated on the catheter itself plus 4 or 5 mL. *Because the fluid must fill the tube leading to the balloon, as well as the balloon itself, you will need this extra amount, and manufacturers indicate that balloons will not overinflate or rupture from using this amount. If you use too little fluid, the catheter may slip out. Check the security of the catheter* by gently pulling it until you feel resistance.

14. In most indwelling catheter sets, the bag is attached to the catheter. If it is not, connect the bag at this time. Be sure to maintain the sterility of the ends of the tubing at the connecting point. Place the tubing over the top of the thigh, *so the leg does not occlude the tubing.*

Hang the bag on the bed frame below the level of the bladder to avoid any return of urine through the tubing. Make sure the bag does not touch the floor.

15. Tape the catheter to the patient *to prevent pull on the neck of the bladder as the patient moves* (Fig. 37–7).

For a man or boy, tape the catheter without tension to the side of the lower abdomen *to prevent the formation of a fistula at the penile-scrotal angle.* For a woman or girl, tape the catheter to the inner thigh (Fig. 37–8). Some physicians prefer that the catheter not be taped. Coil excess tub-

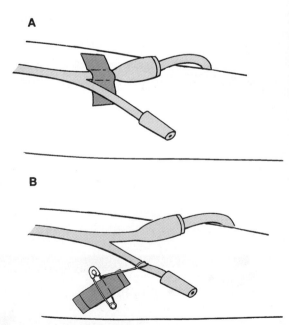

Figure 37–7. Taping a catheter. **(A)** To decrease the chance of the tape pulling loose, the catheter is secured in a loop of tape before the ends are taped to the patient. **(B)** Alternately, the catheter may be attached by using a combination of tape, a safety pin, and a rubber band.

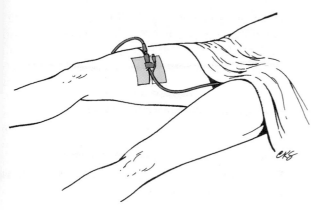

Figure 37–8. A cloth/Velcro peel-off patch or leg straps are also available commercially to secure the catheter and tubing.

ing flatly on the bed, *so that drainage is not impeded. Urine collecting in the tube provides a medium for bacteria to multiply and ascend.* Attach the tubing to the side of the bed with a plastic catheter clamp (which may be included in the set) or with a rubber band and safety pin. Wrap the rubber band around the tubing and pin it to the sheet.

16. Assist the patient to a comfortable position, straighten and lower the bed, and open the curtains. The patient may have further questions or concerns. This is a good time to teach the patient

about the indwelling catheter. Tell the patient that the balloon will hold the catheter in place and that it is all right to move. Stress the need for fluids (if the patient's medical condition permits) *to maintain adequate kidney function. Because of the pressure of the balloon,* the patient with an indwelling catheter usually feels as though he or she needs to void. Explain that this feeling will pass as the tissue becomes less sensitive to the constant stimulation. Understanding this helps the patient to tolerate the discomfort.

17. Gather and discard disposable equipment properly. If you have used nondisposable equipment, follow your hospital's procedure for cleaning.

18. Wash your hands *for infection control.*

Evaluation

19. Evaluate using the following criteria:
    a. Indwelling catheter draining properly or straight catheter inserted and removed without discomfort or other difficulty
    b. Patient comfortable

Documentation

20. Document the following:
    a. Date and time of catheterization
    b. Type and size of catheter inserted
    c. Whether a specimen was obtained and sent to the laboratory

DATE/TIME	
2/14/99 1600	# 6 Fr. indwelling catheter inserted per order, 600 ml, clear, pale yellow urine obtained. Spec. to Lab. Patient stated, "slight discomfort." *S. Holtz, RN*

Example of Nursing Progress Notes Using Narrative Format.

DATE/TIME	
4/19/99 0800	Perineal discomfort: S "I feel like I have to go all of the time and I itch down there." O Perineum reddened and catheter feels gritty when compressed between fingers. Urine dark amber in color, cloudy, and contains white sediment. A Catheter collecting sediment and causing patient discomfort and risk for infection. P Obtain order for replacement of indwelling catheter. Increase fluid intake to 2500 ml/24h. *R. Sanders, RN*

Example of Nursing Progress Notes Using SOAP Format.

d. Amount of urine drained (add to the output record if appropriate)

e. Description of the urine

f. Patient's response to the procedure

CARING FOR A PATIENT WITH AN INDWELLING CATHETER

The urinary tract is normally sterile. *The introduction of organisms through the catheter is a common cause of urinary tract infection.* Various measures are used *to decrease the risk of infection.*

1. Place the patient on intake and output measurement *to assess the functioning of the catheter.*

2. Encourage the patient to increase fluid intake. *Large intake causes a constant flow of urine out of the kidneys and bladder, which tends to inhibit the upward movement of microbes.* By increasing fluid intake, the system is being irrigated internally. Up to 3,000 mL fluids per day (for the patient without circulatory problems and with no fluid restriction) is best. This quantity may be unrealistic for an elderly patient or child, but encourage any increase.

3. Maintain the closed system. *Every time the system is opened, microorganisms can enter.* Carry out all procedures so that the system is uninterrupted if possible. (See Module 11, Collecting Specimens and Performing Common Laboratory Tests, for a method of obtaining urine specimens without interrupting the system.)

4. Maintain external cleanliness around the catheter. *Secretions that build up are an optimum location for bacterial growth, which could ascend the outside of the catheter.* Wash thoroughly with soap and water.

5. Keep the catheter drainage bag below the level of the bladder at all times. *This prevents potentially contaminated urine from draining back into the bladder.* Some brands of collecting bags have one-way valves to prevent backflow.

6. Keep the tubing coiled by the patient's side. *Tubing that hangs off the bed in loops allows urine to sit in the tubing, creating a possible reservoir for microbes, which could then ascend.*

7. Keep the drainage bag off the floor. *If it touches the floor, the outside picks up microorganisms that can then move up the outside of the bag and the catheter.*

8. Tape or coil the catheter in a way that prevents pulling. *Pull irritates the patient's urethra and can actually dislodge the catheter and inflated balloon. In*

addition to causing the patient trauma and discomfort, irritation and inflammation predispose the tissue to infection. Take extra care when moving or ambulating a patient. Watch the position of the tubing and bag at all times *to prevent pulling.*

9. Observe for irritation at the meatal area. If any is found, provide catheter care to the area more frequently.

10. Empty the bag at regular intervals (usually every 8 hours) *so that it does not overfill and cause urine backup in the tubing.* Empty more frequently *if large amounts of urine are being excreted.*

PROCEDURE FOR REMOVING AN INDWELLING CATHETER

Assessment

1. Verify the order to discontinue the indwelling catheter.

2. Determine whether a urine specimen is needed.

Planning

3. Wash your hands *for infection control.*

4. Obtain the necessary equipment:
   a. Several paper towels for wrapping the soiled catheter after removal
   b. A 10-mL syringe
   c. Padding and a small container to catch the fluid
   d. Clean gloves

Implementation

5. Identify the patient *to be sure you are performing the procedure on the correct patient.*

6. Explain to the patient that the catheter is to be removed and that the procedure is not painful. Health teaching should include the following four points:
   a. A mild burning sensation may accompany urination for a short time *because of the irritation caused by the catheter.* If this persists, it should be reported to the physician.
   b. Voiding may be more frequent and in smaller amounts than normal at first *because the bladder has been kept empty and may have to relearn how to respond to a sensation of fullness.* Again, if this persists, it should be reported to the physician *because it may indicate infection.*
   c. For the first 24 hours after the catheter is removed, the nurse should be called *to measure each voiding to facilitate assessment.* If the patient can go to the bathroom, explain how measurement is carried out. Resnick (1993)

recommends daytime removal *to give the patient ample time to void during the day when there are more staff on duty for assistance and assessment.*

   d. It is essential to continue increased fluid intake *to maintain proper kidney and bladder function.*

7. Close the door or draw curtains and prepare the patient. Raise the bed and drape the covers back to expose the catheter. Put on clean gloves.
8. Grasp catheter near the meatus and gently withdraw the catheter.
   a. Place paper towels under the catheter.
   b. Use the syringe *to remove sterile water from the balloon.* In some facilities, nurses cut the balloon-filling tube of the catheter with scissors *to remove the sterile water.* This is unwise, *because there is always some chance that the balloon will not deflate with this method.* If this occurs, the physician will have to introduce a special instrument *to deflate the balloon so that the catheter can be removed.*
   c. Pinch the catheter *to prevent leakage* and pull it out smoothly. This action should not cause discomfort but will be felt. Ask the patient to breathe in and out through the mouth *to relax* while you withdraw the catheter.
   d. With your free hand, wrap the end of the catheter in paper towel while you keep the catheter itself pinched closed.
   e. Hold the end of the catheter up *to allow urine to drain from the tubing into the bag.*
9. Assist the patient to a comfortable position, and straighten and lower the bed.
10. Measure urine output.
11. Dispose of the equipment.
12. Remove gloves and wash your hands.

Evaluation
13. Evaluate using the following criteria:
    a. Catheter removed without difficulty.
    b. Patient voiding in adequate amounts (ap-

proximately 250 mL each time) at regular intervals.
   c. Patient increases fluid intake to 2,400 to 3,000 mL each 24 hours.

Documentation
14. On the patient's record, document the time the catheter was removed, the amount of urine output, and the patient's response to the procedure.

TEACHING THE PROCEDURE FOR INTERMITTENT SELF-CATHETERIZATION

Intermittent self-catheterization is performed using clean rather than sterile technique. Conscientious handwashing is essential *to prevent infection.* Regular emptying of the bladder is another factor *for avoiding urinary tract infections.* The procedure is performed every 2 to 3 hours during the day and once during the sleeping hours, if necessary.

Assessment
1. Check the order to be sure that self-catheterization has been ordered for the patient.
2. Identify the medical diagnosis and whether the patient is learning the procedure for purposes of temporary or permanent urinary drainage.
3. Assess the patient's knowledge of own anatomy and any feelings of anxiety *that may interfere with learning.*

Planning
4. Wash your hands *for infection control.*
5. Collect the following equipment:
   a. A 14 or 16 French straight catheter (two or more)
   b. Lubricating jelly
   c. Small hand mirror (for the female patient)
   d. Small clean pan, container, or leakproof plastic bag

Example of Nursing Progress Notes Using Focus Format.

DATE/TIME	
7/21/99 2000	D: Indwelling catheter removed at 1615. Patient appears anxious regarding ability to void.
	A: Encouraged patient to take fluids. Reassured patient that any initial burning on voiding is normal. Instructed patient to call for assistance if feels need to void.
	R: Voided 250 mL at 1830. Appears relaxed. Visiting with family. G. Raymond, RN

e. Additional clean plastic bag for storing catheter.

Implementation

6. Identify the patient *to be sure you are teaching the procedure to the correct patient.*
7. Review the equipment you have selected with the patient, identifying each item, explaining its use, and answering any questions.
8. Review the steps of the procedure in detail.
9. Have the patient wash hands and clean the perineal area with soap and water.
10. Position the patient. If the patient is female, have her assume the dorsal recumbent position with the legs spread. Later, when the female patient has learned to perform catheterization without the use of a mirror, she can sit on a chair or on the toilet. A male patient can sit on a chair, toilet, or commode.
11. Elevate the female patient's head and position the mirror so that the patient can see the perineum. Spread the labia. You can point to the meatus with a sterile cotton-tipped applicator to help the patient identify the structure. The male patient is taught to retract the foreskin with one hand and elevate the penis with the other so that it is at a right angle to the body.
12. Lubricate the catheter with either lubricating jelly or clean water.
13. The lubricated catheter is introduced through the meatus, 2 to 3 inches for the female, 6 to 10 inches for the male, or until urine begins to flow into the clean pan or a leak-proof plastic bag.
14. When the flow stops, the patient pinches the catheter *to prevent further drainage* and withdraws the catheter.
15. The patient can wipe away any urine that is on the perineum with a tissue, stand up, and re-clothe.
16. The urine collected in the bag can be discarded in the toilet.
17. The patient washes the catheter in warm water with soap and rinses it thoroughly.
18. The catheter is dried then stored in a clean leak-proof plastic bag until its next use.

Evaluation

19. Evaluate according to the following criteria:
    a. Patient understands the procedure and carries out the skill.
    b. Patient empties bladder completely.
    c. Patient maintains clean technique.
20. Have the patient repeat the demonstration of the skill at least one more time.

Documentation

21. Document the following:
    a. Patient performed self-catheterization.
    b. Patient's degree of understanding and proficiency.
    c. Any problems with performing the procedure.

PROCEDURE FOR CATHETERIZATION OF A URINARY DIVERSION

The procedure for catheterizing the stoma of a urinary diversion is similar to that used for the Procedure for Intermittent Self-Catheterization (above), but with some modifications. We have included completely the modified steps as well as references to the Procedure for Intermittent Self-Catheterization that remain the same.

A clean technique is used for this procedure. *The mucous membrane of the ileal pouch is fairly resistant to infection caused by microorganisms that may be introduced to the urinary tract. Also, the time between catheterizations allows the patient's immune system to remain active in fighting off infection.* It must be remembered that resistance to pathogens is not as active in persons who are ill or debilitated.

Assessment

1.–3. Follow the steps of the Procedure for Intermittent Self-Catheterization.

Planning

4. Wash your hands *for infection control.*
5. Collect appropriate equipment. You will not need a mirror for the female patient.

Implementation

6.–8. Follow the steps of the Procedure for Intermittent Self-Catheterization.
9. Have the patient sit in a comfortable position; this could be on a straight-backed chair or on the toilet or commode.
10. Instruct the patient to wash hands and the peristomal area.
11. Lubricate the catheter with either lubricating jelly or clean water.
12. Have the patient introduce the catheter through the urinary diversion stoma 2 to 3 inches or until the urine begins to flow into a small pan or a leak-proof plastic bag.
13. When the flow stops, instruct the patient to pinch the catheter to prevent further drainage and withdraw the catheter.

14. The patient can wipe away any urine that is on the skin with a tissue.
15. The urine collected in the bag can be discarded in the toilet.
16. The patient washes the catheter in warm water with soap and rinses it thoroughly.
17. The catheter is then stored in a leak-proof plastic bag until its next use.

Evaluation
18. Evaluate using the following criteria:
    a. Patient empties the pouch completely.

    b. Patient maintains clean technique.

Documentation
19. Document the following:
    a. Patient performed catheterization of a urinary diversion.
    b. Patient's degree of understanding and proficiency.
    c. Any problems with performing the procedure.

LONG-TERM CARE

Some of the residents in long-term care facilities *have problems with incontinence* that necessitate their having a permanent indwelling catheter. Adaptations may have to be made when performing the catheterization procedure on women of advanced age *because they have difficulty maintaining the dorsal recumbent position for an extended period.*

Certainly, providing privacy is always essential for any patient being catheterized. But for the elderly, this issue is particularly sensitive. An additional problem for older residents who have an indwelling catheter inserted is the increased potential for developing urinary tract infections (Nicolle, 1993). This increased risk may be *caused by a less active immune system. Other reasons for urinary tract infections are poor hygiene and enlargement of the prostate in the male, which partially obstructs drainage of the bladder.* Researchers have found that half of institutionalized elderly people develop urinary tract infections at some time; this is particularly true in those with indwelling catheters.

To decrease the chance of urinary tract infection, the nurse in long-term care can see that perineal hygiene is properly done, that fluid intake is adequate, and that continual assessment for the presence of infection is provided.

HOME CARE

Because more chronically ill persons are being cared for in the home, the presence of persons with indwelling urinary catheters in the home is becoming more common. The person may be discharged with a catheter in place, or the home health nurse may insert one. In either case, meticulous care should be provided *to prevent complications.* It is recommended that clients be showered if possible. Showers do not carry any risk of infection and so are preferable to tub baths. The policy in most long-term care settings and in the home is that the catheter should be changed every 30 days or *more often if there is evidence of sediment, crustations, or leakage.*

If the client is able to be up in a chair or ambulating, the drainage system should be appropriate to the specific patient. Researchers have noted that the drainage system for the person who is not bedridden should be one that does not use rubber straps, is leakproof, eliminates lengthy tubing, maintains correct positioning of the drainage bag, and is suited to the domestic environment.

For reasons of patient safety and comfort, the home healthcare nurse should provide ongoing assessment and advisement.

CRITICAL THINKING EXERCISES

• Your elderly, confused, female patient has an order for catheterization. As you enter her room to make an assessment, she is shouting and flailing her arms. Specify four to five nursing actions that could be taken to ensure her safety and identify at what step in the procedure these actions should be taken.

• An 18-year-old woman who has had surgery has not been able to void for 9 hours. On assessment, you find that her bladder is very distended. She has an order for catheterization, but she adamantly states she does not want to be catheterized. The responses listed below might be given to persuade her that the procedure is necessary. Evaluate each response, explaining why it is appropriate or inappropriate.

"Your doctor has written the order for the procedure."

"It won't hurt at all and will only take a minute."

"I had this procedure once and it went fine."

"We catheterize patients all the time after surgery."

"If you're worried about privacy, we will close the door."

"Your bladder can only hold so much urine and it is dangerous not to drain it."

• Compose two responses that would be appropriate to give this patient.

References

Nicolle, L. E. (1993). Urinary tract infections in long-term care facilities. *Infection Control Hospital Epidemiology, 14*(4), 220–225.

Resnick, B. (1993). Retraining the bladder after catheterization. *American Journal of Nursing, 93*(11), 46–47.

PERFORMANCE CHECKLIST

Procedure for Catheterization	Needs More Practice	Satisfactory	Comments
Assessment			
1. Assess the patient and check the order.			
2. Determine if the procedure is to be a straight or indwelling catheterization.			
3. Assess need for collection of a specimen.			
Planning			
4. Wash your hands.			
5. Select specific type and size of catheter.			
6. Collect appropriate equipment, including catheterization set, light source, bath blanket or sheet for draping, and extra equipment as individually determined.			
Implementation			
7. Identify the patient.			
8. Explain the procedure. Answer any questions.			
9. Draw bed curtains, and position and drape the patient. a. Pediatric patient or confused patient—seek an assistant.			
b. Female patient in dorsal recumbent position, with knees flexed, or in Sims' position.			
c. Male patient in supine position.			
10. Set up the equipment. a. Arrange the lamp.			
b. Open catheterization set and arrange sterile field.			
c. Set up receptacle for soiled cleansing swabs.			
d. If drainage bag is in separate package, open it and attach to bed.			
e. If sterile drape is on top of set, grasp drape by side that is to be nonsterile and place under patient. Then put on sterile gloves.			

(continued)

Procedure for Catheterization *(Continued)*	Needs More Practice	Satisfactory	Comments
f. If sterile gloves (not drape) are on top of set, put them on. Then grasp drape by side that is to be sterile and place under patient, protecting your gloves.			
g. Place second drape to enlarge sterile field.			
h. Open cleansing solution and pour over swabs.			
i. Open lubricant and place it on end of catheter.			
j. For an indwelling catheter, attach syringe and test balloon by instilling all of the sterile water and then deflating balloon by withdrawing water. Leave syringe attached.			
k. Set the specimen container and its cap upside down.			
l. If drainage bag is in set, connect distal end of catheter to drainage tubing.			
11. Catheterize the patient. **a.** Use nondominant hand to expose the meatus.			
b. After meatus is identified, cleanse the area surrounding the meatus, using swabs held in forceps. Use circular motion on males. Swab from anterior to posterior on females. Discard swabs away from sterile field.			
c. Use sterile hand to move tray containing catheter close to patient, and to pick up catheter.			
d. Insert catheter 2–3 inches into female or 6–9 inches into male, holding the penis at a 45° angle, until urine returns.			
12. If using a straight catheter, obtain a specimen and drain the bladder.			
13. If using an indwelling catheter, fill the balloon.			
14. Connect the bag to the catheter.			
15. Tape the catheter to the patient—for a male, to the lower abdomen; for a female, to the thigh or loosely over the leg without taping.			

(continued)

Procedure for Catheterization *(Continued)*	Needs More Practice	Satisfactory	Comments
16. Assist patient to comfortable position.			
17. Gather and discard disposable equipment. Clean nondisposable equipment.			
18. Wash your hands.			
Evaluation			
19. Evaluate using the following criteria: **a.** Indwelling catheter draining properly or straight catheter inserted and removed without discomfort.			
b. Patient comfortable.			
Documentation			
20. Document the following: **a.** Date and time.			
b. Type and size of catheter.			
c. Whether a specimen was obtained.			
d. Amount of urine.			
e. Description of urine.			
f. Patient's response to procedure.			
Caring for a Patient With an Indwelling Catheter			
1. Place patient on intake and output.			
2. Encourage increased fluid intake.			
3. Maintain closed system.			
4. Maintain external cleanliness around catheter.			
5. Keep catheter drainage bag below level of bladder.			
6. Keep tubing coiled by patient's side.			
7. Keep drainage bag off the floor.			
8. Tape catheter to prevent pulling.			
9. Observe for irritation at meatus.			
10. Empty bag at regular intervals.			

(continued)

Procedure for Removing an Indwelling Catheter	Needs More Practice	Satisfactory	Comments
Assessment			
1. Verify the order.			
2. Determine whether a urine specimen is needed.			
Planning			
3. Wash your hands.			
4. Obtain necessary equipment: a. Paper towels			
b. A syringe to remove the fluid from balloon			
c. A small container to catch urine			
d. Clean gloves.			
Implementation			
5. Identify the patient.			
6. Explain that catheter is to be removed and what to expect.			
7. Prepare patient by proper draping. Put on clean gloves.			
8. Withdraw the catheter. a. Place paper towels under catheter.			
b. Use syringe to remove fluid from balloon.			
c. Pinch catheter and pull it out smoothly.			
d. Wrap catheter in paper towel.			
e. Hold end of catheter up to allow urine to drain from tubing.			
9. Assist patient to comfortable position.			
10. Measure urine output.			
11. Dispose of the equipment.			
12. Remove gloves and wash your hands.			
Evaluation			
13. Evaluate using the following criteria: a. Catheter removed without difficulty			
b. Patient voiding adequate amounts (250 mL) at regular intervals			

(continued)

Procedure for Removing an Indwelling Catheter *(Continued)*	Needs More Practice	Satisfactory	Comments
c. Patient is continuing to increase fluid intake.			
Documentation			
14. Document time of catheter removal, urine output, and patient's response.			
Teaching the Procedure for Intermittent Self-Catheterization			
Assessment			
1. Check the order.			
2. Identify the medical diagnosis.			
3. Assess patient's knowledge.			
Planning			
4. Wash your hands.			
5. Collect appropriate equipment, including a mirror for the female patient.			
Implementation			
6. Identify the patient.			
7. Review equipment, explaining use and answering questions.			
8. Review steps of procedure.			
9. Have patient wash hands and clean perineal area.			
10. Position patient: female in dorsal recumbent, male sitting.			
11. Position female so she can see perineal area in mirror. Have male retract foreskin and elevate penis so it is at right angle to the body.			
12. Lubricate the catheter.			
13. Have patient insert lubricated catheter 2–3 inches (female) or 6–10 inches (male) through the meatus until urine flows into a small pan or leakproof plastic bag.			
14. When urine stops flowing, have patient pinch catheter and remove.			
15. Instruct patient to dry perineum with tissue and to reclothe.			

(continued)

Teaching the Procedure for Intermittent Self-Catheterization *(Continued)*	Needs More Practice	Satisfactory	Comments
16. Discard collected urine in toilet.			
17. The patient washes catheter in warm water with soap and rinses it thoroughly.			
18. Dry catheter and store in clean leakproof plastic bag for future use.			
Evaluation			
19. Evaluate according to the following criteria: **a.** Patient understands the procedure and carries out the skill.			
b. Patient empties bladder completely.			
c. Patient maintains clean technique.			
20. Have patient repeat procedure one time later.			
Documentation			
21. Document the following: **a.** Patient performed self-catheterization.			
b. Degree of understanding and proficiency.			
c. Any problems performing procedure.			
Performing Catheterization of a Urinary Diversion			
Assessment			
1.–3. Assess as in Checklist steps 1–3 of the Procedure for Intermittent Self-Catheterization (check order, identify diagnosis, assess patient's knowledge).			
Planning			
4. Wash your hands.			
5. Collect equipment; you will not need a mirror for the female patient.			
Implementation			
6.–8. Implement as in Checklist steps 6–8 of the Procedure for Intermittent Self-Catheterization (identify patient, review equipment, review procedure steps).			
9. Have patient sitting in a comfortable position.			

(continued)

Performing Catheterization of a Urinary Diversion (Continued)	Needs More Practice	Satisfactory	Comments
10. Instruct patient to wash hands, and peristomal area.			
11. Lubricate catheter.			
12. Have patient insert catheter 2–3 inches until urine flows.			
13. When flow stops, patient pinches catheter and withdraws it.			
14. Have patient wipe away any urine on the skin with a tissue.			
15. Discard the urine collected in the bag in the toilet.			
16. The patient washes the catheter in warm water with soap and rinses thoroughly.			
17. Catheter is stored in clean, leakproof, plastic bag until next use.			
Evaluation			
18. Evaluate using the following criteria: a. Patient empties the pouch completely.			
b. Patient maintains clean technique.			
Documentation			
19. Document the following: a. Patient performed catheterization of urinary diversion.			
b. Degree of understanding and proficiency.			
c. Any problems performing procedure.			

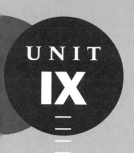

Supporting Oxygenation

MODULE

38

ADMINISTERING OXYGEN

MODULE CONTENTS

PREREQUISITES

Successful completion of the following modules:

VOLUME 1

OVERALL OBJECTIVE

To administer oxygen to patients, using equipment appropriately in a safe and effective manner.

SPECIFIC LEARNING OBJECTIVES

Know Facts and Principles	Apply Facts and Principles	Demonstrate Ability	Evaluate Performance
1. Patients who need oxygen			
List general conditions that necessitate oxygen administration	Give rationale for oxygen administration when assigned a patient.	In the clinical setting, identify a patient's need for supplemental oxygen.	Evaluate patient's need for supplemental oxygen with instructor.
2. Methods of administration			
Name five methods of oxygen administration.	Describe appropriate situation for use of each method. Determine methods used in a given facility.	In the clinical setting, identify appropriate method for a patient.	Evaluate choice of method with instructor.
3. Psychologic support			
Know impact of fear and anxiety on breathing.	Assess level of anxiety in patient.	In the clinical setting, reassure and give adequate explanations to patient.	Evaluate patient's emotional status in terms of relaxation and decreased anxiety.
4. Administering oxygen			
State hazards of oxygen.	Prepare room properly to prevent fire.	In the clinical setting, implement oxygen administration with emphasis on patient's comfort and safety.	Evaluate own performance using Performance Checklist.
5. Assessment of oxygenation			
Describe purpose of pulse oximetry.	Describe a situation in which the use of pulse oximetry would be appropriate.	In the clinical setting, measure oxygen saturation.	Evaluate patient's oxygenation and your own technique using Performance Checklist.
6. Self-inflating Breathing bag (Ambu bag)			
Describe purpose of self-inflating breathing bag.	Identify situations in which a self-inflating breathing bag would be used.	In the clinical setting, use a self-inflating breathing bag.	Evaluate using the Performance Checklist.
7. Documentation			
Know essential information to be documented.	Given a situation, indicate patient's potential physical and psychologic responses that should be documented.	In the clinical setting, document correctly.	Evaluate own performance with instructor.

LEARNING ACTIVITIES

1. Review the Specific Learning Objectives.
2. Read the section on oxygenation in Ellis and Nowlis, *Nursing: A Human Needs Approach,* or comparable material in another textbook.
3. Look up the module vocabulary terms in the glossary.
4. Read through the module as though you were preparing to teach these skills to another person. Mentally practice the skills.
5. In the practice setting, if oxygen equipment is available:
   a. Inspect and handle the equipment.
   b. Practice applying a mask and a nasal cannula for a partner.
   c. Have your partner apply the mask and nasal cannula for you.
   d. If a pulse oximeter is available, measure oxygen saturation on your partner and then have your partner measure your oxygen saturation.
6. In the clinical setting:
   a. Become familiar with the oxygen equipment used in your clinical facility.
   b. Locate the pulse oximeter and read the directions for the particular brand.
   c. Talk with a patient who is receiving oxygen, and assess what he or she has been taught regarding oxygen therapy if it is not uncomfortable for the patient to talk.
   d. Review the records of patients who are receiving oxygen. Note the medical diagnosis, the orders, the therapy, and any laboratory or diagnostic tests. In a small group, compare and contrast the situations of different patients.
   e. Observe the administration of oxygen and the measurement of oxygen saturation for a specific patient. Were all safety precautions observed?
   f. Under supervision, plan and initiate oxygen therapy, pulse oximetry, or both, as ordered for a patient.
   g. Document the procedure properly, and share your notes with your instructor.

VOCABULARY

ambient	dyspnea	liter	tidal volume
cannula	flowmeter	lumen	uvula
catheter	humidifier	oximetry (pulse	
claustrophobia	hypoxemia	oximetry)	
combustion	hypoxia	prongs	

Administering Oxygen

Rationale for the Use of This Skill

Oxygen is essential to life. An optimum level of oxygen must be maintained in the blood to sustain cellular functioning. Hypoxemia is the state in which the level of oxygen in the blood is lowered. In such cases it may be essential to administer additional oxygen to increase its concentration in the blood. However, pure oxygen is a therapeutic agent, which can have adverse effects when given improperly. Therefore, the nurse must be familiar with the indications for oxygen use and the various types of equipment for oxygen delivery as well as possess skill in its use.[1]

▼ NURSING DIAGNOSIS

Oxygen therapy is used most often for the patient with the nursing diagnosis of "Impaired Gas Exchange," which may be related to a variety of factors, including excessive secretions in the lungs; hypoventilation; a disease process that decreases the gas exchange surfaces in the lungs; or a condition that decreases circulation of blood through the lungs.

Not all conditions producing hypoxemia are alleviated by oxygen administration alone. For oxygen to be effective, unoxygenated blood must be circulated through the lungs, alveolar membranes must be capable of gas exchange, and the oxygen delivery method must succeed in increasing the percentage of oxygen in the alveolar air.

METHODS OF ADMINISTRATION

Oxygen administration can be divided into two classifications. *Low-flow oxygen systems* provide only part of the patient's total inspired air. Generally, these systems are more comfortable for the patient, but oxygen delivery varies with the patient's breathing pattern. *High-flow oxygen systems* provide the total inspired atmosphere to the patient. There is consistent oxygen delivery, which can be regulated precisely and does not vary with the patient's breathing pattern.

[1]Rationale for action is emphasized throughout the module by the use of italics.

PROBLEMS FOR THE PATIENT RECEIVING OXYGEN

A variety of psychological and physical problems may be caused by oxygen administration.

Psychological Problems

Oxygen administration, although a common procedure, may make some patients anxious, which may increase difficulty in breathing. Some perceive oxygen administration as a lifesaving measure and are reassured by the therapy. Others perceive it as an indication that they are seriously ill and are made anxious by it. Still others find a mask oppressive and experience claustrophobia when a mask is in place. By explaining the procedure (in simple terms) to the patient and the patient's family, as well as by maintaining a calm attitude, *you can help to allay many unnecessary fears. For this reason, even semicomatose patients should be given explanations.*

Safety

Certain dangers are inherent in oxygen administration.

Fire Hazards

Although oxygen itself is not explosive, it supports combustion. This means that extremely rapid burning takes place in the presence of high oxygen concentration, almost as if the oxygen itself were explosive. Thus, it is essential to prevent sparks or fire in an environment where oxygen is being used. Observe these precautions:

1. Prominently display a "no smoking" sign on the patient's door, *which cautions all persons in the room—including the patient—not to smoke.* Currently, most healthcare institutions have a "no smoking" policy, which may make enforcement of this restriction easier. It is prudent to remove matches, lighters, and cigarettes from the bedside when oxygen is in use and warn visitors of safety precautions.
2. Inspect all electrical equipment in the patient's immediate vicinity *because frayed cords and defective plugs could cause sparks.* All electrical equipment should meet the safety standards of the health care facility.
3. Do not allow the patient to use electrical equipment, including such items as electric razors or personal radios, while oxygen is being administered *because they may malfunction, creating sparks.*

Hospital electric beds provide special safeguards from electrical sparks that protect the patient receiving oxygen.

4. Avoid using wool blankets, *because they produce static electricity, another cause of sparks.*

5. Do not give electric or friction toys to children receiving oxygen.

Pressure Hazards

Oxygen can be stored in several ways. Most acute care facilities have a piped-in system, with outlets on the wall beside the bed; gas flow is adjusted by means of a flowmeter that attaches to the wall outlet. This oxygen comes from a large holding tank that is usually located outside the building.

When oxygen is not piped in, facilities may use tanks that hold oxygen as a compressed gas at more than 2,000 lb pressure per square inch. *Because of the extreme pressure,* these tanks should be handled with great care. Large tanks are chained to stands *to prevent falling and possible rupture of the valve.* Smaller, portable tanks of liquid oxygen are available and are largely replacing the older compressed air tanks in homes and long-term care settings that do not have piped-in oxygen. Oxygen in this form is safe *because of its low pressure.* Storage and transport savings have made liquid oxygen an economical method of oxygen delivery. These tanks are light and can be easily moved by caregivers. Small containers can be moved by the patient using a small wheeled cart or a shoulder strap.

Malfunctioning Equipment

Regardless of the method or appliance used, oxygen should always be turned on and checked before you administer it to a patient. *Regulators and flowmeters do malfunction, so each time oxygen is to be started on a patient, check all equipment first.*

Loss of Stimulus for Breathing

When individuals with chronic pulmonary disease have experienced impaired gas exchange for a long time they often have increased blood carbon dioxide. Their respiratory mechanisms may adapt to this abnormal state. The normal stimulus to breathing that changing CO_2 levels creates is lost. *In these individuals, the low oxygen level becomes the major stimulus for breathing. Abruptly changing the oxygen level without altering the CO_2 level may result in the loss of the stimulus for breathing, and the patient experiences decreased respiratory rate and may even progress to apnea.* Therefore,

oxygen is initially administered at low levels and with caution for those who have chronic pulmonary disease.

Drying of Respiratory Membranes

The nasal mucosa is well designed to moisten air that moves through the nose to the lungs. Any time that oxygen is administered through a tracheostomy or through an endotracheal tube, bypassing the normal moistening mechanism, humidification of the inspired air and oxygen is essential.

The question of when additional moistening of inspired air or oxygen is necessary is an important one. Some experts believe that when oxygen is administered through the normal breathing route, such as by nasal cannula or mask, humidification is unnecessary. Others believe that humidification is always important as a precautionary measure *to decrease the drying effect on the oronasal mucosa.* Follow the policy in your facility when planning initial administration. If humidification is not routinely used, be sure to assess the patient for drying of mucous membranes.

OXYGEN EQUIPMENT

Flowmeter

A flowmeter is a device that attaches to the oxygen outlet *to adjust the amount of oxygen being delivered* (Fig. 38–1).

Two types of flowmeters are available: mercury ball and gauge. Both types register the number of liters of oxygen delivered per minute.

Regulator

An additional device, called a regulator, is attached to the valve of a tank of compressed gas (oxygen or air) *to reduce the pressure to a safe, functional working level.* The amount of gas registers on the gauge in pounds per square inch or psi. When the tank is almost empty, the needle points to a red area, *warning that the tank must be replaced shortly.*

Humidifier

Humidification is provided by containers of sterile water, which may be prefilled and are disposable. They are attached to the oxygen delivery equipment. Oxygen flows through them and picks up moisture. The water must be sterile *to prevent infec-*

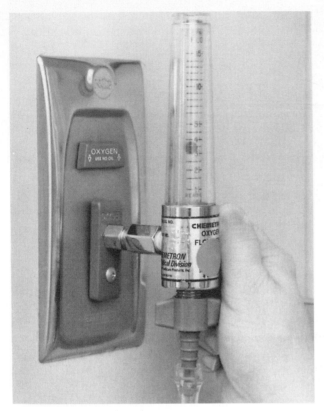

Figure 38–1. Oxygen flowmeter. The nurse adjusts the flowmeter, which registers the number of liters delivered per minute.

tion from organisms that can grow in a moist environment. Sterile water is used because stagnant water is a medium in which the microorganisms present in tap water may begin to multiply. These organisms can then pose a significant infection hazard to the ill person. Each facility has a policy on how frequently the container and the water are changed. Changing the container every 24 hours is common. Sterile water is added whenever the water level is low.

Nasal Cannula

The nasal cannula (also called nasal prongs) is a plastic tubing that has two small open prongs to be positioned over the patient's face under the nose (Fig. 38–2). It is the most common method of administering oxygen, *because it is effective, easy to apply, and comfortable for the patient. The patient receiving oxygen through a nasal cannula is able to communicate easily, to eat, and to engage in activities of daily living. These are all important factors in choosing this method of administration.* The nasal cannula is a low-flow system.

Although patients commonly mouth-breathe and appear as if they are not receiving the oxygen, they do receive a consistent supply. *The oxygen flows into the nose, and the entire upper airway (nose, oronasal*

pharynx, and mouth) becomes a reservoir for oxygen. In addition, some of the oxygen tends to flow down over the mouth, because it is heavier than air. Thus, when the patient breathes in, the inspired air provides a significant oxygen concentration even if the patient breathes through the mouth.

Oxygen by nasal cannula may be given at 1 to 6 L/min and provides 22% to 50% oxygen in the inspired air. An excess of 6 L/min does not increase the oxygen delivery. It does increase the drying of mucous membranes and air swallowing, however. Oxygen by nasal cannula is most commonly used in low flow rates of 2 or 3 L/min. The exact concentration inspired is determined by the interaction of the liter flow of oxygen, the respiratory rate and pattern, and the volume of each inspired breath. Therefore, the patient must be assessed for oxygenation to determine the adequacy of the oxygen delivery.

Nasal Catheter

The nasal catheter is a plastic tubing with perforations through which oxygen can flow. It is inserted into the nasopharynx through the nostril. It provides a low-flow oxygen system. The nasal catheter is rarely used *because it can irritate a patient's nostrils, is unpleasant to have inserted, and must be changed every 8 hours.*

Oxygen Masks

Oxygen masks cover the nose and mouth, are sealed around the edges, and provide the most consistent, effective method of oxygen delivery. Masks are the

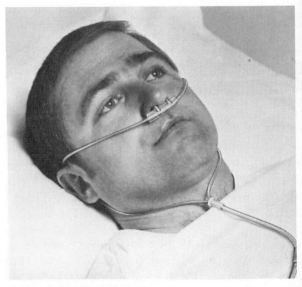

Figure 38–2. Nasal cannula. The patient can communicate easily, eat, and engage in activities of daily living while receiving oxygen. (Courtesy Ohio Medical Products, Madison, Wisconsin)

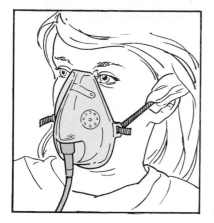 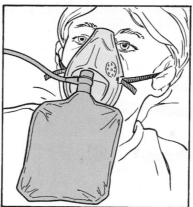 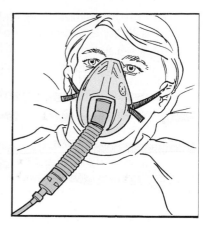

Figure 38–3. Oxygen masks. **(A)** Simple mask. **(B)** Nonrebreathing mask. **(C)** Venturi mask.

only method to reliably deliver a high level of oxygen and thus are preferred in critical care situations. There are, however, several disadvantages to their use. The mask interferes with the patient's ability to communicate. It must be removed when eating, drinking, and taking medications, and it makes some individuals claustrophobic. In addition, *because masks are uncomfortable for many patients,* they are not consistently left in place, thus making it impossible to guarantee the percentage of oxygen actually received by the patient (Fig. 38–3).

The *simple mask* (or rebreathing mask) is a low-flow system. It has side vents and provides a reservoir over the face into which oxygen flows, so the patient breathes in air with a higher concentration of oxygen. It is usually used on a short-term basis when an oxygen concentration of 30% to 60% is desired. (Oxygen dose is often abbreviated as FIO_2, which means fraction of inspired oxygen. Guidelines for estimating FIO2 with simple masks are shown in Table 38–1.)

This requires a flow rate of 6 to 8 L/min. The actual percentage of oxygen received by the patient depends on the patient's tidal volume, respiratory rate, and the fit of the mask as well as the liter flow. *Because the patient breathes out into the same reservoir,* the carbon dioxide content of the inspired air tends to increase. The flow rate of 6 to 8 L/min assists in flushing CO2 from the mask, so for most patients this is not a concern. The slightly higher CO2 may actually stimulate respirations. However, *if the patient retains excess carbon dioxide,* this type of mask is contraindicated.

The *nonrebreathing mask,* a high-flow system, has a bag attached to the bottom and can deliver 50% to 100% oxygen. The oxygen flows into the bag and accumulates there as a reservoir. When the patient breathes out, a special valve between the bag and the mask closes, and exhaled air exits through the vents in the side of the mask. When the person breathes in, the valve opens so that the inspired air comes from the bag and has a high oxygen concentration. This overcomes the problem of excess carbon dioxide in the inspired air and prevents room air from diluting the oxygen. A flow rate of 12 to 15 L/min may be needed to keep the bag inflated.

The *Venturi or air entraining mask,* another high-flow system, is designed to deliver oxygen at a specific percentage between 24% and 40%. Pure oxygen delivered at a high rate flows past special vents, and the "Venturi effect" causes this oxygen to mix with the room air at a predictable level. The patient, therefore, receives a constant oxygen concentration, regardless of the rate or depth of respiration. A Venturi mask can be used with or without humidification. These are the most common type of mask used for the critically ill person.

Oxygen/Humidity Tents

Tents are seldom used now, except for pediatric patients, because of their several disadvantages. Some patients experience an unpleasant closed-in feeling when they are in an oxygen tent; they cannot move about freely in bed without disturbing the tucked edges. Tents require much more oxygen to maintain the desired concentration than other methods and

Table 38–1. Guidelines for Estimating FiO_2 With Oxygen Masks	
100% Oxygen Flow Rate in Liters	**FiO_2**
5–6	40%
6–7	50%
7–8	60%

are therefore more hazardous and costly to operate. Also, it is difficult to maintain a comfortable temperature for a patient in the tent. In addition, tents are difficult to clean, although disposable canopies are now available.

For infants and young children, however, oxygen and humidity tents are commonly used. The mist tent or croup tent delivers cool saturated air *to keep the respiratory tract well hydrated* and is typically used for patients with croup, pneumonia, or other upper respiratory diseases. There are several varieties of equipment. For larger children, the "tent" consists of a transparent plastic canopy that is suspended from a frame. A high-output pneumatic nebulizer and reservoir and a high-pressure hose with an oxygen or compressed air adapter are attached. A flowmeter and tubing may be needed for "bleeding in" oxygen, and sterile distilled water will be necessary to moisturize the air or the oxygen. For small babies and infants, a smaller piece of equipment constructed of hard plastic with transparent sides is used for the same purpose. One brand name is Croupette. Follow the manufacturer's instructions for the specific equipment used in your facility.

Transtracheal Oxygen Catheters

A transtracheal catheter is a very small diameter plastic tubing with several openings near the tip. It is inserted into the trachea under local anesthesia. When individuals need oxygen on a long-term basis, the problems associated with having a facial mask or nasal cannula become a greater concern. The transtracheal oxygen catheter provides an alternative means of oxygen delivery.

This device has advantages over the use of nasal prongs or masks:

1. *Because the oxygen runs directly into the trachea,* a low flow rate is satisfactory, so the therapy is less costly; in addition, there is no oxygen flow into the ambient air, making safety issues less of a problem.
2. *The catheter can be completely or partially covered by clothing,* so the therapy is more socially acceptable and aesthetically pleasing.

The catheter does need to be irrigated on a daily basis with normal saline. This removes any secretions on the inside of the tubing. It is then flushed with air *to dry it.* The small insertion site is routinely cleaned in the bath or shower. Any secretions can be removed with a cotton-tipped applicator moistened with hydrogen peroxide.

Oxygen Extension Tubing

Tubing that may be used to connect the delivery device to the oxygen source is usually long enough to accommodate the patient in bed or seated in a chair near the oxygen source. When a patient needs to move about the room, an extension tubing provides for oxygen delivery at longer distances. Some homebound patients use tubing that allows them to go around a bedroom and into the bathroom without moving the oxygen tank. In the care facility, a patient may be able to ambulate around the room and into a bathroom while receiving oxygen from the piped-in wall source near the bed.

GENERAL PROCEDURE FOR ADMINISTERING OXYGEN

Assessment

1. Check the physician's order. The physician usually writes an order for oxygen that includes the date and time, the flow or concentration of oxygen to be delivered, and the type of equipment to be used. If at any time you assess that a patient is experiencing acute hypoxemia, you can administer oxygen without a doctor's order and notify the physician as soon as possible. Such a decision requires skilled nursing judgment. If a patient's condition makes this a possibility, a physician may order oxygen prn (as needed), so that the nurse can start or discontinue administration according to the patient's needs. This order may be written to give a variable amount of oxygen (ie, up to 5 L) to maintain hemoglobin oxygen saturation at a specific level (ie, 92%). In this instance, the nurse would measure hemoglobin saturation using pulse oximetry (see below). Then the oxygen would be started, increasing the flow rate at intervals until the desired hemoglobin saturation is reached.

   If the patient's respiratory status is such that he or she is in danger, proceed with administering oxygen and obtain an order as soon as possible. Be cautious in administering oxygen to a patient with chronic obstructive pulmonary disease. A flow rate of greater than 2 L/min may cause the patient to stop breathing.
2. Assess the patient's immediate respiratory status. If the patient is anxious, have someone stay with him or her while you assess equipment availability.
3. Identify the types of oxygen equipment and oxygen source in your facility.

Planning

4. Wash your hands *for infection control.*

5. Plan for any assistance needed. Typically, patients who are "oxygen hungry" become extremely restless and even disoriented. You may need a person to assist you *to ensure the patient's safety.*

6. Choose the appropriate equipment for the method of oxygen administration ordered. In an emergency, choose the method that best meets the patient's needs. For example, in some situations a breathing mask is necessary, whereas in others, when the patient is alert and in mild distress, a nasal cannula is sufficient and more comfortable. Obtain a flowmeter if one is not already attached to the wall outlet or tank. A long extension tubing may be needed.

7. Check the immediate environment carefully for any potential source of fire or sparks. Eliminate any possible risk or, if necessary, move the patient to an area that is safer for oxygen administration.

Implementation

8. Identify the patient *to be sure you are performing the procedure for the correct patient.*

9. Carefully and calmly explain what you are going to do. Assure the patient that your actions will provide more comfort and that trying to relax and breathe more slowly and deeply helps.

10. Attach the oxygen supply tube to the cannula, catheter, or mask. Then turn on the oxygen and test the flow.

11. Follow the specific procedure for the equipment you are using.

12. Assess the effectiveness of the oxygen delivery. Assess both the patient's breathing and the functioning of the equipment. Check the position of the cannula, catheter, or mask, and make any necessary adjustments.

13. Explain safety precautions to the patient and any family or visitors present (review the section on safety, above.)

14. Assess the patient's nose and mouth, and provide oronasal care. *Because oxygen dries the mucous membranes,* it is good nursing practice to administer frequent oronasal care to any patient receiving oxygen therapy. You can do this before

you initiate oxygen therapy if the patient's respiratory status allows.

15. Stay with the patient until you are sure the proper flow rate is maintained and the patient is calm enough to be left alone safely. Holding the patient's hand is often very useful and comforting.

16. Post an "oxygen in use" sign on the patient's door.

17. Wash your hands.

Evaluation

18. Evaluate using the following desired outcomes as criteria:
   a. Breathing pattern regular and at normal rate
   b. Pink color in nail beds, lips, conjunctiva of eyes
   c. No disorientation, confusion, difficulty with cognition
   d. Patient resting comfortably
   e. Laboratory measurement of arterial oxygen concentration (PaO_2) or hemoglobin oxygen saturation (HgSat) within normal limits.

Documentation

19. Document the following in a narrative progress note or on a flow sheet:
   a. Date and time oxygen started
   b. Method of delivery
   c. Specific oxygen concentration or flow rate in liters per minute
   d. Subjective and objective observations of patient
   e. Notification of the physician if appropriate.

20. Add oronasal care to the Nursing Care Plan.

SPECIFIC PROCEDURES FOR ADMINISTERING OXYGEN

For each specific procedure discussed, some steps of the General Procedure may be modified. We have included completely the modified steps as well as references to the steps of the General Procedure that remain the same.

DATE/TIME	
2/14/99 8:00 AM	*Complained of mild dyspnea on ambulation. Respirations 34 and shallow after 30 min rest. O_2 at 3 L/min. started by cannula per standing order. Dr. Wilson notified.* —*S. Lester, SN*

Example of Nursing Progress Notes Using Narrative Format.

DATE/TIME	
3/7/99	Impaired gas exchange: Dyspnea on exertion.
1215	S "Walking makes me short of breath."
	O Respirations 34 and shallow after 30 min rest period.
	A Dyspnea unrelieved by rest.
	P Administer O₂ 3 L/min by cannula per standing order.
	Dr. Wilson notified.
	———— J. Hampton, SN

Example of Nursing Progress Notes Using SOAP Format.

Administering Oxygen by Nasal Cannula

Assessment
1.–3. Follow the steps of the General Procedure.

Planning
4.–7. Follow the steps of the General Procedure.

Implementation
8.–10. Follow the steps of the General Procedure.

11. After attaching the oxygen supply tube to the distal end of the nasal cannula, proceed as follows:

a. Allow 3 to 5 L oxygen to flow through the tubing *to make certain the equipment is working properly.* Use a humidifier with flow rates over 4 L/min.

b. Hold the cannula to the patient's face and gently insert the prongs into the nostrils.

c. Adjust straps either behind the head or around the ears and under the chin and tighten to comfort (see Fig. 38–2).

d. Adjust the flow rate to the ordered level.

e. Pad the area where the straps rub the top of the ears, if necessary.

12.–17. Follow the steps of the General Procedure.

Evaluation
18. Follow the General Procedure.

Documentation
19.–20. Follow the steps of the General Procedure.

Administering Oxygen by Nasal Catheter

Assessment
1.–3. Follow the steps of the General Procedure.

Planning
4.–7. Follow the steps of the General Procedure.

Implementation
8.–10. Follow the steps of the General Procedure.

11. After attaching the oxygen supply tube to the distal end of the nasal catheter, proceed as follows:

a. Allow 3 to 5 L oxygen to flow through the tubing *to make certain the equipment is working properly.* Use a humidifier with flow rates over 4 L/min.

b. Ensure that the tip of the nasal catheter rests in the nasopharynx. Measure from the tip of the patient's nose to the earlobe *to determine how far to insert the tube.* Lubricate the catheter with water-soluble lubricant and gently insert it along the floor of the nasal passage.

c. Tape the nasal catheter to the nose to hold it in place.

d. Adjust the flow rate to the ordered level.

12.–17. Follow the steps of the General Procedure.

Evaluation
18. Follow the General Procedure.

Documentation
19.–20. Follow the steps of the General Procedure.

Administering Oxygen by Mask

Assessment
1.–3. Follow the steps of the General Procedure.

Planning
4.–7. Follow the steps of the General Procedure.

Implementation
8.–10. Follow the steps of the General Procedure.

11. After attaching the oxygen supply tube to the mask, proceed as follows:

a. Regulate the oxygen flow. With the nonrebreathing mask, be sure the bag is inflated before placing the mask over the patient's mouth and nose.

b. Place the mask against the face, over the mouth and nose, and fit it securely, shaping the metal band on the mask to the bridge of the nose *to prevent leakage.*

c. Adjust the elastic band around the patient's head and tighten. If the mask is not snug against the face, you may need to place gauze pads over the cheek area *to ensure a tight fit.*

12.–17. Follow the steps of the General Procedure.

Evaluation

18. Follow the General Procedure.

Documentation

19.–20. Follow the steps of the General Procedure.

Administering Oxygen by Oxygen/Humidity Tent

Assessment

1.–3. Follow the steps of the General Procedure.

Planning

4.–7. Follow the steps of the General Procedure.

Implementation

8.–10. Follow the steps of the General Procedure.

11. Prepare the "tent" by attaching the metal frame to the bedsprings of the crib and suspending the canopy from the frame. Be certain that all access ports are closed.

    a. Tuck all sides of the canopy securely under the crib mattress.

    b. Ensure that the ice trough is filled with ice and the water jar with sterile water up to the indicator lines.

    c. Attach the tent to the oxygen or compressed air source.

    d. Turn on the oxygen and adjust the flow rate to 15 L/min for about 5 minutes.

    e. Open the valve that controls the mist output. Check the doctor's orders to see if it is to be left open continuously or partially or opened intermittently.

    f. Adjust the oxygen flow rate to the ordered level of oxygen after 5 minutes.

    g. Place the child in the tent.

12.–17. Follow the steps of the General Procedure.

Evaluation

18. Follow the General Procedure.

Documentation

19.–20. Follow the steps of the General Procedure.

Change damp bed linen and clothing as needed *to prevent the child from chilling.* Monitor the equipment and the child's response to treatment on a regular basis. Follow the policies and procedures in your facility.

USING OXIMETRY FOR ASSESSMENT

Oximetry, sometimes referred to as pulse oximetry, is a noninvasive means of measuring the oxygen saturation of hemoglobin (Fig. 38–4).

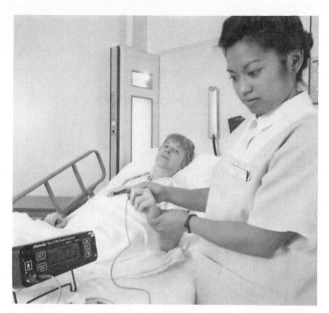

Figure 38–4. Oxygen saturation may be checked with the pulse oximeter.

Oxygen saturation is the percentage of oxygen attached to the hemoglobin that the molecule is capable of holding. Normal hemoglobin is 95% to 98% saturated. The color of the hemoglobin changes depending on the amount of oxygen versus the amount of carbon dioxide it contains. A very sensitive meter can register the differences in color of the hemoglobin and translate that into the percentage of oxygen saturation. The oximetry device, through the use of diodes, measures the reflectance of light off the hemoglobin molecules in the capillaries close to the surface in the ear lobe or fingertip and provides a reading of the oxygen saturation value. Oximetry is widely used in healthcare facilities *to monitor any patient who is at risk of hypoxemia.*

Although a laboratory measurement of the actual level of dissolved oxygen in the arterial blood (PaO_2) provides a more exact measure of the person's level of oxygenation, that laboratory test requires a sample of arterial blood to be drawn and immediately analyzed by an appropriate technician. This is painful, requires a high level of skill and is expensive. The oxygen saturation can be used as a general indicator of oxygenation when exact measurement of blood oxygen is not required. A further explanation of these relationships can be found in a physiology or medical-surgical nursing text.

The physician may order oximetry monitoring as a separate order or as a part of oxygen therapy, or the procedure may be done at the discretion of the nurse to monitor the patient's response to care. The saturation (often abbreviated "sat.") may be used as the determining factor in the amount of oxygen to be given. The order may read "Oxygen per nasal prongs up to 6 L/min to maintain saturation at 92%." This means that the nurse makes sure the oxygen saturation is measured and the oxygen adjusted appropriately. In many hospitals, when the measurement is critical, the oxygen saturation is measured by the respiratory therapist.

Equipment

A pulse oximetry meter is a small-battery operated device that can be hand-held or placed on the bedside table. There is an on-and-off switch, a screen where the oxygen saturation reading appears, and clip-on finger or ear probe attached to the device by a cord (see Fig. 38–4).

PROCEDURE FOR USING OXIMETRY TO MEASURE OXYGEN SATURATION

Assessment

1. Check the patient's record for orders relative to oxygen therapy, oximetry, and respiratory status.
2. Review the procedure and the directions for the equipment used in the facility.
3. Assess the patient, focusing especially on factors that might affect the patient's ability to cooperate or to undergo the procedure, special needs, and knowledge base regarding the test.

Planning

4. Wash your hands *for infection control.*
5. Obtain the oximetry device and review the directions for the specific brand.

Implementation

6. Identify the patient *to be sure you are carrying out the procedure for the correct patient.*
7. Explain to the patient what you will be doing.
8. Carry out the procedure as follows:
   a. Attach the probe to the patient as directed, either to the finger or the ear lobe. Be sure the light-emitting diode is directly opposite the light-receiving diode. *If the light does not have a direct path, an inaccurate reading will result.* Do not fasten the probe so tightly that it impedes blood circulation. *A probe that is fitted too tightly can also cause inaccurate readings* (AJN Clinical News, 1993).
   b. Turn on the meter and read the scale when the numbers have stabilized. The patient should remain still while you are taking the reading. *Excessive movement of the body, a pulse below 20, and a blood pressure below 30 mm Hg (such as occur in shock) all create inaccurate readings* (AJN Clinical News, 1993).
   c. Remove the probe from the finger or ear lobe.
   d. Note the oximetry reading.
9. Clean the equipment according to the facility procedure.
10. Wash your hands.
11. Return equipment to appropriate storage place.

Evaluation

12. Evaluate the results in light of norms for oxygen saturation and the patient's previous readings.

Documentation

13. Document the oximetry reading on the patient's record either on the appropriate flowsheet or in a narrative note.

SELF-INFLATING BREATHING BAG AND MASK

The self-inflating breathing bag and mask (Ambu bag) can be used for rescue breathing, as part of cardiopulmonary resuscitation, or to provide deep breaths of high oxygen concentration before suctioning. This device may also provide temporary artificial ventilation (such as during transport) to the person who is in respiratory arrest or is dependent on a ventilator for breathing.

The device is composed of a face mask that covers the mouth and nose and has a soft rim to make an airtight seal. The mask is attached to a firm rubber or plastic bag that has a connector that may be attached to an oxygen source if a high concentration of oxygen is needed. Manual compression of the bag forces air into the patient's nose and mouth. Humidification is not usually used with this method (Fig. 38–5).

PROCEDURE FOR USING A SELF-INFLATING BREATHING BAG AND MASK

Assessment

1. Assess patient for need for breathing assistance or for hyperoxygenation before suctioning.

Planning

2. Wash your hands for asepsis.
3. Obtain the rebreathing bag and an oxygen connector tubing.
4. Obtain assistance if needed.

Implementation

5. Identify the patient *to be sure you are carrying out the procedure for the correct patient.*
6. Explain to the patient what you are doing. Even

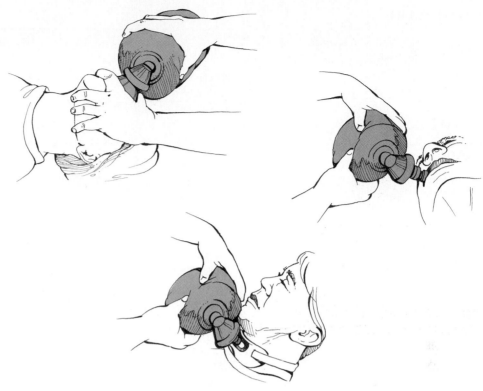

Figure 38–5. The self-inflating breathing bag can be used for rescue breathing, as part of CPR, or to provide deep breaths of high oxygen concentration before suctioning.

in an emergency a patient may feel panic if something is placed over the mouth and nose.

7. Connect the mask to the oxygen supply and turn on to highest flow rate that does not cause the device to stick or jam. In emergency situations, the highest concentration possible is needed.

8. Apply the mask snugly over the patient's nose and mouth *to form an occlusive seal*. Either hold the mask in place manually or fasten straps behind the patient's head.

9. Compress the bag as completely as possible to force air into the patient's nose and mouth.

10. Release the bag to allow expiration. Count 1, 2, 3, 4 *to allow adequate time for expiration and for the bag to reinflate*.

11. Repeat steps 9 and 10 in a rhythmic pattern to provide ventilation at a rate of 12 breaths/min or for the desired number of deep breaths.

Evaluation

12. Evaluate in relationship to the following criteria:
    a. Rise and fall of chest
    b. Skin color
    c. Change in oxygen saturation as indicated by pulse oximetry (if available)

Documentation

13. Document the following:
    a. Assessment indicating need for artificial ventilation
    b. Patient's response

(See Module 30, Emergency Resuscitation Procedures, for complete directions for emergency resuscitation.)

LONG-TERM CARE

Residents in long-term care facilities may also require oxygen therapy—some continuously and some intermittently. Portable oxygen units can be attached to wheelchairs for residents who are not ambulatory and require constant oxygen. Exercise care to prevent fatigue and maintain mobility for the resident. Techniques to decrease exertion might include the use of a bedside commode, small meals, assistance with feeding, and a calm, low-stress environment. The same safety considerations apply in long-term care as in acute care.

HOME CARE

Many persons require oxygen therapy at home. These persons or a family member must be taught how to administer oxygen as well as care for the equipment. A "no smoking" sign should be posted on the outside door. However, it may be more difficult to get people to cooperate with this restriction in the home than in a healthcare facility. Most people receiving oxygen at home use nasal prongs, but some will have had the option to choose transtracheal oxygen therapy.

CRITICAL THINKING EXERCISES

• You are caring for a patient who has a physician's order that states: "Oxygen per nasal prongs to maintain sat. at 87%. Call me if more than 6 L/min. needed." The night nurse informs you that the patient was comfortable all night and the O_2 sat. remained at 88% with O_2 given at 4 L/min. As you plan for care during the day, identify the times when it is most important to measure oxygen saturation. When would you expect to need to increase the oxygen? What events might increase the need for oxygen?

• Mr. Smith, who is on long-term oxygen therapy at home, uses compressed oxygen in a tank. He states that he cannot go anywhere without his oxygen on, so he stays in the bedroom, uses a commode, and bathes at the bedside. Considering the various ways to deliver oxygen, identify at least two alternative plans for oxygen therapy that might allow Mr. Smith to leave his bedroom. Determine what other considerations—besides the method of oxygen delivery—that may need to be addressed in relationship to this patient's situation. Explain how the nurse might manage these concerns.

Reference

AJN Clinical News: Pitfalls of pulse oximetry. (1993). *American Journal of Nursing, 94*(9), 9–10.

PERFORMANCE CHECKLIST

General Procedure for Administering Oxygen	Needs More Practice	Satisfactory	Comments
Assessment			
1. Check physician's order or proceed in an emergency.			
2. Assess immediate respiratory status.			
3. Identify oxygen equipment and source.			
Planning			
4. Wash your hands.			
5. Plan for any assistance needed.			
6. Choose appropriate equipment for patient's specific needs.			
7. Check environment for safety.			
Implementation			
8. Identify the patient.			
9. Explain what you are going to do.			
10. Attach oxygen supply tube to device you are using, turn on oxygen, and test flow.			
11. Follow procedure for equipment you are using.			
12. Assess patient's breathing and adjust equipment if necessary.			
13. Explain safety precautions to patient and family or visitors present.			
14. Assess condition of nose and mouth and provide oronasal care if needed.			
15. Stay with patient until safe to leave.			
16. Post an "oxygen in use" sign on the patient's door.			
17. Wash your hands.			
Evaluation			
18. Evaluate using the following criteria: a. Breathing pattern regular and at normal rate			
b. Pink color in nail beds, lips, conjunctiva of eyes			

(continued)

General Procedure for Administering Oxygen *(Continued)*	Needs More Practice	Satisfactory	Comments
c. No disorientation, confusion, difficulty with cognition			
d. Patient resting comfortably			
e. Laboratory measurement of arterial oxygen (PaO_2), or hemoglobin oxygen saturation within normal limits			
Documentation			
19. Record on the patient's chart: **a.** Date and time oxygen started			
b. Method of delivery			
c. Specific oxygen concentration or flow rate in liters per minute			
d. Subjective and objective observations of patient			
e. Notification of the physician, if appropriate.			
20. Add oronasal care to Nursing Care Plan.			
Administering Oxygen by Nasal Cannula			
Assessment			
1.–3. Follow Checklist steps 1–3 of the General Procedure for Administering Oxygen (check physician's order, assess respiratory status, and identify oxygen equipment and source).			
Planning			
4.–7. Follow Checklist steps 4–7 of the General Procedure (wash your hands, plan for any assistance needed, choose appropriate equipment, and check environment for safety).			
Implementation			
8.–10. Follow Checklist steps 8–10 of the General Procedure (identify the patient, explain what you are going to do, and connect cannula to oxygen supply).			
11. After attaching oxygen supply tube to distal end of nasal cannula: **a.** Allow 3–5 liters oxygen to flow through tubing.			

(continued)

Administering Oxygen by **Nasal Cannula** *(Continued)*	Needs More Practice	Satisfactory	Comments
b. Hold cannula to patient's face and gently inset prongs into nostrils.			
c. Adjust straps and tighten to comfort.			
d. Adjust flow rate.			
e. Pad top of ears as needed.			
12.–17. Follow Checklist steps 12–17 of the General Procedure (assess patient's breathing and adjust equipment if necessary, explain safety precautions, assess condition of nose and mouth and provide oronasal care, stay with patient until safe to leave, post an "oxygen in use" sign, and wash your hands).			
Evaluation			
18. Evaluate, using the criteria in Checklist step 18 of the General Procedure (breathing pattern, skin color, mental status, comfort, and oxygenation).			
Documentation			
19.–20. Document as in Checklist steps 19 and 20 of the General Procedure (date and time oxygen started, method of delivery, specific oxygen concentration or flow rate in liters per minute, subjective/objective observations of patient, notification of physician if appropriate, and add oronasal care to the Nursing Care Plan).			
Administering Oxygen by Nasal Catheter			
Assessment			
1.–3. Follow Checklist steps 1–3 of the General Procedure for Administering Oxygen (check physician's order, assess respiratory status, and identify oxygen equipment and source).			
Planning			
4.–7. Follow Checklist steps 4–7 of the General Procedure (wash your hands, plan for any assistance needed, choose appropriate equipment, and check environment for safety).			

(continued)

Administering Oxygen by Nasal Catheter *(Continued)*	Needs More Practice	Satisfactory	Comments
Implementation			
8.–10. Follow Checklist steps 8–10 of the General Procedure (identify the patient, explain what you are going to do, and connect catheter to oxygen supply).			
11. After attaching oxygen supply tube to distal end of nasal catheter: **a.** Allow 3–5 liters oxygen to flow through tubing.			
b. Lubricate and insert catheter.			
c. Tape catheter in place.			
d. Adjust flow rate.			
12.–17. Follow Checklist steps 12–17 of the General Procedure (assess patient's breathing and adjust equipment if necessary, explain safety precautions, assess condition of nose and mouth and provide oronasal care, stay with patient until safe to leave, post an "oxygen in use" sign, and wash your hands).			
Evaluation			
18. Evaluate, using the criteria in Checklist step 18 of the General Procedure (breathing pattern, skin color, mental status, comfort, and oxygenation).			
Documentation			
19.–20. Document as in Checklist steps 19 and 20 of the General Procedure (date and time oxygen started, method of delivery, specific oxygen concentration or flow rate in liters per minute, subjective/objective observations of patient, notification of physician if appropriate, and add oronasal care to the Nursing Care Plan).			
Administering Oxygen by Mask			
Assessment			
1.–3. Follow Checklist steps 1–3 of the General Procedure for Administering Oxygen (check physician's order, assess respiratory status, and identify oxygen equipment and source).			

(continued)

Administering Oxygen by Mask *(Continued)*	Needs More Practice	Satisfactory	Comments
Planning			
4.–7. Follow Checklist steps 4–7 of the General Procedure (wash your hands, plan for any assistance needed, choose appropriate equipment, and check environment for safety).			
Implementation			
8.–10. Follow Checklist steps 8–10 of the General Procedure (identify the patient, explain what you are going to do and connect mask to oxygen supply).			
11. After attaching oxygen supply tube to mask: **a.** Regulate oxygen flow.			
b. Fit mask over mouth and nose.			
c. Adjust elastic band around patient's head.			
12.–17. Follow Checklist steps 12–17 of the General Procedure (assess patient's breathing and adjust equipment if necessary, explain safety precautions, assess condition of nose and mouth and provide oronasal care, stay with patient until safe to leave, post an "oxygen in use" sign, and wash your hands).			
Evaluation			
18. Evaluate, using the criteria in Checklist step 18 of the General Procedure (breathing pattern, skin color, mental status, comfort, and oxygenation).			
Documentation			
19.–20. Document as in Checklist steps 19 and 20 of the General Procedure (date and time oxygen started, method of delivery, specific oxygen concentration or flow rate in liters per minute, subjective/objective observations of patient, notification of physician if appropriate, and add oronasal care to the Nursing Care Plan).			

(continued)

Administering Oxygen by Oxygen/Humidity Tent	Needs More Practice	Satisfactory	Comments
Assessment			
1.–3. Follow Checklist steps 1–3 of the General Procedure for Administering Oxygen (check physician's order, assess respiratory status, and identify oxygen equipment and source).			
Planning			
4.–7. Follow Checklist steps 4–7 of the General Procedure (wash your hands, plan for any assistance needed, choose appropriate equipment, and check environment for safety).			
Implementation			
8.–10. Follow Checklist steps 8–10 of the General Procedure (identify the patient and explain what you are going to do, considering the child's age and developmental level).			
11. Prepare the tent (attach metal frame to crib, suspend canopy from frame, close access ports). **a.** Tuck all sides of canopy under mattress.			
b. Fill ice trough and water jar to indicator lines.			
c. Attach tent to oxygen or compressed air source.			
d. Turn on oxygen and adjust flow rate to 15 L/min for 5 minutes.			
e. Open valve that controls mist output and follow doctor's orders.			
f. Adjust oxygen flow rate to ordered level.			
g. Place child in tent.			
12.–17. Follow Checklist steps 12–17 of the General Procedure (assess patient's breathing and adjust equipment if necessary, explain safety precautions, assess condition of nose and mouth and provide oronasal care, stay with patient until safe to leave, post an "oxygen in use" sign, and wash your hands).			

(*continued*)

Administering Oxygen by Oxygen/Humidity Tent *(Continued)*	Needs More Practice	Satisfactory	Comments
Evaluation			
18. Evaluate using the criteria in Checklist step 18 of the General Procedure (breathing pattern, skin color, mental status, comfort, and oxygenation).			
Documentation			
19.–20. Document as in Checklist steps 19 and 20 of the General Procedure (date and time oxygen started, method of delivery, specific oxygen concentration or flow rate in liters per minute, subjective/ objective observations of patient, notification of physician if appropriate, and add oronasal care to the Nursing Care Plan).			
Procedure for Using Oximetry			
Assessment			
1. Check for orders.			
2. Review the procedure for the equipment.			
3. Assess the patient.			
Planning			
4. Wash your hands.			
5. Obtain the oximetry device.			
Implementation			
6. Identify the patient.			
7. Explain oximetry to patient.			
8. Carry out procedure. a. Attach probe according to device directions.			
b. Turn on device, wait for reading to stabilize, and read meter.			
c. Remove probe.			
d. Note the oximetry reading.			
9. Clean equipment.			
10. Wash your hands.			
11. Return equipment to appropriate storage place.			

(continued)

Procedure for Using Oximetry *(Continued)*	Needs More Practice	Satisfactory	Comments
Evaluation			
12. Evaluate results in light of norms for oxygen saturation and previous readings.			
Documentation			
13. Document the oximetry reading on the patient's record.			
Self-Inflating Breathing Bag and Mask			
Assessment			
1. Assess patient for need for breathing assistance.			
Planning			
2. Wash your hands.			
3. Obtain the rebreathing bag and oxygen connector tubing.			
4. Obtain assistance if needed.			
Implementation			
5. Identify the patient.			
6. Explain procedure to patient.			
7. Connect mask to oxygen supply and turn on to highest flow rate.			
8. Apply mask snugly to form occlusive seal.			
9. Compress bag to force air into patient's lungs.			
10. Release bag, counting to 4.			
11. Repeat steps 9 and 10 in a rhythmic pattern at a rate of 12 breaths/minute.			
Evaluation			
12. Evaluate in relation to: **a.** Rise and fall of chest			
b. Skin color			
c. Change in oxygen saturation			
Documentation			
13. Document the following: **a.** Assessment indicating need for ventilation			
b. Patient's response			

MODULE

39

RESPIRATORY CARE PROCEDURES

MODULE CONTENTS

PREREQUISITES

Successful completion of the following modules:

VOLUME 1

*A review of the anatomy and physiology of the respiratory system, paying special attention
to the physiology of the cough reflex.*

OVERALL OBJECTIVE

To assist patients effectively with deep breathing, coughing, postural drainage, percussion, and vibration as necessary in their individual situations.

SPECIFIC LEARNING OBJECTIVES

Know Facts and Principles	Apply Facts and Principles	Demonstrate Ability	Evaluate Performance
1. Deep breathing State reasons for deep breathing. Identify patient situations in which deep breathing is needed. Describe procedure for deep breathing. State purposes for incentive and spirometer and intermittent positive pressure breathing.	Given a patient situation, identify when deep breathing is needed.	In the clinical setting, assist patient to deep breathe effectively.	Evaluate effectiveness of deep breathing by checking depth of patient's respiration (identifying extent of rise and fall of abdomen and chest as breath is taken).
2. Coughing Define *cough*. State reasons for encouraging patient to cough. Identify patient situations in which coughing is needed. Describe procedure for effective coughing.	Given a patient situation, identify when coughing is needed.	In the clinical setting, assist patient to cough effectively.	Evaluate effectiveness by checking for movement of secretions.
3. Postural drainage Define *postural drainage*. Identify patient situations in which postural drainage is used. Describe positions used for postural drainage for all lung areas. Describe common problems of postural drainage.	Given a patient situation, identify which position for postural drainage would be most effective. Given a patient situation, identify problems occurring.	In the clinical setting: a. Assist patient in postural drainage. b. Recognize problems occurring during postural drainage and decide appropriate course of action related to problem.	Evaluate effectiveness of postural drainage by auscultation of lungs. Validate decision with instructor.

(continued)

SPECIFIC LEARNING OBJECTIVES (continued)

Know Facts and Principles	Apply Facts and Principles	Demonstrate Ability	Evaluate Performance
4. *Percussion and vibration*			
State purpose of percussion and vibration. Describe procedure for percussion and vibration.	Identify situations where percussion and vibration might be helpful.	In the clinical setting, perform percussion and vibration correctly.	Evaluate own performance using Performance Checklist. Evaluate by checking amount of secretions raised.
5. *Documentation*			
State information to be recorded regarding respiratory care procedures.		Record appropriate information when doing respiratory care procedures.	Evaluate with instructor.

LEARNING ACTIVITIES

1. Review the Specific Learning Objectives.
2. Read the material on oxygenation and the chapter on health teaching in Ellis and Nowlis, *Nursing: A Human Needs Approach*, or comparable chapters in another text.
3. Look up the module vocabulary terms in the glossary.
4. Read through the module and mentally practice the skills.
5. Using the module directions as a guide:
    a. Practice deep breathing until you can do deep abdominal breathing easily.
    b. Practice coughing until you can create an effective cough.
    c. Practice postural drainage at home on your own bed.
        (1) Use pillows to position yourself in a moderately slanted position.
        (2) Try the jackknife position.
        (3) Consider the fatigue and discomfort caused by these positions.
6. In the practice setting: Obtain a partner. Each of you, in turn, will be the patient while your partner is the nurse. Practice each skill as though you were instructing a patient with no previous knowledge or skill. The person representing the patient should do exactly as told, not what he or she knows to be correct.
    a. Teach one another deep breathing.
    b. Evaluate one another, using the Performance Checklist.
    c. Teach one another to cough effectively.
    d. Evaluate one another, using the Performance Checklist.
    e. Assist one another with postural drainage.
    f. While the "patient" is in each position, use percussion and vibration over the area being drained.
    g. When you can perform all skills correctly, ask your instructor to evaluate your performance.
7. In the clinical setting:
    a. Seek an opportunity to observe respiratory care being given.
    b. Seek opportunities to use these skills.

VOCABULARY

abdominal (diaphragmatic) breathing	cough	inspiration	nebulizer
	diaphragm	intermittent	percussion
	expectorate	lingula	postural hypotension
alveoli	expiration	lobe	segment
atelectasis	gatched bed	lung	sputum
auscultation	hyperventilation	mucous	Trendelenburg position
bronchiole	hypoventilation	mucus	vibration

Respiratory Care Procedures

Rationale for the Use of This Skill

Respiratory care procedures are used to prevent and treat respiratory complications that may occur as a result of bed rest, immobility, and a variety of illnesses. They are effective because they assist in inflating all alveoli and in removing secretions that are a place for microbial growth and that might interfere with gas exchange. Respiratory care personnel may be responsible for some of this care, but the nurse is always responsible for assessing, monitoring, and evaluating the patient's respiratory status and may be responsible for all respiratory care, including teaching these measures.[1]

▼ NURSING DIAGNOSIS

These procedures are used for the patient who has "Risk for altered respiratory function." This reflects a general category rather than a specific nursing diagnosis within the NANDA framework, but it may be appropriate to use for the individual who does not yet have a specific nursing diagnosis, but who is at risk of developing one of several respiratory-related nursing diagnoses. The nursing diagnosis Ineffective Airway Clearance may be present in the individual who needs these procedures.

GENERAL PROCEDURE FOR GIVING RESPIRATORY CARE

Assessment

1. Count the individual's respiratory rate and assess for depth and chest expansion.
2. Auscultate the patient's lungs, especially noting areas where there are diminished breath sounds and areas where moisture is present.
3. Assess the individual's activity pattern.
4. Identify whether the patient is at risk for respiratory problems because of bed rest, inactivity, or surgical treatment.
5. Check the patient for pain or other factors *that may limit respiratory effort.*

Planning

6. Plan for pain relief, if necessary, before performing any respiratory care procedure. *A patient who has a surgical wound feels pain when moving the muscles that were cut during surgery. You can minimize this pain by holding the incisional area firmly, decreasing movement.* This is called *splinting.* Splinting can be accomplished by spreading your hands and holding them firmly over the incision, or the patient can hold the incision with his or her own hands, or a pillow can be held firmly over the incisional area to splint it. It may also be necessary to arrange for pain medication. Make sure that you allow enough time for the medication to take effect before you begin the procedure.
7. Choose the appropriate respiratory care procedure. Some procedures require a physician's order. Deep breathing and coughing may be initiated by the nurse.
8. Plan an appropriate time for performing the procedure as well as how often the procedure should be repeated. The times may be spaced throughout the day. It is preferable to choose a time when the patient is rested.

Implementation

9. Wash your hands *for infection control.*
10. Identify the patient *to be sure you are performing the procedure on the correct patient.*
11. Explain to the patient why you are concerned about his or her respiratory status in a way that does not increase anxiety. Tell the patient which measures are necessary *to prevent or alleviate problems.*
12. Carry out planned pain relief measures.
13. Carry out the specific procedure as outlined below.

Evaluation

14. Evaluate, using the following criteria:
    a. Respiratory rate equal to or less than rate before procedure.
    b. Chest expansion equal to or greater than before procedure.
    c. Lungs clear to auscultation.
    d. Patient resting comfortably.

Documentation

15. On a flow sheet or in the nurses' progress notes, document the respiratory care procedure performed. A simple flow sheet is most often used to document respiratory care procedures themselves.
16. Document the patient's response as evaluated on the appropriate assessment form in the chart. If there is no specific form, complete a narrative progress note providing the pertinent information.

---

[1] Rationale for action is emphasized throughout the module by the use of italics.

For each respiratory care procedure discussed, some steps of the General Procedure may be modified. We have included completely the modified steps as well as references to the steps of the General Procedure that remain the same.

ASSISTING THE PATIENT WITH DEEP BREATHING

All alveoli are not equally expanded during each breath taken. Normal respiration includes occasional deep breaths *that serve to fully expand all alveoli and encourage the movement of secretions.* Whenever a person is bedridden or otherwise immobile, continuous shallow respirations are common. This tends to encourage the retention of secretions and the collapse of alveoli (atelectasis).

Deep breathing is a planned part of the nursing care of every immobilized patient, especially those who have had increased secretions (persons who have inhaled respiratory anesthetics or who have respiratory disease).

For patients who have undergone abdominal or chest surgery, deep breathing may be difficult and even painful. These patients may require a great deal of assistance and support when you help them to deep breathe.

PROCEDURE FOR ASSISTING THE PATIENT WITH DEEP BREATHING

Assessment
1.–5. Follow the steps of the General Procedure for Giving Respiratory Care.

Planning
6.–8. Follow the steps of the General Procedure.

Implementation
9.–12. Follow the steps of the General Procedure.
13. Assist the patient with deep breathing as outlined below:
   a. Instruct the patient. *Because the patient must carry out the procedure, he or she must understand* what should be done and why. *A person who understands and accepts the importance of deep breathing is more likely to cooperate and participate in the exercise.* As part of the instruction, demonstrate proper deep breathing for the patient. Remember to use the principles of health teaching as you plan for the patient's instruction.
   b. Position the patient *for maximum expansion of the lungs.* To accomplish this, the chest should not be constricted. Having the patient sit on the edge of the bed or in a chair is ideal, but deep breathing can be done in any position necessitated by the patient's condition.
   c. Have the patient inspire slowly. *This allows for more comfortable alveolar expansion. (Slow movement usually creates less discomfort than rapid movement does.)* It is helpful if you count slowly to two during inspiration.
   d. *Because normal expiration is twice as long as inspiration,* have the patient expire slowly while you count to four. *This preserves the normal inspiratory–expiratory ratio and encourages maximum filling and emptying of the alveoli.*
   e. Watch the patient for chest and abdominal expansion. *Maximum expansion of the lungs occurs when both abdomen and chest expand during inspiration.* This is called *abdominal, or diaphragmatic, breathing. The expansion of the abdomen is caused by the diaphragm moving downward, displacing abdominal contents to allow complete lung expansion.* Observe the patient's breathing *to see whether complete lung expansion occurs.*
   f. Correct the patient's breathing technique as necessary *to encourage complete lung expansion.*
   g. Repeat the procedure, for a total of 10 deep breaths.

Evaluation
14. Follow the General Procedure.

Documentation
15.–16. Follow the steps of the General Procedure.

DATE/TIME	
4/19/99	Pneumonia
	S "I've been feeling so short of breath and my chest is tight."
	O Decreased breath sounds on left. Crackles scattered throughout lung fields. R-32.
	A Impaired gas exchange related to pneumonia.
	P Increase deep breathing to hourly. Encourage pt. to alternate any activity with rest periods.
	W. Madson, NS

Example of Nursing Progress Notes Using SOAP Format.

Mechanisms for Encouraging Deep Breathing

Incentive Spirometers

Physicians often order an incentive spirometer (IS) *to encourage the patient to breathe deeply.* Several models of incentive spirometers are available, and *all have been developed to encourage the patient to deep breathe.* The volume-oriented or electronic device is set so that a signal is activated when the patient achieves a prescribed inspiratory volume. The patient is instructed in deep breathing, with particular emphasis on the long inspiratory effort. The patient expires normally, and then places the mouthpiece in the mouth and inspires only through the machine. If the inspiratory volume meets the preset amount, the signal is activated. Most incentive spirometers have counters to indicate the number of deep breaths taken.

The flow-oriented or mechanical incentive spirometer has plastic chambers with movable balls similar to ping-pong balls. The patient inhales through the nose, exhales through the mouth, and then inhales through the mouthpiece, attempting to keep the balls at the top of the chambers for 3 seconds (Fig. 39–1). The patient is usually encouraged to do this exercise 10 times every 1 or 2 hours.

The incentive spirometer is based on the learning theory that immediate objective feedback about performance increases motivation to learn and results in quicker learning. When volume-oriented incentive spirometers are used, the achievement signal is set low at first, allowing the patient to master that level before moving higher. This also allows the patient to progress gradually. Spirometers are quite effective, in that many patients do far more deep breathing using them.

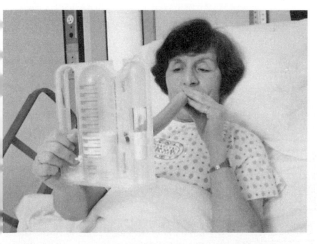

Figure 39–1. A mechanical incentive spirometer. The patient attempts to keep the balls at the top of the chambers for 3 seconds.

Intermittent Positive Pressure Breathing (IPPB)

The IPPB machine uses positive pressure to increase inspiration and to deliver nebulized moisture (with or without medication) deep into the lungs. Most often, IPPB is used for the patient with respiratory disease who needs to have a medication delivered to the lungs. A treatment usually lasts 5 to 10 minutes or as long as it takes to get all of the ordered medication delivered. In some cases, a short rest period may be needed during the treatment.

The actual procedure is specific to the brand of machine. The manufacturer provides a manual giving directions for use.

TEACHING THE PATIENT TO COUGH PRODUCTIVELY

Coughing is always combined with deep breathing, but deep breathing may be done without coughing. *Deep breathing fully expands the alveoli and enhances the normal respiratory function. Coughing raises respiratory secretions so they do not plug the bronchioles (causing atelectasis) or provide a medium for bacterial growth. However, coughing when the patient has no secretions to raise may collapse alveoli* and therefore is not recommended.

PROCEDURE FOR TEACHING THE PATIENT TO COUGH PRODUCTIVELY

Assessment
1.–5. Follow the steps of the General Procedure for Giving Respiratory Care.

Planning
6.–8. Follow the steps of the General Procedure.

Implementation
9.–12. Follow the steps of the General Procedure.
13. Teach the patient to cough productively as outlined below:
  a. Explain the reasons for coughing. *A patient who understands and accepts the reason for an activity is more cooperative in performing that activity.*
  b. Place the patient in a sitting position if possible. *This is normally the most effective position for coughing.* Other positions can be used, depending on the patient's needs.
  c. Splint, as described above in the General Procedure for Giving Respiratory Care, step 6, if necessary.
  d. Have the patient deep breathe, following steps 13.c. and 13.d. as in the Procedure for Assisting with Deep Breathing.

e. After the third deep breath, have the patient inspire and hold the breath 3 seconds.

f. Have the patient expire forcefully against the closed glottis and then release the air abruptly while flexing forward. *Exhaling against the closed glottis builds up pressure, which tends to create a force that raises secretions. Flexion forward exerts abdominal pressure against the diaphragm, which increases the force of the expired air sufficiently to carry secretions.* (Use simpler language when explaining this to the patient. For example, instead of "Exhale against the closed glottis," say, "Hold your breath and then try to breathe out when your throat is closed.")

g. Repeat for three deep coughs if possible, or repeat until mucus is expectorated. Do not prolong deep breathing and coughing, *because these actions can cause hyperventilation.* Watch for dizziness and tingling of the extremities, the most common symptoms of hyperventilation. Wear gloves only if the patient cannot manage his or her own secretions.

h. Check the lungs by auscultation.

i. Offer oral hygiene. *Sputum often leaves a disagreeable taste in the mouth.*

j. Repeat deep breathing and coughing hourly as needed to clear the lungs of secretions, or as ordered.

Evaluation
14. Follow the General Procedure.

Documentation
15.–16. Follow the steps of the General Procedure.

POSTURAL DRAINAGE

When a large volume of secretions is present in the lungs, raising all of them by deep breathing and coughing may be impossible. *Postural drainage—positioning the patient so that the force of gravity helps drain the lung secretions*—may be required.

For most individuals, moderately slanted positions are successful in draining lungs. *Because of the branching structure of the lungs,* however, a variety of positions must be used *to drain all the lung segments adequately.*

When postural drainage is used for a patient with chronic respiratory problems but no current acute difficulty, each position needs to be held for only 15 seconds *to drain the lung segments adequately.* For a person with an acute problem, it is recommended that 5 minutes be spent initially in each position. When you have determined the position in which most of the secretions are raised, you can shorten the time the patient spends in some positions and lengthen the time in others. Not all positions are necessary for every patient—*only those that drain specific affected areas.*

Postural drainage is best tolerated if done between meals, at least 2 hours after the patient has eaten, *to decrease the possibility of vomiting.* This will also allow the patient time to rest before the next meal. Even if you are not responsible for carrying out the postural drainage, you *are* responsible for coordinating all aspects of care in the patient's best interests.

The positions in the following procedure are moderate. Certain lung segments do not drain in these positions, but if the entire sequence is used, most do.

PROCEDURE FOR PERFORMING POSTURAL DRAINAGE

Assessment
1. Check the chart for a physician's order, which is needed to perform postural drainage.

2. Identify the specific segments of the lung to be drained. This may be part of the physician's order, or the areas with excessive secretions may be identified by the physician in the progress notes. The areas with excessive secretions may also be identified through auscultation or by checking the chest x-ray report.

DATE/TIME	
2/09/99	D: Coughing frequently. Gurgles and crackles heard throughout lung fields. Unable to cough up sputum.
	A: Taught techniques of effective coughing and encouraged to cough up secretions.
	R: Coughing more effectively and raising small amounts of sputum. N. Tillots, RN

Example of Nursing Progress Notes Using Focus Format.

Most often, the lower lobes are drained. It is assumed that *most of the upper lobes drain in normal daily activity, but this would not be true for a severely immobilized patient. The complex sequence is tiring* and can be done with rest periods between positions. Pay particular attention to elderly patients with heart disease who may experience difficulty with the procedure.

Planning

3. Wash your hands *for infection control.*
4. Plan how you will place the patient in the various positions. Some beds can be "gatched" (raised in the middle) *to provide the correct position for postural drainage.* Some beds that cannot be gatched do have a foot section that can be lowered, in which case you can position the patient with his or her head at the foot of the bed and use the foot drop to achieve the desired position. Most electric beds can be placed in a head-down (Trendelenburg) position. You can use this position for postural drainage, but *raising the patient's feet may increase fatigue and is not essential to the procedure's effectiveness.* If the bed cannot be positioned properly, you will need one large or two small pillows to place under the patient's hips to provide the correct position. You will also need another pillow to support the patient in the side-lying position.
5. Obtain pillows and a sputum cup and tissues for the patient to use for expectorated secretions. Obtain clean gloves if the patient is unable to manage his or her own secretions.

Implementation

6. Identify the patient *to be sure you are performing the procedure for the correct patient.*
7. Explain to the patient the purpose and method of postural drainage, using the basic principles of health teaching.
8. Position the patient.
9. Drain the upper lobes.
   a. Have the patient sit up if possible. (Sitting in a fairly straight chair is ideal.) You can also raise the head of the bed to its maximum height.
   b. Have the patient lean to the right side (45° angle for 5 minutes *to drain the left aspect of both upper lobes.* Support the patient with pillows if necessary.
   c. Then have the patient lean to the left side (45° angle) for 5 minutes *to drain the upper right lobes.* Again, support the patient with pillows if necessary.
   d. Have the patient lean forward at a 30° to 45° angle and stay in this position for 5 minutes. *This position drains the posterior segments of the*

upper lobes. Let the patient brace the elbows on the knees to maintain this position. Or you can pad an overbed table and place it in front of the patient to lean on.
   e. Have the patient lean backward at a 30°–45° angle for 5 minutes. *This position drains the anterior segments of the upper lobes.* Help the patient maintain the position by having him or her lean back in bed, with the headrest at the proper height.
   f. Have the patient lie on the abdomen, back, and both sides while horizontal *to drain the remaining segments* of the upper lobes.
10. Drain the lower lobes.
   a. Place the patient in the left side-lying position in bed. Use pillows or adjust the bed so that the patient's head and thorax are 30° to 45° down from the horizontal position. *The 30° position is less tiring and creates fewer adverse circulatory effects than the 45° position does.*
   b. Remember that there are six positions. Each can be achieved if the patient starts out lying on one side and gradually turns like a rotisserie. Use the same sequence of positions each time *to help you remember them easily. To identify which lung segments are drained with each position,* refer to the drawings in an anatomy text, which outline various lung segments. The patient should remain in each position for 5 minutes.
      (1) Have the patient lie on the left side, with the shoulders perpendicular to the bed. *This position drains the lateral basal segment of the right lower lobe* (Fig. 39–2). Use pillows to support the patient, and place a small pillow under the head if essential to comfort.
      (2) Turn the patient halfway onto the back, so the shoulders are at a 45° angle to the bed (Fig. 39–3). *This position drains the right middle lobe.* Again, use pillows to support this position.
      (3) Turn the patient flat on the back (Fig. 39–4). *This position drains the anterior basal segments of the right and left lower lobes.*
      (4) Turn the patient halfway to the right side, so the shoulders are at a 45° angle to the bed (Fig. 39–5). *This position drains the lingula of the left lower lobe.*
      (5) Turn the patient completely onto the right side, so the shoulders are again at a 90° angle to the bed (Fig. 39–6). *This position drains the lateral basal segments of the left lower lobe.*

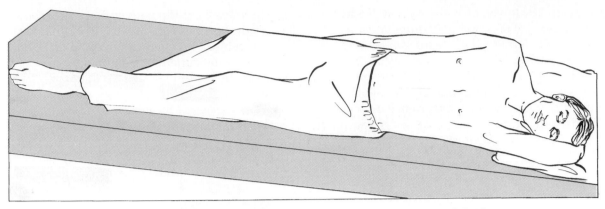

Figure 39–2. Draining the lateral basal segment of the right lower lobe. The patient lies on the left side with the head and thorax 30° to 45° down from the horizontal.

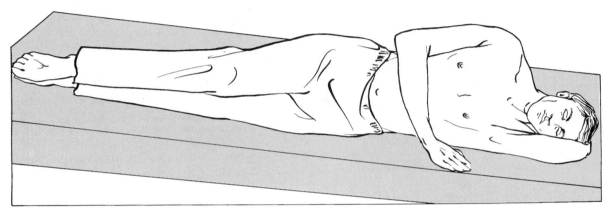

Figure 39–3. Draining the right middle lobe. The shoulders are at a 45° angle to the bed.

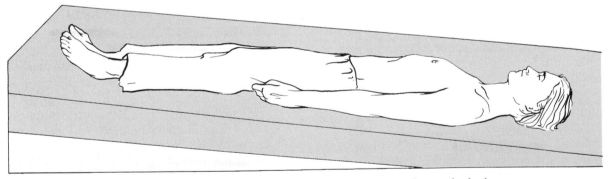

Figure 39–4. Draining the anterior basal segments of both lungs. The patient is flat on the back (supine) with thorax 30° to 45° down from the horizontal position.

(6) Have the patient turn onto the abdomen, with the head turned to the side (Fig. 39–7). *This position drains the posterior basal segments of the lower lobes.* It is usually used last, *because secretions are often easier to cough out when the patient is on the abdomen.*

11. Have the patient cough forcefully (lying on the abdomen) *to expel secretions.*

12. Return the patient to a comfortable position, offer mouth care, and allow for a rest period.

Evaluation
13. Evaluate, using the following criteria:
   a. Lungs clear to auscultation.
   b. Patient resting comfortably.

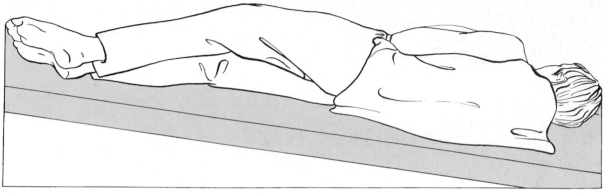

Figure 39–5. Draining the lingula of the left lower lobe. Pillows are used to support the shoulders at a 45° angle to the bed.

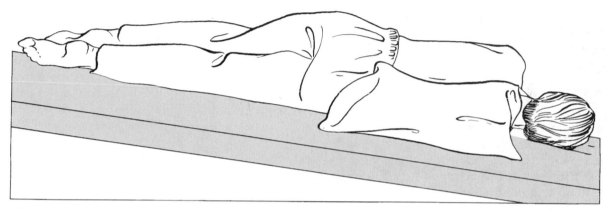

Figure 39–6. Draining the lateral basal segments of the left lower lobe. The shoulders are at a 90° angle to the bed.

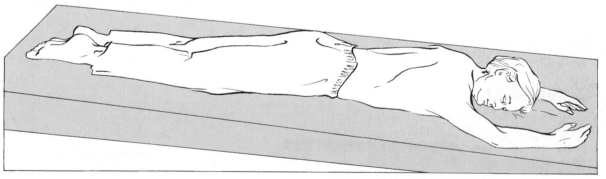

Figure 39–7. Draining the posterior basal segments of the lower lobes. This position is also used for coughing out secretions.

Documentation

4. On a flow sheet or in the nurses' progress notes document:
   a. Positions used for postural drainage
   b. Secretions produced
   c. Any changes in respiratory status

Problems Associated With Postural Drainage

Falling because of dizziness or fainting is a common concern when the patient is placed in postural drainage. Although this problem can occur when the patient is in the head-down position, it is more likely to occur

DATE/TIME	
3/31/99	*Respirations shallow with crackles in the bases bilaterally.*
	Encouraged to use incentive spirometer hourly.
	M. Jacobs, NS

Example of Nursing Progress Notes Using Narrative Format.

when the patient is returning to the normal position, *because of postural hypotension*. By changing the patient's position slowly, *you can help alleviate this problem. To protect the patient,* raise the side rails and make frequent observations during the procedure. Some patients cannot be left alone during the procedure, so use careful nursing judgment.

If a large volume of secretions is mobilized from the alveoli and small bronchioles at one time, a larger airway may be temporarily blocked, causing severe respiratory distress, anxiety, and fear. This experience may be so upsetting that the patient may resist future attempts at postural drainage. Explain what is happening and help the patient cough out the secretions. Support the patient with your continued presence and reassurance.

Sometimes it is necessary to use percussion (or clapping) and vibration (see below) to remove secretions. If the blockage is severe, suctioning may be required.

PERCUSSION AND VIBRATION

Percussion

Percussion is the manual application of light blows to the chest wall. These blows are transmitted through the tissue and *help loosen secretions in the lung segment immediately below the area struck*. Percussion is done over areas that need to be drained. Percuss over a patient gown or other light clothing, not against the bare skin *to decrease friction.*

1. Place the patient is in the postural drainage position of choice.
2. Cup your hands.
3. Clap them over the chest wall (Fig. 39–8).

Correctly done, this action should produce a hollow sound and should not be painful for the patient. Instruct the patient to take slow deep breaths during percussion *to prevent tensing of the chest and to assist with the mobilization of secretions.*

Mechanical percussion devices that deliver percussion at a set force and rate are used by respiratory therapists. These devices are not commonly available in nursing departments.

Vibration

Vibration is performed for the same purpose as percussion and is as effective as percussion if done correctly. Ask the patient to exhale after a deep inspiration and vibrate as the patient exhales.

1. Position the patient in the appropriate position for postural drainage.
2. Using flat hands, place your hands firmly against the chest wall, one over the other.
3. Keeping your arms and shoulders straight, vibrate your hands back and forth rapidly while the patient exhales (Fig. 39–9). *The vibration is transferred through the tissues and loosens mucus.*

Mechanical vibrators also loosen secretions by transferring vibrations though the chest wall. Read the directions for the particular brand and model o

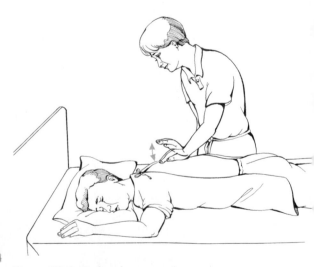

Figure 39–8. Performing percussion.

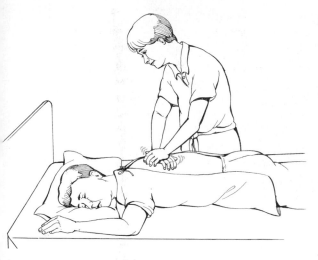

Figure 39–9. Performing vibration.

vibrator available (generally you place the vibrating head firmly against the chest wall over the area where secretions are retained).

LONG-TERM CARE

Respiratory care procedures may be needed by those in long-term care facilities as well as by those in acute care. Treatments are the same, but may need to be modified for the older adult. For example, the resident may not be able to stay in a position for postural drainage as long, and you may need to use a gentler touch with percussion and vibration techniques.

HOME CARE

Patients may need to continue respiratory care procedures at home after discharge from the hospital, or those with chronic respiratory problems may need to carry them out on a long-term basis. In any event, you will need to assess the home setting *to facilitate teaching* the patient as well as the family or care provider, to supervise the treatments, and to evaluate their effectiveness.

CRITICAL THINKING EXERCISES

• Mabel Thomas, age 73, is being seen in the outpatient clinic for a respiratory infection that has been causing a severe cough. The coughing has interfered with her sleep, but it has not been productive. How will you determine what teaching this patient needs in regard to deep breathing and coughing? Identify the special concerns that might exist for this patient.

• Jonathan Jordan, age 8, has cystic fibrosis. He was hospitalized for a respiratory infection and will be returning home with a regular regimen of postural drainage, vibration, and clapping to remove secretions. His parents will be performing these procedures at home. Identify the nursing role in relationship to his discharge planning and teaching. Determine the specific actions the nurse should take in this situation.

PERFORMANCE CHECKLIST

General Procedure for Giving Respiratory Care	Needs More Practice	Satisfactory	Comments
Assessment			
1. Count respiratory rate and assess depth and chest expansion.			
2. Auscultate the patient's lungs.			
3. Assess the individual's activity pattern.			
4. Identify whether the patient is at risk for respiratory problems.			
5. Check the patient for pain or other factors that may limit respiratory effort.			
Planning			
6. Plan for pain relief.			
7. Plan what respiratory care procedure is appropriate.			
8. Plan an appropriate time and frequency for the procedure.			
Implementation			
9. Wash your hands.			
10. Identify the patient.			
11. Explain to the patient why you are concerned and tell him or her which respiratory measures are to be used.			
12. Carry out pain relief measures.			
13. Carry out the specific procedure.			
Evaluation			
14. Evaluate, using the following criteria: a. Respiratory rate equal to or less than rate before procedure.			
b. Chest expansion equal to or greater than before procedure.			
c. Lungs clear to auscultation.			
d. Patient resting comfortably.			

(continued)

General Procedure for Giving Respiratory Care *(Continued)*	Needs More Practice	Satisfactory	Comments
Documentation			
15. Record the respiratory care procedure on the flow sheet or nurses' progress notes.			
16. Document patient's response as evaluated.			
Assisting the Patient With Deep Breathing			
Assessment			
1.–5. Follow Checklist steps 1–5 of the General Procedure for Giving Respiratory Care. (Count respiratory rate and assess depth and chest expansion, auscultate lungs, assess activity pattern, identify whether the patient is at risk for respiratory problems, and check for pain or other factors that may limit respiratory effort.)			
Planning			
6.–8. Follow Checklist steps 6–8 of the General Procedure. (Plan for pain relief, plan what respiratory care procedure is appropriate, and plan an appropriate time and frequency for the procedure.)			
Implementation			
9.–12. Follow Checklist steps 9–12 of the General Procedure. (Wash your hands, identify the patient, explain which respiratory measures are to be used and why, and provide pain relief.)			
13. Assist the patient with deep breathing as outlined below: **a.** Instruct patient, demonstrating if necessary.			
b. Position patient.			
c. Have patient inspire while counting slowly to two.			
d. Have patient expire while counting slowly to four.			
e. Observe patient for chest and abdominal expansion.			
f. Correct patient's technique as necessary.			
g. Repeat for total of 10 deep breaths.			

(continued)

Assisting the Patient With Deep Breathing
(Continued)

	Needs More Practice	Satisfactory	Comments
Evaluation			
14. Evaluate, using the following criteria: 　**a.** Respiratory rate equal to or less than rate before procedure.			
b. Chest expansion equal to or greater than before procedure.			
c. Lungs clear to auscultation.			
d. Patient resting comfortably.			
Documentation			
15.–16. Follow Checklist steps 15 and 16 of the General Procedure. (Record the procedure on the flow sheet or nurses' progress notes and document patient's response as evaluated.)			
Teaching the Patient To Cough Productively			
Assessment			
1.–5. Follow Checklist steps 1–5 of the General Procedure for Giving Respiratory Care. (Count respiratory rate and assess depth and chest expansion, auscultate lungs, assess activity pattern, identify whether the patient is at risk for respiratory problems, and check for pain or other factors that may limit respiratory effort.)			
Planning			
6.–8. Follow Checklist steps 6–8 of the General Procedure. (Plan for pain relief, plan what respiratory care procedure is appropriate, plan an appropriate time and frequency for the procedure.)			
Implementation			
9.–12. Follow Checklist steps 9–11 of the General Procedure. (Wash your hands, identify the patient, explain to the patient why you are concerned which respiratory measures are to be used and provide pain relief.)			
13. Teach the patient to cough productively as outlined below: 　**a.** Explain the reasons for coughing.			

(continued)

Teaching the Patient to Cough Productively *(Continued)*	Needs More Practice	Satisfactory	Comments
b. Position patient (in sitting position, if possible).			
c. Splint if necessary.			
d. Have patient deep breathe.			
e. After third deep breath, have patient inspire and hold breath 3 seconds.			
f. Have patient expire forcefully against closed glottis and then release air abruptly while flexing forward.			
g. Repeat for three deep coughs or until mucus is expectorated. Use gloves if indicated.			
h. Auscultate lungs.			
i. Offer oral hygiene.			
j. Repeat hourly or as needed to clear lungs of secretions.			
Evaluation			
14. Evaluate, using the following criteria: **a.** Respiratory rate equal to or less than rate before procedure.			
b. Chest expansion equal to or greater than before procedure.			
c. Lungs clear to auscultation.			
d. Patient resting comfortably.			
Documentation			
15.–16. Follow Checklist steps 15 and 16 of the General Procedure. (Record on the flow sheet or nurses' notes and document patient's response as evaluated.)			
Procedure for Performing Postural Drainage (Moderate Positions)			
Assessment			
1. Check for physician's order.			
2. Identify specific lung segments to be drained.			
Planning			
3. Wash your hands.			

(continued

Procedure for Performing Postural Drainage (Moderate Positions) *(Continued)*	Needs More Practice	Satisfactory	Comments
4. Plan how to place the patient in appropriate positions.			
5. Obtain pillows, sputum cup, tissues, and gloves, if necessary.			
Implementation			
6. Identify the patient.			
7. Instruct patient.			
8. Position patient.			
9. Drain upper lobes. **a.** Have patient sit up if possible.			
b. Have patient lean right (45° angle) for 5 minutes.			
c. Have patient lean left (45° angle) for 5 minutes.			
d. Have patient lean forward (30°–45° angle) for 5 minutes.			
e. Have patient lean backward (30°–45° angle) for 5 minutes.			
f. Have patient lie on abdomen, back, and both sides while horizontal.			
10. Drain lower lobes. **a.** Place patient in left side-lying position in bed. Use pillow or bed gatch to elevate hips higher than head. (Head should be approximately 30°–45° below horizontal level.)			
b. Have patient lie in each of the following six positions for 5 minutes, breathing deeply. (1) On left side with shoulders perpendicular to bed			
(2) On left side with shoulders slanted backward at a 45° angle from bed			
(3) On back			
(4) On right side with shoulders slanted backward at a 45° angle from bed			
(5) On right side with shoulders perpendicular to bed			
(6) On abdomen with head turned to side			

(continued)

Procedure for Performing Postural Drainage (Moderate Positions) *(Continued)*	Needs More Practice	Satisfactory	Comments
11. While still on abdomen, have patient cough to raise secretions.			
12. Return patient to comfortable position and allow to rest.			
Evaluation			
13. Evaluate, using the following criteria: **a.** Lungs clear to auscultation.			
b. Patient resting comfortably.			
Documentation			
14. Document			
a. Positions used for postural drainage.			
b. Secretions produced.			
c. Changes in respiratory status.			
Percussion			
1. Place patient in appropriate position for postural drainage.			
2. Use cupped hands.			
3. Clap rapidly over area being drained.			
Vibration			
1. Place patient in appropriate position for postural drainage.			
2. Use flat hands placed firmly against chest wall.			
3. Vibrate hands against chest while patient exhales.			

MODULE

40

ORAL AND NASOPHARYNGEAL SUCTIONING

MODULE CONTENTS

PREREQUISITES[1]

Successful completion of the following modules:

[1]For tracheostomy suctioning, see Module 41, Tracheostomy Care and Suctioning.

OVERALL OBJECTIVE

To suction patients of all ages safely and effectively using the oral or nasopharyngeal route.

SPECIFIC LEARNING OBJECTIVES

Know Facts and Principles	Apply Facts and Principles	Demonstrate Ability	Evaluate Performance
1. Patient explanation State information included in explaining suctioning to alert patient.	Given a patient situation, give adequate explanation.	In the clinical setting, explain procedure to alert patient.	Evaluate effectiveness with instructor.
2. Equipment Know variety of equipment available for suctioning adults and infants.	Given a patient situation, select appropriate equipment.	In the clinical setting, select appropriate equipment for suctioning patient.	Evaluate selection with instructor.
3. Routes for suctioning Name two routes for suctioning.	Given a patient situation, assess need for procedure and determine appropriate route.	In the clinical setting, determine appropriate route for suctioning.	Validate choice with instructor.

4. Procedure
  a. Sterile technique
  b. Patient position
  c. Inserting catheter
  d. Applying suction
  e. Safety
Describe correct patient position and method to suction patient safely.
	Given a patient situation, describe patient position and correct procedure for suctioning, using sterile technique and observing safety precautions.	In the clinical setting, carry out procedure safely on alert or comatose adult or an infant.	Evaluate performance with instructor using Performance Checklist.

5. Assessment List assessments made before, during, and after suctioning.	Given a patient situation, identify specific assessment needed.	In the clinical setting, make significant observations.	Evaluate performance with clinical instructor.
6. Documentation State information to be documented.	Given a patient situation, document procedure and results correctly.	In the clinical setting, record data on patient's progress record.	Evaluate charting with clinical instructor.

LEARNING ACTIVITIES

1. Review the Specific Learning Objectives.
2. Read the section on respiration in Ellis and Nowlis, *Nursing: A Human Needs Approach,* or comparable material in another textbook.
3. Look up the module vocabulary terms in the glossary.
4. Read through the module as though you were preparing to teach the contents to another person. Mentally practice the skills.
5. Review the Performance Checklist.
6. In the practice setting:
   a. Familiarize yourself with the suctioning equipment available.
   b. Using the available equipment and a manikin, simulate oral and nasopharyngeal suctioning.
   c. Again, with available equipment and an infant manikin, perform the bulb method and DeLee suction as used on an infant.
   d. Have your partner evaluate your performance, using the Performance Checklist.
   e. Compare your own evaluation with that of your partner.
   f. Reverse roles, and repeat steps b through e.
   g. Practice assessing and recording the suctioning procedure.
   h. When you feel you have practiced the procedure adequately, have your instructor evaluate your performance.
7. In the clinical setting:
   a. Consult with your clinical instructor regarding an opportunity to suction an alert adult, a comatose adult, and an infant.

VOCABULARY

aeration	cough reflex	mucous	pharynx
amniotic	cyanotic	mucus	saliva
aspirate	hypoxia	nasopharynx	secretions
bronchial	inspiration	oropharynx	trachea

Oral and Nasopharyngeal Suctioning

Rationale for the Use of This Skill

An abnormal increase in respiratory secretions can result from a variety of conditions. Among the more common causes are lung and bronchial infections, central nervous system depression, and exposure to anesthetic gases. In the newborn, saliva and amniotic fluid may be present in the mouth and throat in amounts the infant cannot expectorate. The premature newborn has an absent or decreased cough reflex and may be unable to raise secretions. In such situations the secretions must be removed mechanically to facilitate breathing.

In the conscious, alert adult, the cough reflex is activated when respirations are compromised, and secretions are then expectorated. Newborn, unconscious, or very ill patients are incapable of coughing and must rely on the nurse and the nurse's familiarity with the equipment and various techniques for suctioning to carry out this function for them.[2]

▼ NURSING DIAGNOSES

These procedures may be needed for the patient with a nursing diagnosis of Ineffective Airway Clearance. This diagnosis may be related to the patient's inability to cough effectively when copious secretions are present. Another nursing diagnosis is that of Anxiety. The procedure itself can produce an anxious state *because normal breathing may be temporarily compromised.*

STERILE TECHNIQUE

Because the respiratory tract is continuous and moist, pathogens can readily move downward from the area being suctioned. The bronchi and lungs of an ill person *are particularly susceptible to infection,* so sterile technique should be used for suctioning, whether performed orally or nasopharyngeally. If the suctioning route is changed for any reason (such as an obstruction), you must obtain a new sterile catheter.

Use sterile gloves to perform suctioning. One gloved hand holds the sterile portion of the catheter, which is in contact with the patient, while the other hand operates the machine or clean pieces of equipment. This hand is considered contaminated and is not used to touch sterile equipment.

Sterile water or saline is used *to flush the catheter and tubing. Tap water contains microorganisms that are not harmful to the well person but may cause infection of the respiratory tract in the ill person.*

When a patient is taught self-care suctioning, clean technique instead of sterile technique is sometimes used. However, the patient is carefully monitored for signs of infection and is often on maintenance antibiotics.

SUCTION CATHETERS

Suction catheters are available with two types of tips (Fig. 40–1). Each has special advantages. The *open-ended catheter* has a large opening at the end of the catheter and two opposite eyes. This type is effective when the mucus is very thick and tenacious, but it does have a tendency to pull at tissue unless it is used carefully. The *whistle-tip catheter* has a large oblique opening in the end, *which has less tendency to grab or pull tissue.*

With any catheter, the system must be closed *to obtain suction, or pull.* Suctioning is easily controlled by using a Y-tube connector and placing the thumb over the open end of the Y *to close the system.* A button-type connector is also available. To use it, place the thumb over the opening in the protruding button (Fig. 40–2).

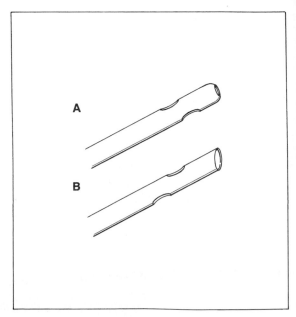

Figure 40–1. Suction catheters. **(A)** Open-ended catheter. **(B)** Whistle-tip catheter.

[2]Rationale for action is emphasized throughout the module by the use of italics.

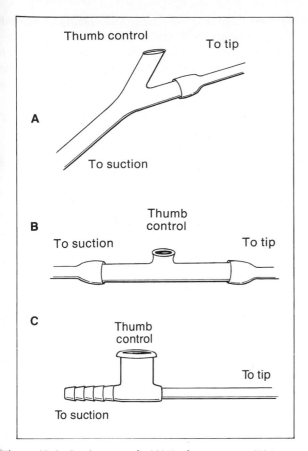

Figure 40–2. Suction controls. **(A)** Y-tube connector. **(B)** Button-type connector attached to catheter. **(C)** Button-type connector as part of suction catheter.

SUCTION SOURCE

In many healthcare facilities, each room has a suction outlet on the wall. Only a length of clean tubing, a wall outlet control, and a reservoir are needed to connect to the outlet (Fig. 40–3). If wall suction is not available, a portable suction machine (Fig. 40–4) may be obtained from the central processing department.

The equipment should be tested before the procedure. To be effective, suction tubing must be tightly fastened to the outlet *to maintain a closed system.* The nurse should inspect all plugs and cords on portable units to make sure they are in good repair, *to prevent sparks. Remember that sparks can be hazardous when oxygen is in use, and often the patient who is ill enough to require suctioning is also receiving oxygen.*

ROUTES FOR SUCTIONING

The suction catheter may be inserted orally (through the mouth to the back of the throat) or nasopharyngeally (through one of the nostrils). Nasopha-

ryngeal suctioning, particularly if done frequently, can cause irritation and even bleeding of the nares. For an infant, suctioning is done orally, *because the nostrils are too small for the introduction of a suction catheter.* With oral suctioning, you can easily assess the length of catheter needed to aspirate the back of the throat (Fig. 40–5).

When using the nasopharyngeal route, the length for depth of insertion is generally the distance from the tip of the nose to the tip of one ear lobe, or about 5 inches for an adult.

Tracheal or deep suctioning is done by a respiratory therapist, a critical care nurse, or an experienced and skilled staff nurse who can perform this more complicated procedure safely. In tracheal suctioning, the catheter is introduced past the glottis, deep into the trachea. *This route is used when the secretions are deep in the respiratory tract, are interfering with ventilation, and cannot be suctioned by another route.*

The cough reflex can be stimulated using either route. Although unpleasant for the conscious patient, *coughing raises deeper secretions, which can then be removed by suctioning.*

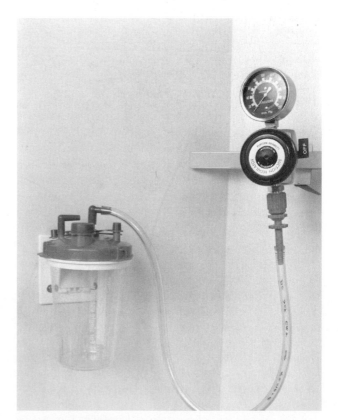

Figure 40–3. Wall outlet suction device. In many healthcare facilities, each patient unit has a suction unit on the wall to which suction equipment can be attached.

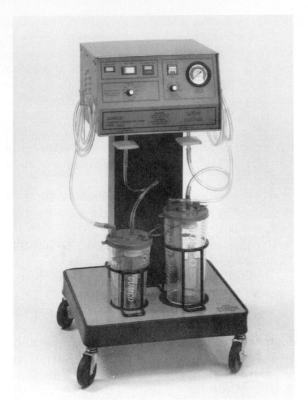

Figure 40–4. Portable suction machine. When wall suction is not available, a portable suction machine may be used. (Courtesy Allied Health Care Products, Inc., St. Louis, Missouri)

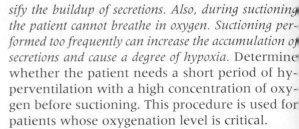

PROCEDURE FOR ORAL AND NASOPHARYNGEAL SUCTIONING

Assessment

1. Check for a doctor's order for suctioning, if this is your facility's policy. But keep in mind that most facilities do not require a doctor's order for suctioning. When it is written, it is usually done as a prn order. Suctioning can be performed at the discretion of the nurse who assesses the need for suctioning the patient. *If the patency of the patient's airway is threatened,* an emergency exists and you should promptly proceed with suctioning *to prevent respiratory obstruction.*

2. Carefully assess the patient before you proceed with suctioning unless the patency of the patient's airway is threatened. In such a situation, proceed without delay. Assess by listening to chest sounds and to sounds of the higher respiratory tract. You can sometimes hear gurgling sounds from the back of the throat. A patient with severely compromised respirations from the presence of copious secretions may appear cyanotic and have labored breathing. You must be thoughtful about the decision to suction a patient, *because the irritation of the catheter may inten-*

sify the buildup of secretions. Also, *during suctioning the patient cannot breathe in oxygen. Suctioning performed too frequently can increase the accumulation of secretions and cause a degree of hypoxia.* Determine whether the patient needs a short period of hyperventilation with a high concentration of oxygen before suctioning. This procedure is used for patients whose oxygenation level is critical.

3. Be familiar with the suctioning equipment available and the details of the procedure prescribed by the facility.

Planning

4. Wash your hands *for infection control.*

5. Plan for any needed assistance from another staff person. Suctioning can cause the patient to become agitated *because of the feeling that breathing is being interfered with.*

6. Choose the appropriate equipment for the route of suctioning you plan. If you are not sure which route will be used, select two catheters for possible change of route (see Sterile Technique above). Most healthcare facilities have prepared suction kits available that contain the following equipment (Fig. 40–6):

   a. Sterile catheter (sizes vary)
   b. Sterile gloves
   c. Sterile container or basin
   d. Tear packet of sterile water or saline.

   Add the following:

   a. Sterile water or sterile saline (if not in set)
   b. Wall suction connector or portable suction machine (if wall suction is not available)
   c. Tongue depressor (for oral suctioning)
   d. Suction trap, if a sputum specimen is needed (see Fig. 41–8, page 220)
   e. Face mask *for protection if patient coughs*

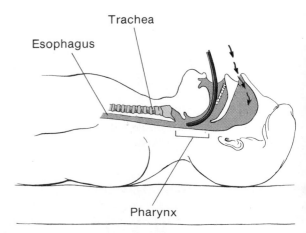

Figure 40–5. Oral suctioning. Placement of suction catheter in pharynx.

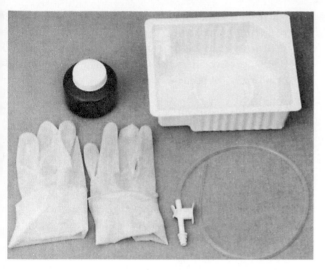

Figure 40–6. Commercial suction catheter set. The sterile water is in a container and ready to use, so no pouring is required.

  f. Eye protection (goggles provide front and side protection, but most people who wear eyeglasses believe they provide adequate protection).

Implementation

7. Identify the patient *to be sure you are performing the procedure on the correct patient.*

8. Explain what you are going to do. Suctioning can be threatening to any patient. It is natural to resist foreign objects that enter the respiratory tract. *This is, in fact, the basis for our protective cough reflex.* You can alleviate the patient's fear and gain increased cooperation *by adequately explaining the procedure and the reasons for it.*

   Tell the patient that you will insert the catheter gently, and that you will stop the procedure if the patient wishes. Ask the patient to relax as much as possible. Inform the patient that coughing may be induced, but explain that this *may help to raise the secretions to a level where they can be suctioned.*

9. Secure adequate lighting *so you can see properly and suction safely.* If the room lighting is inadequate, obtain additional lighting.

10. Position the patient appropriately:

    a. For oropharyngeal suctioning, place the patient in semi-Fowler's position with the head turned slightly toward you.

    b. For nasopharyngeal suctioning, place the patient in semi-Fowler's position with the neck hyperextended *to promote smooth insertion of the suction catheter.*

    c. Place the unconscious patient in the lateral position facing toward you *to promote drainage of secretions and prevent aspiration.*

11. Place the drape (from a suction catheter kit) or a clean towel across the patient's chest *to protect the gown.* If prior oxygenation is needed, do so at this time. Follow the procedure for using the self-inflating breathing bag and mask in Module 38, Administering Oxygen. It is good practice to routinely have the patient take two to three deep breaths before you start suctioning.

12. Open the suction kit, maintaining sterile technique. Use the wrapper as a sterile field. If you are not using a kit, use the inner surface of the sterile glove package *to provide a sterile field.*

13. If the sterile solution and container are not in the suction kit, set up the sterile container and open and pour the sterile solution into it at this time.

14. Connect the tubing to the wall or portable suction source.

15. Turn on the wall suction mechanism or the suction machine and test by placing thumb over the end of the suction tubing (Fig. 40–7).

16. Put on sterile gloves. Kits contain two sterile gloves *so that both hands are protected from contact with respiratory secretions and the patient is protected from microorganisms.* Reserve the sterile glove on your dominant hand for contact with the suction catheter, and use the other hand for any other needs. *This action protects the patient from contact with microorganisms.* Fill the container in the kit with sterile solution.

17. Pick up the catheter with your gloved dominant hand and attach the connector end to the suction tubing, which is held in your nondominant hand. Do not touch the tubing with the dominant hand *to avoid contamination.*

18. Again, test the equipment by suctioning a small amount of saline or water once through the tubing and catheter. (*The water also serves to lubricate the catheter.*)

19. Insert the catheter either:

    a. Through the mouth, using a tongue blade if necessary *to hold the tongue aside for visibility.* Slide the catheter along the side of the mouth to the oropharynx. Do not apply suction at this time; *the tip may adhere to the tissues so that secretions cannot be suctioned or the tissue may be damaged.*

    b. Through the nostrils. (If you detect an obstruction in one nostril, try the other side.) Slide the catheter gently along the floor of the unobstructed nostril to the nasopharynx. No suction should be applied during this step. Use a catheter only for a single route. If you

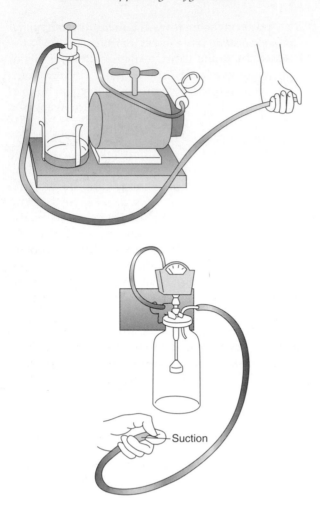

Figure 40–7. Testing the suction pressure by turning on the equipment and placing the thumb over the open end of the tubing.

must change the route, obtain a new sterile catheter. For example, if you have attempted to suction a patient orally and have met with resistance, and then decide to proceed with the nasopharyngeal approach, discard the first catheter and obtain a second. If you are not using a kit, open separate sterile packs and proceed. Some facilities allow using the same catheter for oral and nasopharyngeal suctioning if the oral suctioning is done last. This practice should be discouraged because it is possible that microorganisms can be transmitted from the patient's nose to the throat.

20. Holding your thumb over the opening in the catheter, apply suction for no longer than 15 seconds. As a beginner, practice holding your breath during the suctioning period to help you remember *that the patient is not receiving oxygen or inspiring while you suction.*

When suctioning orally, suction carefully in the cheeks, *where secretions tend to pool.*

21. Withdraw the catheter under suction with a rotating motion. *This action aspirates the secretions protruding from the catheter's tip.*
22. Flush the catheter *to remove secretions.*
23. Using the nondominant hand, turn off the suction *to listen to the patient's breath sounds and assess the need for repeated suctioning.* If the patient's breathing is not clear, repeat steps 18 through 21, allowing the patient to rest 20 to 30 seconds between suctioning periods. It is also good practice to have the patient deep breathe and cough between suctioning periods *to get the secretions up where they can be reached by suctioning.* When the patient's breathing sounds clear, stop suctioning. You should never apply suction more than three times. Sometimes you will stop *because you have not been successful in reaching the secretions. At other times you may be forced to stop because the patient is actively resisting the procedure.* Knowing when to stop suctioning requires good nursing judgment. Remember that this procedure can be tiring, as well as frightening, for the patient.
24. Detach the catheter from the tubing.
25. With your nondominant hand, grasp the cuff of the sterile glove and pull it downward over the used catheter in your gloved hand. Dispose of it safely in a receptacle. *This method neatly encloses the used catheter in the glove, making disposal more sanitary* (Fig. 40–8).

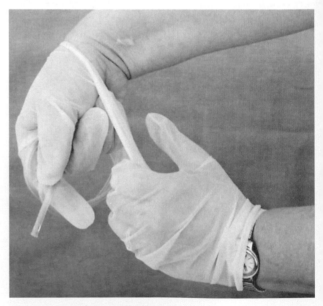

Figure 40–8. Disposing of the suction catheter. The nurse grasps the cuff of the glove and pulls it downward over the used catheter.

26. Reposition the patient *for comfort.*
27. Provide oral hygiene.
28. Wash your hands.

Evaluation
29. Evaluate, using the following criteria:
  a. Breath sounds clear
  b. Vital signs stable
  c. Patient comfortable and calm

Documentation
30. Record the procedure on the patient's chart. Include date, time, and the amount and character of secretions removed. Also note the patient's tolerance of the procedure.

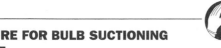

PROCEDURE FOR BULB SUCTIONING AN INFANT

Most infants have minimal secretions and are able to cough, *which effectively clears their air passages.* But *when amniotic fluid in the newborn's passages or in-* *creased mucus production in the infant's lungs causes breathing to become labored,* suctioning must be done to maintain a patent airway.

Assessment
1. Note that usually you do not need a doctor's order for bulb suctioning an infant.
2. Assess the rate and depth of the infant's respirations, as well as breath sounds and chest movements. Note also the pulse rate and skin color. Check the mouth and nose for the presence of secretions.

Planning
3. Wash your hands *for infection control.* Good medical asepsis is all that is necessary in this procedure, *because you are suctioning only in the mouth and nostrils.* Deeper suctioning is usually performed in the nursery by specially prepared nurses.
4. Gather the necessary equipment.
  a. Sterile bulb syringe. (You should begin with a sterile syringe. If frequent suctioning is needed, rinse the bulb well and place it in a clean

DATE/TIME	
8/20/99 4:20 AM	Unresponsive to painful stimuli. Gurgling sounds with respirations. Nasopharyngeal suctioning done with moderate amount thick green mucus obtained. ———— K. Jones, RN

Example of Nursing Progress Notes Using Narrative Format.

DATE/TIME		
8/20/99 0420		Ineffective airway clearance ————
	S	
	O	Unresponsive to painful stimuli. Gurgling sounds with respirations. Moderate amount thick green mucus obtained by nasopharyngeal suctioning. ————
	A	Unable to cough up secretions independently. ————
	P	Recheck respirations hourly and suction prn. ———— K. Jones, RN

Example of Nursing Progress Notes Using SOAP Format.

DATE/TIME		
6/12/99 1020	D:	Patient coughing and pointing to throat. Dusky color. Nods "yes" when asked if wants to be suctioned. ————
	A:	Oral suction performed. ————
	R:	Moderate amount of white tenacious secretions obtained. Patient more relaxed and sleeping. Breathing comfortably with no audible sounds. ———— S. Alton, RN

Example of Nursing Progress Notes Using Focus Format.

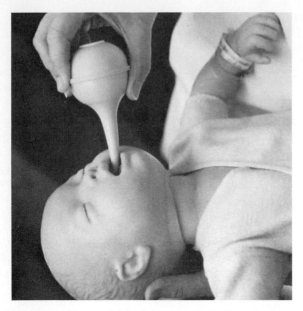

Figure 40–9. The mother is demonstrating bulb suctioning an infant.

towel at the side or foot of the crib for further use. *This is often done for convenience and to decrease response time when suctioning is needed.*)

b. Clean diaper or towel to place under the infant's chin *to protect chest area.*

c. Small container *as a waste receptacle for secretions.*

d. Clean gloves.

Implementation

5. Put on clean gloves *to protect against contact with respiratory secretions.*

6. Wrap the infant in a warm blanket *to prevent chilling.*

7. Position the infant. You can swaddle, or wrap, the infant with a small sheet if necessary (see Module 19, Basic Infant Care). The infant's head should be flat on the surface of the crib. A new-

born can be held "football" fashion, with the head slightly downward. *Gravity will help move secretions from the back of the throat to the mouth, where they can be suctioned more readily.* If the infant is held during the suctioning, swaddling *for restraint* is usually not necessary.

8. Compress the bulb before inserting the syringe tip into the infant's mouth. *Any compression with the syringe tip in the mouth may force secretions deeper into the respiratory tract.*

9. Insert the syringe tip into the mouth and release the bulb to aspirate (Fig. 40–9).

10. Remove the syringe and compress the bulb, expressing the contents into the basin.

11. Repeat steps 8 through 10 until the infant's cheeks and mouth are clear.

12. Carefully suction the nostrils, placing the syringe tip just at each opening. You can use the same syringe, *because it is not entering the nasal passages.*

13. Remove gloves and discard them.

14. Place the infant on the side after suctioning *so any remaining secretions can drain freely.*

15. Wash your hands.

Evaluation

16. Evaluate, using the following criteria:
    a. Breath sounds clear.
    b. Mouth and nose free of secretions.

Documentation

17. Bulb suctioning the infant—particularly the newborn—is often a routine procedure and is not recorded each time it is performed. In some facilities, suctioning is included in a checklist for the infant. If your facility uses such a checklist, enter "bulb" in the method column. Enter any significant observations (unusual color or amount of secretions) in the nursing progress notes.

DATE/TIME	
4/1/99	*Ineffective airway clearance*
1115	*S*
	O Frequent coughing and restlessness. Mildly dusky. Turning head with cough and "spitting" moderate amounts of mucus.
	A Increased secretions, partially interfering with aeration. Possible upper respiratory infection.
	P Observe q 15min and bulb suction prn.
	M. Schultz, RN

Example of Nursing Progress Notes Using SOAP Format.

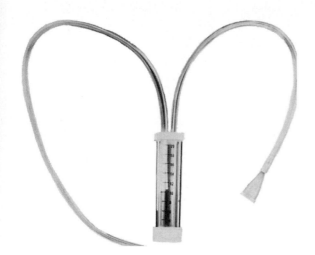

Figure 40–10. DeLee infant aspirator. This device uses mouth suction to achieve the suction pressure. (Courtesy Sherwood Medical, St. Louis, Missouri)

DELEE INFANT ASPIRATOR

A device called a DeLee infant aspirator has traditionally been used to suction newborn infants. This device uses mouth suction applied to a tubing to achieve the suction pressure (Fig. 40–10). Secretions fall into a small receptacle attached to the tubing. The same general procedure used for bulb suctioning can be used for the DeLee infant aspirator.

The DeLee suction method is commonly used in the labor and delivery unit to identify whether amniotic fluid has been aspirated by the infant during the birth process. Although the secretions do not reach the mouth of the nurse who is aspirating, *air passes through the secretions and could potentially transmit microorganisms.* It is prudent practice not to use this device on any infant suspected of having an infection.

CLEANING THE SUCTION APPARATUS

Empty the receptacle for suction secretions frequently, *because it has the potential for growing many pathogenic microorganisms. In addition, it is aesthetically unpleasant for staff, patients, and visitors.* Emptying after each use is recommended. When emptying the suction secretion container, empty it into the toilet in the room or take it to a utility sink. Do not empty it into a sink in the patient's room *because the secretions tend to stay in the sink and are difficult to rinse away.* Always rinse the container with cold water *because hot water tends to coagulate protein and make the secretions more difficult to rinse off.* Wear clean gloves while emptying the container *to protect yourself from contact with the secretions.* Replace the container frequently; check your facility's policy to determine frequency.

CRITICAL THINKING EXERCISES

When assessing a semicomatose patient, you identified that the patient needed suctioning. You attempted to provide nasopharyngeal suctioning through the left nostril, but found you were unable to pass the catheter. You changed to the oral route, but the agitated patient bit on the suction catheter. Analyze this situation. What other assessment data could you have used before you began? What data should you collect at this time? What nursing actions might effectively assist in clearing this patient's airway? Explain how you might involve others in your planning.

✔ PERFORMANCE CHECKLIST

Procedure for Oral and Nasopharyngeal Suctioning	Needs More Practice	Satisfactory	Comments
Assessment			
1. Check for doctor's order if this is facility's policy.			
2. Carefully assess patient's need for suctioning before proceeding.			
3. Be familiar with equipment available and details of procedure as performed in the facility.			
Planning			
4. Wash your hands.			
5. Plan for any needed assistance.			
6. Choose appropriate equipment for route of suctioning planned.			
Implementation			
7. Identify the patient.			
8. Explain what you are going to do.			
9. If room lighting is inadequate, secure additional lighting.			
10. Position patient. a. Oropharyngeal suctioning: Semi-Fowler's with head toward you.			
b. Nasopharyngeal suctioning: Semi-Fowler's with neck hyperextended.			
c. Unconscious: Lateral position facing you.			
11. Place drape or clean towel across patient's chest and hyperoxygenate the patient if needed.			
12. Provide a sterile field.			
13. Set up sterile container and pour solution (if not in kit).			
14. Connect tubing to suctioning equipment.			
15. Turn on suction mechanism and test by placing thumb over end of tube.			
16. Put on sterile gloves.			

(continued)

Procedure for Oral and Nasopharyngeal Suctioning *(Continued)*	Needs More Practice	Satisfactory	Comments
17. Pick up catheter with dominant hand and using nondominant hand, attach connector end to suction tubing.			
18. Test equipment by suctioning water through tubing and catheter.			
19. Insert catheter, using either the oral or the nasopharyngeal route and described procedure.			
20. Apply suction by closing the system.			
21. Withdraw catheter.			
22. Flush catheter with sterile water to remove secretions.			
23. Turn off suction and listen to patient's breath sounds. Repeat suctioning if needed.			
24. Detach catheter from tubing and discard it.			
25. Pull glove downward over used catheter, enclosing it for disposal.			
26. Reposition patient for comfort.			
27. Provide oral hygiene.			
28. Wash your hands.			
Evaluation			
29. Evaluate, using the following criteria: a. Breath sounds clear			
b. Vital signs stable			
c. Patient comfortable and calm			
Documentation			
30. Document procedure and pertinent observations.			
Procedure for Bulb Suctioning an Infant			
Assessment			
1. Note that doctor's order usually not needed.			
2. Assess rate and depth of infant's respirations, breath sounds, and chest movements. Check pulse rate, skin color, and mouth and nose for secretions.			

(continued)

Procedure for Bulb Suctioning an Infant *(Continued)*	Needs More Practice	Satisfactory	Comments
Planning			
3. Wash your hands.			
4. Gather necessary equipment.			
Implementation			
5. Put on clean gloves.			
6. Wrap infant in warm blanket.			
7. Either swaddle infant or hold "football" fashion for stability.			
8. Compress bulb before inserting syringe tip in infant's mouth.			
9. Insert syringe tip into mouth and release bulb to aspirate.			
10. Remove syringe and compress bulb, expressing contents into basin.			
11. Repeat steps 8–10 until tract is clear.			
12. Carefully suction nostrils, placing tip just at each opening.			
13. Remove gloves and discard them.			
14. Place infant on his or her side.			
15. Wash your hands.			
Evaluation			
16. Evaluate, using the following criteria: **a.** Breath sounds clear			
b. Mouth and nose free of secretions			
Documentation			
17. Record any pertinent observations or according to the facility's policy.			

MODULE

41

TRACHEOSTOMY CARE AND SUCTIONING

MODULE CONTENTS

PREREQUISITES

Successful completion of the following modules:

1996 by Lippincott-Raven Publishers

OVERALL OBJECTIVE

To care for patients with tracheostomies appropriately and to perform suctioning through the tracheostomy safely and effectively.

SPECIFIC LEARNING OBJECTIVES

Know Facts and Principles	Apply Facts and Principles	Demonstrate Ability	Evaluate Performance
1. General considerations			
a. Definition			
Define *tracheostomy*.			
b. Indications for tracheostomy			
State two reasons for tracheostomy.	Given a patient situation, state rationale for tracheostomy.	In the clinical setting, state why a patient has a tracheostomy.	Evaluate with instructor.
c. Types of tracheostomy tubes			
Name two types of tracheostomy tubes and advantages and disadvantages of each.	In the practice setting, identify various types of tubes.	In the clinical setting, identify type of tube in use for a patient.	Evaluate own performance with instructor.
d. Safety factors			
State three important safety measures and rationale for each.	Given a patient situation, state safety measures appropriate to that situation.	In the clinical setting, carry out measures safely with patient.	Evaluate performance with instructor.
2. Tracheostomy suctioning			
a. Equipment			
Describe equipment used in tracheal suctioning.	In the practice setting, select and adapt equipment correctly.	In the clinical setting, use appropriate equipment in manner described.	Evaluate with instructor.
b. Procedure			
State information to be given to patient. Know correct positioning. Explain use of sterile technique. State distance catheter is inserted for shallow or deep suctioning. Describe method and how long to apply pressure.	In the practice setting, role play appropriate patient teaching and nurse–patient interaction. In the practice setting, correctly plan and carry out tracheostomy suctioning on a manikin.	In the clinical setting, carry out appropriate nurse–patient interaction and patient teaching. In the clinical setting, correctly suction the patient with a tracheostomy.	Evaluate interaction with instructor. Evaluate own performance with instructor using Performance Checklist.

(continued)

SPECIFIC LEARNING OBJECTIVES (continued)

Know Facts and Principles	Apply Facts and Principles	Demonstrate Ability	Evaluate Performance
c. Documentation State what needs to be documented.	Given a patient situation, identify pertinent information to be documented.	In the clinical setting, record accurately on patient's record.	Evaluate documentation format and content with instructor.
3. Cleaning and dressing *a. Equipment* Name equipment needed for cleaning and dressing tracheostomy.	Given a specific situation, select and assemble equipment correctly.	In the clinical setting, correctly use equipment and materials.	Evaluate with instructor.
b. Procedure State explanation to be given to patient. Know correct positioning. Explain use of sterile equipment. List steps in cleaning and dressing procedure.	In the practice setting, correctly clean and dress a tracheostomy.	In the clinical setting, carry out cleaning and dressing procedure.	Evaluate own performance with instructor using Performance Checklist.
c. Documentation State items to be documented.	Given a patient situation, identify pertinent information to be documented.	In the clinical setting, record accurately on patient's chart.	Evaluate documentation format and content with instructor.

LEARNING ACTIVITIES

1. Review the Specific Learning Objectives.
2. Read the section on the respiratory system in the chapter on basic vital functions in Ellis and Nowlis, *Nursing: A Human Needs Approach,* or comparable material in another textbook.
3. Look up the module vocabulary terms in the glossary.
4. Read through the module as though you were preparing to teach the contents to another person. Mentally practice the skills.
5. Review the Performance Checklist.
6. In the practice setting, do the following:
   a. Examine the various tracheostomy tubes available.
   b. Select and gather the equipment for suctioning a tracheostomy.
   c. If a tube can be attached to a manikin, use the Performance Checklist as a guide and practice suctioning the tracheostomy.
   d. Gather the equipment for cleaning a tube and changing a dressing.
   e. Following the Performance Checklist, practice cleaning the tube and changing the dressing.
   f. When you think you are prepared to demonstrate the skills, ask your instructor to evaluate your performance.
7. In the clinical setting, consult with your instructor for an opportunity to care for and suction a patient with a tracheostomy.

VOCABULARY

Ambu bag	catheter	hypoxia	respirator
apnea	clockwise	inflatable cuff	sordes
asphyxiation	counterclockwise	lumen	suction
aspirate	dead-air space	mucus	trachea
bronchi	fenestrated	necrosis	tracheal ring
button	tracheostomy tube	obturator	tracheostomy
cannula	hydrogen peroxide	prophylactic	

Tracheostomy Care and Suctioning

Rationale for the Use of This Skill

Because patients with tracheostomies are commonly cared for in a variety of healthcare settings, the nurse must be familiar with the special care required and the variations needed for suctioning such patients. Normally, the upper respiratory passages protect the trachea, filtering out foreign material and providing some protection from microorganisms. Because the tracheostomy opens directly into the trachea, which is highly susceptible to infection, the nurse must have a thorough knowledge of sterile technique to care for and suction a tracheostomy. In addition, a patent airway must be maintained constantly.[1]

▼ NURSING DIAGNOSES

Risk for Infection is always present in the patient with a tracheostomy *because the protection of the upper respiratory tract has been disrupted.* Much of the care described in this module is directed toward preventing infection by using correct technique when caring for a tracheostomy.

Suctioning is needed for an individual with a nursing diagnosis of Ineffective Airway Clearance. The tracheostomy tube irritates the respiratory tract and causes an increase in secretions. If the patient is not able to cough these secretions out effectively, this nursing diagnosis is present, and you will need to suction the patient *to remove secretions.*

Risk for Aspiration related to tracheostomy tube placement is an appropriate nursing diagnosis for people using ventilation devices that *may obstruct the respiratory tract.*

The patient with a tracheostomy tube in place is unable to speak except when a fenestrated tube is used or when the regular tracheostomy tube is "buttoned" or occluded. This is because the vocal cords are above the tracheostomy opening. For this reason, the nursing diagnosis of Impaired Verbal Communication is often appropriate.

Another appropriate nursing diagnosis is Body Image Disturbance, *because any alteration in what is considered normal functioning by the patient and others can produce stress.*

[1]Note that rationales for action are emphasized throughout the module by the use of italics.

TRACHEOSTOMY

A tracheostomy is a surgical incision into the trachea *to insert a tube through which the patient can breathe more easily and secretions can be removed.* At one time, the procedure was performed only as an emergency measure *to allow a critically ill patient to breathe when life was imminently threatened by respiratory obstruction.* In current practice, a tracheostomy is performed more commonly *as a prophylactic procedure so that secretions in the respiratory tract can be removed more effectively before a patient's breathing is severely compromised.* A tracheostomy may also be performed *to decrease the amount of dead-air space in the airway and thus reduce the effort of breathing.* In some instances, the procedure is done *so that a ventilator can be used to breathe for the patient.* Another purpose is to provide an effective airway when swelling is expected, such as after surgery on the neck.

The surgeon usually performs the tracheostomy in the operating room or the critical care unit. In emergency situations, it may be performed in the emergency room or even on a patient care unit. A small, horizontal incision is made just below the first tracheal ring, and a tracheostomy tube is inserted. In most cases, this is a temporary measure. Once the patient can tolerate temporary closure (sometimes referred to as "buttoning"), starting with short periods and gradually moving to longer ones, the tracheostomy tube is removed, and the incision heals.

Tracheostomy Tubes

Tracheostomy tubes are composed of three parts: an outer cannula, an inner cannula, and an obturator. The outer cannula (tube) fits through the tracheostomy opening and should rest comfortably on the surrounding tissue but never so tightly that it causes erosion or irritation. This cannula is curved and has a flange near the upper opening, which rests against the surface of the neck. Ties attached to this flange secure the cannula to the patient's neck. Inside the outer cannula is an inner cannula, which has a slightly smaller diameter. A latch usually holds this cannula securely and allows it to be removed for cleaning of both cannulas. An obturator with a smooth, oval end fits inside the inner cannula and protrudes from the end. *This makes it easier for the physician to insert the tracheostomy tube through the opening into the trachea* (Fig. 41–1), and it is removed once the tube is in place.

The size of the tube used is usually the choice of the physician who performs the procedure and inserts the tube. Most tubes are available in standard sizes: 0 to 12 or French 24 to 44.

DATE/TIME		
11/8/99 *1000*	*D:*	*Patient has cuffed 32 French tracheostomy tube in place.*
		Appears anxious, attempting to talk.
	A:	*Touched patient, indicated that it is the tube that prevents*
		talking. Obtained paper and pencil for patient.
	R:	*Smiling, wrote phone number of son and his wishes to have son*
		visit.
		D. Martinez, RN

Example of Nursing Progress Notes Using Focus Format.

Tracheostomy tubes are most commonly made of plastic, but silver tubes also are available. The plastic tube has a larger lumen and is softer than the metal tube. It molds more easily to the trachea, so *it causes less irritation and is more comfortable for the patient.* Plastic tracheostomy tubes are disposable; metal tubes may be cleaned, sterilized, and reused by that patient.

Most tracheostomy tubes used today are cuffed plastic tubes. These have a foam or inflatable cuff that surrounds the outer cannula. A cuffed tracheostomy tube is required if the patient is ventilated *to provide a closed system.* The cuff also *prevents air leaks and aspiration of secretions or vomitus from the upper airway into the lungs* (Fig. 41–2).

If a patient has a tube with a firm inflatable cuff, the cuff can be deflated *to prevent pressure necrosis or erosion of the tracheal lining.* The cuff is usually deflated for 10 minutes of each hour or as the physician orders. Any accumulated oral secretions should be suctioned before the cuff is deflated *to prevent them from going deeper into the trachea when the cuff is deflated.* While the cuff is deflated, take special precautions to ensure that the tapes are secure and the tracheostomy tube is in the proper position *so that it is not coughed out.* This is not a problem if the tube has a double cuff, *because one cuff remains inflated while the other is deflated, providing alternating pressure areas and preventing necrosis.* Many tubes have soft, pliable cuffs that can remain inflated. Other cuffs are inflated with atmospheric pressure.

The nurse should inspect the equipment for the type of cuff and follow the procedure recommended by the manufacturer or the facility. It is essential to check the cuff pressure frequently. A pressure gauge, available through most respiratory therapy departments, is attached to a port on the cuff. By turning a stop-cock mechanism on the gauge, the nurse can see the number on the gauge, indicating the amount of pressure in the cuff.

A fenestrated tracheostomy tube is designed with openings that allow air to pass through the larynx and into the upper airway from the lungs. A fenestrated tube allows an individual to talk while the tracheostomy is in place. It can also be used as a step toward removal of the tracheostomy (Fig. 41–3).

One approach to determining whether an individual can function without a tracheostomy tube in place is to close the tube, usually with a "button," which requires air to move around the sides of the tracheostomy tube (or through the fenestration) as it passes from the upper airway to the lungs and then exits (Fig. 41–4).

Safety Measures

Preventing infection to the wound and to the bronchi and lungs is crucial when caring for a tracheostomy. If a patient has a new or recent tracheostomy, sterile tech-

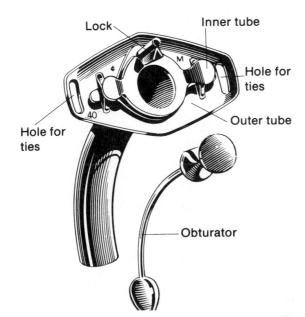

Figure 41–1. The parts of a tracheostomy tube. (Courtesy Pilling Company, Fort Washington, Pennsylvania)

Lock
Inner tube
Hole for ties
Hole for ties
Outer tube
Obturator

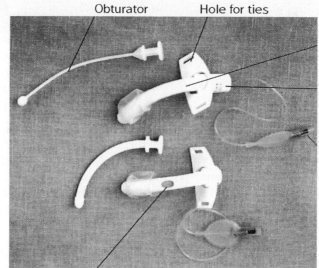

Obturator   Hole for ties

Outer tube with cuff
and inflating tube

Inner cannula

Inflating tube

Opening in fenestrated tube

Figure 41–2. Two types of plastic cuffed tracheostomy tubes.

nique is used when cleaning the tracheostomy or changing the dressing. In home settings and some long-term care facilities, good handwashing and clean technique are used when cleaning or dressing a long-standing tracheostomy. Regardless of how long a patient has had the tracheostomy, sterile technique is always used when suctioning.

Emergency equipment should be kept at the bedside *in case the tracheostomy tube becomes dislodged or is coughed out, allowing the opening to close.* Many acute care facilities have a policy requiring that an extra tracheostomy set be kept at the bedside of a patient with a new tracheostomy. During the acute care period, if the tube becomes accidentally dislodged, the opening may close, occluding breathing. This set contains a clamp *that can quickly be inserted into the opening to maintain patency.* If it is not the policy to have a complete set at the bedside, a sterile clamp and a tube of the correct size and type should be kept there. A new sterile tube is then inserted. If a tube is dislodged or coughed out by a person with a well-established tracheostomy, the opening usually remains patent because healing has taken place.

If cloth material or gauze is used in tracheostomy care, it must be lint-free *to avoid the possibility of aspirating particles into the respiratory tract.* For this reason, the nurse should not use cut cloth or cut gauze for tracheostomy care.

A patient with a tracheostomy must be constantly and carefully watched. Although the person is unable to speak, an alert patient can summon help

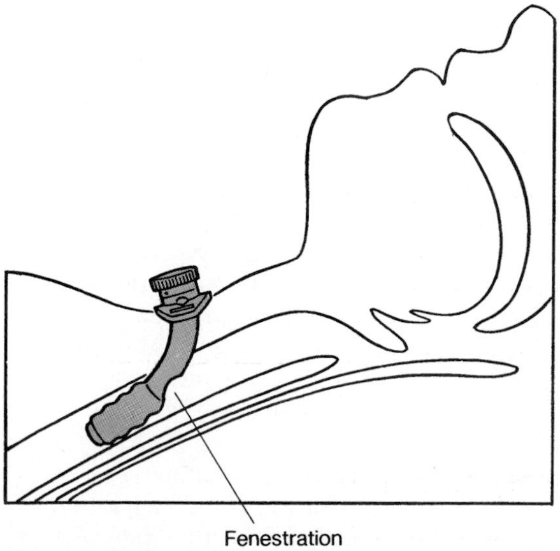

Fenestration

Figure 41–3. A fenestrated tracheostomy tube (often called a "talking trach").

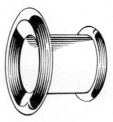

Figure 41–4. Tracheostomy button. When a "button" is in place, air passes from the upper airway to the lungs and back out, moving around the sides of the tracheostomy tube. (Courtesy Pilling Company, Fort Washington, Pennsylvania)

by using a call bell placed within easy reach. This action *provides safety*.

PROCEDURE FOR SUCTIONING THE TRACHEOSTOMY

The procedure for tracheal suctioning is similar to that described for nasopharyngeal suctioning in Module 40, Oral and Nasopharyngeal Suctioning. If the patient with a tracheostomy is on a ventilator, the procedure is more complex and requires advanced skills not included in this module.

Suctioning the trachea and bronchi decreases the oxygen available to the lungs and causes collapse of alveoli. The result is hypoxemia (a lowered blood oxygen level). *To prevent hypoxemia*, you must hyperventilate the patient with 100% oxygen immediately before and after suctioning. Many ventilators can be set to provide hyperventilation when it is needed, or you can use a breathing bag, commonly referred to as an Ambu bag, attached to oxygen. Some equipment is structured so that the breathing bag can be attached directly to the tracheostomy or endotracheal tube. In other cases, the breathing bag is attached to a T-shaped piece on the tracheostomy tube.

To use the breathing bag effectively and still maintain sterility of the suction catheter, two people should work together on tracheostomy suctioning, although an experienced, skillful individual may be able to do this procedure effectively alone. The procedure presented here is for two people working together. The individual handling the suction equipment is designated person 1, and the individual handling the breathing bag is designated person 2. All steps are done by person 1 except those that specify person 2.

When the patient is very stable, hyperventilation may be omitted. If you are not using hyperventilation, omit the steps that refer to person 2.

Assessment

1. Assess the needs of the patient with a tracheostomy for suctioning and cleaning. *This assessment is especially critical because many of these patients are comatose, and most conscious patients cannot talk because of the tracheal opening.*

If suctioning, cleaning, and a dressing change are all needed, suction first *so that the tube and dressing will remain clean.* While giving care, always observe the incision for redness and swelling, which *can be symptoms of infection or irritation. Suctioning removes oxygen, causes tissue irritation, and increases secretions,* so use discretion when performing this procedure. Also, for tra-

cheostomies, do not suction longer than 10 seconds at any one time.

To assess the patient, listen to the breath sounds. These should be quiet, not labored. If the respirations are labored and you hear the movement of secretions (a gurgling sound), the patient needs suctioning. You can also observe the condition of the tubes.

Planning

2. Wash your hands *for infection control.*
3. Obtain the necessary equipment. Some items may already be at the bedside. Commercial suctioning kits, which contain the essential items you will need, are available. If the kits are not used in your facility, gather the following:
   a. Sterile gloves
   b. Sterile suction catheter
   c. Sterile basin
   d. Sterile water or sterile normal saline
   e. Sterile syringe and normal saline if saline is to be instilled
   f. Sterile gauze squares
   g. Portable suction machine if wall suction is not available
   h. Self-inflating breathing bag (Ambu bag)
   i. Eye protection (goggles or eyeglasses)
   j. Mask
   k. Suction trap, if a sputum specimen is needed

Implementation

4. Identify the patient *to be sure you are performing the procedure on the correct patient.*
5. Provide privacy.
6. Explain the procedure. If the patient is responsive, it is imperative to explain the procedure carefully. *Without proper psychological preparation, the patient may fear choking or hemorrhaging.* An explanation should also be given to the unresponsive patient, *because the patient often understands even though unable to respond.* The responsive patient should be asked to cough to raise secretions *so they are more easily suctioned.*
7. *Because the patient with a tracheostomy usually cannot speak,* establish a way of communicating. *Being able to communicate greatly relieves the patient's feeling of helplessness.* Provide a slate or pencil and paper for the alert patient so he or she can respond to you during the procedure. If the patient cannot write, establish a yes or no signal system.

Tell the patient *that the tracheal opening prevents air from reaching the vocal cords, so speech is not possible.* Later, the patient will be able to speak by placing a button or finger over the opening, thus forcing air around the tube.

8. Test the suction apparatus.
  a. Turn on either the wall suction or the portable suction machine.
  b. Place your thumb over the end of the un-sterile tubing that is attached to the suction equipment and test for "pull."
  suction regulated to a range of effi-sually low to medium.
  tient supine or in mid-Fowler's position. Turn the patient's head slightly toward you *so that the chin is out of the way and you can see better.* Place the unconscious patient in the lateral position facing you.
10. Put on eye protection and mask *to prevent contact with secretions.*
11. Prepare 5 mL sterile saline in a syringe, if this is the policy. *The properties of normal saline may help liquefy thickened respiratory secretions,* although this is not supported by research. Remove the needle *for safety.*
12. Open the sterile suction set, and prepare the equipment.
  a. Place the drape from the kit or a clean towel over the patient's chest to *protect the gown or clothing.*
  b. Most kits contain a packet of saline solution, sterile gloves, the sterile suction catheter, and sterile gauze squares. If your kit contains all this equipment, first put on the sterile gloves.
  c. Pour the saline into the basin.
  d. Hold the catheter in your dominant hand, and use the nondominant hand to hold the suction tubing, to control the suction, and to handle any other nonsterile object. *The nondominant hand is now contaminated* and cannot touch the catheter. *The glove will protect you from contact with secretions and protect the patient from microorganisms.*
    If the solution is not in the kit, you will need to set up the basin carefully, touching only the outside, and move the glove package to one side. Pour the saline from the original container into the basin, and then put your sterile gloves on and proceed. Rinse the catheter in the normal saline solution.
13. Person 2 attaches the breathing bag to the oxygen source and prepares to ventilate the patient.
14. Person 2 attaches the breathing bag to the tracheostomy tube and provides three deep breaths coordinated with the patient's breathing pattern.
15. Instill the normal saline into the tracheostomy if this is the policy.
16. Control the suction with your unsterile gloved hand while suctioning with your sterile hand.

  a. Insert the catheter 4 to 5 in into the tracheostomy without occluding the port on the suction catheter so that suction is not being applied. *Suctioning at this time would further deprive the patient of oxygen.*
  b. Apply suction by closing the system. This is usually done by placing your thumb over the port or side opening at the base of the catheter. The patient may cough in response to the irritation caused by the catheter, *which helps to raise secretions.* Persistent coughing *can indicate tracheal spasm,* in which case you should stop the procedure.
  c. Apply suction for only 10 seconds (per entry). *Remember that the patient cannot breathe during the procedure.* (You can hold your own breath while suctioning *to help you time the procedure.*) If oxygen is ordered, administer after each period of suctioning.
  d. Withdraw the catheter, rotating it gently while you continue suctioning, *so higher secretions are removed and are not tracked through the lumen of the tracheostomy.*
  e. Rinse the catheter with sterile water or normal saline.
  f. Person 2 provides ventilation immediately after the suction catheter is removed *to supply needed oxygen.*
17. Observe the patient for dyspnea and skin color changes.
18. If these symptoms of hypoxia occur, person 2 immediately provides additional deep breaths of oxygen *to reverse hypoxia.*
19. Turn off the suction and listen for clear breath sounds.
20. If breathing is not clear, repeat steps 16a through e.
21. If the breathing sounds clear, person 2 uses the breathing bag to provide three or four deep breaths of oxygen *to oxygenate the patient fully.*
22. Disconnect the catheter from the suction tubing.
23. Grasp the cuff of the sterile glove, and pull the glove down over the used catheter. *This method makes disposal of the equipment more sanitary.* Remove eye protection and mask.
24. Discard all disposable equipment, and take nondisposable equipment to the appropriate location for cleaning.
25. Wash your hands.
26. Provide oral hygiene.

Evaluation
27. Evaluate, using the following criteria:
  a. Tracheostomy tube securely in place
  b. Respiratory rate and depth normal

DATE/TIME	
10/2/99 9:15 AM	*Respirations noisy and labored. Not coughing. Tracheostomy* *suctioned. 5 ml normal saline instilled. Mod am't thick, white* *mucus obtained. Respirations quiet after suctioning. Vital signs* *remained stable. Skin reddened around tube. —— B. Cook, RN*

Example of Nursing Progress Notes Using Narrative Format.

   c. Breath sounds clear
   d. Patient resting comfortably

Documentation

28. Document the procedure and your observations on the patient's chart. Some facilities have a flow sheet for this purpose. The entry should include the amount and description of secretions and the patient's response to the procedure.

PROCEDURE FOR ADMINISTERING TRACHEOSTOMY CARE

Assessment

1. Check the tracheostomy frequently *because the opening can become obstructed by secretions.* Never allow the patient to reach the point of labored breathing. Clean by necessity, not by a definite schedule *because some patients have more secretions than others.* For example, cleaning and dressing the tracheostomy once per shift may be adequate for some patients, but more frequent care (two or three times per shift) may be necessary for others.

Planning

2. Wash your hands *for infection control.*
3. Gather the equipment you will need. Commer-

cial tracheostomy care kits that contain the necessary items are available (Fig 41–5). If your facility does not use such kits, obtain the following equipment:

   a. Sterile gloves, if the tracheostomy has recently been performed, *to prevent the wound from becoming infected*
   b. 4 × 4 gauze squares
   c. Cleansing solution (often a hydrogen peroxide mixture or saline)
   d. Basin
   e. Tracheostomy brush, pipe cleaners, or swabs *to clean the cannula surfaces*
   f. Sterile water. If you plan to change the tracheostomy dressing at this time, you will also want to obtain the equipment for that procedure *to avoid making another trip out of the room for needed supplies.* Add the equipment listed in step 3 of the Procedure for Changing the Tracheostomy Dressing, page 218.

Implementation

4. Identify the patient *to be sure you are performing the procedure on the correct patient.*
5. Provide privacy.
6. Explain what you are going to do. *Many patients are afraid the tube may become dislodged during care.*

DATE/TIME	

10/2/99
9:15 AM
	Ineffective airway clearance ——
	S
	O *Respirations noisy and labored. Not coughing up secretions.*
	    Tracheostomy suctioning with 5 mL normal saline instilled
	    to liquefy secretions produced mod am't thick, white sputum.
	    Respirations quieted. Vital signs remained stable. Skin
	    reddened around tube. ——
	A *Continues unable to clear airway. Secretions decreasing in*
	    amount. Irritation around stoma increasing. ——
	P *Increase frequency of changing tracheostomy dressing to*
	    q4h. Notify Dr. Ryan of increasing irritation. Continue plan
	    for tracheostomy suctioning. —— B. Cook, RN

Example of Nursing Progress Notes Using SOAP Format.

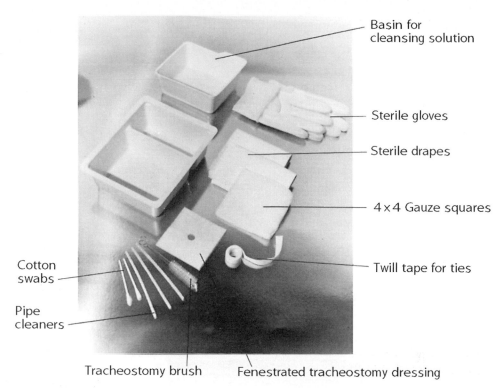

Basin for cleansing solution

Sterile gloves

Sterile drapes

4 × 4 Gauze squares

Twill tape for ties

Cotton swabs

Pipe cleaners

Tracheostomy brush

Fenestrated tracheostomy dressing

Figure 41–5. A commercially prepared tracheostomy care kit. (Courtesy Sherwood Medical, St. Louis, Missouri)

By demonstrating competence, you can reassure the patient.

7. Provide a slate or pencil and paper to the alert patient *for communication.*
8. Place the patient supine or in mid-Fowler's position *to promote comfort and visibility.*
9. Set up the supplies.
10. Put on sterile or clean gloves as necessary.
11. To clean a cannula-type tracheostomy tube:
    a. Hold the outer tube carefully in place with one hand as you turn the lock clockwise with your other hand *to unfasten the inner cannula.*
    b. Slide out the inner cannula by curving it toward you.
    c. Place the inner cannula in the basin.
    d. Immerse the cannula in normal saline or a cleansing solution for a few minutes *to soften dried secretions.*
    e. Apply friction to the cannula with brush, pipe cleaners, or swabs to remove any residue.
    f. Rinse the cannula well in cold sterile water or saline.
    g. Dry the cannula thoroughly with sterile, lint-free gauze or towel.
    h. If the patient's secretions are copious or if the patient coughs while you are cleaning the inner cannula (so that the secretions come in contact with the inside surface of the outer cannula), remove the secretions, and thoroughly dry the inner surfaces as described in step 11g *to prevent the surfaces of the two cannulas from adhering.*
    i. Hold the outer cannula, and replace the clean inner cannula.
    j. Turn the lock counterclockwise *to secure.*
    k. Test to make sure the inner cannula is firmly in place by gently pulling with the fingers.
12. If a plastic tube with no inner cannula is being used, carefully clean the inner surfaces with pipe cleaners or swabs dampened, but not saturated, with normal saline *to prevent aspiration.*
13. If you are planning to change the tracheostomy dressing, move on to step 6 of the Procedure for Changing the Tracheostomy Dressing. If not, complete this procedure.
14. Dispose of the equipment.
15. Wash your hands.

Evaluation

16. Evaluate, using the following criteria:
    a. Tracheostomy tube securely in place
    b. No secretions present
    c. Breath sounds clear

Documentation

17. The procedure is usually documented in conjunction with the dressing change that follows

(see Procedure for Changing the Tracheostomy Dressing below).

PROCEDURE FOR CHANGING THE TRACHEOSTOMY DRESSING

Changing the tracheostomy dressing is usually done at the time of cleaning, but in some situations, it may be needed more frequently.

Assessment

1. *Because a tracheostomy is prone to infection,* dressings should always be clean and intact. Change the dressing routinely after giving tracheostomy care. At other times, assess the patient for any appreciable amount of drainage or soiling of the dressing, which indicates the need for changing.

Planning

2. Wash your hands *for infection control.*
3. Obtain a tracheostomy care kit, or gather the following items:
   a. 4 × 4 gauze squares or special tracheostomy dressings
   b. Twill tape ties
   c. Scissors
   d. Swabs
   e. Cleansing solution
   f. Oral care equipment
   g. One pair of clean gloves and one pair of sterile gloves
   h. Bag for soiled dressings

Implementation

4. Identify the patient *to be sure you are performing the procedure on the correct patient.*
5. Provide privacy.
6. Explain what you are going to do.
7. Put on clean gloves, and remove the soiled dressing and discard it.
   a. Hold the tube in place while you remove the soiled dressing.
   b. To do this, place one hand gently around the tube *to keep it secure* as you carefully remove the soiled gauze.
8. Remove contaminated gloves. Place gloves and soiled dressing in a plastic bag, and wash hands.
9. Put on sterile gloves.
10. With sterile swabs moistened in saline or hydrogen peroxide solution, clean around the edges of the tracheostomy opening.
11. Note any redness or swelling of the wound margins.
12. Prepare the dressing. Use a precut tracheostomy dressing or a 4 × 4 gauze square.

a. Open the first fold of a 4 × 4 gauze square if you are using plain gauze squares.
b. Fold it in half lengthwise.
c. Fold each end toward the center (Fig. 41–6). This type of dressing eliminates the need to cut the material, *which could expose the patient to free lint that could be inhaled.*

13. Apply light pressure to the tube *to prevent dislodging it;* while you cut the soiled tape, remove it and discard.
14. Carefully slip the prepared dressing, ends extending up, around the tube. With the tube held in place, apply tapes (Fig. 41–7).
   a. Thread the tape through the flange on one side of the tube.
   b. Bring the tape around the back of the patient's neck.
   c. Thread the loose end through the remaining flange. It is possible to develop the dexterity to hold the tracheostomy tube with the nondominant hand and use the dominant hand to remove the old tape and fasten the new. After you have attached both new tapes, hold the ties firmly while you tie them

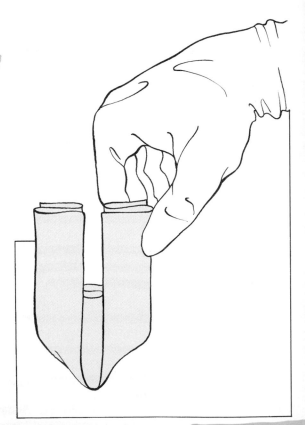

Figure 41–6. Tracheostomy dressing. Open a 4 × 4 gauze square, fold it in half lengthwise, and place it around the tube with ends up.

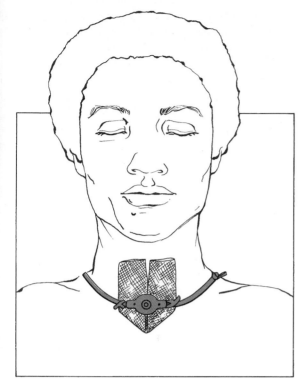

Figure 41–7. Tapes holding the tracheostomy tube in place. The tape is tied to the side to prevent pressure when the patient is supine.

enough so there is not undue pressure on tissues. It is helpful for you or the patient to hold a finger under the tape as it is tightened *to allow for slack.*

15. Check the placement of the tube.
16. Perform oral care, following the guidelines in Module 18, Hygiene. *Because a patient with a tracheostomy has a changed breathing pattern (without air moving freely through the mouth), the oral cavity becomes dry and there is a build-up of sordes and bacteria. This condition can cause odor, which is distressing to the patient and to those providing care. Because the patient needs meticulous oral care frequently, make this procedure part of the general tracheostomy care so that it is neither forgotten nor neglected.*
17. Dispose of the equipment.
18. Remove your gloves, and wash your hands.

Evaluation

19. Evaluate, using the following criteria:
    a. Tracheostomy tube securely in place
    b. No redness or swelling present
    c. No secretions present
    d. Dressing and tapes clean and dry
    e. Absence of stale or foul-smelling breath

Documentation

20. Document the procedure and any observations, such as status of the surrounding skin and the amount and type of drainage.

around the neck. The knot should be to the side *to prevent discomfort when the patient is supine.*

d. Tie the tapes at the side of the neck *tightly enough so the tube is held securely but loosely*

DATE/TIME	
9/17/99 2:15 PM	Tracheostomy stoma cleaned with H₂O₂. Clean drsg applied. Small amount of serosanguineous exudate noted on old drsg. Skin around stoma intact with no redness or edema. S. Burns, NS

Example of Nursing Progress Notes Using Narrative Format.

DATE/TIME	
9/17/99 1415	Impaired skin integrity: new trach stoma
	S
	O Small amount serosanguineous exudate on old drsg. Stoma cleaned with H₂O₂ and clean drsg applied. Skin around stoma intact with no redness or edema.
	A Stoma healing.
	P Continue with cleansing and drsg changes q4h. S. Burns, NS

Example of Nursing Progress Notes Using SOAP Format.

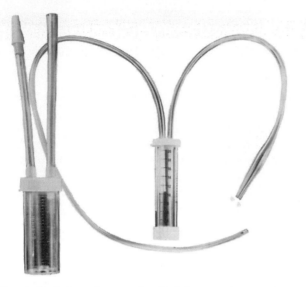

Figure 41–8. A suction trap for obtaining a sputum specimen. (Courtesy Sherwood Medical, St. Louis, Missouri)

OBTAINING A SPUTUM SPECIMEN THROUGH A TRACHEOSTOMY

A sputum specimen may be obtained when you are suctioning a tracheostomy. Use a special suction trap (Fig. 41–8) with two outlets. One outlet is attached to the suction catheter, and the other is attached to the tubing from the suction source. As the sputum is suctioned, a specimen is collected in the container. The entire container is then sent to the laboratory. *This protects the specimen from the possibility of outside contamination, and it protects healthcare workers from contact with the sputum.*

LONG-TERM CARE

The same general procedures for suctioning, caring for, and changing a tracheostomy dressing are used in long-term care settings and acute care settings. You may use clean technique when cleaning or changing a dressing for a tracheostomy that has been in place for a long time. Always use sterile technique for suctioning.

HOME CARE

Caring for the client who returns home with a tracheostomy requires that the client and family members be taught not only how to perform the various aspects of care, but also how to recognize reportable signs and symptoms and how to respond in an emergency. Initially, the client and family members may feel inadequate to the task. However, with complete written instructions and opportunities to observe the nurse and practice the skills, they can provide competent and knowledgeable care.

CRITICAL THINKING EXERCISES

• Your alert, 61-year-old patient has been transferred from the critical care unit with a tracheostomy. Identify the risks and concerns for care that are present because of the tracheostomy. With each risk or concern identified, describe the nursing actions that may prevent the patient from being placed at risk or those that are appropriate for alleviating patient concerns.

• Your patient who has a tracheostomy is to return home. Imagine you are the staff nurse teaching the care provider how to care for and dress the tracheostomy. Identify which specific teaching instructions you should give. Use this scenario as a health teaching exercise.

✔ PERFORMANCE CHECKLIST

Procedure for Suctioning the Tracheostomy	Needs More Practice	Satisfactory	Comments
Assessment			
1. Assess needs of patient for suctioning by listening to breath sounds and involving patient.			
Planning			
2. Wash your hands.			
3. Obtain a tracheostomy suctioning kit or gather the following: **a.** Sterile gloves			
b. Sterile suction catheter			
c. Sterile basin			
d. Sterile water or sterile normal saline			
e. Sterile syringe and normal saline if saline is to be instilled			
f. Sterile gauze squares			
g. Portable suction machine if wall suction is not available			
h. Self-inflating breathing bag (Ambubag)			
i. Eye protection			
j. Mask			
k. Suction trap, if needed			
Implementation			
4. Identify the patient.			
5. Provide privacy.			
6. Explain procedure carefully to the patient.			
7. Establish a way patient can communicate.			
8. Test suction apparatus.			
9. Position the patient: Supine or mid-Fowler's with head slightly toward you if conscious; lateral position facing you if unconscious.			
10. Put on eye protection and mask.			
11. Prepare 5 mL sterile saline in a syringe; remove needle.			

(*continued*)

Procedure for Suctioning the Tracheostomy *(Continued)*	Needs More Practice	Satisfactory	Comments
12. Open kit and prepare equipment. **a.** Place drape or towel over patient's chest.			
b. Put on gloves.			
c. Open and pour saline.			
d. Attach catheter to suction tubing, and moisten catheter in normal saline solution.			
13. Person 2 attaches breathing bag to oxygen source.			
14. Person 2 attaches breathing bag to tracheostomy tube and provides three breaths.			
15. Instill saline into tracheostomy.			
16. Suction: **a.** Insert catheter 4–5 in without applying suction.			
b. Close system to apply suction.			
c. Apply suction for 10 seconds.			
d. Rotate catheter while withdrawing it.			
e. Rinse catheter in sterile water or normal saline.			
f. Person 2 provides ventilation immediately after suction catheter removed.			
17. Observe for dyspnea and skin color changes.			
18. If necessary, person 2 provides additional deep breaths.			
19. Turn off suction and listen to respirations.			
20. If breathing is not clear, repeat steps 16a–e.			
21. When breathing is clear, person 2 provides three or four deep breaths.			
22. Disconnect the catheter from the suction tubing.			
23. Pull sterile glove over catheter to cover it, and remove eye protection and mask.			
24. Discard disposable equipment, and take nondisposable equipment to appropriate place for cleaning.			
25. Wash your hands.			

(continued)

Procedure for Suctioning the Tracheostomy *(Continued)*	Needs More Practice	Satisfactory	Comments
26. Perform oral hygiene.			
Evaluation			
27. Evaluate, using the following criteria: **a.** Tracheostomy tube securely in place			
b. Respiratory rate and depth normal			
c. Breath sounds clear			
d. Patient resting comfortably			
Documentation			
28. Document procedure and observations.			
Administering Tracheostomy Care			
Assessment			
1. Check condition of tracheostomy and need for cleaning.			
Planning			
2. Wash your hands.			
3. Obtain tracheostomy care kit or gather: **a.** Sterile gloves (or clean gloves for long-standing tracheostomy in long-term care facility)			
b. 4 × 4 gauze squares			
c. Cleansing solution, according to policy of facility			
d. Basin			
e. Tracheostomy brush, pipe cleaners, or swabs			
f. Sterile water			
Implementation			
4. Identify the patient.			
5. Provide privacy.			
6. Explain what you are going to do.			
7. Provide method of communication for patient.			
8. Place patient supine or in mid-Fowler's position.			

(continued)

Administering Tracheostomy Care *(Continued)*	Needs More Practice	Satisfactory	Comments
9. Arrange supplies.			
10. Put on sterile or clean gloves.			
11. To clean cannula-type tube: **a.** Hold outer tube with one hand, and turn lock clockwise with other hand.			
b. Slide inner cannula out by sliding toward you.			
c. Place cannula in basin.			
d. Immerse in saline or cleansing solution for several minutes.			
e. Apply friction with brush, pipe cleaners, or swabs.			
f. Rinse well in sterile water.			
g. Dry thoroughly.			
h. If necessary, carefully clean and dry inner aspect of outer cannula.			
i. Hold outer cannula, and replace inner cannula.			
j. Turn lock counterclockwise to engage.			
k. Test to make sure cannula is secure.			
12. If plastic tube does not have an inner cannula, clean inner surfaces of tube.			
13. If you plan to change dressing, move to step 6 of procedure for changing tracheostomy dressing. If not, complete this procedure.			
14. Dispose of equipment.			
15. Wash your hands.			
Evaluation			
16. Evaluate, using the following criteria: **a.** Tracheostomy tube securely in place			
b. No secretions present			
c. Breath sounds clear			
Documentation			
17. Document procedure in conjunction with dressing change.			

(continued)

Procedure for Changing the Tracheostomy Dressing	Needs More Practice	Satisfactory	Comments
Assessment			
1. Although done routinely after tracheostomy care, assess the patient's dressing for drainage or soiling.			
Planning			
2. Wash your hands.			
3. Obtain tracheostomy care kit or gather the following items: **a.** 4 × 4 gauze squares			
b. Twill tape ties			
c. Scissors			
d. Swabs			
e. Cleansing solution			
f. Oral care equipment			
g. One pair clean gloves and one pair sterile gloves			
h. Bag for soiled dressings			
Implementation			
4. Identify the patient.			
5. Provide privacy.			
6. Explain what you are going to do.			
7. Put on clean gloves, and remove old dressing and discard. **a.** Hold tube while you remove dressing.			
b. Place your fingers around tube while you remove dressing.			
8. Remove gloves and wash hands.			
9. Put on sterile gloves.			
10. With sterile, moistened swabs, clean around edges of tracheostomy opening.			
11. Note any redness or swelling.			
12. Prepare the dressing using precut or 4 × 4 gauze squares: **a.** If 4 × 4 gauze, open first fold.			
b. Fold in half lengthwise.			
c. Fold each end toward center.			

(*continued*)

Procedure for Changing the Tracheostomy Dressing *(Continued)*	Needs More Practice	Satisfactory	Comments
13. Secure the tube by gently holding in place. Cut and remove soiled tape.			
14. Position new dressing. **a.** Thread tape through flange on one side.			
b. Bring tape around back of patient's neck.			
c. Pass tape through opposite flange.			
d. Tie tape securely at side of neck.			
15. Check tube placement.			
16. Perform oral care.			
17. Dispose of equipment.			
18. Remove gloves, and wash your hands.			
Evaluation			
19. Evaluate, using the following criteria: **a.** Tracheostomy tube securely in place			
b. No redness or swelling present			
c. No secretions present			
d. Dressing and tapes clean and dry			
e. Absence of stale or foul-smelling breath			
Documentation			
20. Document procedure and any observations, such as status of surrounding skin and amount and type of drainage.			

MODULE

42

CARING FOR PATIENTS WITH CHEST DRAINAGE

MODULE CONTENTS

PREREQUISITES

Successful completion of the following modules:

Review of the anatomy and physiology of the respiratory system, especially the dynamics of breathing.

O V E R A L L   O B J E C T I V E

To assist in the placement and removal of chest tubes; to care for patients with chest drainage safely and appropriately, ensuring proper functioning of the chest drainage system.

S P E C I F I C   L E A R N I N G   O B J E C T I V E S

Know Facts and Principles	Apply Facts and Principles	Demonstrate Ability	Evaluate Performance
1. Rationale for chest tube insertion			
State three reasons for insertion of chest tube(s).	Given a patient situation, state the reason for the placement of the chest tube(s).	In the clinical setting, identify the reason(s) for the placement of chest tube(s) in a designated patient.	Evaluate with instructor.
2. Anatomy and physiology			
Describe the anatomy of the pleural space.	Given a patient situation, identify the type of chest tube.		
Differentiate between pleural and mediastinal chest tubes.			
Describe what happens when the negative pressure in the pleural space is disturbed.			
3. Hemothorax, pneumothorax, and hemopneumothorax			
Define hemothorax, pneumothorax, and hemopneumothorax.	Given a patient situation, state which of these is the problem.		Evaluate with instructor.
Differentiate between open pneumothorax and closed, or tension, pneumothorax.			
Explain the reason for location of a pleural tube to remove air versus one to remove fluid.	Given the location of a chest tube in a hypothetical situation, state the probable reason for its insertion.	In the clinical setting, identify the reason for a chest tube, according to its location.	Using facility procedure, evaluate with instructor.
State two reasons why it is preferable to connect chest tubes to individual drainage systems when two are placed in a single patient.		In the clinical setting, connect chest tubes appropriately.	Evaluate with instructor.
4. Insertion of chest tubes			
List equipment that might be needed for chest tube insertion on the clinical unit.	Adapt equipment list to your assigned clinical facility.	Select appropriate equipment for chest tube insertion in your clinical facility.	Evaluate using Performance Checklist and facility procedure.

(continued)

SPECIFIC LEARNING OBJECTIVES (continued)

Know Facts and Principles	Apply Facts and Principles	Demonstrate Ability	Evaluate Performance
5. *Waterseal drainage*			
Describe how waterseal drainage works.		Keep waterseal drainage system below the level of the patient's chest at all times.	Evaluate with instructor.
State two reasons for locating waterseal drainage system *below* the level of the patient's chest.			
a. One-container system			
Describe the one-container system of waterseal drainage. State the function of the two pieces of glass tubing.	Explain why the vent must be kept open at all times.	In the practice or clinical setting, set up one-container water seal correctly.	Evaluate with instructor using diagrams.
b. Two-container system			
Describe the two-container system of waterseal drainage. Identify one advantage of the two-container system when fluid is being drained from the pleural space.		In the practice or clinical setting, set up two-container chest drainage correctly.	Evaluate with instructor using diagrams.
c. Three-container system			
Describe the function of the third container in the three-container system of waterseal drainage.		In the practice or clinical setting, set up three-container chest suction correctly.	Evaluate with instructor using diagrams.
		In the clinical setting, check any chest drainage systems to be sure they are set up correctly.	
d. Commercial waterseal chest drainage systems			
Identify the purpose of each chamber of the commercial waterseal system.		In the clinical setting, set up a commercial waterseal system correctly.	Evaluate with instructor.

(continued)

Know Facts and Principles	Apply Facts and Principles	Demonstrate Ability	Evaluate Performance
6. Care of patients with chest tubes			
Know facts and principles related to the care of patients with chest tubes connected to chest drainage.	Given a patient situation, identify appropriate action(s) for that situation.	Under supervision, care for patients with chest tubes.	Evaluate performance with instructor.
7. Stripping or milking the tubing			
State rationale for not stripping tubing. State rationale for milking tubing gently and only when necessary.	In the practice setting, practice the technique for milking chest tubing.	In the clinical setting, milk chest tubing gently and only as ordered.	Evaluate with instructor.
8. Assisting with the removal of chest tubes			
List equipment that might be needed for chest tube removal on the clinical unit. Discuss items that would be included in your explanation to a patient about to undergo chest tube removal. Name two things for which you would observe after the removal of chest tubes.	Adapt equipment list to your assigned facility.	Select appropriate equipment for chest tube removal in your clinical facility. Given an opportunity in the clinical setting, prepare a patient for the removal of chest tubes. Make appropriate observations after chest tube removal.	Evaluate with instructor.
9. Documentation			
State information and observations that need to be documented with the insertion, maintenance, and removal of a chest tube.	Given a patient situation, record data as though on a chart.	Document procedure and observations accurately.	Evaluate with instructor.

LEARNING ACTIVITIES

1. Review the Specific Learning Objectives.
2. Read the material on thoracentesis in Appendix J in Ellis and Nowlis, *Nursing: A Human Needs Approach*, or comparable material in another textbook.
3. Look up the module vocabulary terms in the glossary.
4. Read through the module as though you were preparing to teach the information to another person.
5. Mentally practice the specific procedure.
6. In the practice setting, do the following:
   a. Examine any chest tube insertion materials available, for example, trocars of various sizes and rubber and plastic chest tubes.
   b. Using your partner as a patient, simulate the explanation and positioning appropriate for chest tube insertion. Have your partner evaluate your performance.
   c. Examine any chest tube drainage containers or systems available.
   d. Explain to a partner how each of the above systems works.
7. In the clinical setting, do the following:
   a. Consult with your instructor for an opportunity to assist with the insertion or removal of a chest tube and to care for a patient with a chest drainage in place.

VOCABULARY

atelectasis	mediastinum	rubber-shod	thoracentesis
fibrin	parietal pleura	stab wound	tidaling
hemopneumothorax	pleural space	subcutaneous	trocar
hemothorax	pleural tube	emphysema	visceral pleura
mediastinal tube	pneumothorax	tension pneumothorax	waterseal drainage

Caring for Patients With Chest Drainage

Rationale for the Use of This Skill

The most common type of chest tube, the pleural tube, is used to drain air or fluid from the pleural cavity and to restore the normal negative intrapleural pressure, making lung expansion possible after surgery or trauma to the chest cavity. Another type of chest tube, the mediastinal tube, is used to drain fluid from the mediastinal space after cardiac surgery or other surgery in the mediastinum. The nurse should be able to anticipate the needs of the patient and physician during the insertion and removal of chest tubes and care safely for the patient with any type of chest drainage system.[1]

TYPES AND PURPOSES OF CHEST TUBES

Pleural Tubes

The pleural space is a *potential* space formed by the visceral and parietal pleura. It contains only enough lubricating fluid to allow the two surfaces to slide smoothly over each other during inhalation and exhalation. On inspiration, the negative pressure is approximately −8 cm water and remains negative on expiration but somewhat less so, at about −4 cm water. The pleural space does not normally contain air or fluid except for the small amount of lubricating fluid.

When the chest has been opened, there will be some drainage from the wound (the amount will depend on the extent of surgery or trauma). There will also be air in the pleural space that causes collapse of the lung. A collection of blood in the pleural space is a *hemothorax.* An accumulation of air in the pleural space is a *pneumothorax.* The presence of blood and air is a *hemopneumothorax.* The air and fluid must be removed *for the lung to reexpand and healing to occur.*

If additional air enters the space or any fluid accumulates, breathing is compromised *because the space normally occupied by the expanded lung is filled with the air or fluid.* If too much space is occupied by fluid or air and the pressure exerted is great enough, *the lung may collapse completely.*

In an *open pneumothorax,* breathing is compromised by the air entering the pleural space from the outside of the chest. This most commonly occurs be-

cause of surgery on the chest or trauma to the chest wall, either of which may allow air to enter the chest, thus collapsing the lung.

In a *closed* or *tension pneumothorax, air enters the pleural space from the lung (usually because an alveolus has ruptured) and cannot escape. This leads to a build-up of pressure in the pleural space with each inspiration, which in turn collapses the lung and pushes the structures in the mediastinum toward the opposite side of the chest (mediastinal shift). This condition can result in the collapse of the other lung and can rapidly compromise respiratory function. This increased pressure in the pleural space may also interfere with the filling of the ventricles of the heart, leading to circulatory problems.*

The insertion of the chest tube or tubes *permits removal of the air or bloody fluid and allows for reexpansion of the lung and restoration of the normal negative pressure in the pleural space. Because air rises,* a chest tube inserted to remove air is usually placed anteriorly through the second intercostal space. A chest tube inserted to remove fluid is placed posteriorly in the eighth or ninth intercostal space *because fluid tends to flow to the bottom of the pleural space.* If both air and fluid are in the pleural space, two chest tubes may be inserted. Sometimes both tubes are inserted through a stab wound—a small surgical cut made in the chest after the skin has been anesthetized—low on the chest. The end of one tube is threaded high in the pleural cavity *to remove air.*

A chest tube inserted at surgery may be brought out of the chest through the incision or through a separate stab wound near the incision. Although two chest tubes can be connected to each other with a Y connector and drain to the same waterseal collection device, it is preferable to leave the chest tubes separate for two reasons: 1) *Fluid or air and drainage returning through each tube may be observed and measured individually.* 2) *One tube can be removed without disturbing the other tube or the rest of the waterseal setup.*

Mediastinal Tubes

The mediastinal space surrounds the heart. After cardiac surgery, there will be some serosanguineous drainage. Mediastinal tubes are placed *to ensure that fluid does not accumulate and put pressure on the heart but instead drains to facilitate healing. If the fluid begins to accumulate in the mediastinal space, the pressure exerted on the heart will interfere with cardiac filling and thus decrease cardiac output.* Therefore, maintaining appropriate drainage is critical to the patient's well-being.

---

[1]Note that rationale for action is emphasized throughout the module by the use of italics.

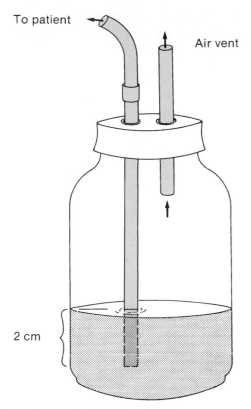

Figure 42–1. One-bottle system (note vent). The drainage will combine with the waterseal.

CHEST DRAINAGE CONTAINERS

The chest tube (or tubes) is connected to plastic or rubber tubing, which is attached to a plastic drainage container that has several compartments. Although commercial plastic chest drainage sets are almost always used, you may on occasion see glass bottles used as containers for chest drainage systems. All drainage containers function on the same principles. Therefore, this module explains the principles and provides drawings of bottles and of plastic drainage containers to help you clearly see how they function.

Waterseal Container

A waterseal at the end of a chest tube is essential *to allow air to escape through the tube* (Fig. 42–1) *but prevent air from traveling back up the tube and into the pleural space.* The waterseal drainage system is placed *below the level of the patient's chest, taking advantage of the force of gravity to promote drainage and prevent backflow of bottle contents into the pleural space.*

To create a waterseal in a bottle, a long glass or plastic tube is inserted through a rubber stopper and submerged about 2 cm in the sterile water or saline.

Air from the chest passes through the chest tube and bubbles out through the water into the bottle. Also inserted through the rubber stopper is a short tube, which acts as an escape valve or vent and allows air to escape from the waterseal bottle, *thus preventing pressure build-up in the bottle. Increased pressure could back up the water or saline in the bottle toward the chest.*

A plastic drainage set has a separate compartment in the center that is labeled as the waterseal chamber. Water is instilled to the marked depth. The container has a molded plastic tube that opens under the water of the waterseal compartment.

A one-bottle system provides waterseal drainage using gravity to promote drainage from the pleural space (see Fig. 42–1). Because only one bottle is in place, it is also a drainage container.

Because the single bottle is serving a dual purpose, it must be marked at the original (2 cm) fluid level and again at the end of each shift *to keep track of the amount of drainage.* A long strip of tape can be attached vertically to the bottle for this purpose (Fig. 42–2). *When the amount of fluid in the bottle is increased by drainage, more of the tube is submerged, creating more resistance to drainage.* For this reason, some physicians use the one-bottle system for pneumothorax only.

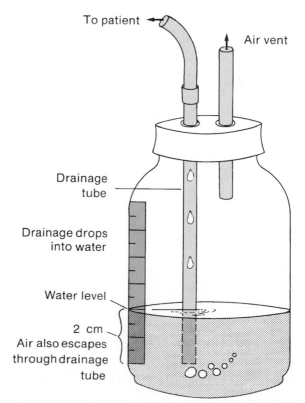

Figure 42–2. One-bottle system with vertical tape to measure drainage. Tape can be marked hourly or by the shift to check the amount of drainage.

In an emergency, such as a cracked chest drainage system, you may be able to create a waterseal chest bottle quickly by immersing the end of a chest tube approximately 2 cm into a sterile water or saline bottle at the bedside. Some facilities routinely keep a sealed bottle of sterile saline at the bedside of an individual who has a chest tube in place *to be used if an emergency situation occurs.*

Drainage Container

The amount and type of drainage may be observed and described more accurately if drainage accumulates in a separate container from the waterseal container. The simplest way to set this up is with a two-bottle system consisting of a bottle for the waterseal described above and a second bottle to collect drainage (Fig. 42–3).

Gravity drainage or suction may be used. If suction is used, the air vent tube on the waterseal bottle is attached to a suction source. The suction level is regulated by a wall gauge or a gauge attached to the suction machine.

In a plastic chest tube container, the first compartment is a drainage compartment. It is usually divided into three sections. As one section fills, it spills over into the second section, which then fills. This chamber has markings to indicate the amount of drainage that has been collected.

Suction Control Container

Even though the suction is set to a certain level, *it is possible for a higher level of suction to be reached at the end of the attached tubing if the tubing is blocked. To prevent this,* a suction control container *that limits the amount of suction that can be applied to the chest tube by the suction source is used.*

The amount of suction applied is determined by the depth to which the long tube from the suction source is submerged in the sterile water or saline (Figs. 42–4 and 42–5). Mechanical suction is responsible for the negative pressure but will not rise above the amount of suction (usually 10–20 cm) necessary to pull air through the water and into the suction tube. A suction control container is most of-

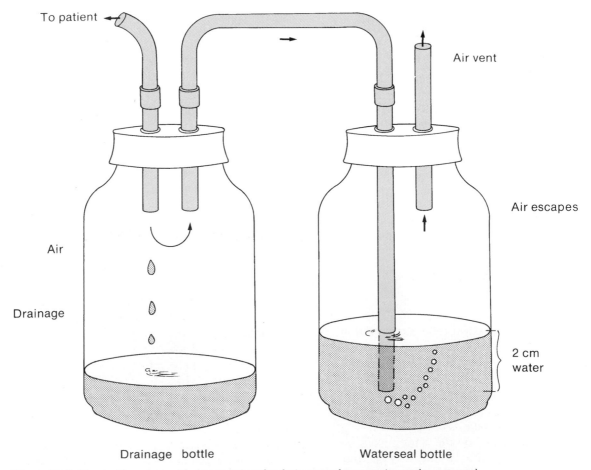

Figure 42–3. Two-bottle system with one container for drainage and one serving as the waterseal.

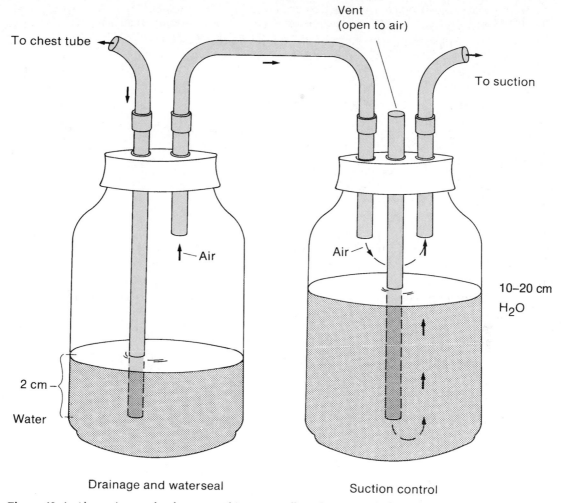

Figure 42–4. Alternative two-bottle system. This system collects drainage with the waterseal and has a suction control container.

ten added to a system containing a waterseal container and a drainage container. However, a suction control container may be added to a one-container system in which the waterseal and drainage are in the same container.

Commercial Chest Drainage Units

Two of several plastic, disposable chest drainage units available commercially are the Pleur-Evac (Fig. 42–6) and the Atrium units. The Pleur-Evac is essentially a three-container system, with a positive pressure release valve *to prevent the build-up of excessive pressure in the system*. The Atrium unit is similar to the Pleur-evac but does not have the same type of pressure release valve (Fig. 42–7). In these units, separate plastic chambers serve the purpose of each container as previously described. The units are lightweight, not easily broken, and can hang from the bed frame for convenience. Settings for suc-

tion level and for measuring drainage are clearly marked.

ALTERNATIVE TO CHEST TUBES

An alternative to chest tubes for the treatment of pneumothorax is to insert a chest catheter, which can be used to withdraw air. This process can provide immediate relief of symptoms and correction of the underlying problem. The distal 3 in of the catheter has multiple perforations *to allow air to flow into the tubing*. A Luer-Lok connector at the proximal end allows staff to connect a three-way stopcock after the chest catheter is inserted and to remove the air from the pleural space with a 50-mL syringe.

After the air has been withdrawn as much as possible, the Luer-Lok end of the catheter is then connected to a Heimlich drainage valve, which permits a one-way flow of air away from the pleural cavi-

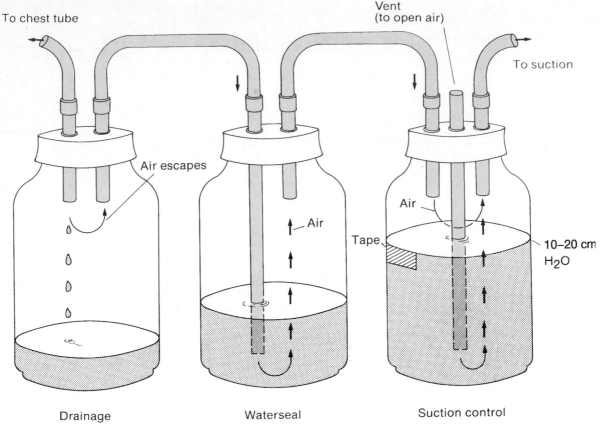

To chest tube

Vent (to open air)

To suction

Air escapes

↓

Air

Tape

Air

10–20 cm H₂O

Drainage   Waterseal   Suction control

Figure 42–5. Three-bottle system. One bottle is for drainage, one for waterseal, and a third for suction control.

ty (Fig. 42–8) and does not allow air to reenter the pleural space. This system can be connected to waterseal drainage or suction if necessary. The pneumothorax catheter is not recommended for patients who have large amounts of fluid or hemorrhage *because its small internal diameter may easily be occluded.*

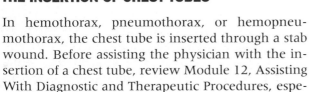

PROCEDURE FOR ASSISTING WITH THE INSERTION OF CHEST TUBES

In hemothorax, pneumothorax, or hemopneumothorax, the chest tube is inserted through a stab wound. Before assisting the physician with the insertion of a chest tube, review Module 12, Assisting With Diagnostic and Therapeutic Procedures, especially noting the procedure for thoracentesis.

Assessment

1. Check the physician's order.
2. Check to see if the patient has signed a consent form. If not, notify the physician who is to perform the procedure.

3. Assess the patient's status and abilities with emphasis on vital signs and respiratory status.

Planning

4. Wash your hands *for infection control.*
5. Obtain equipment, including the following:
   a. Chest tube tray. This usually contains the trocar, sterile drapes, antiseptic solution, syringes, gauze dressing materials, and chest tubes. After you have determined which items are included on the tray in your clinical setting, you can add other needed items.
   b. Chest drainage set. If two drainage tubes will be maintained separately, you will need to prepare two drainage sets. You will need sterile water to fill the waterseal section. Review the directions on the specific set to determine how to fill it. Sterile covers should remain over the connectors until they are ready to be connected to the chest tube.
   c. Other supplies, which may include sterile water, local anesthetic, antiseptic, suture materials, and sterile gloves. Knowing the specific preferences of the physician inserting the tube

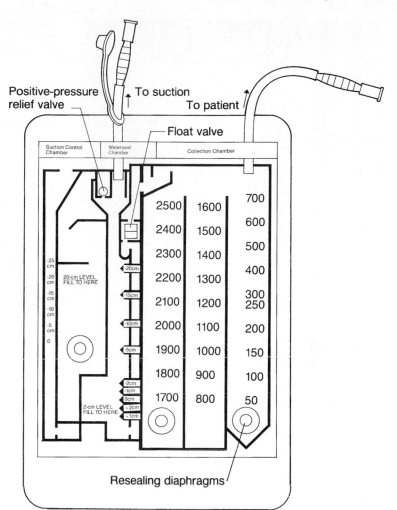

Figure 42–6. Pleur-Evac. A commercial chest drainage system with three containers molded into the plastic: suction control container on the left, waterseal in the center, and drainage container to the right.

is useful and will help the procedure go more smoothly.

Implementation

6. Identify the patient *to be sure you are performing the procedure on the correct patient.*

7. Explain the procedure to the patient in general terms.

8. Prepare the unit, including privacy and setting up the equipment on a sterile field.

9. Prepare the patient.

   a. Administer pain medication or sedative as ordered. Follow the procedure in Module 47, Administering Medications: Overview.

   b. Assist the patient to the upright position *so that the pull of gravity consolidates the chest fluid in the lower portion of the affected lung.* This positioning may be accomplished in any of the following ways:

      (1) Pad the back of a straight chair *for comfort,* and have the patient straddle the chair, leaning the arms on the padded back.

      (2) Have the patient sit upright in bed and lean forward, resting on the overbed table.

      (3) Have the patient sit at the edge of the bed, leaning on the overbed table.

10. Assist with the procedure, and assess, reassure, and support the patient. Carefully assess for skin color, diaphoresis, respiratory status, and chest pain. You may be asked to assist in any of the following ways:

    a. Pour antiseptic over the cotton balls.

    b. Hold the vial of local anesthetic as the physician withdraws the proper dosage.

    c. Apply an occlusive dressing or dry sterile gauze and tape to the tube insertion site(s). Wear sterile gloves if you will be handling sterile dressing materials.

    d. Set up the requested drainage system.

    e. Make sure a chest film is ordered following the procedure *to check proper placement of the chest tube.*

11. Conclude the procedure.

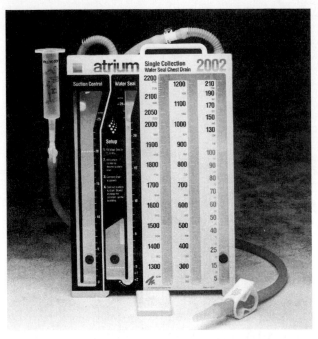

Figure 42–7. Atrium waterseal suction container.

a. Return the patient to a comfortable position.
b. Restore the unit.
c. If a specimen of fluid is obtained, label it and send it to the laboratory.
d. Care for the equipment appropriately. Most will be disposable.
e. Recheck pulse, respirations, and blood pressure, and notify the physician of any significant changes.
f. Wash your hands.

Evaluation

12. Evaluate, using the following criteria:
   a. Patient vital signs stable.
   b. Patient comfortable.
   c. Chest tube system functioning properly.
   d. Patient states understanding of situation.

Documentation

13. Document appropriate data, including the physician's name, before-and-after vital signs, type of drainage system in use, amount of suction, and the response of the patient.

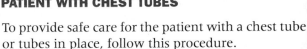

PROCEDURE FOR CARING FOR THE PATIENT WITH CHEST TUBES

To provide safe care for the patient with a chest tube or tubes in place, follow this procedure.

Assessment

1. Check the order to determine the type of chest tube(s) in place, the suction ordered, and any specific assessment plans.
2. Review appropriate procedures and protocols for your facility.

Planning

3. Wash your hands.
4. Obtain supplies, including clean gloves, sterile saline or water as needed for containers, and sterile gloves and dressing materials if needed. Clean gloves will be needed only if you come in contact with body fluids, but you should be prepared for that possibility.

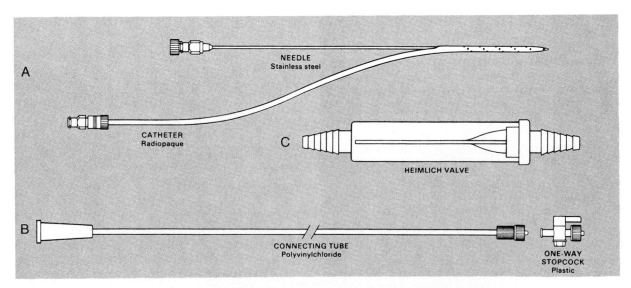

Figure 42–8. Pneumothorax catheter set. **(A)** A trocar with a catheter for insertion. **(B)** A connecting tube to attach the catheter and valve. **(C)** The Heimlich valve. (Courtesy Cook Critical Care, Bloomington, Indiana.)

DATE/TIME	
5/21/99 1400	*Chest tube inserted in left lower chest by Dr. Martin and attached to low suction under waterseal. Breath sounds decreased in left lower lobe. Respirations 28, shallow but regular. See parameter sheet for record of vital signs. Patient resting comfortably and states only slight discomfort at insertion site.* *——— S. O'Riley, RN*

Example of Nursing Progress Notes Using Narrative Format.

Implementation

5. Assess and adjust the drainage system. Be sure to put on gloves before manipulating any part of the system in a way that might expose you to body secretions.

   a. Check the entire length of the tubing, from the patient to the container. Make sure it is positioned correctly. The tubing between the patient and the waterseal bottle should be long enough *to allow the patient to move and turn* (usually about 6 ft). It should be coiled and fastened to the bed (or chair if the patient is up) so that it does not form dependent loops or kinks *that would inhibit free drainage.* There should be no obstructions on the tube.

   b. Check the chest tube container to ensure that the waterseal is intact and the vent is open. A vent must be present *to allow air to escape.* Except for this vent, the system should be airtight *to prevent air from entering the pleural space.* Fluctuation (tidaling) of the water level will occur in a waterseal container that is not connected to suction. The water level rises when the patient inhales and falls when the patient exhales. Shallow breathing results in slight fluctuation. When the patient must work harder to breathe—for example, when secretions are retained—negative pressure in the chest is higher and therefore fluctuation is greater. *Continuous bubbling in the waterseal bottle can mean either persistent leakage of air from the lung or a leak in the system.* When a chest tube is connected to suction, the suction obscures the tidaling in the waterseal container.

   Position the chest tube container 2 to 3 ft below the patient's chest *to facilitate drainage in the tubing and to prevent any backflow of fluid from the container into the pleural space.* If the drainage container is accidentally raised above the level of the patient's chest, lower it immediately, encourage the patient to deep breathe, and observe the patient for signs of further lung collapse and mediastinal shift. If

indications of these are seen (see section on complications), notify the physician. If the drainage container is on or near the floor, be careful not to lower a high-low bed or side rail onto it, because this could break the container and disrupt the entire waterseal drainage system.

   c. Secure connections, and retape them if needed. In many facilities, the policy is to tape all connections and to check the system on a routine basis *to be sure that all connections are intact.* Adhesive or plastic tape is used *because it is impervious to air.* Paper tape is not suitable for this purpose *because it will admit air.*

   d. Observe the amount, character, and rate of accumulation of drainage *to identify excessive bleeding, beginning infection, or tube blockage.* This observation is usually made hourly immediately after chest tube insertion and less often thereafter—at least every 8 hours.

   e. Check the suction level set on the suction device. If suction is ordered, the level must be kept at the amount ordered at all times. *An inadequate level may delay lung reexpansion. The water in the suction control section protects the lung from excess suction.*

   Suction should not be applied to chest drainage without a suction control chamber to protect the lung. A piece of tape placed at the level of solution in the suction control bottle or at the ordered levels on a gauge can be a helpful reminder. If a suction control container is used, check for gentle, continuous bubbling. *Gentle bubbling indicates that suction is constantly reaching the desired level but cannot go higher. If the bubbling is very vigorous,* the fluid will evaporate more rapidly. The fluid level in the container should be checked periodically *to be sure it is the proper depth to provide the amount of suction ordered.* If it is not the proper depth, sterile water or saline must be added. Likewise, sterile water or saline is added if the physician orders the amount of suction increased. The higher the fluid level, the more suction develops before the seal is broken and the bottle bubbles.

f. Problem solve and correct any difficulties.

g. Keep two large rubber-shod hemostats or Kelley clamps at the bedside. *These are used to clamp the chest tube(s) if necessary.* A chest tube is clamped *to determine the cause of an air leak when there is bubbling in the waterseal bottle and the patient is on chest suction.* It is also necessary to clamp a chest tube *to empty the collection bottle or replace a broken or cracked container in the system.* Do not leave the tubes clamped for more than a few minutes. *If the lung is leaking air into the pleural space, air can accumulate there, collapsing the lung and causing pressure on the mediastinum.*

When clamps are used, be careful not to cover them with the sheet or blanket to avoid the possibility of the chest tube(s) being clamped and forgotten. If clamps are forgotten and left in place for too long, *pressure can build up in the pleural space, causing a tension pneumothorax.*

h. Keep petrolatum (Vaseline) gauze at the bedside *to provide an airtight dressing in case the chest tube is inadvertently pulled out of the chest cavity.*

6. Examine the wound, and change the dressing if needed. Protect the chest tube insertion site with a sterile dressing. The dressing is removed and the site inspected for signs of infection unless the protocol in use indicates that the physician will change the dressing. Redress the wound according to the procedure in Module 35, Wound Care (Fig. 42–9).

7. Complete essential physical assessment.

a. Lung assessment is essential for the person with a chest tube. The areas in which breath sounds are heard and the presence of adventitious sounds are important.

b. Temperature measurement will assist in monitoring for the potential of infection.

c. Blood pressure and pulse measurement are essential when monitoring for complications related to the presence of chest tubes.

8. Assist the patient with moving and positioning. Position the patient in good alignment, and encourage him or her to change positions frequently *to prevent complications of immobility, such as hypoventilation, venous stasis, and postural hypotension.* When the patient is lying on the affected side, *the tubing can be occluded by the patient's weight.* You can prevent this by placing rolled towels beside the tubing.

9. Assist the patient with coughing and deep

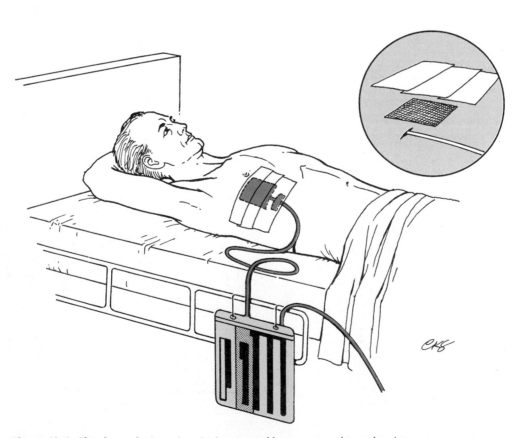

Figure 42–9. The chest tube insertion site is protected by a gauze and tape dressing.

breathing. Encourage the patient to cough and deep breathe at least once hourly *to prevent atelectasis and to assist in removing air or fluid from the pleural space.*

10. Transport or ambulate the patient. You should not clamp chest tubes to transport a patient to another department or to ambulate the patient. When transporting or ambulating a patient, you must do the following:
    a. Disconnect the tubing from the suction device.
    b. Keep the waterseal container upright *so that the waterseal is maintained.*
    c. Keep the container(s) below the level of the patient's chest *to prevent backflow into the chest.*
    d. Maintain an airtight system *to prevent air from entering the system or the chest.*
    e. Keep the vent open *to ensure that pressure does not build up in the system.*

Evaluation

11. Evaluate the patient's status based on the following:
    a. Respiratory rate and lung sounds
    b. Pain and anxiety
    c. Integrity of system
    d. Drainage type and amount
    e. Condition of the wound

Documentation

12. Document information regarding the chest tubes, including the following:
    a. Time system checked
    b. Amount and description of drainage
    c. Suction level
    d. Equipment status
    e. Condition of the wound

f. Patient's respiratory status, pain, and anxiety. For an example of a chest tube parameter flow sheet, see Figure 42–10.

PROBLEMS AND COMPLICATIONS RELATED TO CHEST DRAINAGE

1. *The drainage is copious and bright red.* Bleeding of more 100 mL/h is considered heavy bleeding. Take vital signs, assess patient's physical status, and immediately call the physician.
2. *The drainage quickly fills the collection chamber.* Obtain a new sterile drainage container. Fill the waterseal section with sterile water. Briefly clamp the tube and connect to a new sterile system. Remove clamp, reinstate the suction, and dispose of old container.
3. *Fluctuations and drainage stop.* Mediastinal tubes will not fluctuate and will usually have minimal drainage. A gradual cessation of fluctuation or drainage in a pleural tube could indicate that the lung has reexpanded. In any type of tube, drainage stopping may indicate kinking of the tube, the patient lying on the tube, or a blood or fibrin clot within the tube.
    a. Ensure that the tubing is free of external obstructions.
    b. If the patient has atelectasis or retained secretions, be aware that respirations may be shallow and may not create tidaling. Auscultate the chest to determine lung function. Have the patient deep breathe and cough. This may restore drainage.
    c. When clots are seen in the drainage and they

DATE/TIME	
4/29/99	*Chest Tube on Left*
	D: Respirations 26, shallow, symmetrical. Lung sounds decreased on left. System checked 0930. Drainage in container is dark red, approximately 60 mL. Pain 3 on 1–5 scale. Chest drainage container intact, bubbling continuously with suction at 22 cm; no leaks in system. Dressing dry and intact.
	A: Pain medication administered (see MAR). Patient encouraged to deep breathe and cough and change position frequently.
	R: Patient expresses understanding of need for deep breathing, coughing, and exercise. Pain decreased to 1–2 level 30 min after medication.
	M. Williams, RN

Example of Nursing Progress Notes Using Focus Format.

Suction Device ___Waterseal___

Location of chest tube A. (L) lower lobe

B. ___——___

Key

1. Character of resp: normal, symmetry, shallow, deep labored
2. Sputum: character, amount, color
3. Drainage: character, amount, color
4. Pain scale: 0=non; 1=mild; 2, 3=moderate; 4,5=severe
5. Anxiety: none, minimal, moderate, severe
6. Air leak: none, small, medium, large bubbling
7. Dressing: dry, intact, loose, reinforced
8. Equipment function: yes/no, check q8°

*Document in nursing progress notes any notable changes & q8° evaluative statement.

Date	Time	lung assessment	character of respirations	character of sputum	drainage	dressing	level of suction	equipment function	air leak	pain	anxiety		init.
6/10/99	0700	↓ LLL	reg.	sm. white	mod.	change	20 cm	✓	Ø	1 +	min		J.B.
6/10	1500	↓ LLL	reg.	mod. white	mod	——	20 cm	✓	Ø	2	min	medi-cated	SW
6/10	2300	——	——	⌣	——	change	——	✓	Ø	1	Ø		SW
6/11	0200	↓ LLL	——	sm. white	mod.	——	20 cm	✓	Ø	1	Ø	sleeping	DD

Identify Initials with Signature:	4.	8.
1. *Jean Bennett, RN*	5.	9.
2. *Sue Williams, RN*	6.	10.
3. *Donna Davis, RN*	7.	11.

ADDRESSOGRAPH:

WARNER, Steven   M

754 56 2354   27

SWEDISH HOSPITAL MEDICAL CENTER
Seattle, Washington

Figure 42–10. Chest drainage observations can be made by the nurse on a special parameter sheet.

have the potential to obstruct the tubing, remove them into the drainage chamber by "milking" the tubing. Milking may be done in various ways, but basically it means compressing the tubing and then releasing it. This same motion is used in subsequent sections of the tubing, moving away from the patient's chest toward the drainage container. *Because milking may create high negative pressure on the lung,* it should be done only if there is evidence of clots in the tubing that may obstruct drainage. If the tubing is in place to remove air, there is no logical reason to milk the tube.

Another procedure called "stripping" was used in the past to clear chest tubes. This involved compressing the tubing and then sliding the fingers down the tubing toward the drainage container. *Research indicates that negative pressures created by stripping are considerably higher than the suction pressures of* -15 *to* -20 cm water usually applied to chest drainage systems. Researchers have found that stripping *has produced negative pressures as high as* -350 cm water. Therefore, stripping is now not recommended *to prevent potential tissue injury.* When air alone is being evacuated from the chest, there is no logical reason to strip the tubing *because there is no potential for obstruction.*

d. If the lung is not reexpanded and drainage is not restored, notify the physician.

4. *The drainage bottle or plastic system has broken.* Prepare a new sterile drainage container. Clamp the tubing close to the patient, and replace as described previously.

5. *The chest tube has pulled out.* You must know whether air is entering the chest from inside the lung.

a. If air is *not* entering from the lung, immediately place an occlusive dressing, such as a sterile petrolatum gauze (which should be available in the room), over the site *to prevent room air from entering the pleural space.* Cover the petrolatum gauze with a dry dressing and tape the dressing on all four sides *to form an occlusive seal.*

b. If air is entering from the lung, make sure that this air can exit *to prevent tension pneumothorax.* Place the dressing over the wound, tape loosely on three sides, and allow the fourth side to be open. *When the patient inhales, the dressing will be pulled against the wound, preventing room air from entering the chest. When the patient exhales, the dressing will be pushed away from the wound by the air exiting the chest.*

c. Assess the patient's respiratory status, and immediately notify the physician that the tube has pulled out.

6. *Bubbling is increased with inspiration and expiration.* This is usually caused by a leak in the system. To identify a leak, do the following:

a. Check the connections to be sure that they are firm. Retape connections if necessary.

b. If the leak continues after connections are tight, there may be a crack in the drainage container or a pinhole leak in the tubing. To identify the location of the leak, place one of the clamps on the tubing close to the chest. If the excess bubbling continues, the leak is distal to the clamp. Gradually move the clamp toward the container. When the bubbling stops after placing the clamp, you know that the leak is between where the clamp is currently placed and the last placement of the clamp. A leak in the tubing may often be sealed with occlusive tape. If the leak is in the drainage container, the container must be changed.

7. *The patient's anxiety increases.* Lack of oxygen creates a physiologic basis for anxiety. First, assess the patient's respiratory status. Next, check the drainage system for problems, and correct any that you may find. If the system is working properly and respiratory status is stable, spend time with the patient. Explain how the drainage system works and why the sounds of the suction are important and beneficial.

8. *Patient experiences moderate pain when moving.* Medicate the patient based on the physician's order to provide pain relief adequate for easy movement. The patient must decide what level of pain relief is essential. Consult with the physician if ordered medications are not providing adequate pain relief.

PROCEDURE FOR ASSISTING WITH THE REMOVAL OF CHEST TUBES

To assist the physician with the removal of a chest tube, you should refer to Module 12, Assisting With Diagnostic and Therapeutic Procedures. The physician may order an analgesic premedication, or you can give the patient the ordered pain relief medication about 30 minutes before the chest tube is removed.

Assessment
1. Check the physician's order.
2. Note that a signed permission form is not needed for removal. The permission to insert chest tubes implies permission to remove them.
3. Assess the patient's status with emphasis on vital signs (pulse, respirations, and blood pressure) to use as a baseline. Also assess the need for premedication.

Planning
4. Wash your hands *for infection control.*
5. Gather the following equipment:
a. Sterile gloves
b. Suture set (or sterile scissors and sterile forceps)

DATE/TIME	
2/25/99 1400	*Interim Note*
	S "I'm glad to have that out."
	O *Chest tube removed by Dr. Martinez. Stab wound sutured and covered with petrolatum gauze and occlusive dressing. Portable chest film ordered. VS stable. Breath sounds clear bilaterally. No respiratory difficulty.*
	A *Chest tube removed without difficulty.*
	P *Continue to assess respiratory status.*
	J. Ross, RN

Example of Nursing Progress Notes Using SOAP Format.

c. Sterile petrolatum gauze

d. Skin closure material

e. Dressing material

f. Wide tape

Implementation

6. Identify the patient *to be sure you are performing the procedure on the correct patient.*

7. Explain the procedure to the patient in general terms.

8. Prepare the unit by providing privacy and setting up equipment.

9. Assist the patient to the proper position—either sitting at the edge of the bed or lying on the unaffected side.

10. Assist the physician as indicated. The physician first removes any dressing materials and then cuts the sutures. The patient is asked to take a deep breath and bear down (Valsalva maneuver) *to raise intrathoracic pressure and prevent air from entering the chest* while the physician quickly pulls out the tube. Alternatively, the tube may be removed during expiration, *to prevent air from being pulled back into the pleural space during the removal of the tube.* After the tube is removed, the wound may be sutured or clipped closed and covered with the petrolatum gauze and dressing material, which is securely taped in place. Alternatively, the wound may simply be covered with petrolatum gauze and an occlusive dressing, *which forms an airtight seal to prevent air from entering the chest.* Usually a chest film is ordered when the procedure is complete *to be sure the lung is expanded and that no air has entered the pleural space.* Reassure and observe the patient throughout the procedure. Be sure to put on gloves before handling any equipment that might expose you to body secretions.

11. When the procedure is complete, reassess the patient:

a. Recheck vital signs.

b. Auscultate breath sounds, and watch for indications of pneumothorax (dyspnea, tachypnea, chest pain) and subcutaneous emphysema (air trapped in the subcutaneous tissue that crackles when palpated) *to identify complications that must be reported to the physician.*

c. Properly care for equipment.

d. Wash your hands.

Evaluation

12. Evaluate, using the following criteria:

a. Patient vital signs stable.

b. No indication of pneumothorax or subcutaneous emphysema.

c. Patient comfortable.

Documentation

13. On the patient's chart, document appropriate data, including physician's name, before-and-after vital signs, the patient's response, and any other significant observations.

CRITICAL THINKING EXERCISES

• William Morrison, who had surgery to the lower lobe of his left lung, returned from the postanesthesia recovery unit at 1500. He has a chest tube in place on the left. The tube is attached to 20 cm of suction. You note that there is no drainage in the container. Analyze what might be the cause of this. Determine what assessments you should make and what actions you might take.

• Maud Raines had heart surgery yesterday. She has a mediastinal tube in place. You note that there has been only 10 mL of drainage from the tube and that there is no evidence of tidaling in the waterseal section of the drainage container. Explain the significance of these observations, and then determine what actions you should take.

✔ PERFORMANCE CHECKLIST

Assisting With the Insertion of Chest Tubes	Needs More Practice	Satisfactory	Comments
Assessment			
1. Check the physician's order.			
2. Check to see if consent form has been signed.			
3. Measure vital signs.			
Planning			
4. Wash your hands.			
5. Obtain equipment. a. Chest tube tray			
b. Chest drainage set			
c. Other supplies			
Implementation			
6. Identify the patient.			
7. Explain the procedure.			
8. Prepare the unit.			
9. Prepare the patient. a. Administer mild sedation, if ordered.			
b. Assist patient to one of the following up-right positions: (1) Patient straddles chair, leaning on the padded back.			
(2) Patient sits upright in bed, resting on overbed table.			
(3) Patient sits at edge of bed, leaning on overbed table.			
10. Assist with the procedure, assessing and re-assuring patient. a. Pour antiseptic over cotton balls.			
b. Hold vial of local anesthetic as physician withdraws proper dosage.			
c. Apply an occlusive dressing to tube insertion site(s).			
d. Have requested drainage system available.			
e. Make sure chest film is ordered to check tube placement.			

(continued)

Assisting With the Insertion of Chest Tubes *(Continued)*	Needs More Practice	Satisfactory	Comments
11. Conclude the procedure. **a.** Return patient to a comfortable position.			
b. Restore the unit.			
c. Label and send specimen to laboratory.			
d. Care for equipment.			
e. Recheck vital signs.			
f. Wash your hands.			
Evaluation			
12. Evaluate, using the following criteria: **a.** Patient vital signs stable			
b. Patient comfortable			
c. Chest tube system functioning properly			
d. Patient states understanding of situation.			
Documentation			
13. Document appropriate data, including physician's name, vital signs, response of patient.			
Caring for the Patient With Chest Tubes			
Assessment			
1. Check order for type of chest tube, suction, and specific assessment ordered.			
2. Review procedures and protocols.			
Planning			
3. Wash your hands.			
4. Obtain supplies: clean gloves, sterile saline or water, sterile gloves, and dressing materials if needed.			
Implementation			
5. Assess and adjust drainage system. **a.** Check tubing to be sure it is coiled on bed and draining.			
b. Check chest tube container, and position it 2–3 ft below patient's chest.			
c. Secure connections: retape as needed.			
d. Observe amount, character, and rate of drainage.			

(continued)

Caring for the Patient With Chest Tubes *(Continued)*	Needs More Practice	Satisfactory	Comments
e. Check suction level and water level in suction control chamber			
f. Problem-solve and correct any difficulties.			
g. Keep two large rubber-shod clamps at the bedside.			
h. Keep petrolatum gauze at the bedside.			
6. Examine the wound, and change dressing as needed.			
7. Complete essential physical assessment, including the following: **a.** Lung assessment			
b. Temperature measurement			
c. Blood pressure and pulse measurement			
8. Assist patient with moving and positioning.			
9. Assist patient with coughing and deep breathing.			
10. Transport or ambulate patient. **a.** Disconnect the tubing from suction.			
b. Keep waterseal upright.			
c. Keep container below chest.			
d. Maintain airtight system.			
e. Keep vent open.			
Evaluation			
11. Evaluate patient's status" **a.** Respiratory rate and lung sounds			
b. Pain and anxiety			
c. Integrity of system			
d. Drainage type and amount			
e. Condition of chest wound			
Documentation			
12. Document the following: **a.** Time system checked			
b. Amount and description of drainage			
c. Suction level			

(continued)

Caring for the Patient With Chest Tubes *(Continued)*	Needs More Practice	Satisfactory	Comments
d. Equipment status			
e. Condition of the wound			
f. Patient's respiratory status, pain, and anxiety.			
Assisting with the Removal of Chest Tubes			
Assessment			
1. Check the physician's order.			
2. Note that no permission form needed.			
3. Assess patient's status.			
Planning			
4. Wash your hands.			
5. Gather equipment. **a.** Sterile gloves			
b. Suture set (or sterile scissors and sterile forceps)			
c. Sterile petrolatum (Vaseline) gauze			
d. Skin closure material			
e. Dressing material			
f. Wide tape			
Implementation			
6. Identify the patient.			
7. Explain the procedure.			
8. Prepare the unit.			
9. Assist patient to proper position—either sitting at edge of bed or lying on unaffected side.			
10. Assist physician by opening sterile packages, having suture materials ready, applying petrolatum gauze and occlusive dressing, and checking to see if chest film is ordered. Reassure and observe patient throughout procedure.			

(continued)

Assisting With the Removal of Chest Tubes *(Continued)*	Needs More Practice	Satisfactory	Comments
11. Reassess patient. **a.** Recheck vital signs, and report any significant changes.			
b. Observe patient for indications of pneumothorax and subcutaneous emphysema.			
c. Care for equipment.			
d. Wash your hands.			
Evaluation			
12. Evaluate, using the following criteria: **a.** Patient vital signs stable.			
b. No indication of pneumothorax or subcutaneous emphysema.			
c. Patient comfortable.			
Documentation			
13. Document appropriate data, including physician's name, before-and-after vital signs, response of patient, and any other significant obnservations.			

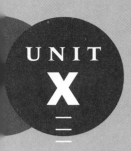

UNIT

X

Special Therapeutic and Supportive Procedures

MODULE

43

NASOGASTRIC INTUBATION

MODULE CONTENTS

PREREQUISITES [1]

Successful completion of the following modules:

[1]For nasogastric irrigation, see Module 46, Irrigations: Bladder, Catheter, Ear, Eye, Nasogastric Tube, Vaginal, Wound. For feeding through a nasogastric tube, see Module 29, Tube Feeding.

OVERALL OBJECTIVES

To insert nasogastric tubes to feed, instill medications, irrigate the stomach, or initiate gastric suction and to remove them safely.

SPECIFIC LEARNING OBJECTIVES

Know Facts and Principles	Apply Facts and Principles	Demonstrate Ability	Evaluate Performance
1. Types and uses of tubes Identify characteristics of nasogastric tubes.	Know when to ice tubes and how to lubricate.	Ice tube if needed. Lubricate tube correctly.	Evaluate own performance with instructor.
2. Equipment Recognize type of equipment needed and whether it should be clean or sterile.		Select appropriate equipment, and assemble tray.	Evaluate own performance with instructor.
3. Psychological support Know importance of preparing patient for procedure.	Given a patient situation, identify psychological problems present.	In the clinical setting, explain procedure, and elicit cooperation from patient.	Review interaction with instructor.
4. Inserting tube Describe placement of tube in pharynx and esophagus. Explain how to ascertain correct distance to insert tube.	Given a patient situation, identify appropriate nursing action in response to patient problems during nasogastric tube insertion.	Under supervision, insert nasogastric tube.	Evaluate using Performance Checklist.
5. Placing tube properly List three methods for determining proper placement.	Identify which method is most reliable.	Use a reliable method to determine correct placement. Do not proceed until sure.	Evaluate placement of tube with instructor.
6. Attaching suction equipment Know types of suction equipment used in facility.	Take safety factors into account when planning.	Attach suction equipment only after testing.	Have procedure checked by staff nurse or instructor.
7. Carrying out irrigation State purposes of gastric irrigation.	Select proper solution and equipment.	Instill solution slowly, and aspirate with care.	Evaluate own performance with instructor.
8. Documentation State observations to be made and data to be included when documenting the procedure.	List data for documenting specific patient situation.	Make routine data entries and specific observations for given patients.	Have instructor review entries.

LEARNING ACTIVITIES

1. Review the Specific Learning Objectives.
2. Read the section on the effects of immobility in the chapter on activity and rest and the section on the essentials of nutrition in the chapter on nutrition in Ellis and Nowlis, *Nursing: A Human Needs Approach,* or comparable material in another textbook.
3. Look up the module vocabulary terms in the glossary.
4. Review the anatomy of the upper gastrointestinal tract.
5. Read through the module and mentally practice the skill. Read as though you were preparing to teach the information to another person.
6. In the practice setting, do the following:
   a. Inspect the various nasogastric tubes available. Note the differences in length and size of lumen.
   b. After carefully reading over the procedure and the Performance Checklist, simulate an insertion, irrigation, and removal of a nasogastric tube, using a manikin.
   c. Give instructions and explanations to the manikin as if it were an actual patient.
7. In the clinical setting, do the following:
   a. Observe the insertion, irrigation, and removal of a nasogastric tube if possible by either your instructor or a staff nurse. Were the steps followed precisely? What was the patient's response?
   b. Familiarize yourself with the kind of nasogastric suction used in your facility. If the patient in step 7a is to have suction applied, observe how this is done.
   c. When you are ready and with your instructor's supervision, perform the following activities in the clinical setting:
      (1) Insert a nasogastric tube.
      (2) If ordered, attach it to suction.
      (3) If ordered, irrigate the tube.
      (4) Remove a nasogastric tube.
   d. After performing each procedure, again review the Performance Checklist, and evaluate your skills.
   e. Consult your instructor regarding any problems you encounter.

VOCABULARY

asepto syringe	gastric sump tube	mercury	sternum
aspirate	gavage	nasogastric tube	stylet
dyspnea	intubation	peristalsis	trachea
enteral	lavage	pharynx	xiphoid process
enteric	Levin tube	pylorus	
gag reflex	lumen	silicone	

Nasogastric Intubation

Rationale for the Use of This Skill

Nasogastric tubes are inserted to instill liquid feedings and medications for the patient who cannot swallow without aspirating or who cannot eat by mouth, to decompress the abdomen before or after surgery, or to wash out (lavage) the stomach.

Because many patients cannot take food orally after surgery or during a chronic illness, continual tube feeding in the long-term care facility or in the home is sometimes necessary. Physical and muscular debilitation caused by stroke or cerebrovascular accident or by other conditions may necessitate tube feeding for a long time.

Nausea and general discomfort can occur after surgery. Distention is not only uncomfortable, but it can place tension on an abdominal suture line. To prevent these conditions, physicians may order a nasogastric tube inserted. A nasogastric tube can be attached to suction to prevent nausea and vomiting when peristalsis is absent due to illness or gastric or bowel surgery. When suction is applied to the tube, gastric secretions and any accumulated gas are removed, leaving the patient more comfortable. A nasogastric tube is also used if a patient has ingested toxic substances and the stomach must be emptied through washing (lavage).

Most facilities consider the use of the nasogastric tube a routine procedure, but it can be frightening and unfamiliar to patients. It is the nurse's responsibility to help patients overcome their anxieties about the tube's insertion and removal and to make these procedures as comfortable as possible. All patients with nasogastric tubes in place for treatment should be put on intake and output monitoring.[2]

TYPES OF NASOGASTRIC TUBES

Several types of nasogastric tubes are available. They may be made of rubber, plastic, or silicone. Diameters also vary. Lumen sizes range from small to quite large.

Several tubes are designed with a stylet or fine metal wire that threads through the center of the tube. *This makes the tube more rigid and easier to pass. Stylets are also radiopaque and can be viewed by x-ray to verify placement.* The distal ends of some nasogastric tubes are weighted *so that when secretions or gas collect, they settle in the lower portion of the stomach.* If necessary, weighted tubes can pass further down the alimentary tract into the small intestine. This module discusses several of the common tubes.

[2]Note that rationale for action is emphasized throughout the module by the use of italics.

Nasogastric Tubes

The nasogastric tube may be used for either decompressing the stomach by suctioning gastric contents or administering medications or tube feedings. Often called a Levin tube, it comes in a variety of sizes from 5 French (very small) to 18 French (very large). All are approximately 50 in long. Sizes 5 through 12 are customarily used for children, and sizes 12 through 18 are used for adults. Most facilities carry only one or two sizes. The portion inserted into the stomach has a large opening at the tip and several side openings located near the end. The external end is slightly funnel shaped to allow easy connection to a suction tubing or to a feeding set (Fig. 43–1). All are disposed of after use.

All nasogastric tubes cause some irritation to the nares and to the throat through which they pass. When being inserted, they may also cause gagging and even vomiting. If this occurs, the patient should be placed in high Fowler's position *to prevent regurgitation of stomach contents into the esophagus, which can possibly be aspirated into the lungs.*

The most common type of tube is made of rigid, clear plastic with a number of measured black circular marks to denote the appropriate tube length for insertion. Red rubber tubes of the same design also are available. Some physicians prefer them *because they cause less irritation in the back of the throat and the nose due to their softness.* Red rubber tubes are more expensive, and in the past, were cleaned and resterilized. Many nurses find the red rubber tubes easier to insert if they are chilled in a pan of ice for 15 to 20 minutes before insertion. *This makes them more rigid and less likely to coil in the back of the throat when they are being inserted.*

Pediatric-sized nasogastric tubes with a smaller lumen may be used for some adults *because they are less irritating.* The smaller lumen tubes may also be used for unconscious adults, *but these tubes tend to coil rather than move down smoothly,* and insertion is often difficult. To facilitate passage of a small lumen tube

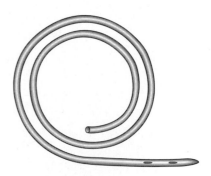

Figure 43–1. Levin tube.

into an unconscious adult patient, first obtain a small and a standard nasogastric tube. Also obtain half of an empty gelatin capsule. Fill the empty capsule half full with water-soluble lubricant (*in case the patient aspirates*) and insert the ends of both tubes into the capsule. Pass both tubes together into the patient. *The large tube facilitates passage of the small tube.* After the tubes are in the stomach, the gelatin capsule will dissolve. Then the large tube can be withdrawn, leaving the small tube in place.

Gastric Sump Tubes (Salem, Ventrol)

The gastric sump tube is a variation of the nasogastric tube that is especially designed for gastric suctioning. The gastric sump tube has a double lumen, with two distinct tube "tails" at the distal portion. Its advantage is that its smaller, open end (color-coded blue) is open to room air, *allowing equalization of pressure and therefore continuous, steady suction without pull on the tissues. Suction pull above the level of capillary fragility, which can cause damage to tissues, is prevented* (Fig. 43–2).

One nursing precaution you should take is to position the open end of the air-vent tube above the patient's midline *to prevent leakage of stomach contents* when low suction is on and the pull pressure is not

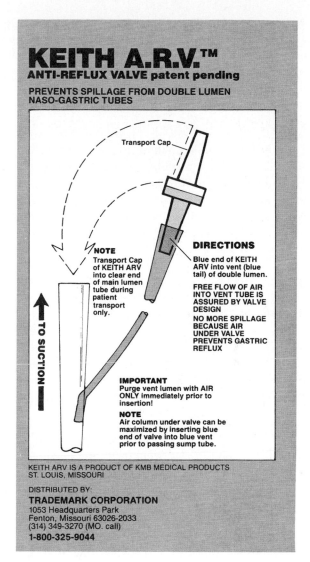

Figure 43–3. Antireflux valve. (Courtesy Trademark Corp., Fenton, Missouri.)

sufficient to maintain flow through the drainage tube. An antireflux valve device *that allows the Salem sump tube to be equalized by air but prevents leakage of gastric secretions* is available (Fig. 43–3).

The nurse should always irrigate the tube using the larger or primary tube, because the vented air tube *may become occluded with the irrigation solution or secretions.* If it is necessary to irrigate the vent lumen to clear secretions, always follow the solution with a small amount of air to restore the open vent.

Small-Bore, Silicone Rubber Feeding Tubes

A variety of small-bore, silicone rubber feeding tubes are available. Their soft material and small size decrease the irritation of nose and throat. In

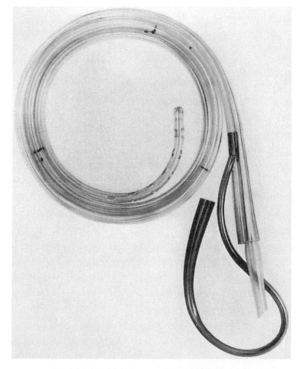

Figure 43–2. Salem sump tube with second lumen to provide air vent.

addition, the cardiac sphincter closes more tightly around them, lessening the possibility of regurgitation and aspiration. Although the softness and small size make them desirable for the patient, they are more difficult to insert.

Keofeed Tube

The Keofeed tube is small in diameter and made of soft Silastic (silicone rubber) with a weighted end. The tube comes from the manufacturer with a firm metal stylet threaded through its lumen *to facilitate insertion.* Final positioning is usually verified by x-ray with the stylet in place. Then the stylet is removed. The stylet should be saved because the tube might be removed or pulled out and have to be reinserted. Lubricating the stylet well with water-soluble lubricant *facilitates its reinsertion so the tube can be reinserted into the patient.*

Because the end of the tube is weighted, it will move with peristalsis into the small intestine if the tube is not taped with tension to the nose. This feature makes it especially suitable for delivering enteral or tube feedings (see Module 29, Tube Feeding).

Duo-Tube

Another variation of a weighted tube is the Duo-Tube. This clear vinyl tube surrounds a silicone radiopaque catheter. The silicone catheter comes with either a silicone weight *for gastric feeding* or a mercury weight *if passage into the pylorus is desired for diagnostic or feeding purposes.* After lubrication with a water-soluble lubricant, the Duo-Tube is inserted into the stomach in the same manner as other nasogastric tubes. The inner tube is advanced approximately 2 in by attaching a water-filled bulb (which comes with the set) to the distal end of the tube and compressing it. This maneuver can be repeated until the tube is inserted the desired length. The clear tube is then carefully withdrawn. It remains attached to the inner tube and forms a continuous long tube. It can be attached to a feeding set or shortened. The inner tube, then, directly attaches to the feeding set (Fig. 43–4).

Dobbhoff Tube

Another type of weighted tube is the Dobbhoff tube, which is made of soft plastic material and coated on both its inner and outer surfaces with a water-soluble lubricant. The stylet is hollow *so that air can be injected through it to check tube placement before the stylet is removed.* The distal end of the tube is weighted with tungsten rather than mercury. If a rupture occurs (which is rare), *tungsten is considered less hazardous to*

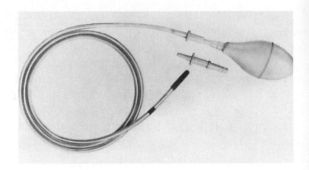

Figure 43–4. Duofeed tube with bulb to advance inner tube. (Courtesy Argyle Division of Sherwood Medical, St. Louis, Missouri.)

the patient than mercury. The Dobbhoff tube is designed to be passed from the stomach into the small intestine, minimizing the chance of regurgitation, which can lead to aspiration.

Special Purpose Tubes

Some tubes are used for special functions other than routine suctioning or feeding. These include the Ewald, Cantor, and Miller-Abbott tubes.

Ewald Tube

The Ewald tube has a very large lumen. It ranges in size from 26 to 30 French and is *used for lavage, usually for a patient who has ingested poisonous agents.* The Ewald tube is also used for diagnostic tests. Its use is uncommon on the general nursing unit.

Cantor Tube

The Cantor tube is a long, single-lumen rubber tube with a rubber bag attached to its distal tip (Fig. 43–5).

Just before insertion, medical personnel inject approximately 30 mL mercury into the bag, using a needle and syringe. Insertion of this tube is uncomfortable, *because the bag is large.* This tube is usually inserted by a physician, who uses a topical anesthetic in the nose and posterior pharynx *to make insertion more tolerable for the patient.* The weight of the mercury *facilitates passage of the tube into the small bowel and may help overcome an obstruction.* When the Cantor tube is removed, a flashlight is used *to observe the back of the throat.* When the bag reaches that level, a pair of forceps is used to grasp the bag and pull it out through the mouth. The bag is then cut off and the tube pulled out through the nose. *This prevents the possibility of this large, heavy bag damaging the inside of the nose.* When the Cantor tube is used, a safety consideration should be *to protect the patient and the*

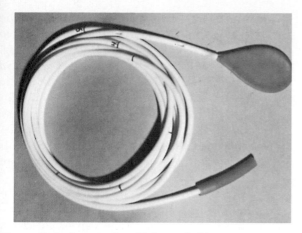

Figure 43–5. Cantor tube with bag to hold mercury. (Courtesy American Hospital Supply Corp., McGaw Park, Illinois.)

nurse from the mercury, which can cause poisoning through skin absorption, inhalation of mercury vapor, and ingestion. The container should be kept covered, and the mercury should not be spilled. Do not touch the mercury with bare hands. Before the mercury is inserted, inspect the bag for holes. When the tube is removed, do not throw the mercury away, but return it in a sealed container through appropriate hospital channels for correct disposal. *Mercury is very expensive,* so it should not be wasted.

Miller-Abbott Tube

The Miller-Abbott tube is a long, double-lumen rubber tube. One lumen leads to a rubber bag at the tube's end. This lumen can be filled with air or fluid *to provide a larger object at the end so that peristalsis can advance the tube into the small intestine.* The other lumen is used for suction and irrigation. The Miller-Abbott tube is inserted in the same manner as a conventional nasogastric tube. Once the tube is positioned in the stomach, the bag is inflated with air or fluid through its lumen. If the tube is not secured with tape to the patient's nose, it will gradually advance into the small bowel. This is desirable when small bowel obstruction is suspected. It is important to keep the openings to each lumen clearly marked *so suction is attached correctly.*

PROCEDURE FOR INSERTING AND IRRIGATING A NASOGASTRIC TUBE

Assessment

1. Check the physician's orders *to determine the type of tube to be inserted and the reason (feeding, suction).*
2. Assess the patient's capabilities for cooperating with the procedure.

3. Determine where the needed equipment is located. Some items may be kept on the unit; others may need to be ordered from central services.

Planning

4. Wash your hands *for infection control. Because the gastrointestinal tract is not sterile,* it is acceptable to use clean but not sterile technique.
5. Gather the equipment. If the tube is to be used for feeding or suction, also obtain the appropriate feeding set or suction apparatus. In addition to the tube, you will need clean gloves and a water-soluble lubricant, which, if aspirated, *will not cause aspiration pneumonia.* An emesis basin, tape, tissues, a towel, a glass, a straw, a stethoscope, and a large syringe with an adapter or an asepto syringe should also be available. A rubber band and safety pin are commonly used to attach the tube to the patient's gown.
6. If it is necessary, plan for any assistance. Even though the patient may be alert and able to participate, another person's support during the procedure may be appreciated by the patient.
7. If a special or weighted tube is being used, review the manufacturer's directions for insertion. If an unweighted tube is to be inserted, continue with the next steps.

Implementation

8. Identify the patient *to be sure you are performing the procedure for the correct patient.*
9. Explain the procedure to the patient and why it is needed. *Because the patient is apt to be anxious,* do not explain the procedure too far in advance. Tell the patient that the procedure will not be painful but may be uncomfortable. Explain how the patient can participate. For example, *relaxation is important,* so ask the patient to breathe deeply, and explain as you proceed. *Your confidence will also help the patient to relax.*
10. Place the patient in high Fowler's position if possible *so gravity aids insertion of the tube.* Put a clean towel over the patient's chest *to protect the linen.* If the patient's skin is oily, you may use an alcohol swab to cleanse the nose for later tape application. A skin preparation may also be used on the nose to increase tape adherence.
11. Some manufacturers mark the length for insertion for pediatric and adult use on the tube. If the tube you are using is not marked, stand to the patient's right, if you are right-handed, and measure the portion of tube to be inserted by extending it from the tip of the patient's nose to the earlobe and from the earlobe to the xiphoid process.

Experience has shown that in tall people, it may be necessary to add 2 in to the length of the tube *to ensure entrance into the stomach*. If you are measuring the nasogastric tube for an infant, extend it from the tip of the nose to the earlobe and then from the earlobe to a point halfway between the xiphoid process and the umbilicus *because the body proportions are different in infants and adults*. Mark the tube with a piece of tape.

12. Put on gloves, and lubricate the tube with a water-soluble lubricant. Lubricate the portion of the tube from tip to marking *to avoid damaging the nasopharyngeal mucosa when you insert the tube*.

13. Flex the patient's head slightly forward. *In this position the tube is less likely to pass into the trachea because the glottis closes the trachea in this position.* Grasp the tube with your right hand, about 3 in from the end, and gently insert it into the nostril, guiding it straight back along the floor of the nose.

14. Have a basin in the patient's lap and tissues handy. If orders allow, have the patient sip water and swallow while you gently but steadily advance the tube. There may be some temporary gagging, *caused by the gag reflex*, but this should subside as the tube is progressed. If any coughing persists or dyspnea occurs, remove the tube immediately *because you may have entered the trachea*.

15. Using tape, secure the tube to the patient's nose.

Place a vertical strip down the bridge of the nose. Cut the lower end of the tape into two "tails" and wrap them around the tube (Fig. 43–6). *This method is comfortable for the patient and prevents irritation of the side of the nostril.* Fasten the length of tube to the patient's gown with a rubber band and safety pin, *so the patient can move freely in bed without pulling or dislodging the tube*.

Flexible tape bandages may also be used to attach the tube to the nose. Figure 43–7 gives an example of one type.

16. Check to see if the end of the tube is in the stomach. *If it is curled in the back of the throat, it is uncomfortable and ineffective*. You can easily check this by asking the patient to open the mouth or by holding down the tongue with a tongue depressor. Using a flashlight, you can see if the tube is curled in the back of the throat. *The possibility that it is partially in the trachea, so that fluids would enter the lungs and cause serious complications, is more dangerous*. You can check the tube's position in several ways; some are more reliable than others.

In a conscious patient who is able to swallow a nasogastric tube, identifying incorrect tube placement is usually quite uncomplicated. If the patient swallows the tube voluntarily, the

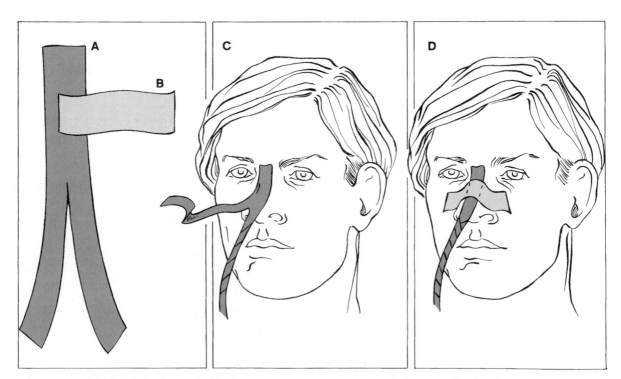

Figure 43–6. Securing the nasogastric tube. **(A)** Tape torn lengthwise for several inches to be placed lengthwise on nose, with tails hanging beyond end of nose. **(B)** Second tape to be placed crosswise over bridge of nose. **(C)** Tape A in place, one tail spiraled around tube. **(D)** Second tail spiraling in opposite direction; tape B over bridge of nose secures tape A.

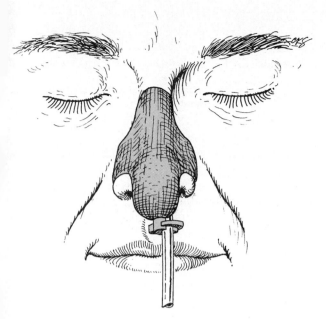

Figure 43–7. Commercial nasogastric suction tube attachment device.

epiglottis closes over the tracheal opening, preventing the tube from entering the trachea. Although the patient may gag or vomit *from the stimulation of the pharynx by the tube,* this is usually easy to differentiate from the coughing and choking that occur if the tube does enter the trachea. The patient will be unable to talk *because the tube will interfere with vocal cord movement.* The general skin color may change, becoming dusky *as the person does not receive enough oxygen.* You should immediately withdraw the tube if these indications occur. These indications of tube misplacement may be completely absent in the unconscious patient or in the patient with neurologic deficits. Verifying accurate tube placement (ie, clearly with the end in the stomach or small intestine as desired) is much more difficult, and many different bedside methods have been used by nurses throughout the years. Most of these methods have not been confirmed by research data. If the tube will be used only for suction, these bedside methods may be considered adequate and the tube simply repositioned if it is not functioning adequately.

The only positive method of guaranteeing correct placement is through x-ray. Even though tubes with stylets are initially verified by x-ray, they should be checked at the bedside each time a feeding is given *because they can become dislodged after verification. Instilling feedings where they might be aspirated is a serious danger.* Several bedside methods can be used, as follows:

a. **Aspirating visually recognizable gastrointestinal secretions.** This is considered an excellent method *because in most instances, gastric secretions are clearly identifiable by their greenish brown, mucoid appearance.* This method is less reliable if the patient has had bleeding in the respiratory tract, making respiratory secretions dark, or if the patient has been receiving dilute tube feedings that might give a frothy white appearance to gastric contents, which are mistaken for respiratory secretions. This method may not work with tubes with a small lumen (small-bore) *because they often collapse when suction pressure is applied.* Sometimes the stomach is empty, and it is not possible to aspirate any fluid.

b. **Auscultating air insufflated through the nasogastric tube.** The nurse auscultates over the epigastrium as 10 to 15 mL of air is introduced into the tube with a syringe. *The air makes a gurgling, bubbling noise that can be heard clearly if the tube is placed correctly.* This is more discernable through a large-bore tube. Through a small tube, the sound may be muffled, and it may be difficult to distinguish between air in the stomach and air in the esophagus.

c. **pH testing of aspirates.** This method may be valuable. *The pH of the stomach is low (very acid) and the pH of the small intestine is higher (more alkaline).* This method might help to identify when the tube entered the stomach and then when it was passed into the duodenum. However, no reliable data are available clearly documenting the pH. *Some factors may need to be considered, such as the administration of drugs that lessen gastric acidity, the recent administration of other drugs that affect gastric pH, and the effect of tube feedings.* This method does rely on the ability to obtain secretions when aspirating.

d. **Observing for coughing and choking.** As previously discussed, this method is useful for identifying misplacement when working with an alert patient who has all neurologic responses intact. It is not reliable for an unconscious or neurologically impaired patient. This method does not verify whether the end of the tube is placed in the esophagus, stomach, or duodenum.

e. **Testing for ability to speak.** This method has worked with large lumen (large-bore) tubes placed in alert, neurologically intact patients. However, there are reports of patients with small silicone rubber tubes in the

DATE/TIME	
2/14/99 1430	*Salem sump tube inserted. Attached to low intermittent suction. Resting quietly with no discomfort. —— T. Kent, SN*

Example of Nursing Progress Notes Using Narrative Format.

trachea who could still talk. It is not useful for the unconscious or nonalert patient. Again, it may identify misplacement but will not verify correct placement.

In the past, some nurses have observed for bubbling when the tip of the tube is placed under water. This method is unreliable *because air bubbles may come from the stomach and from the respiratory tract. Also, the patient who has shallow breathing may not be able to force air out of the tube through the water and so would not create bubbles even if the tube were in the lungs.*

17. *To prevent air from entering the stomach, which could cause distention,* keep the free end of the tube plugged at all times except when checking position, feeding, or irrigating.
18. To irrigate the tube, do the following:
    a. Slowly instill 10 to 20 mL solution, usually water or normal saline, with a syringe. The physician may order a larger volume to be used for irrigation.
    b. Gently aspirate. If any bleeding is apparent, stop the aspiration, and report your observations to the physician. Carefully measure all gastric secretions, which must be considered output.
19. To suction, do the following:
    a. Turn on the equipment *before* attaching it to the nasogastric tube. This way, *if the suction is too strong or the device malfunctions, the patient is not harmed.* Test the suction by placing your finger over the suction tube opening and feeling the amount of pull. Unless otherwise ordered, always begin with the low setting

when applying suction *so tissues are not damaged.*
    b. Attach the suction to the patient's nasogastric tube, using an adapter.
    c. Check the equipment regularly *to make sure suction is occurring, and the proper suction level is being maintained.*
20. Help the patient to a comfortable position.
21. Provide frequent oronasal care. *This is because the tube irritates the nostrils and the back of the throat, producing a drying condition. Also, the mouth becomes particularly dry because the patient is mouth breathing and is neither eating nor taking fluids.*
22. Dispose of gloves, and wash your hands.

Evaluation

23. Evaluate using the following criteria:
    a. Patient comfortable.
    b. No irritation at nostrils.
    c. Normal breathing rate and rhythm.
    d. No indications of nausea or regurgitation.
    e. Tube properly placed.

Documentation

24. Initiate an intake and output patient record.
25. Document the following on the patient record:
    a. Type and size of tube inserted
    b. Amount and characteristics of any drainage returned
    c. Suction pressure applied
    d. Patient response to procedure
26. Add to the Nursing Care Plan information pertinent to care needed.

DATE/TIME		
8/17/99 0930	D:	*Salem sump tube in place. Air-vent tube in low position with drainage soiling gown. Patient appears anxious and fearful.*
	A:	*Inserted antireflux device into air-vent tube. Provided hygiene and clean gown. Reassured patient. ——*
	R:	*Patient stated, "I feel so much better now." —— K. Ryan, RN*

Example of Nursing Progress Notes Using Focus Format.

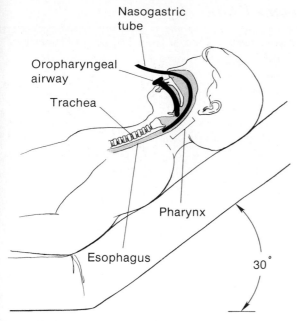

Figure 43–8. Nasogastric intubation of an unconscious patient. The oropharyngeal airway prevents the nasogastric tube from coiling forward, so the tube passes easily into the esophagus.

INTUBATING THE UNCONSCIOUS PATIENT

An unconscious patient may require insertion of a nasogastric tube *to relieve gastric distention or to receive liquid feedings.*

Observe all the principles described in the previous procedure, with the following important adaptations. Place the patient in low to mid-Fowler's position, again with the head flexed forward slightly *to facilitate passage past the trachea. The main danger is the possible insertion of the tube through the bronchus into the lung. The unconscious patient may have lost gag and cough reflexes,* so you may not accurately know the position of the tube *because the patient will not cough if the tube is positioned incorrectly.* An easy but effective way to avoid this problem is to insert an oropharyngeal airway into the patient's mouth. *The distal end of the airway acts as a guide,* moving the tube smoothly down into the esophagus (Fig. 43–8). Even if you have used an airway, carefully check tube placement. When you are sure the location is correct, remove the airway.

PROCEDURE FOR REMOVING A NASOGASTRIC TUBE

Assessment
1. Verify that the tube is no longer needed and that the physician has ordered its removal.

Planning
2. Wash your hands *for infection control.*
3. Obtain clean gloves and a towel *for handling and covering the soiled tube.*

Implementation
4. Identify the patient *to be sure you are performing the procedure for the correct patient.*
5. Explain to the patient that although removing the tube will be uncomfortable, it will be over quickly.
6. If suction is operating, turn it off, and disconnect the tube. If suction is on while you are removing the tube, *patient discomfort may be increased.*
7. Put on gloves, and pinch the tube closed or plug it *to prevent secretions from leaking into the esophagus and pharynx.* The secretions in the tube are stomach acids and therefore are irritating.
8. Withdraw the tube smoothly in a continuous motion. Any nausea and gagging that occur are increased by pulling the tube too slowly, *which stimulates the posterior pharynx.*
9. Place the soiled tubing in the towel and cover it, *because it is aesthetically unpleasant.*
10. Provide comfort, and give mouth care.
11. Measure secretions in the collection container.
12. Dispose of the equipment and gloves properly.
13. Wash your hands.

Evaluation
14. Evaluate using the following criteria:
    a. Patient comfortable.
    b. No abdominal distention present.

Documentation
15. In the manner prescribed by your facility, document the time the tube was removed, the amount and description of material in the collection container, and the patient's response to the procedure.

DATE/TIME	
2/17/99 2200	*Nasogastric tube removed per order. 1,100 mL cloudy, light green drainage in suction bottle. Abdomen soft, bowel tones present.* — *T. Kent, SN*

Example of Nursing Progress Notes Using Narrative Format.

LONG-TERM CARE

Inserting and removing a nasogastric tube is a skill that is frequently used by the nurse in the long-term care setting. The purpose is commonly to introduce nutrients (tube feeding) on a temporary or permanent basis for residents who are unable to eat a diet normally. Because of this, the types of tubes used in long-term care are generally those used for tube feeding rather than those used for gastric decompression or diagnostic determinations. On occasion, a resident may have suffered a stroke and is not conscious; therefore, the directions for inserting a feeding tube in the unconscious person are useful. Maintaining safety while performing these skills is an extremely important consideration for the nurse practicing in any setting. The same precautions must be taken so that the tube is positioned correctly and does not become dislodged. Some long-term care settings obtain a portable x-ray to validate proper placement. Using a mobile x-ray unit is costly but may be necessary if the policy of your facility requires this safeguard. Another cost is the reinsertion of a nasogastric tube when the one in place is no longer patent. The nurse can often irrigate or unclog a tube so that replacement is unnecessary.

The nurse may also be responsible for teaching assessment techniques regarding the presence of a nasogastric tube to other staff members and act as a resource person. Nurses working in long-term care who interact with families may answer questions regarding the presence and necessity of a feeding tube.

HOME CARE

People who at one time would have remained in the acute or chronic care setting for convalescence are receiving care in the home. The insertion of a nasogastric tube may be ordered for the purpose of introducing tube feeding.

This procedure may be frightening for the client or the care providers and family. By demonstrating expertise and following all safety precautions, the home care nurse can reassure everyone. Depending on the agency, an x-ray may be required for checking placement. It is therefore important that the home health nurse review the policies and procedures of the agency.

Clear explanations of all steps of the procedure to the client and others giving care also are important. Teaching what data are needed for continual assessment to these people aids the nurse in responding to concerns that arise. Ongoing evaluation is a process that can be shared with the client and care providers in the home.

CRITICAL THINKING EXERCISES

An 82-year-old, alert woman in long-term care has refused to eat for the last 5 days. Her physician ordered the insertion of a nasogastric tube for the purpose of tube feeding. The resident pulled out the tube, stating that it made her nose and throat uncomfortable. Identify additional assessment data that are important for you to collect. Describe what steps you might take to determine whether or not the tube is to be reinserted. Depending on what you determine, relate how you would interact with the resident.

✔ **PERFORMANCE CHECKLIST**

Inserting and Irrigating a Nasogastric Tube	Needs More Practice	Satisfactory	Comments
Assessment			
1. Check the physician's order.			
2. Assess patient's capabilities for cooperating.			
3. Determine availability of equipment.			
Planning			
4. Wash your hands.			
5. Gather equipment.			
6. Plan for any assistance necessary.			
7. If weighted or special tube is to be used, review manufacturer's directions for insertion.			
Implementation			
8. Identify the patient.			
9. Explain the procedure to the patient.			
10. Place patient in high Fowler's position with head flexed forward. (Prepare nose skin for tape.)			
11. Determine length of tube to be inserted and mark.			
12. Put on gloves, and lubricate tube.			
13. Flex patient's head slightly forward, and gently insert tube into nostril.			
14. Using prescribed procedure, advance tube.			
15. Secure tube to bridge of nose.			
16. Check to see if tube is in stomach.			
17. Plug end of tube.			
18. If irrigating, follow directions.			
19. If applying suction, follow directions.			
20. Make patient comfortable.			
21. Give oronasal care.			
22. Dispose of gloves, and wash your hands.			

(continued)

Inserting and Irrigating a Nasogastric Tube (Continued)	Needs More Practice	Satisfactory	Comments
Evaluation			
23. Evaluate using the following criteria: a. Patient is comfortable.			
b. No irritation at nostrils.			
c. Normal breathing.			
d. No indications of nausea or regurgitation.			
e. Tube properly placed.			
Documentation			
24. Initiate an intake and output record.			
25. Document the following on the patient record: a. Type and size of tube inserted			
b. Amount and characteristics of any drainage returned			
c. Suction pressure applied			
d. Patient response to procedure			
26. Add information to the nursing care plan relative to care needed.			
Removing a Nasogastric Tube			
Assessment			
1. Verify that tube is to be removed.			
Planning			
2. Wash your hands.			
3. Obtain clean gloves and a towel for handling and covering tube.			
Implementation			
4. Identify the patient.			
5. Explain procedure to patient.			
6. If suction is on, turn it off.			
7. Put on gloves and pinch tube closed.			
8. Withdraw tube rapidly and smoothly.			
9. Place soiled tube in towel and cover.			
10. Make patient comfortable, and provide oral care.			

(continued)

Removing a Nasogastric Tube *(Continued)*	Needs More Practice	Satisfactory	Comments
11. Measure any output and record.			
12. Dispose of equipment and gloves.			
13. Wash your hands.			
Evaluation			
14. Evaluate using the following criteria: **a.** Patient is comfortable.			
b. No abdominal distention present.			
Documentation			
15. Document time of procedure, amount of any drainage, and patient's tolerance.			

PREOPERATIVE CARE

MODULE CONTENTS

PREREQUISITES

Successful completion of the following modules:

(continued)

PREREQUISITES (continued)

Module 5   Documentation
Module 6   Introduction to Assessment Skills
Module 7   Temperature, Pulse, and Respiration
Module 8   Blood Pressure
Module 11   Collecting Specimens and Performing Common Laboratory Tests
Module 13   Admission, Transfer, and Discharge

VOLUME 2
Module 39   Respiratory Care Procedures

The following modules are not essential, but their successful completion will allow you to carry out more complete care for selected patients.

VOLUME 1
Module 12   Assisting With Diagnostic and Therapeutic Procedures
Module 28   Administering Enemas

VOLUME 2
Module 37   Catheterization
Module 43   Nasogastric Intubation
Module 46   Irrigations: Bladder, Catheter, Ear, Eye, Nasogastric Tube, Vaginal,
            Wound
Module 47   Administering Medications: Overview
Module 48   Administering Oral Medications
Module 50   Giving Injections

OVERALL OBJECTIVE

To prepare patients physically and psychologically for all phases of the perioperative experience: the preoperative, intraoperative (anesthesia and surgery), and postoperative phases.

SPECIFIC LEARNING OBJECTIVES

Know Facts and Principles	Apply Facts and Principles	Demonstrate Ability	Evaluate Performance
1. Initial preoperative planning and care			
a. Interview			
List information to be obtained through preoperative interview.	Given a patient situation, identify information indicating potential problem.	Carry out preoperative interview effectively.	Evaluate own performance using Performance Checklist.
b. Teaching			
State information to be included in preoperative teaching.	Adapt teaching plan to meet individual patient's concerns.	Carry out preoperative teaching appropriately.	Evaluate own performance using Performance Checklist.
2. Preoperative skin preparation			
State three objectives of preoperative skin preparation.			
a. Bath			
State rationale for bathing/showering before surgery and for using an antimicrobial agent.	Explain to patient rationale for preoperative bath or shower.	Assist patient with preoperative bath or shower.	Evaluate with instructor.
b. Scrub of surgical site			
State rationale for scrub of the surgical site before selected surgeries.	Explain to patient rationale for scrub of surgical site.	Carry out preoperative scrub of surgical site when ordered.	Evaluate with instructor.
c. Hair removal			
(1) Timing of hair removal			
State rationale for timing preoperative shave.	Given a time schedule for surgery, identify appropriate time for shave preparation.		
(2) Wet versus dry shave			
List advantages and disadvantages of wet and dry shaving.			
(3) Depilatories			
List advantages and disadvantages of using chemical depilatories.			

SPECIFIC LEARNING OBJECTIVES (continued)

Know Facts and Principles	Apply Facts and Principles	Demonstrate Ability	Evaluate Performance
d. Shaving procedure List equipment needed for preoperative shave.	Given a patient situation, describe correct area to be shaved by naming perimeters.	Correctly and safely complete preoperative shave.	Evaluate shave by checking skin with strong light for hair removal and irritation. Evaluate own performance using Performance Checklist.
3. Immediate preoperative care List aspects of physical care given during immediate preoperative period.	In the practice setting, simulate immediate care of patient.	Carry out immediate care of preoperative patient.	Evaluate own performance using Performance Checklist.
4. Checklist State information included on preoperative checklist.	In the practice setting, complete preoperative checklist.	In the clinical setting, complete patient's preoperative checklist.	Evaluate with instructor.

LEARNING ACTIVITIES

1. Review the Specific Learning Objectives.
2. Read the chapters on health teaching, hygiene and the experience of surgery; and the section on anxiety in the chapter on mental health in Ellis and Nowlis, *Nursing: A Human Needs Approach*, or comparable material in another textbook.
3. Review the material in your medical-surgical nursing textbook that relates to preoperative care.
4. Look up the module vocabulary terms in the glossary.
5. Read through the module as though you were preparing to teach the skills and procedures to another person. Mentally practice the skills.
6. In the practice setting, do the following:
   a. Using a partner as a patient, practice performing the assessment interview. Include preoperative teaching, and document your data.
   b. Have your partner evaluate your performance using the Performance Checklist.
   c. Reverse roles, and have your partner interview you and perform preoperative teaching.
   d. Evaluate your partner's performance.
   e. Observe the equipment used for the preoperative shave.
   f. Again, with your partner, role-play the immediate preoperative period using the Performance Checklist as a guide.
   g. Have your partner evaluate your performance.
   h. Reverse roles, and repeat step 6f.
   i. Evaluate your partner's performance.
   j. Demonstrate making a postoperative bed.
7. In the clinical setting, do the following:
   a. Perform initial preoperative planning and care.
      (1) Review your facility's procedure manual for initial preoperative planning and care.
      (2) Consult your instructor when you are ready to perform initial preoperative planning and care.
   b. Perform preoperative skin preparation.
      (1) Review your facility's procedure for preoperative skin preparation, paying special attention to the areas to be shaved for designated surgeries.
      (2) Ask for an opportunity to observe a preoperative shave.
      (3) Consult with your instructor regarding an opportunity to do a preoperative shave. (Shaving for abdominal surgery is a wise choice for beginning experience.)
   c. Perform immediate preoperative care.
      (1) Review your facility's procedure for giving immediate preoperative care.
      (2) Examine the checklist used.
      (3) Request an opportunity to give immediate preoperative care, including the completion of the checklist.

VOCABULARY

ambulatory surgery	antimicrobial	epithelial	perineal
anesthesia	aspirate	inpatient	perioperative
anesthesiologist	complete blood count	intraoperative	postanesthesia care
anesthetic	depilatory	laparotomy	unit (PACU)
anesthetist	diuretic	NPO	TEDs
antiembolic stockings	endotracheal tube	outpatient	thoracotomy

Preoperative Care

Rationale for the Use of This Skill

Perioperative nursing practice includes activities performed by the registered nurse during the preoperative, intraoperative, and postoperative phases of the patient's surgical experience. An important factor that contributes to a safe and successful perioperative experience and an uneventful convalescence is the conscientious and individualized preparation of the patient by the registered nurse. Remember that the patient is traumatized not only by the surgical procedure, but also by exposure to anesthetic agents. In addition, surgery is emotionally stressful, causing degrees of fear and anxiety. Preoperative care, therefore, must include appropriate health teaching, physical preparation, and psychological support. Although portions of preoperative care may be undertaken by other members of the health-care team, overall coordination and implementation remain the nurse's primary responsibilities.[1]

PLANNING PREOPERATIVE CARE

Traditionally, patients entered the hospital at least 1 day before a scheduled surgery to ensure adequate time for preoperative care. These same patients were expected to stay several days after surgery for recovery. Surgeries scheduled in advance are called *elective* surgeries. In some instances, such as those in which complex preparations must begin the evening before surgery, patients still enter the hospital the day before the scheduled surgery.

However, to limit hospital costs by decreasing the length of stay, many patients now enter the hospital the morning of surgery. "AM admission" often results in limited time for preoperative care. Nurses working in units with morning surgical admissions have to develop excellent organizational skills and plan carefully to complete all the preoperative care described in this module. Typically, more than one task is accomplished at the same time.

When patients have day surgery, also referred to as ambulatory surgery, they commonly enter the hospital the day of surgery and are discharged later that same day. This increases the importance of the patient's preoperative preparation about postoperative care, because that care must be performed independently by the patient and family.

Preadmission outpatient visits are used in some hospitals to allow adequate time for preoperative care.

This is especially true for patients scheduled for major surgery involving lengthy recovery periods and for children undergoing surgery. During these visits, the initial patient or family interview, laboratory work, and consent forms are completed. In addition, the nurse begins preoperative teaching. This may be done on a one-to-one basis, or special programs may be structured for groups of patients undergoing similar procedures. Family members may also be included.

These programs are directed and instructed by nurses with special surgical and teaching skills. Patients receive health teaching regarding what to expect preoperatively, intraoperatively, and postoperatively and how to participate in regaining independence. With the help of booklets and visual aids, they are taught deep-breathing exercises, leg and foot exercises, how to move in bed, and how to get in and out of bed. They are also shown equipment that may be used. Some programs include a tour of the surgical unit and introductions to the staff. *Such programs are helpful in reducing anxiety and decreasing complications after surgery.*

If the patient has not participated in a preadmission outpatient visit, the patient entering the preoperative unit has probably already been to the laboratory, where blood and urine samples have been collected for laboratory studies, such as a complete blood count (CBC) and urinalysis (UA). In some settings, patients have no laboratory studies before surgery unless there is a recognized problem. The consent-for-surgery form may have been signed and witnessed in the admitting office. If it has not, the physician or nurse will ask the patient to sign the form on the unit. (See Module 13, Admission, Transfer, and Discharge, for general admitting procedure.)

When a patient needs emergency surgery (a surgery not scheduled in advance), the nurse will need to determine which parts of preoperative care are essential for this particular situation and which parts can be omitted or abbreviated. Sometimes several hours elapse from the time an emergency surgery is scheduled until it is performed. On other occasions, the patient moves from the emergency department directly to the operating room.

Preoperative care varies from facility to facility. At points throughout the module, you may have to check the policies of the facility in which you practice and adapt your care to those policies.

Role of the Anesthesiologist

The *anesthesiologist* is a medical doctor whose specialty is administering local, regional, and general anesthetic agents. Many also have expertise in pain control procedures.

---

[1]Note that rationale for action is emphasized throughout the module by the use of italics.

An *anesthetist* is a nurse with advanced education and skills to administer anesthetics under the supervision of an anesthesiologist. One of these people will visit the patient before surgery—usually the evening before or morning of surgery. The purpose of the visit is to assess the patient for the dosage and appropriate anesthetic to be used, give the patient information about the anesthetic that is to be given and answer any questions, and write the orders for the preoperative medication.

Role of the Surgeon

When surgery is planned, the surgeon is responsible for obtaining informed consent for the procedure. This may be done before the patient enters the hospital. If not, the patient will sign a consent for surgery in the hospital, and a nurse may witness that signature. The nurse in this situation is not responsible for informing the patient about the surgery; that remains the surgeon's responsibility. The nurse should notify the surgeon if assessment reveals that the patient is not adequately informed.

Because surgery is a highly technical and complex field that changes rapidly, the surgeon has the ultimate responsibility for determining what preoperative care is needed specific to the surgery itself. Although every facility will have certain routine procedures, the individual surgeon may alter these. Therefore, the nurse working on a surgical unit must have a close collaborative relationship with the surgeons to ensure that the patient receives the best possible care.

Role(s) of the Nurse

The nurse is responsible for the following aspects of preoperative care:

• Preoperative assessment interview
• Preoperative teaching
• Various preoperative interventions
• Aspects of skin preparation (in some settings)
• Immediate preoperative care (ie, care given just before the patient leaves the patient care unit for the operating room)

PREOPERATIVE INTERVIEW

The initial step in preoperative care is the preoperative interview. If the patient has not been admitted to the hospital before beginning your preoperative interview, you will also need to perform an admission physical assessment (see Module 6, Introduc-

tion to Assessment Skills, and Module 13, Admission, Transfer, and Discharge).

PROCEDURE FOR PREOPERATIVE INTERVIEW

Assessment
1. Verify the type of surgery, the date and time surgery is scheduled, and the name of the surgeon. You can do this by checking the operative schedule form that comes to the unit from the operating room or one that is entered into the computer. A specific time will usually be listed, or the abbreviation TF may be used. This means your patient's surgery is "to follow" a previous procedure, and the exact time is undetermined.
2. Check the preoperative orders *to determine your responsibilities regarding preparing the patient for surgery.* Some surgeons use a stamp for their routine orders on a specific procedure and add any special orders for the individual patient.

Planning
3. Consult the procedure book of your facility regarding the type of surgery, the preparation needed, and the surgeon's preferences. Some facilities maintain a Kardex or file listing surgeons' preferences.
4. Check the patient's chart for the history and physical (H&P) and the signed consent form. A CBC or a UA (or both) may be ordered by the physician if indicated by the patient's status. The H&P and the completed consent form must be on the record before surgery *to protect the patient, the physician, and staff.* Depending on the patient's health and type of surgery, other tests may also be performed. In some facilities, it is permissible to proceed with the surgery if the H&P is not on the record but has been performed and dictated. You may need to investigate this. Surgery cannot proceed (except in a life-threatening emergency) without a properly completed consent form. Know your facility's policy regarding consent.
5. Arrange to complete the forms and procedures listed in step 4 if they are not on the record. Inform the laboratory or physician about any missing data.
6. Plan sufficient uninterrupted time to carry out the preoperative interview.

Implementation
7. Using the appropriate form, interview the patient, making sure to include the following areas:
   a. *Verification of patient's identity. To practice safely,*

always validate the patient's identity by comparing the wristband to the name and hospital number on the chart. At a preoperative outpatient visit, the patient will not have a wristband. Ask the patient to spell his or her name *to ensure correct identification.* If the patient is confused or very young, verify his or her identity with a close family member or caretaker.

b. *General appearance and physical condition.* A description of the patient's general appearance and physical condition is considered objective data. Record the patient's height and weight, *which is sometimes used to compute the amount of anesthetic agent to be administered.*

c. *Anxiety level.* Communication with the patient during the interview *will usually give you an indication of the patient's anxiety level.* Look for restlessness, fidgeting, rapid respirations and pulse, and statements indicating anxiety.

d. *Knowledge level regarding current surgery.* Ask the patient what he or she knows about the surgery. The physician may have adequately explained the procedure. If not, you should give a general explanation. As with all health teaching, direct any necessary explanation to the patient's level of understanding. *Explicit details or unfamiliar terminology can raise the patient's anxiety level.* Any questions regarding specific points of the surgical procedure or expected results of surgery should be directed to the physician.

e. *Previous surgeries.* List all previous surgeries. *These may have physical and psychological consequences for the current surgery.* Never assume that the patient who has had multiple surgeries needs less preparation. He or she may still be anxious and have inadequate knowledge. A previous negative experience may cause the patient to be even more anxious.

f. *Chronic illnesses.* Inquire about any chronic illness the patient may have. Some illnesses, such as chronic lung disease, hypertension, kidney disorders, or liver disease, may have implications for other aspects of care, including choice of anesthetic(s), medications ordered for pain and sleep, and respiratory care.

g. *Smoking habits.* Note whether the patient is a smoker or nonsmoker. *The lung tissue of a patient who smokes is more sensitive to anesthetic gases because of mild irritation.* Discourage smoking just before surgery. Many hospitals are nonsmoking environments, and not being able to smoke may increase anxiety in some smokers.

h. *Drug, alcohol, and caffeine intake.* List all medications the patient is taking, including vitamin preparations, birth control pills, and nonprescription drugs. Some patients do not think to mention long-term medications, such as diuretics or daily birth control pills. Emphasize the importance of a complete list *because anesthetic agents and other medications ordered may interact with the medications the patient is already taking.* Certain medications (for example, anticonvulsant drugs) will be continued throughout the operative period *because interruption would cause adverse effects for the patient.*

A reliable alcohol history also is essential. *Heavy use of alcohol has multiple effects on the body that can change the patient's response to anesthesia, surgery, and recovery.*

Knowledge of the patient's usual daily caffeine intake may be helpful, especially during the immediate preoperative and postoperative phases. *Some patients will experience severe headaches related to the sudden absence of caffeine intake.*

i. *Support system data.* It is important to list on the form the names and relationships of close family members and friends along with telephone numbers *because the family and significant others are concerned about the patient, may be involved in the health teaching, and often care for the patient after discharge.*

8. Encourage the patient to ask questions about the procedure, the policies of the hospital, or aspects of care. If you do not know the answers to specific questions, consult the appropriate resource person.

9. Provide emotional support. Convey a sense of confidence. Use touch as appropriate *to provide reassurance.*

Evaluation

10. Evaluate your interview by reviewing the data for completeness. If you need more information in any area, return to the patient and clarify.

Documentation

11. Attach the interview form to the patient's chart where you and others can refer to it as you begin the written plan of care.

Rationale for Preoperative Teaching

Well-planned, individualized preoperative teaching prepares the patient for intelligent participation in the activities surrounding the surgery and results in fewer postoperative complications and a smoother postoperative course, according to research. Incorporate your knowledge of the principles of teaching and learning into your facili-

ty's routines and with the physician's orders to plan a teaching strategy to best meet the patient's needs and ensure the best outcome. *If the surgery is an emergency, and time for teaching is short, you may be able to include only priority information.*

PROCEDURE FOR PREOPERATIVE TEACHING

Assessment

1. Carefully review the preoperative orders *so that you can give appropriate information.*
2. Assess the patient's language level, educational background, and anxiety level. If you interviewed the patient, you have some knowledge of these areas. If you have not previously met the patient, spend some time assessing these specific areas.

Planning

3. Allow considerable uninterrupted time *so that you will not be hurried in your instruction, and the patient will feel more relaxed.*
4. If family members or significant friends are present, ask the patient if he or she would like to have them included in the preoperative teaching. Parents or guardians of small children should always be included. *During the postoperative period, these people can often reinforce what has been taught.*

Implementation

5. Provide a quiet, nonstressful environment in which to teach. This includes providing comfortable chairs for those present, turning off the television set, and using an empty day room or conference room if the teaching could disturb a roommate.
6. You may design your own teaching plan or use one provided in your clinical setting (Fig. 44–1), but be sure to include these points as appropriate to the specific surgery planned:
   a. *Preoperative routines.* Outline the routines for the patient in clear, understandable terms. You may do this by system, describing preoperative care of the gastrointestinal tract, skin, and so on, or by going through the preparation sequentially.
   b. *Postoperative routines.* Explain what will be done, with what frequency, and why.
      (1) *Vital signs.* Blood pressure, pulse, and respiration are checked every 15 minutes *for early identification of any problems.*
      (2) *Dressing checks.* These are made to observe the kind and amount of drainage.

(3) *Progressive surgical diet.* List the usual progression—from ice chips, to clear liquids, to full liquids, to a soft diet, and finally to a regular diet. *The surgical patient can regain normal eating patterns sooner if this progression is followed.* For some less extensive surgeries, the full progression will not be used.
(4) *Special procedures.* Specific procedures (irrigation, respiratory therapy, casting, brace fitting) may be necessary for particular surgeries. Explain any special or unusual procedures that will be ordered *so the patient will know what to expect.*
   c. *Pain management.* All surgical patients want to be as free from pain as possible after surgery. By encouraging the patient before the surgery to participate in planning for pain management, *you help to relieve the patient's fear that pain will not be controlled.* Tell the patient about available pain medications. Instruct the patient to alert a nurse before the pain becomes moderate or acute. *Avoiding pain medication "peaks" and "troughs" consistently results in more effective pain management.* It is difficult to control pain that has become severe. Allay possible fears of medication overuse by explaining that after the first few postsurgical days, the pain will subside and large doses of injectable medications will no longer be necessary. The physician will then order oral pain medications *so the patient can maintain a comfort level that will help increase mobility.*

   A patient-controlled analgesia (PCA) pump may be ordered for postoperative pain control. In this case, the patient should be told how the unit functions and what he or she needs to do to self-medicate. See Module 53, Administering Intravenous Medications, for a more detailed explanation of PCA.
   d. *Postoperative appliances, tubes, and equipment.* Inform the patient of any equipment or appliances that will be in place after surgery. These might include a catheter, an IV infusion, a nasogastric tube, or a suction apparatus.
   e. *Deep breathing and coughing.* If the patient is going to have a general anesthetic, *the medication and the immobility of surgery will cause secretions to build up in the lungs.* Therefore, teach the patient how to breathe deeply and cough. (For instructions, consult Module 39, Respiratory Care Procedures.) In some hospitals, this teaching and that regarding the use of the incentive spirometer or other special equipment are done by a respiratory therapist.

TEACHING MAY INCLUDE: Pathophysiology, Treatments, Nutrition, Medications, Side Effects, Procedures, Symptoms to report, Home Management, Preventative Health, etc.

TEACHING CONTENT PRE-OPERATIVE TEACHING	PATIENT RESPONSE			
	Indicates Understanding	Needs Reinforcement	Return Demonstration	Able to Perform Independently
1. Understands surgical procedure and expected outcome.	3/14 PB			
2. Immediate Post-op				
a. Recovery room	3/14 PB			
b. Frequent monitoring of vital signs	3/14 PB			
c. Return to floor/ICU	3/14 PB			
3. Diet				
a. Pre-op (i.e., clear liquids)	3/14 PB			
b. NPO after midnight	3/14 PB			
c. Progression after surgery	3/16 JE	3/14 PB		
4. Medications				
a. Sedation at H.S.	3/14 PB			
b. Pre-op medication day of surgery	3/14 PB			
c. Post-op medications (analgesics, antibiotics, other)	3/14 PB			
5. Pre-op Preparation				
a. Skin prep	3/14 PB			
b. Bowel prep				
c. Other				
6. Equipment				
a. Intravenous	3/14 PB			
b. Foley catheter	3/14 PB			
c. Naso-gastric tube				
d. Drains				
e. Dressings	3/14 PB			
f. Cast/splints				
g. Other				
7. Activity Post-Op				
a. Positioning				
b. Exercise	3/16 JE	3/14 PB	3/14 PB 3/16 JE	3/16 JE
c. Restrictions				
8. Pulmonary Care				
a. Turn, cough, deep breathe	3/14 PB		3/14 PB	3/14 PB

Identify Initials with Signature:	2. J. Ellison, R.N.	4.	6.
1. P. Boyd, R.N.	3.	5.	7.

ADDRESSOGRAPH:

THE SWEDISH HOSPITAL MEDICAL CENTER
SEATTLE, WASHINGTON

Figure 44–1. Patient education flow sheet.

f. *Methods for moving.* These methods include moving in bed and getting in and out of bed, as appropriate for the patient's postoperative condition and expected physician's orders. *The purpose of teaching the patient to move with as little discomfort as possible is to encourage mobility.* Turning in bed and getting in and out of bed *prevent circulatory problems, stimulate the respiratory system, and decrease discomfort from gas.* Review your medical-surgical text for the use of pillows for splinting, side rails for support, and body mechanics adaptations.

g. *Leg exercises. These exercises facilitate venous return in the lower extremities and prevent stasis and clot formation.* They are often augmented by the use of antiembolic stockings or sequential compression devices, *which provide continuous support to the veins, decreasing venous stasis and promoting venous return.* Three exercises are most commonly taught:

(1) *Calf pumping.* Instruct the patient to alternately dorsiflex and plantar flex the foot. *This causes the calf muscles to contract and relax.*

(2) *Quadriceps setting.* Instruct the patient to alternately contract the anterior thigh muscles and allow them to relax.

(3) *Gluteal setting.* Instruct the patient to alternately contract the posterior thigh and gluteal muscles and allow them to relax.

h. These exercises should be done 10 times each hour as soon as possible after surgery. If appropriate to the patient's surgery, active range-of-motion exercises can be substituted for these isometric exercises. When teaching steps 6e through g, first *explain* what you want the patient to do and why it is important. Then *demonstrate* for the patient. Finally, ask the patient to *return the demonstration.* Give positive feedback to the patient when the return demonstration is correct, and encourage the patient if extra practice is needed.

Evaluation

7. Evaluate the effectiveness of your health teaching by asking the patient to summarize with you the points you have covered. You may also involve the family and significant others. Clarify any false information, or reemphasize points missed or misunderstood.

Documentation

8. Some facilities have a preoperative form that provides space for noting preoperative teaching (see Fig. 44–1). If your facility does not have such a form, make an entry in the nurses' progress notes.

PROCEDURE FOR PREOPERATIVE INTERVENTIONS

Depending on the operative procedure planned, various preparatory interventions appropriate to that procedure may be ordered. For example, bowel preparation is routinely ordered for many abdominal procedures. The following approach to planning and carrying out preoperative interventions applies to most common interventions.

Assessment

1. Check to see if any new preoperative orders have been written, and if so, incorporate them into your care plan.
2. Assess the patient's readiness for procedures. You may wish to delay a procedure briefly if the patient has visitors but may need to ask the visitors to step out *to allow adequate time for all aspects of care necessary.* It may be appropriate for a parent or spouse to stay during some procedures.

Planning

3. Plan time for carrying out the tasks ordered.
4. Review a manual or any modules necessary to carry out any ordered procedures, such as Module 28, Administering Enemas, and Module 46, Irrigations.
5. Wash your hands *for infection control.*

Implementation

6. Identify the patient *to be sure you are performing the procedure for the correct patient.*
7. Carry out the ordered procedure.

Evaluation

8. Evaluate using the following criteria:
   a. Patient comfortable.
   b. Patient states questions were answered.
   c. Procedure completed successfully.

Documentation

9. Consult the appropriate modules, and document as indicated.

PREOPERATIVE SKIN PREPARATION

The effective preparation of the skin before an operation *is an important aspect of preventing infection in the postoperative patient. Because the skin—the first line of defense against invasion by microorganisms—will be opened, additional measures to prevent the invasion of microbes are necessary.*

DATE/TIME	
4/16/99 10:30 AM	*Preoperative teaching done, including coughing and deep breathing, moving in bed, leg exercises, and pain management. Return demonstrations and clarification of questions show good patient understanding. Family present. ———— M. Davies, RN*

Example of Nursing Progress Notes Using Narrative Format.

The main objective of preparing the skin is *to remove dirt, oils, and microorganisms.* A second objective is *to prevent the growth of microorganisms that remain.* A third objective is *to leave the skin undamaged, with no irritation from the cleansing and hair removal procedure.*

Bath

In most facilities, the preoperative patient is asked to shower or bathe, using an antimicrobial cleansing agent, on the evening before or the morning of surgery. If possible, the patient should shampoo at the time of the bath. *Bathing removes gross contamination and soil and reduces colonization of typical wound pathogens. The antimicrobial agent leaves a residue on the skin that decreases the overall bacterial count.*

Scrub of the Surgical Site

Sometimes a surgeon orders that a surgical site be scrubbed for a predetermined length of time (for example, 5 minutes) daily for several days before the surgery. This is most commonly done for elective orthopedic (bone) surgery *because of the high risk of infection. The process results in a significantly lower bacterial count on the surgical site at the time of surgery.* Because the procedure is so time consuming and infection is not as frequent and serious in other kinds of surgeries, it is not performed routinely for most surgeries. A scrub procedure may also be ordered after the preoperative hair removal.

Hair Removal

Because microorganisms are found in large concentrations on hairs, the removal of skin hair at and near the operative site reduces the number of these organisms. The smooth skin can then be cleaned more completely. However, *because shaving with a razor can potentially injure skin and* thereby increase the risk of infection, clipping hair, using a depilatory, or no shaving at all has been suggested. Consult the policy or procedure book in your facility.

Timing of Hair Removal

Although the timing can be ordered by the surgeon, it may be determined by hospital routine. If you have an opportunity to participate in the planning, you should understand the differences in infection rates that result from changes in timing of preoperative hair removal in relation to the time of surgery. *Any time interval between the hair removal and the actual surgery allows hair to begin to regrow and microorgan-*isms *to multiply.* Therefore, preoperative hair removal is carried out as close to the time of surgery as possible. In some hospitals, hair removal is done on the nursing unit early in the morning on the day scheduled for surgery. Increasingly, hospitals are going a step further: Preoperative hair removal is being done immediately before the surgery in a special preparation area or in the induction room in the operating room suite. Not all hospitals have the facilities to make this type of change in procedure, but when it is possible, it is wise practice.

Depilatories

Depilatories are chemicals that destroy the hair below the skin level, *causing the hair to break off and leaving the skin cut-free and freer of hair than is possible with a razor.* If a patient is not sensitive to depilatories, using them is a safer method of hair removal than shaving. To use a chemical depilatory, read the instructions carefully, and follow them exactly.

Wet Versus Dry Shaving

Wet shaves are done using warm water and lather; dry shaves are done on dry skin. Most patients feel that the wet shave is more comfortable. *The water and lather are lubricants to the razor, decrease the pull, and lessen the chance of nicks or cuts. In addition, the use of antibacterial soap is one more technique to decrease the skin count of microorganisms.*

Recent evidence indicates that fewer epithelial cells are removed by using a dry shave. Also, the skin is clearly visible, making a very close shave possible. When you perform a dry shave, it is imperative to use a sharp razor *to avoid nicks and cuts.* In fact, you may have to change the blade during the procedure *if you are cutting thick hair.* You can use powder as a lubricant. Some facilities specify that clippers are to be used for a dry shave. Usually, hospital policy determines whether a wet or dry shave is used, but the surgeon may also decide.

PROCEDURE FOR WET SHAVING

Assessment

1. Verify the surgeon's order. Do not perform a shave preparation unless it has been ordered by a surgeon. The order may indicate the specific area to be "prepped," although in many facilities, a standard routine is followed unless the surgeon specifically describes another preparation area. If the order simply reads, "Prep for gastric surgery,"

you will have to refer to your facility's procedure book to identify the exact area to be prepped.

2. Assess the patient's readiness for the procedure.

Planning

3. Wash your hands *for infection control.*
4. Obtain the necessary equipment. In most settings, the preoperative shave is done using disposable equipment that is originally sterile. Although the procedure itself is a clean procedure, *starting with sterile equipment ensures that new microorganisms from the hospital environment are not introduced to the patient's skin at this critical time.* If disposable equipment is not available, carefully clean the reusable items, and send them to the central processing department for resterilization.
   a. Bath blanket to drape the patient. Top linen is sometimes substituted for the bath blanket, but it can cause subsequent discomfort if small hairs drop in the bed or if the linen becomes wet or soiled.
   b. Shaving equipment. A prepackaged shave preparation kit usually contains most of the necessary items, but be sure to check the label. If you are not using a prepackaged kit, obtain the following:
      (1) Clean gloves
      (2) Small basin of warm water
      (3) Antibacterial soap for lather
      (4) Razor with a new blade
      (5) Sterile gauze squares
      (6) Antibacterial cleansing agent
      (7) Cotton swabs
   (If the prepackaged kit in your facility does not include clean gloves, wear them *to protect yourself from exposure to blood or other body secretions.*)
   c. If the instructions for the shave preparation in your facility include covering the area with a sterile towel after shaving, include one in the equipment.
5. Plan the area to be shaved. Obviously, you will include the area of the incision itself, but you will also include a large area beyond the incisional site. *This decreases the possibility that microorganisms will move from unprepared areas to the surgical site. In addition, this provides a safeguard if the physician must enlarge the surgical area during the surgery beyond what was originally planned.*

Implementation

6. Identify the patient *to be sure you are performing the procedure for the correct patient.*
7. Explain the procedure to the patient. *Because a patient might be upset at the idea of the shave preparation,* carefully explain the exact nature and extent of the preparation.

8. Provide for the patient's privacy. To do a thorough job, you will have to expose the patient, but make sure that the window drapes and door are closed.
9. Arrange for adequate lighting.
10. Drape the patient with a bath blanket *to provide as much warmth and privacy as possible.* Base the draping technique on the area to be exposed.

   The areas to be shaved presented here are the long-standing, wide preparation approach that has been used for many years. Some surgeons prefer a smaller area of preparation because it is more comfortable for the patient, and there is little evidence to document a difference in infection rates between widely prepared areas and more limited prepared areas. Use the areas presented here as a general guideline, but follow the policy in your facility or the specific orders of the surgeon.
   a. *Head and neck surgeries.* If the scalp must be shaved, it is best to wait until the person has been anesthetized. *Shaving the head can be psychologically traumatic.* If it must be done earlier, provide a head covering *to lessen the patient's embarrassment. Because a patient may wish to keep the hair that is removed,* especially if it is long, be sure to ask the patient about this in advance.

   Do not shave the eyebrows unless expressly ordered by the surgeon. *Eyebrows may not grow back in or may grow in irregularly. This can significantly alter a patient's appearance* and should be avoided unless it is essential.

   The prepared area extends from above the eyebrows over the top of the head and includes the ears and both anterior and posterior areas of the neck (Fig. 44–2). The face is not shaved.
   b. *Lateral neck surgery.* The prepared area extends from the midline of the back, from the scapula to a line level with the top of the ear, around the operative side, across the front of the neck, and to the top of the opposite shoulder. Anteriorly, the preparation area slants down from the top of the ear on the operative side across the chin line, and extends down below the clavicle across the thorax (Fig. 44–3).
   c. *Chest surgery.* For a lateral thoracotomy, prepare the chest from the center of the sternum, extending from the neck to the bottom of the rib cage. Continue to the posterior side to the center of the back at the same level. The arm on the operative side is also prepared to the middle of the forearm. In some

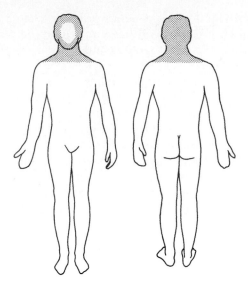

Figure 44–2. Preparation area for head and neck surgery.

instances, the preparation is extended across the entire back and chest (Fig. 44–4A).

For a midline or sternal incision, the preparation extends from the neck to the pubic bone and to the midaxillary line on each side (see Fig. 44–4B).

For access to the femoral artery, extend the preparation to include the area prepared for femoral artery surgery on the designated side (see Fig. 44–4C).

d. *Abdominal surgery.* The abdomen is prepared from a line level with the axillae to the pubic bone. The area extends on each side to the midaxillary line (Fig. 44–5).

e. *Perineal surgery.* The perineal preparation in-

cludes shaving all the pubic area. The area begins above the pubic bone in the front and extends beyond the anus posteriorly. Shave the inner thighs approximately one-third of the way to the knees (Fig. 44–6).

f. *Cervical spine surgery.* Prepare the back from the line level with the bottom of the ears down to the waist. Include the shoulders. The back area is prepared to the midaxillary line on each side (Fig. 44–7).

g. *Lumbar spine surgery.* Prepare the back from a line level with the axillae, down onto the buttocks, to the midgluteal level. The area extends to the midaxillary line on each side (Fig. 44–8).

h. *Rectal surgery.* Shave the buttocks from the il-

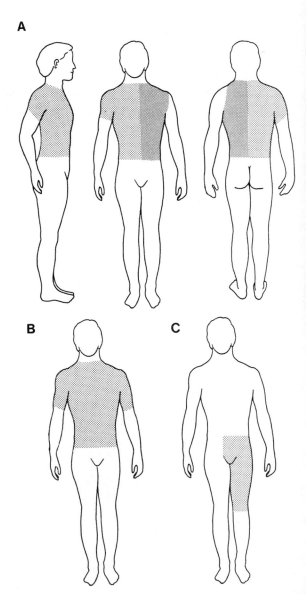

Figure 44–4. Preparation area for chest surgery. **(A)** Lateral thoracotomy. **(B)** Sternal incision. **(C)** Femoral artery access needed.

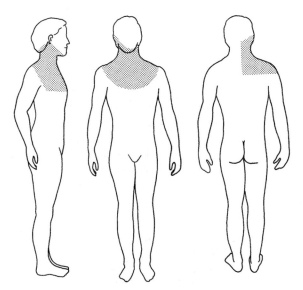

Figure 44–3. Preparation area for lateral neck surgery.

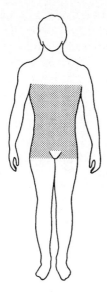

Figure 44–5. Preparation area for abdominal surgery.

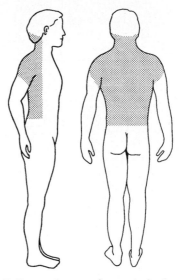

Figure 44–7. Preparation area for cervical spine surgery.

iac crest down the posterior thigh, to a line one-third of the way to the knee. Include the anal area. The area extends to the midline on each side (Fig. 44–9).

i. *Flank incision.* Prepare from just beyond the midline anteriorly, around the designated side, to beyond the midline posteriorly. Include the axilla, from the upper level at the nipple line in the front to the scapula in the back. Shave the back down to the middle of the buttocks. In the front, the pubic area and the upper thigh are shaved (Fig. 44–10).

j. *Hand and forearm surgery.* Prepare the entire circumference of the arm to the axilla (Fig. 44–11).

k. *Entire lower extremity surgery.* Prepare the entire leg, including the toes and the foot. Extend posteriorly up over the buttocks and anteriorly over the pubis up to the umbilicus (Fig. 44–12).

l. *Lower leg surgery.* Prepare the leg and foot, extending the area to midthigh (Fig. 44–13).

11. Shave the area as follows:

a. Make sure the water is warm. *Warm water is more comfortable for the patient, produces better lather, and helps soften the hair.* Lather the area well. *The suds soften the hair and provide lubrication so that the razor moves easily.*

b. Shave carefully. Hold the skin taut *to prevent nicks* and shave by stroking in the direction of

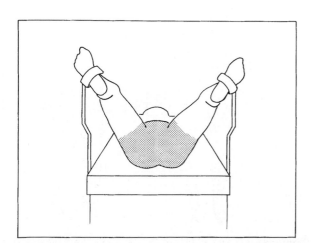

Figure 44–6. Preparation area for perineal surgery.

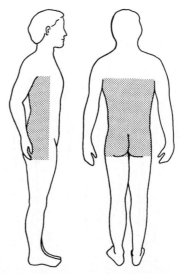

Figure 44–8. Preparation area for lumbar spine surgery.

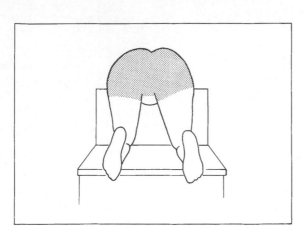

Figure 44-9. Preparation area for rectal surgery.

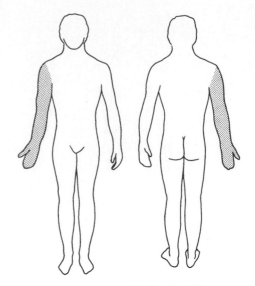

Figure 44-11. Preparation area for hand and forearm surgery.

hair growth. Use short strokes, *which are more easily controlled.*

c. Rinse the razor frequently *to remove hairs that have accumulated on the blade. These hairs could interfere with the cutting action of the razor.*

d. Wipe off excess hair from the skin as it is removed *to allow you to see the skin clearly and the razor to operate more freely.*

e. After all the hair has been removed, scrub the area with an antibacterial cleaner. In some settings, the cleansing agent is left in contact with the skin for 5 minutes *to kill or inhibit more adherent, deep, resident flora.* Check your facility's procedures *because some omit this step.*

f. Clean any body orifice or crevice in the preparation area (the umbilicus, the ear canals, under the fingernails), using cotton swabs.

g. Rinse the area with clean water.

h. Blot the skin dry—do not rub vigorously. *Vigorous rubbing can traumatize the skin.*

i. Observe the general condition of the skin. Any abnormal skin irritation, infection, or break in the skin's integrity on or near the operative site should be reported to the surgeon, *because it might be a contraindication to surgery.*

j. Cover the area with a sterile towel if necessary.

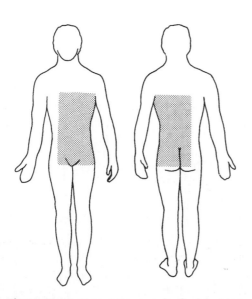

Figure 44-10. Preparation area for flank incision.

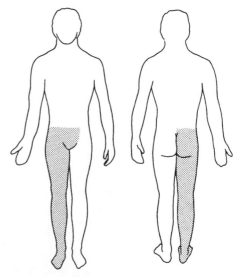

Figure 44-12. Preparation area for entire lower extremity surgery.

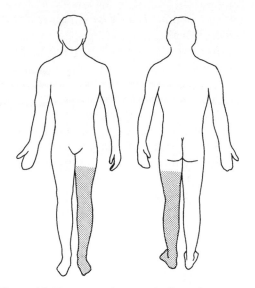

Figure 44–13. Preparation area for lower leg surgery.

k. Remove the bath blanket carefully *to prevent small hairs from dropping into the bed and causing discomfort.* Replace top linen.
12. Make the patient comfortable.
13. Dispose of the equipment.
14. Wash your hands.

Evaluation

15. Evaluate using the following criteria:
   a. Skin free of hair.
   b. Skin free of nicks and cuts.
   c. Skin shows no evidence of irritation.

Documentation

16. Document the procedure either on a flow sheet or the progress notes, according to the policy of your facility.

THE NIGHT BEFORE SURGERY

Understandably, many patients are anxious the night before surgery. Plan to spend time with the patient, and allow the patient to share any feelings or fears about the procedure. A quiet time with the patient, after visitors have left, *can be reassuring and supportive.*

Administer any sleeping medication ordered. *It is important for the patient to understand that unfamiliar surroundings and thoughts of the impending surgery may prevent a good night's rest before surgery.* Explain that the patient will not be given anything by mouth for some period of time prior to surgery. For many years patients have been kept NPO after midnight *to ensure that the stomach is free of contents that could be vomited and aspirated.* Recent research indicates that allow-

ing patients undergoing elective surgery to ingest clear liquids up to two hours before surgery does not alter the volume or pH of stomach contents nor increase the likelihood of postoperative vomiting (Schreiner, 1994; Moon, 1995). In both pediatric and adult patients, shorter periods of fasting resulted in greater patient comfort. As a result, many facilities have now liberalized their policies to allow consumption of clear liquids up to two to three hours before elective surgery. In some cases, intake of coffee is also permitted. It is still recommended that adults avoid solid foods and all liquids other than clear ones on the day of surgery. Pediatric guidelines suggest that infants up to 6 months of age can safely be fed breast milk, formula, or pureed food up to four hours before surgery (Moon, 1995; Glauber, 1994). Follow the policies in your facility. At the appropriate time, remove the water pitcher and glass from the patient's bedside and post an NPO sign. If the patient is to be admitted to the facility the morning of surgery, he or she is given responsibility for carrying out these activities.

PROCEDURE FOR IMMEDIATE PREOPERATIVE CARE

Assessment

1. Determine the precise time scheduled for the surgery.
2. Check the chart for any changes or additions in orders.
3. Check to be certain that the operative permit has been signed. If it has not, obtain consent as soon as possible *because this must be done before the patient receives any preoperative sedation.* If the patient's sensorium is clouded by medications, such as narcotics, or if he or she does not know the essential information pertaining to the surgery, he cannot give valid consent for it (Atkinson, 1992).

   The patient has the right to withdraw consent after it is given. Contact the surgeon if this occurs.

Planning

4. Plan ample time to complete the tasks necessary before the patient leaves the unit for surgery.

Implementation

Consult individual modules for specific procedures.

5. Record the patient's vital signs. Blood pressure, pulse, and respirations may be increased *because of anxiety,* but if the patient's temperature is even slightly elevated, report this to the surgeon at once. *An elevated temperature can mean an infec-*

tion, and the surgeon will have to decide whether to proceed with the surgery. By recording the vital signs, *you also establish a baseline for future measurements.*

6. Administer or assist the patient with oral care. *Oral care is necessary because the mouth tends to dry during the unconscious period with the administration of anesthetic gases.* Caution the patient not to swallow water, but only to rinse the mouth. You may have to perform oral care for some patients.

7. Insert a nasogastric tube if ordered (see Module 43, Nasogastric Intubation).

8. Have the patient remove all items of clothing, including undergarments, and put on a clean gown, untied. If the gown is untied, *it can be changed or removed easily when the patient is unconscious.*

9. Have the patient void, or insert a Foley catheter if ordered. *The bladder is emptied to avoid incontinence or injury during surgery.* If the surgery is of short duration, voiding is usually sufficient. If a Foley catheter is ordered, consult Module 37, Catheterization. Some physicians prefer to have gastric intubation and catheterization done in surgery after the patient has been anesthetized.

10. Remove colored nail polish *so that the anesthesiologist can observe the nail beds during surgery for circulatory assessment.*

11. Remove any makeup *so that skin color can be assessed during surgery.*

12. Remove hairpins and hairpieces. *These can cause pressure on the patient's scalp during the unconscious period.*

13. Remove all prostheses, such as eyeglasses, contact lenses, hearing aids, and partial or complete dentures, and store them appropriately. Usually patients go to surgery without their dentures in place. Some anesthesiologists, however, prefer that dentures be kept in place *to provide a better seal around the endotracheal tube that delivers the anesthetic agent.* If the patient has natural teeth or is a child, check for loose teeth *that might be dislodged and aspirated during surgery.* Note the presence of crowned or capped teeth or a permanent bridge.

14. Remove and secure the patient's jewelry. Jewelry can be given to the family during surgery. Religious medals are often sent with the patient *for comfort.* If a patient does not want to have a wedding band removed, tape it in place *to guard against loss.* If the ring contains a stone, use a Band-Aid, *so that the stone is in contact with the gauze instead of with the sticky tape.*

15. Put antiembolism stockings (TEDs) on the patient if ordered. *These stockings compress the pe-* ripheral leg tissue, increasing venous return during the immobile period.

16. Determine the location of the patient's family or friends during surgical procedures *so that they can be reached in an emergency or can be informed when the patient moves to the postanesthesia care unit.*

17. Check the chart for the preoperative medication order. Review the preoperative checklist for completion prior to giving the medication.

18. Prepare medications as ordered; administer them and document. More than one medication is usually given, and you must be certain all drugs are compatible and measured accurately (see Module 50, Giving Injections).

19. Caution the patient to remain quiet in bed after medication has been given.

20. Put the side rails up *for safety.* Return the bed to the low position until the stretcher arrives.

21. Place the call bell within the patient's reach.

22. Wash your hands. Complete the preoperative checklist (Fig. 44–14). Check the form used in your facility. You also should record the location of glasses or contact lenses, dentures, and jewelry.

23. Follow the proper procedure for patient identification as the patient leaves the unit. In most facilities, the operating room transport person reads the patient's identifying data from the patient's wristband while another hospital employee checks the chart. *This is a legal precaution to verify identification.*

24. Send the patient's chart and x-rays with the patient. *The surgeon may need to refer to them during surgery.*

Evaluation

25. Evaluate using the following criteria:
    a. All actions or procedures ordered completed on time.
    b. Patient ready for surgery on time.

Documentation

26. Document all pertinent data. *The completed record must be ready to accompany the patient to surgery.*
    a. Preoperative checklist completed and signed
    b. All nursing actions taken to prepare the patient for surgery and the patient's response
    c. Any articles sent with the patient to surgery
    d. Time and mode of transportation to operating room

AMBULATORY SURGERY

Patients having ambulatory surgery—also called short-stay, day, or outpatient surgery—need the same preparation as inpatients. These patients have

	YES	NO	N/A
1. Consent signed and witnessed	*JE*		
2. Time of last oral intake liquids _2400_			
solids _____			
3. Preop lab work CBC _____	*JE*		
Blood Ordered _____	—	*JE*	
Here _____			
Other			
_____			
_____			
_____			
_____			
Urinalysis	*JE*		
4. Preoperative bath or shower	*JE*		
5. Makeup and nail polish removed	*JE*		
6. Bobby pins, combs, hair pieces & wig removed	*JE*		
7. Rings, earrings, jewelry, watch (Disposition) *c̄ husband*	*JE*		
8. Prosthesis artificial eye—in - out contact lens—in - out pacemaker other			*JE*
9. Teeth natural _____ artificial upper _____ lower _____ bridges _____ partial plate _____ loose teeth	*JE*		
10. Describe size and location of any skin lesion, burns, abrasions, etc. *None JE*			
11. Surgical Prep		*JE*	
12. Apparent preop mental condition of patient within normal limits _____ excited _____ depressed _____ apprehensive *JE* irritable _____ other _____			

13. Location of family
Rotunda _____
Home _X - Will return at 1000_
Office _____

14. Allergies   *None*

15. Pre-op vital signs
TPR _98⁴ - 88 - 24_
B/P _136/88_
Wt. _149 #_

16. Voided
Yes _0715_   No _____   NA _____

17. Retention Catheter
Yes _____   No _JE_   NA _____

18. Pre-op Medication
Ordered _None_
Given _____

Form completed by:

X   *Jean Estes R.N.*
Signature

Date _4/22/_

Patient identification on unit
A.   Person from surgery calling for patient
1.   Ask for patient by name & check identification band.
2.   Check patient's chart with nursing personnel on unit according to procedure.

Signature:

X   *Holly Martin LPN*
Nursing Unit

X   *John Peters*
Surgery Personnel

NURSING UNIT PREOPERATIVE CHECK LIST

Figure 44–14. Preoperative checklist.

their history and physical examination, laboratory tests, and other necessary preoperative examinations (such as electrocardiograms) on an outpatient basis, usually 72 to 96 hours before their planned surgery. They are responsible for their own night-before-surgery preparation, which might be as little as remaining NPO for a period of time or might include as much as the administration of special medications, enemas, and so forth. Careful preoperative teaching and instructions are the best insurance for a successful outcome from the surgery.

CRITICAL THINKING EXERCISES

Sylvia Winter, 27 years old, has just been admitted to the hospital for an emergency appendectomy. You are to administer the preoperative medications and do the "essential" preoperative teaching before she leaves your unit for the operating room. Describe how you will proceed. Determine the information that you consider "essential" in this situation.

References

Atkinson, L. J. (1992). *Berry & Kohn's introduction to operating room technique* (7th ed.). New York: McGraw-Hill.

Glauber, D. (1994, May). *Northwest Hospital Department of Anesthesiology NPO guidelines.*

Moon, R. (1995, April 19). Fasting before surgery. *JAMA,273*(15)1171.

Schreiner, M. (1994). Preoperatuve and postoperative fasting in children. *Pediatric Clinics of North America, 41*(1), 111–199.

✔ **PERFORMANCE CHECKLIST**

Procedure for Preoperative Interview	Needs More Practice	Satisfactory	Comments
Assessment			
1. Verify type and exact time of surgery.			
2. Check preoperative orders.			
Planning			
3. Consult facility procedure book regarding specific type of surgery and preparation.			
4. Check patient's chart for history and physical, signed consent form, and results of required laboratory tests.			
5. Complete or secure any information listed above in planning.			
6. Plan sufficient time to carry out preoperative interview.			
Implementation			
7. Using appropriate form, perform interview, including the following areas: a. Verification of patient's identity			
b. General appearance and physical condition			
c. Anxiety level			
d. Knowledge level regarding proposed surgery			
e. Previous surgeries			
f. Chronic illnesses			
g. Smoking habits			
h. Drug, alcohol, and caffeine intake			
i. Family data			
8. Encourage patient to ask questions and answer any inquiries.			
9. Provide emotional support.			
Evaluation			
10. Check data for completeness.			
Documentation			
11. Attach interview form to patient's chart.			

(continued)

Procedure for Preoperative Teaching	Needs More Practice	Satisfactory	Comments
Assessment			
1. Review preoperative orders.			
2. Assess patient's language level, educational background, and anxiety level.			
Planning			
3. Plan considerable uninterrupted time for teaching.			
4. Include family members present if they so wish.			
Implementation			
5. Provide a quiet, nonstressful environment.			
6. Design your own plan but include as appropriate: a. Preoperative routine, including procedures and skin preparation			
b. Postoperative routine and what is included in postoperative care			
c. Principles of pain management			
d. Explanation of postoperative equipment and appliances that may be used			
e. Deep-breathing exercises and coughing			
f. Methods for moving			
g. Leg exercises (Remember to demonstrate and request a return demonstration of such things as breathing and leg exercises and methods for moving postoperatively.)			
Evaluation			
7. Evaluate teaching by asking the patient to summarize points you have covered.			
Documentation			
8. Document on health teaching form or patient's chart, according to policy of your facility.			

(continued)

Procedure for Preoperative Interventions	Needs More Practice	Satisfactory	Comments
Assessment			
1. Check for new orders before proceeding.			
2. Assess patient's readiness for procedures.			
Planning			
3. Plan time for carrying out procedures unhurriedly.			
4. Review manual or modules for any skill you are undertaking.			
5. Wash your hands.			
Implementation			
6. Identify the patient.			
7. Carry out the ordered procedures, such as enema, douche, or irrigations.			
Evaluation			
8. Evaluate using the following criteria: a. Patient comfortable			
b. Patient states questions were answered			
c. Procedure completed successfully			
Documentation			
9. Document as directed by facility policy.			
Procedure for Wet Shaving			
Assessment			
1. Verify surgeon's order to determine area to be prepared.			
2. Assess patient's readiness for shaving.			
Planning			
3. Wash your hands.			
4. Obtain necessary equipment: a. Bath blanket for draping			
b. Shaving equipment: gloves, basin of warm water, soap for lather, razor, sterile gauze squares, cleansing agent, cotton swabs			
c. Sterile towel to cover area after shaving			
5. Plan area to be shaved.			

(continued)

Procedure for Wet Shaving *(Continued)*	Needs More Practice	Satisfactory	Comments
Implementation			
6. Identify the patient.			
7. Explain the procedure to patient.			
8. Provide privacy.			
9. Arrange for adequate lighting.			
10. Drape patient with bath blanket.			
11. Shave area.			
12. Make patient comfortable.			
13. Dispose of equipment.			
14. Wash your hands.			
Evaluation			
15. Evaluate using the following criteria: a. Skin free of hair.			
b. Skin free of nicks and cuts.			
c. No evidence of skin irritation.			
Documentation			
16. Document according to facility policy.			
Procedure for Immediate Preoperative Care			
Assessment			
1. Determine precise time scheduled for surgery.			
2. Check chart for any changes or additions in orders.			
3. Check to see that the operative permit has been signed.			
Planning			
4. Plan ample time to complete tasks before time of surgery.			
Implementation			
5. Record vital signs, and report any unusual findings.			
6. Administer or assist with oral care.			
7. Insert nasogastric tube if ordered.			

(continued)

Procedure for Immediate Preoperative Care (Continued)	Needs More Practice	Satisfactory	Comments
8. Have patient remove all clothing and put on clean gown, untied.			
9. Have patient void, or if ordered, insert Foley catheter.			
10. Remove colored nail polish.			
11. Remove any makeup.			
12. Remove hairpins or hairpieces.			
13. Remove all prostheses, including eyeglasses, contact lenses, hearing aids, and partial or complete dentures, and store them appropriately. Leave dentures in if indicated by anesthesiologist.			
14. Remove jewelry and secure or give to family.			
15. If ordered, assist patient to put on TEDs.			
16. Determine location of family during surgery.			
17. Check orders for preoperative medication.			
18. Prepare, administer and document medications as ordered.			
19. Caution patient to remain quietly in bed after medication is given.			
20. Put side rails in up position after injection of medications.			
21. Place call bell or light within patient's reach.			
22. Wash your hands.			
23. Follow facility policy for final identification of patient before leaving unit for surgical suite.			
24. Send patient's chart and x-rays with patient.			
Evaluation			
25. Evaluate using the following criteria: **a.** All actions or procedures ordered were completed on time.			
b. Patient is ready for surgery on time.			
Documentation			
26. Document all pertinent data. **a.** Preoperative checklist completed and signed			

(*continued*)

Procedure for Immediate Preoperative Care *(Continued)*	Needs More Practice	Satisfactory	Comments
b. Nursing actions taken and patient's response			
c. Any articles sent with patient to surgery			
d. Time and mode of transportation to surgery			

POSTOPERATIVE CARE

MODULE CONTENTS

PREREQUISITES

Successful completion of the following modules:

(continued)

PREREQUISITES (continued)

The following modules are not essential, but their successful completion will allow you to carry out more complete care for selected patients in the postoperative state:

VOLUME 1

Module 23 Caring for Patients With Casts and Braces

Module 24 Applying and Maintaining Traction

Module 28 Administering Enemas

VOLUME 2

Module 33 Sterile Technique

Module 35 Wound Care

Module 37 Catheterization

Module 38 Administering Oxygen

Module 40 Oral and Nasopharyngeal Suctioning

Module 42 Caring for Patients With Chest Drainage

Module 43 Nasogastric Intubation

Module 47 Administering Medications: Overview

Module 48 Administering Oral Medications

Module 50 Giving Injections

Module 52 Preparing and Maintaining Intravenous Infusions

Module 53 Administering Intravenous Medications

Module 54 Caring for Central Intravenous Catheters

Module 56 Administering Blood and Blood Products

Module 57 Administering Parenteral Nutrition

Module 58 Giving Epidural Medications

OVERALL OBJECTIVE

To give comprehensive postoperative care designed to prevent complications when possible; to identify promptly and report complications that occur; and to initiate appropriate interventions rapidly, thereby facilitating the surgical patient's return to health.

SPECIFIC LEARNING OBJECTIVES

Know Facts and Principles	Apply Facts and Principles	Demonstrate Ability	Evaluate Performance
1. Postoperative nursing unit			
Discuss items to be included in postoperative nursing unit.	Given a patient situation, state which items should be included in postoperative nursing unit.	In the clinical setting, prepare unit to receive postoperative patient.	Evaluate with instructor using Performance Checklist.
2. Initial observations			
List observations to be made immediately when postoperative patient arrives from the postanesthesia care unit (PACU).	Given a patient situation, state appropriate initial observations.	In the clinical setting, make complete initial observations on postoperative patient. Document initial observations correctly.	Evaluate with instructor using Performance Checklist.
3. Information from chart			
State information to be obtained from chart after initial observations are made.	Given a sample patient's chart, obtain appropriate information about patient, following PACU period.	In the clinical setting, check chart of postoperative patient for specific items of information after initial observations are made.	Evaluate for completeness of information with instructor.
4. Potential problems			
Discuss observations, preventative actions, and treatment for potential postoperative problems.	Given a patient situation, state appropriate observations and preventive actions.	In the clinical setting, make appropriate observations and take appropriate actions to prevent postoperative problems.	Evaluate own performance with instructor.

LEARNING ACTIVITIES

1. Review the Specific Learning Objectives.
2. Read the chapter on the experience of surgery; the section on hypothermia in the chapter on homeostasis and the section on surgery and sexuality in the chapter on sexuality in Ellis and Nowlis, *Nursing: A Human Needs Approach*, or comparable material in another textbook.
3. Read the material in your medical-surgical nursing textbook that relates to postoperative care.
4. Look up the module vocabulary terms in the glossary.
5. Read through the module as though you were preparing to teach another person about postoperative care. Mentally practice the skills.
6. In the practice setting, do the following:
   a. Set up a postoperative unit using the Performance Checklist.
   b. Using another student as the patient, practice receiving your patient from the postanesthesia care unit (PACU), and make all the appropriate initial observations. Use the Performance Checklist as a guide.
   c. Practice documenting your initial observations, using the format used in your clinical facility.
7. In the clinical setting, do the following:
   a. Ask your instructor for an opportunity to assist a staff member in receiving a patient from the PACU. Notice how the patient is moved. Compare your initial observations with those of the staff person.
   b. Ask your instructor to arrange for you to receive a patient from the PACU under supervision. Compare your initial observations with those of your instructor.

VOCABULARY

atelectasis	hypoventilation	postanesthesia recovery room	second-intention healing
collaborative problem	intensive care unit	pulmonary embolus	shock
dehiscence	paralytic ileus	purulent	singultus
evisceration	pneumonitis	recovery room	thrombophlebitis
hemorrhage	postanesthesia care unit		
Homans' sign			

Postoperative Care

Rationale for the Use of This Skill

Patients who have just returned from the postanesthesia care unit (PACU) are, in most instances, dependent. They may depend on the nurse for all aspects of care after major surgery or for only selected aspects of care after minor surgery. In either situation, the nurse must make frequent and astute observations of these patients to provide for their comfort and safety, to prevent potential problems, and to act appropriately when problems are identified.[1]

POSTOPERATIVE CARE

Immediately after surgery, the patient is usually taken to the PACU, also known as the recovery room or postanesthesia recovery room, where skilled care is provided by experienced nurses until the patient has recovered from the anesthetic or can respond to stimuli. Usually, patients spend at least 1 hour in the PACU, but this time can be considerably longer. Patients who have had complex surgery or who develop complications may be taken to the intensive care unit for several days. This module discusses the care of patients who return to a regular nursing unit. For a complete understanding of the problems mentioned, consult your medical-surgical nursing text.

The nurse caring for any postoperative patient spends a large amount of nursing time teaching the patient and family or other caregivers how to manage at home. Topics might include activity, wound care, diet, hygiene, pain management, signs and symptoms of complications, and how to seek help if any problems arise. Standard instructions are often developed by the nursing staff to facilitate thorough and consistent teaching. When standard instructions are not available, the nurse is responsible for identifying the important teaching areas.

Written instructions are particularly important *because this is a stressful time for those involved, and complex instructions are easily forgotten or misunderstood.* Many hospitals have standardized forms of home care instructions for common surgical procedures. These may be modified for the individual. If standard written instructions are not available, the nurse must write out the necessary information.

[1]Note that rationale for action is emphasized throughout the module by the use of italics.

AMBULATORY SURGERY

The person having ambulatory surgery returns home within 24 hours of admission to the hospital. This is sometimes referred to as *day surgery.* Many hospitals now have a special unit for these patients. Here the patient is admitted, sent to surgery, received back from the PACU, monitored until stable, and discharged home with planned transportation. If complications occur or if the patient remains unstable, he or she is then admitted to the hospital for ongoing care.

The same guidelines for care apply as in inpatient surgery; however, the potential for problems is usually less. In particular, the patient is usually not immobile, so the problems of immobility that follow major surgeries are of less concern.

It is customary for a nurse from the facility to make a follow-up telephone call to the patient the day after the ambulatory surgery *to see if any difficulties are being encountered and to answer questions.*

PREPARING THE POSTOPERATIVE NURSING UNIT

Before you receive a patient from the PACU, prepare the room *to facilitate efficient care.*

1. Make the postoperative bed to receive the patient (see Module 14, Bedmaking).
   a. Provide extra protection at the head, such as a pad or bath towel.
   b. Provide extra protection in the middle (plastic drawsheet, pad, or Chux) *to make changing easier in case of vomiting or soiling.* A turning sheet is also helpful if the patient is going to need assistance with positioning.
2. Obtain the necessary equipment, including the following:
   a. Tissues
   b. Emesis basin
   c. Equipment for taking vital signs
      (1) Thermometer
      (2) Stethoscope
      (3) Blood pressure cuff
      (4) Sphygmomanometer
   d. IV stand
   d. Pencil and paper *for making notes*
   e. Special equipment appropriate to the type of surgery the patient has undergone. This might include traction equipment for a patient who has undergone an orthopedic procedure or a tracheostomy tray for a patient who has had thyroid surgery. Place this equipment in the

room *to prevent disorganization at the time of the patient's arrival.*

PROCEDURE FOR THE IMMEDIATE CARE OF A POSTOPERATIVE PATIENT

You can use this general approach to care for any postoperative patient being received from the PACU. It can be modified as appropriate for the needs of a specific patient.

1. Receive the patient from the PACU nurse. Move the patient carefully from the stretcher to the postoperative bed. *Rough or precipitous handling can contribute to sudden changes in pulse and blood pressure.* Use of a device, such as a sliding board, can make the move safer and more comfortable for the nurse and patient. You may also wish to review Module 20, Transfer. Leave in place the blanket that covered the patient en route to the unit *to help prevent chilling.*

Assessment

2. Receive the report from the PACU nurse. *This report gives you information about the patient's stay there and is a baseline for your own assessment.* In some facilities, PACU personnel telephone a status report to the nursing unit before the patient leaves the PACU to assist the nurse in preparing for the arrival of the patient.
3. Make the following initial observations:
   a. Time of arrival on unit
   b. Responsiveness (to what the patient responds and how he or she responds, for example, to name call)
   c. Vital signs:
      (1) Temperature
      (2) Pulse
      (3) Respirations
      (4) Blood pressure
   d. Skin:
      (1) Color
      (2) Temperature (warmth or coolness)
      (3) Condition (dryness or moisture)
   e. Dressing:
      (1) Clean
      (2) Dry
      (3) Intact
   f. Look and feel under patient to detect pooling of blood.

   g. Presence of an intravenous infusion:
      (1) Type of solution
      (2) Amount left in bottle
      (3) Drip rate
   h. Presence of urinary bladder catheter:
      (1) Unclamped
      (2) Connected to drainage bag or bottle
      (3) Freely draining
      (4) Characteristics and amount of urine
   i. Presence of other drainage tubes:
      (1) Unclamped
      (2) Attached appropriately to bottle or suction
      (3) Tubes not kinked or under patient
      (4) Characteristics and amount of drainage
   j. Safety and comfort:
      (1) Presence of pain, nausea, or vomiting
      (2) Position appropriate for surgical procedure
      (3) Side rails up, bed in low position, and call light within reach
4. Check the chart for the following information (some of which may have been included in the report from the PACU nurse):
   a. Surgical procedure or length of surgery
   b. Postoperative diagnosis
   c. Anesthetic agents used or length of anesthesia
   d. Estimated blood loss
   e. Blood or fluid replacement given during surgery and PACU stay
   f. Type and location of drains
   g. Vital signs when patient left PACU (for use as a baseline)
   h. Medications administered in the PACU:
      (1) Time
      (2) Type
      (3) Amount
      (4) Response of the patient
   i. Output:
      (1) Urine
      (2) Other drainage
      (3) Vomitus
   j. Physician's orders:[2]
      (1) Frequency of vital signs
      (2) Diet
      (3) Activity
      (4) Intravenous orders
      (5) Medications (amount and frequency of pain and other medications)
      (6) Laboratory or respiratory therapy orders
      (7) Orders specific to type of surgery or other problems of patient

Some institutions use a PACU nursing record, which can be very helpful to the nurse who is taking over the care of the patient on the nursing unit (Fig. 45–1).

---

[2]In most facilities, postoperative orders automatically cancel all previous written orders. Previous orders must be reordered by the physician after surgery if still wanted.

Group Health Cooperative
POSTANESTHESIA RECORD

Schwartz, Mabel
000 - 92 - 7654
Dr. Jenkins

ADMISSION 1410	DISCHARGE 1520	ANESTHESIA general

SURGERY cholecystectomy

NURSE I. Hubbard RN

OR TOTAL INTAKE	OR TOTAL OUTPUT	PERTINENT MEDICAL DATA	O₂ L/M 2 LPM
Fluid— 275 mL	EBL— 350 mL	No significant medical history	AIRWAY dcd @ 1430 INTUBATED dcd @ 1420
Blood— Ø	Urine— 100 mL		VENTILATOR Ø

☐ ECG   ☐ 12-LEAD ECG   ☐ ART. LINE   ☐ CVP   ☐ SWAN GANZ   ☐ X-RAY

NO	SOLUTION	VOL.	ADDITIVE	TIME	TOTAL ABSORBED	TUBES	LOCATION DESCRIPTION	INTAKE	OUTPUT
1	D5LR	1,000	—	1200	400 mL	FOLEY CYSTO CATH.	—	—	75 mL
						CBI/IBI			
						HEMOVAC/JP			
						PLEUREVAC/EMERSON			
						NASO GASTRIC Ø			
						EMESIS Ø			
						DRESSINGS Ø			

ALDRETE SCORING

COLOR	AWAKE	VENTILATION	BP	MOVEMENT
2 PINK	2 AWAKE-AWARE	2 DEEP BREATHS & COUGHS	2 BP 20% ANESTH	2 MOVES 3 LIMBS
1 PALE-DUSKY-BLOTCHY	1 ROUSABLE-ORIENTED	1 SHALLOW BREATH AIRWAY	1 BP 20 - 50%	1 MOVES 2 LIMBS
0 CYANOTIC	0 NOT RESPONDING	0 APNEA/OBSTRUCTED	0 BP 50%	0 MOVES 0 LIMBS

ALLERGIES

COLOR:	2	2	2	2	2
AWAKE	0	0	1	1	2
VENTILATION	1	1	2	2	2
BP	1	2	2	2	2
MOVEMENT	0	1	1	2	2

MEDICATIONS

	AMT.	TIME
Demerol	50 mg	1425

VITAL SIGNS (graph)

- PULSE
X CUFF BP
X MONITOR BP

RESP.	14	16	16	18	18
TEMP.	97.6				
SAB					
CVP					
URINE					
PAIN	Ø	Ø	5	5	2

ABGS	PH	PCO²	PO²	% SAT	HCO³	B.E.	TESTS

Figure 45–1. Postanesthesia record.

5. Identify any problems present. Be alert to signs and symptoms that could indicate impending problems.

Planning
6. Plan actions to resolve or monitor problems identified.
7. Wash your hands *for infection control.*
8. Determine the equipment necessary.
9. Assemble the appropriate equipment not already in the room.

Implementation
10. Identify the patient *to be sure you are performing the procedure for the correct patient.*
11. Explain to the patient what you plan to do.
12. Carry out procedure(s) deemed necessary according to assessment.

Evaluation
13. Evaluate, using appropriate criteria.

Documentation
14. Document appropriately on flow sheet(s) or on the narrative record.

ONGOING CARE OF THE POSTOPERATIVE PATIENT

The ongoing care of the postoperative patient is largely preventive. It is presented in Table 45–1 using a human needs approach.

In the first column, the general category of nursing care and the pertinent assessment observations are listed. The second column lists nursing diagnoses and collaborative problems. Nursing diagnoses are patient problems that the nurse is able to identify and treat independently. Collaborative problems are patient problems for which the nurse must assess and report to the physician who orders the treatment. Collaborative problems are stated as "potential complications." The third column lists the defining characteristics for the problem. Defining characteristics indicate that the problem is present. The fourth and fifth columns provide information on selected nursing actions. This is not meant to be an exhaustive list of all possible nursing actions but outlines the most important ones. The actions listed in the fourth column help prevent the patient problem. Actions listed in the fifth column will either correct the problem or refer it for corrective measures.

CRITICAL THINKING EXERCISES

You are caring for a 48-year-old woman who has a history of thrombophlebitis and has undergone a hysterectomy. Identify the potential complication that is of greatest concern for this woman. Determine what physician's orders you would expect relative to this potential complication.

Table 45–1. Ongoing Care of the Postoperative Patient

Human Needs Area	Nursing Diagnosis/ Collaborative Problems	Defining Characteristics	Selected Nursing Actions	
			Prevention	Treatment
1. Circulation Assess: Blood pressure, pulse, color of mucous membranes, peripheral circulation, temperature and color of lower legs, pain, visible bleeding	a. Potential complication: Hypovolemic shock related to blood loss	External or internal hemorrhaging; drop in blood pressure; rapid, weak pulse; cold clammy skin	Avoid sudden movements; get patient up slowly; maintain IVs per physician's orders; keep warm.	Place flat with legs elevated; report changes in patient status to physician immediately; be prepared to administer medications, start oxygen, administer blood or IV fluids per physician's orders.
	b. Potential complication: Thrombophlebitis related to venous stagnation	Localized pain, heat, and swelling, usually in lower extremities; positive Homans' sign	Encourage early ambulation or bed exercises, active or passive; encourage fluids; provide elastic hose per physician's orders.	Provide bed rest; notify physician and prepare to apply hot moist packs; administer drug therapy per physician's orders.
	c. Altered Tissue Perfusion: Peripheral venous stasis related to immobility	Legs immobile, dilated superficial veins, edema	Teach patient the importance of active exercise of legs while in bed and early ambulation; teach value of fluids in maintaining blood viscosity.	Encourage early ambulation or bed exercises, active or passive; encourage fluids; provide elastic hose per physician's orders.
	d. Fluid Volume Deficit related to inadequate fluid intake	Decreased urine output, dry mucous membranes, hypotension, fever, increased urine specific gravity, thirst	Maintain IV fluids at ordered rate; encourage adequate fluid intake as soon as oral intake permissible.	Readjust IV fluids based on policy and physician's orders; offer oral fluids of the patient's choice every hour.
	e. Fluid Volume Excess related to rapid infusion of IV fluids	Rapid, bounding, full pulse; moist sounds on auscultating lungs; puffy areas around eyes, sacrum, ankles	Maintain IV fluids at ordered rate.	Slow IV fluids according to policy or physician's orders; notify physician, and be prepared to administer medications as ordered.

(continued)

Table 45–1. Ongoing Care of the Postoperative Patient (Continued)

Human Needs Area	Nursing Diagnosis/ Collaborative Problems	Defining Characteristics	Selected Nursing Actions	
			Prevention	Treatment
2. *Oxygenation/aeration* Assess: Respiratory rate, depth, chest excursion, respiratory effort, breath sounds, color of mucous membranes, nail beds, and conjunctiva	a. Potential complication; Pulmonary embolism	Rapid respirations, sudden chest pain, shortness of breath, anxiety, shock	Prevent thrombophlebitis (see above); *do not* massage lower extremities.	Notify physician. Administer drug therapy and oxygen per physician's orders; place patient in Fowler's position.
	b. Ineffective Breathing Pattern: Hypoventilation related to pain and immobility	Rapid, shallow breathing; diminished breath sounds	Preoperative teaching regarding the importance of deep breathing; pain management	Encourage turning, deep breathing, and coughing at least every 2 h. Encourage fluids and early ambulation.
	c. Ineffective Airway Clearance: Retained secretions related to painful coughing or decreased cough reflex secondary to narcotics	Presence of adventitious lung sounds; use of accessory muscles for respiration	Preoperative teaching regarding the importance of coughing up secretions; pain management	Increase frequency of turning, deep breathing, and coughing; use suction if patient cannot cough out secretions. Notify physician for possible respiratory therapy.
	d. Potential complication: Atelectasis related to ineffective breathing pattern	Areas of absence of breath sounds, low-grade fever in first 24 h postoperatively; ineffective breathing pattern; ineffective airway clearance	All of the above treatments for ineffective airway clearance and ineffective breathing pattern	Notify physician for possible respiratory therapy; continue with treatment for ineffective airway clearance as above, increasing frequency.
	e. Potential complication: Hypostatic pneumonia	Rapid, noisy respirations; elevated temperature; increased pulse rate; restlessness; pain; cough	All of the above treatments for ineffective airway clearance and ineffective breathing pattern	Administer respiratory therapy and antibiotics per physician's orders.

3. Comfort Assess: Patient subjective statements regarding comfort, willingness to engage in activities of daily living (ADLs), facial expressions, vital signs		
a. Pain related to incision/surgical procedure	Complaint of pain, grimacing; immobility (guarding wound); restlessness; blood pressure drop not accompanied by signs of blood loss	Administer pain medication *before* pain becomes severe; enhance pain medication with nursing measures (change of position, back rub, reassurance, information as to how long it will take pain medication to work); inspect for edema, tight dressings, or tight casts. Administer medication per physician's orders; splint when moving; move slowly.
b. Altered Comfort: Nausea and vomiting related to anesthetic agents, pain medications*	Complaint of nausea; emesis	Position patient on side to prevent aspiration; provide frequent oral care; give antiemetic medication before meals per physician's orders; NPO and nasogastric tube per physician's orders (for persistent vomiting).
c. Altered Comfort: Abdominal discomfort related to retained gas*	Complaint of discomfort; drumlike distention of abdomen (palpate and percuss)	Urge patient to breathe in and out through mouth; keep area well ventilated and free of odors. Continue to encourage active movement and ambulation; encourage hot fluids (ice can increase problem); administer rectal tube, return-flow enema (Harris flush), or medication per physician's orders. Encourage early ambulation.
d. Altered Comfort: Hiccoughs (singultus) related to phrenic nerve stimulation secondary to dilation of the stomach or irritation of the diaphragm*	Complaint of hiccoughs	Have patient rebreathe own carbon dioxide (inhaling and exhaling into paper bag held tightly over nose and mouth); administer medication per physician's orders.

(continued)

Table 45–1. Ongoing Care of the Postoperative Patient (Continued)

Human Needs Area	Nursing Diagnosis/ Collaborative Problems	Defining Characteristics	Selected Nursing Actions	
			Prevention	Treatment
4. *Skin integrity/hygiene* Assess: Wound appearance, temperature of skin around wound, wound drainage	a. Risk for infection related to wound contamination or decreased resistance	Local signs of infection (redness, heat, swelling, pain, purulent drainage); generalized signs of infection (fever, increased pulse and respiratory rate)	Observe wound for signs of poor healing: (wound edges not approximated, excess edema and inflammation).	Administer antibiotics per physician's orders.
			Keep dressing clean and dry; pay conscientious attention to caring for patient's hygiene needs; change linen at least daily; follow strict aseptic technique when changing dressing; administer antibiotics per physician's orders.	
	b. Potential complication: Risk for dehiscence related to delayed healing*	Separation of skin edges	Apply abdominal binder per physician's orders.	Keep sterile dressings over wound; notify physician (surgical reclosure may be needed or the wound may be left open to heal by second intention).
	c. Potential complication: Risk for evisceration related to delayed healing*	Complaint of "giving" sensation in area of incision; sudden leakage of fluid from wound; wound open with abdominal contents protruding	Apply abdominal binder per physician's orders.	Cover open wound with sterile, warm saline packs; keep patient quiet; observe for signs of shock; notify physician; notify surgery (emergency surgical treatment usually required); stay with patient for psychological support.
	d. Impaired Skin Integrity related to surgical wound	Surgical wound not yet intact		Use sterile technique in care of wound, encourage optimum nutrition as permitted.

5. *Elimination*	a. Constipation related to inadequate fluids and bulk, decreased activity, and effects of anesthesia and analgesics	Complaint of no bowel movement or small amounts of hard, dry stool; abdominal discomfort; abdominal distention	Encourage early ambulation, encourage fluids, administer stool softeners per physician's orders.	Administer enema per physician's orders (if no bowel movement in first 4 or 5 d); administer stool softeners per physician's orders.
Assess: Bowel tones, abdominal palpation, passing flatus? stool appearance, urinary output, color and clarity of urine	Potential complication: Paralytic ileus	Abdominal distention and discomfort, no flatus, absence of bowel tones	Encourage early activity and ambulation.	Notify physician; NPO and nasogastric tube per physician's orders (if paralytic ileus exists); administer medication to stimulate peristalsis per physician's orders.
	b. Potential complication: Urinary retention related to recumbent position, effects of anesthetic and narcotics	Urine output (measure); bladder distension (palpate); complaint of discomfort	Encourage early activity and ambulation.	Attempt measures to encourage voiding; pass urinary catheter per physician's orders (if no voiding 8–12 h after surgery).
	Risk for urinary tract infection related to catheterization or urinary stasis*	Elevated temperature; cloudy or dark urine, burning on urination	Maintain adequate fluid intake; if catheter in place, give thorough catheter care.	Encourage fluid intake; administer medications per physician's orders.
6. *Activity and rest*	a. Impaired Physical Mobility related to general muscle weakness secondary to decreased mobility; pain and soreness secondary to surgical procedure	Weakness, dizziness, fatigue	Encourage early ambulation or active or passive range of motion if ambulation not possible; encourage adequate nutrition.	Same as preventive actions.

(continued)

Table 45–1. Ongoing Care of the Postoperative Patient (Continued)

Human Needs Area	Nursing Diagnosis/ Collaborative Problems	Defining Characteristics	Selected Nursing Actions	
			Prevention	Treatment
7. *Psychosocial* Assess: Ability to make decisions, willingness to assume responsibility for selfcare, ability to identify resources for support	a. Ineffective Individual Coping related to diagnosis, physical status, hospitalization	Asocial behavior, malaise, listlessness, sleep disturbance	Encourage early ambulation; assist patient with personal needs; encourage patient's participation as appropriate; keep patient and patient's unit neat and free of odor; be available as listener; perform patient teaching.	Same as preventive actions; also arrange consultation per physician's orders.
Assess: Expression of feelings, facial expressions, and body posture	b. Anxiety related to pain and discomfort or possible outcome of surgery	Rapid pulse and respiration, elevated blood pressure, fidgety movement, states feels anxious or "nervous"	Provide preoperative teaching; stay with patient; encourage presence of significant others who are supportive; meet needs promptly.	Provide explanation, and let patient know anxiety is normal response; encourage expression of feelings; help patient to name feelings; consider previous coping strategies; challenge unrealistic expectations of self; instruct in relaxation methods.
	c. Self-concept Disturbance related to illness, surgery, change in body image, or effect of medications*	Crying, withdrawal, sad appearance, indecision, apathy	Encourage participation in care; encourage use of support people; point out indications of progress; listen to concerns; teach about expected course of recovery.	Encourage activity as possible; point out progress in recovery; spend time with patient; encourage visits from significant others; inform that these feelings are common in postoperative period and resolve as recovery progresses.

*These currently are not North American Nursing Diagnosis Association-approved nursing diagnoses, but have been included because they are commonly encountered by nurses caring for postoperative patients.

PERFORMANCE CHECKLIST

Preparing the Postoperative Nursing Unit	Needs More Practice	Satisfactory	Comments
1. Make postoperative bed. a. Extra protection at head			
b. Extra protection and turn sheet in middle			
2. Obtain necessary equipment. a. Tissues			
b. Emesis basin			
c. For vital signs: (1) Thermometer			
(2) Stethoscope			
(3) Blood pressure cuff			
(4) Sphygmomanometer			
d. Intravenous (IV) stand			
e. Pencil and paper			
f. Special equipment			
Procedure for the Immediate Care of a Postoperative Patient			
1. Receive patient from PACU. Move patient carefully from stretcher to postoperative bed.			
Assessment			
2. Receive report from the PACU nurse.			
3. Make the following observations: a. Time of arrival on unit			
b. Responsiveness			
c. Vital signs: (1) Temperature			
(2) Pulse			
(3) Respirations			
(4) Blood pressure			

(*continued*)

Procedure for the Immediate Care of a Postoperative Patient *(Continued)*	Needs More Practice	Satisfactory	Comments
d. Skin: (1) Color			
(2) Temperature			
(3) Condition			
e. Dressing: (1) Clean			
(2) Dry			
(3) Intact			
f. IV infusion: (1) Type of solution			
(2) Amount left in bottle			
(3) Drip rate			
g. Bladder catheter: (1) Unclamped			
(2) Connected to drainage bag or bottle			
(3) Freely draining			
(4) Characteristics and amount of urine			
h. Other drainage tubes: (1) Unclamped			
(2) Attached appropriately to bottle or suction			
(3) Not kinked or under patient			
(4) Characteristics and amount of drainage			
i. Safety and comfort (1) Pain, nausea, and vomiting			
(2) Appropriate position			
(3) Side rails up; bed in low position; call bell within reach			
4. Check the chart for the following information: **a.** Operation performed			
b. Postoperative diagnosis			
c. Anesthetic agents used			

(continued)

Procedure for the Immediate Care of a Postoperative Patient *(Continued)*	Needs More Practice	Satisfactory	Comments
d. Estimated blood loss			
e. Blood or fluid replacement			
f. Type and location of drains			
g. Vital signs when patient left PACU			
h. Medication administered in the PACU (1) Time			
(2) Type			
(3) Amount			
(4) Response of patient			
i. Output (1) Urine			
(2) Other drainage			
(3) Vomitus			
j. Physician's orders (1) Frequency of vital signs			
(2) Diet			
(3) Activity			
(4) IV orders			
(5) Medications			
(6) Laboratory or respiratory therapy orders			
(7) Orders specific to type of surgery or other problems			
5. Identify any problems present.			
Planning			
6. Plan actions to resolve or monitor problems identified.			
7. Wash your hands.			
8. Determine equipment necessary.			
9. Gather appropriate equipment not already in room.			

(continued)

Procedure for the Immediate Care of a Postoperative Patient *(Continued)*	Needs More Practice	Satisfactory	Comments
Implementation			
10. Identify the patient.			
11. Explain to patient what you plan to do.			
12. Carry out procedure(s).			
Evaluation			
13. Evaluate, using appropriate criteria.			
Documentation			
14. Document appropriately.			

46

IRRIGATIONS: BLADDER, CATHETER, EAR, EYE, NASOGASTRIC TUBE, VAGINAL, WOUND

MODULE CONTENTS

PREREQUISITES

Successful completion of the following modules:

The following may be needed for some irrigations:

OVERALL OBJECTIVES

To know the purpose of an irrigation; to plan the correct technique needed to accomplish that purpose; and to carry out the irrigation safely and correctly.

SPECIFIC LEARNING OBJECTIVES

Know Facts and Principles	Apply Facts and Principles	Demonstrate Ability	Evaluate Performance
1. Purposes			
List two general purposes for irrigation.	In a specific situation, identify purpose of irrigation.	Identify purpose of irrigation before proceeding.	
2. General concerns			
a. Clean versus sterile technique			
Identify irrigations that require sterile technique.	Given an example of an irrigation, determine whether clean or sterile technique is needed.	In the clinical setting, use correct technique for situation.	Evaluate own performance with instructor using Performance Checklist.
b. Safety			
List factors in irrigation that may irritate or damage tissue		Use correct pressure, solution, and temperature for irrigation.	Evaluate safety plans with instructor
Identify measures to protect the nurse from infectious agents.		Choose appropriate protective measures.	
3. Performing irrigations			
State procedures for each irrigation discussed in module	Modify procedure for individual situation.	Carry out specific irrigation correctly.	Evaluate own performance with instructor using Performance Checklist.
	Explain procedure to patient.		
4. Observations			
State important observations to be made during irrigation.	Identify observations that are most critical for particular situation.	Make appropriate observations while performing irrigation.	Evaluate appropriateness of observations with instructor.
5. Documentation			
State what needs to be documented.	Given an example of an irrigation, identify what should be documented.	Document appropriate information on narrative record or flow sheet.	Evaluate using Performance Checklist.

LEARNING ACTIVITIES

1. Review the Specific Learning Objectives.
2. Read the chapter on the collaborative nursing role in Ellis and Nowlis, *Nursing: A Human Needs Approach,* or a comparable chapter in another textbook.
3. Look up the module vocabulary terms in the glossary.
4. Read through the module and mentally practice the specific procedures. Study as though you were planning to teach the skills to another person.
5. Arrange for time to practice irrigations.
6. In the practice setting:
   a. Review the equipment available for irrigations.
   b. Identify the various types of syringes and any prepackaged sets for specific types of irrigations.
   c. Try using each piece of equipment to make sure you understand its function and can handle it.
   d. Review the recording of irrigations in sample situations given in the module.
7. In the clinical setting:
   a. Seek opportunities to observe irrigations done by others.
   b. Perform irrigations with supervision.

VOCABULARY

asepto syringe	concentration of	instill	pinna
canthus	solution	irrigate	Toomey syringe
catheter tip syringe	douche	mucous	
cerumen	exudate	mucus	

Irrigations: Bladder, Catheter, Ear, Eye, Nasogastric Tube, Vaginal, Wound

Rationale for the Use of This Skill

Generally, irrigations are done for two purposes. The first is to clean the passage or body area. Small or large amounts of solution can be used to remove secretions, small clots, foreign material, and microorganisms. The solution used may be one that simply flushes particles away or may contain special cleansing agents.

The second purpose is to instill medication. The medication may be an antibacterial agent, a soothing agent, or an agent that exerts another specific therapeutic effect, such as changing acidity. Sometimes an irrigation serves both purposes at the same time (see Module 49, Administering Medications by Alternative Routes, regarding instilling medications).

The nurse must understand that frequent or excessive irrigation of some body cavities with hypotonic solutions can lead to electrolyte imbalance. Irrigations may be ordered by the physician specific to the needs of the patient. Or in some institutions, there is a standing order for irrigations to be performed at the nurse's discretion. There are many similarities in the way these irrigations are done, but the differences are critical. The nurse must be able to plan an appropriate procedure and to carry it out correctly.[1]

▼ NURSING DIAGNOSES

> Irrigations are often ordered as part of medical therapy. In addition, nurses may initiate irrigations based on standing orders or protocols. A number of nursing diagnoses may benefit from irrigation intervention. Examples are:
>
> Altered Urinary Elimination: Urinary retention related to occlusion of the indwelling urinary catheter due to sediment
>
> Auditory Sensory Alteration: Decreased hearing bilaterally related to increased collection of cerumen in ear canals
>
> Risk for Injury: Left eye, related to presence of small foreign body
>
> Pain: Abdominal distress related to nonfunctioning of nasogastric tube

[1]Rationale for action is emphasized throughout the module by the use of italics.

ASEPSIS

Sterile technique must be used on all areas of the body that are normally sterile. These include the bladder, the kidney pelvis, and open wounds. Sterile technique is also used for irrigations involving the eye *because of the potential for serious injury from even a minor eye infection.*

Clean technique is used for all other irrigations, including irrigations of the throat, ear, vagina, bowel, and stomach. However, if surgery has been performed on any of these organs, sterile technique is necessary *because the surgical incision has broken the intact tissue that provides a barrier to microbes.*

SAFETY

The nurse wears clean gloves when performing most irrigations *to provide protection from the patient's body secretions.* Sterile gloves are worn when it is necessary to touch sterile equipment for irrigating a sterile environment, such as the eye. A moisture resistant gown or apron is needed if irrigant might contact the nurse's uniform. Eye protection (goggles or face shield) are essential if there is potential for splashing irrigant to the eyes.

Most body tissue is sensitive to excessive pressure. Because fluid under pressure can cause spasms of an organ such as the bladder, and actual tissue damage to a structure as sensitive as the eye, use gentle pressure only. If the patient feels discomfort, reduce the pressure. *Remember that by decreasing the height of the container you decrease the pressure.*

Medications or chemicals may also irritate or cause tissue reaction. This is especially true if the wrong concentration is used for a particular tissue. For example, a benzalkonium chloride solution, suitable for use on instruments, is far too strong for mucous membranes. Therefore, carefully check both the type and the concentration of solution used to make sure they are correct.

Most irrigations are done with solutions at room temperature. *To increase the patient's comfort,* warm solutions to body temperature. Do not use extreme temperatures, however. *Very high temperatures can burn tissues. Low temperatures can produce a chilling or even a shocklike reaction as the body attempts to maintain homeostasis.*

If medications are being instilled by irrigation, follow the directions in Module 47, Administering Medications: Overview.

PATIENT TEACHING

Teaching the patient about the procedure and what to expect is essential. *This allows the patient to participate in care as much as possible.* To begin, find out what the patient knows. Then explain what the patient does not understand. If an irrigation has been done previously, it is important to find out what the previous procedure was and the patient's response. It may upset the patient to have each nurse proceed in a different manner. The irrigation technique should be noted in the Nursing Care Plan *to facilitate continuity of care.*

Allow time for the patient to ask questions and to express personal feelings about the procedure. Some persons fear that the irrigation will cause pain. Additionally, many irrigation procedures produce anxiety. You will, therefore, have to take action *to decrease the patient's anxiety by listening and using therapeutic communication techniques.*

OBSERVATION

During an irrigation, it is important that you observe the area being irrigated as much as possible. Of course, certain internal areas cannot be observed directly, but the opening into the area can be observed. Notice any drainage or exudate, and describe the amount, color, consistency, and odor of it. Also, observe the irrigation fluid for secretions that may be washed out with the fluid.

DOCUMENTATION

When recording, note the type of irrigation and time it was performed; the type, concentration, and amount of solution used; appearance of any secretions; results of the procedure; and the patient's response. These are often documented on a flow sheet, but may be included in the narrative, especially if it is a one-time procedure.

All fluid used for irrigating should be returned. If the fluid fails to return, note that fact in the chart according to facility policy and record the amount retained on the intake worksheet.

GENERAL PROCEDURE FOR IRRIGATION

Assessment
1. Verify the following:
   a. Type of irrigation ordered
   b. Amount, temperature, type, and concentration of solution ordered

Planning
2. Decide whether the irrigation is to be clean or sterile.
3. Wash your hands *for infection control.*
4. Identify and gather the equipment needed for the specific irrigation, including:
   a. Solution
   b. Irrigating device (Figs. 46–1 and 46–2)
   c. Receptacle for used irrigating fluid
   d. Protective padding (towels or disposable waterproof pads) *to keep the patient and the environment dry*
   e. Clean or sterile gloves *to protect yourself if body secretions are contacted.* It is also important to protect the patient from microorganisms that you may harbor in small cracks in your skin or on a minor abrasion. Sterile gloves are worn when sterile equipment must be touched. All nurses should become accustomed to wearing gloves while performing irrigations for patients *because there is current evidence that organisms can be transferred during any procedure.*
   f. Gown or apron and eye protection, if needed.

Implementation
5. Identify the patient *to be sure you are performing the procedure for the correct patient.*
6. Explain the procedure to the patient.
7. Provide privacy by closing curtains and adequately draping the patient as appropriate for the specific irrigation *to safeguard the patient's modesty.*
8. Position the patient as needed for the irrigation.
9. Place protective padding where needed.
10. Put on gloves and other protective garb needed and carry out the irrigation according to the specific procedure outlined below.
11. Make sure the patient is dry and comfortable.
12. Dispose of the used equipment following the policy of your facility. If the equipment is

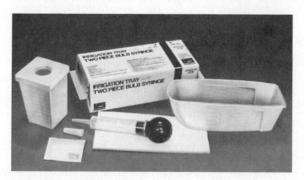

Figure 46–1. A commercial irrigation set consists of a container that holds the solution and bulb syringe, an alcohol wipe, protective pad, and a receptacle for collecting the irrigation. (Courtesy American Hospital Supply Corp., McGaw Park, Illinois)

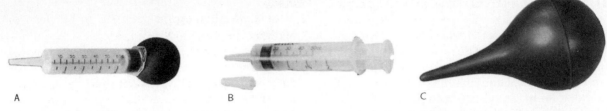

Figure 46–2. Types of syringes used for irrigations. **(A)** Asepto syringe. **(B)** Catheter-tip syringe. **(C)** Bulb syringe. (Courtesy American Hospital Supply Corp., McGaw Park, Illinois)

reusable, you may have to wash it thoroughly or return it to central supply for processing. If it is disposable, you may have to discard it in a specific place.

13. Wash your hands.

Evaluation

14. Evaluate using the following criteria:

    a. Area of irrigation was thoroughly cleaned.

    b. Medication, if used, contacted desired area.

    c. Patient dry and resting comfortably.

    d. Amount of solution returned compared with amount instilled.

Documentation

15. Document the following on either a flow sheet or the narrative in the record:

    a. Type of irrigation and time it was performed

differenc is amou of Solut

DATE/TIME	
2/10/98 1600	3 cm open sacral decubitus ulcer irrigated with 100 ml half-strength hydrogen peroxide. Solution returned with large amount yellow-green exudate. Wound surface still not clear of exudate. States there is no discomfort with irrigation. ——— K. Thorsen, RN

A

DATE/TIME	
2/10/98 1600	Alteration in Skin Integrity: Sacral decubitus ulcer
	S States no discomfort associated with ulcer or irrigation
	O Wound irrigation with 100 ml half-strength hydrogen peroxide returned large amount of yellow-green exudate. Wound surface still not clear of exudate.
	A Infection of decubitus ulcer persists.
	P Continue with irrigations each shift. Keep wound covered with dressing between irrigations. Continue to isolate wound drainage and follow specific isolation procedures. Consult physician regarding treatment of infection. ——— K. Thorsen, NS

B

DATE	Time	Procedure	Result
2/10/98	1600	Irrigation of decubitus ulcer 100 ml 1/2 st H_2O_2.	Large amount of yellow-green drainage.

C

A: Example of Nursing Progress Notes Using Narrative Format.
B: Example of Nursing Progress Notes Using SOAP Format.
C: Example of Flow Sheet

b. Type, concentration, and amount of fluid used

c. Appearance and odor of any secretions washed away

d. Results of the procedure

e. Patient's response to the procedure

SPECIFIC IRRIGATION PROCEDURES

For each specific irrigation procedure discussed below, some steps of the General Procedure may be modified. We have included completely the modified steps as well as references to the steps of the General Procedure that remain the same.

100 cc

30 – 60 cc

BLADDER AND CATHETER IRRIGATION

The terms *bladder irrigation* and *catheter irrigation* are often used interchangeably. However, they are not the same. So when either is ordered, carefully check the purpose of the irrigation. A *catheter irrigation* is performed to keep the catheter patent. A *bladder irrigation* is performed to clean or medicate the bladder itself. Much of the technique is identical for both procedures and both procedures require sterile technique *because the inside of the bladder is sterile.*

An open or closed technique can be used for intermittent irrigations. It is highly recommended that if at all possible, the closed technique be used *so that the system is not interrupted, which could allow microorganisms to enter the sterile environment of the urinary tract.* Today, the closed technique is being used increasingly *to maintain the urinary drainage as a closed system, preventing the introduction of microorganisms that might cause infection.*

To use closed technique, a three-way catheter is used. It then can be hooked to irrigation fluid by one channel and to the drainage bag by another. If a three-way catheter has not been used, it is possible to use a Y-connector to establish a closed system connecting the catheter to both an irrigating fluid container and a drainage bag. See the procedure for three-way irrigation, below. (For a further discussion of catheter care, see Module 37, Catheterization.)

PROCEDURE FOR BLADDER AND CATHETER IRRIGATION: OPEN TECHNIQUE

Assessment

1. Follow the General Procedure for Irrigation.

Planning

2. Use sterile technique.

3. Follow the General Procedure.

4. Gather the necessary equipment described in the General Procedure, plus:

a. Sterile irrigation set (asepto syringe, container for irrigating fluid, drainage receptacle, alcohol wipe)

b. Solution (normal saline is commonly used, but acidifying or antibacterial solutions can also be ordered)

c. Clean gloves

Implementation

5.–7. Follow the steps of the General Procedure.

8. Position the patient so that the connection between the catheter and the drainage tubing is readily accessible.

9. Place the protective padding under the connection site.

10. Put on gloves and carry out the bladder or catheter irrigation:

a. Open the set, maintaining sterile technique. You can touch the exterior of the fluid container, the exterior of the receptacle, and the bulb of the syringe to set them up conveniently *because these areas will not touch the sterile inside surface of the catheter or the sterile fluid.*

b. Pour the solution from the bulk container into the irrigating bottle *to maintain sterility of the original container as you work and to facilitate drawing up the fluid from the irrigating bottle.*

c. *To reduce the possibility of contamination,* clean the junction of the catheter and drainage tubing with an alcohol swab before disconnecting these two items. Some sets contain a sterile cleansing wipe in a foil package for this purpose. If the set does not contain one, obtain separately.

d. Disconnect the catheter from the drainage tubing and hold the catheter end over the drainage fluid receptacle *so the fluid will drain into the receptacle.* Some receptacles have a notched end to hold the catheter firmly *so it does not touch anything and become contaminated.* If the receptacle does not have a notch, position the catheter carefully on the receptacle so the end does not become contaminated.

e. Protect the end of the drainage tubing from contamination *so it will be sterile when reconnected.* You can do this in many ways. For example, you can fold a sterile gauze square over the end of the drainage tubing and secure it with a rubber band. You can slip the end of the drainage tubing inside the foil package that contained the cleansing wipe (it is sterile inside) and secure it with a rubber band. Also, a sterile drainage tubing cap may be included in the set or may be available separately.

f. Instill the fluid.
  (1) For a catheter irrigation:
    (a) Fill the asepto syringe with 30 to 60 mL solution.
    (b) Insert the tip of the asepto into the catheter and instill the fluid with gentle pressure.
    (c) Pinch the catheter closed and hold it closed while you withdraw the syringe *so you do not put suction on the bladder and cause trauma.*
    (d) Allow the fluid to drain into the drainage receptacle.
    (e) Observe the drainage for color and sediment and for amount of solution returned.
    (f) Repeat this procedure until the catheter is clear of sediment. Usually three times is sufficient.

g. Avoid aspirating the fluid into the asepto syringe, *because it can traumatize the bladder lining or even collapse the bladder.*
  (1) For bladder irrigation:
    (a) Instill the ordered fluid into the bladder.
    (b) Clamp the tubing *so the solution remains in the bladder for several minutes.*
    (c) Unclamp the tubing and allow the fluid to drain out.

h. Reconnect the catheter to the drainage tubing.

11.–13. Follow the steps of the General Procedure.

Evaluation
14. Follow the General Procedure.

Documentation
15. Follow the General Procedure.

PROCEDURE FOR BLADDER AND CATHETER IRRIGATION: THREE-WAY AND CLOSED TECHNIQUE

A special three-way catheter is inserted when this type of irrigation is needed (Fig. 46–3). Other names sometimes used for a three-way catheter are "through and through" and "CBI"(continuous bladder irrigation). The catheter has a channel for fluid to be instilled as well as the usual channels for drainage and for inflating the balloon in the bladder.

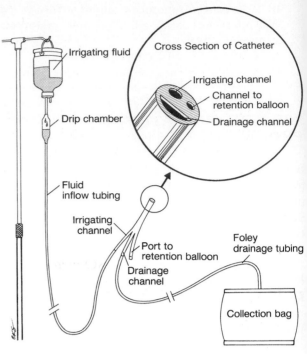

Figure 46–3. Three-way irrigation setup.

This type of irrigation is most frequently done after surgical procedures on the bladder and prostate surgery. The catheter is inserted at the time of surgery.

Assessment
1. Follow the General Procedure for Irrigation.

Planning
2. Use sterile technique.
3. Follow the General Procedure.
4. Gather the following equipment:
  a. IV stand
  b. Solution (normal saline is most commonly used)
  c. Connector tubing
  d. Gloves

Implementation
5.–9. Follow the steps of the General Procedure.
10. Put on gloves and carry out the bladder or catheter irrigation:
  a. Insert the tubing spike into the ordered sterile fluid bag and hang it from an IV pole. This bag looks much like an large IV solution container and usually contains 2,000 to 3,000 mL.
  b. Expel all air from the tubing before you attach it to catheter port, *so air is not instilled into the bladder.* Do this by opening the fluid

clamp and allowing the fluid to flow from the receptacle until it is at the tip of the tubing. Be sure to maintain sterility of the tip *because it will be inserted into the sterile catheter.*

   c. Attach the tubing to the inflow channel of the three-way catheter.

   d. Attach the other channel of the catheter to the drainage tubing and assure that it is open.

   e. Regulate the irrigation as a continuous drip by using the clamp on the tubing.

      (1) For continuous drip, regulate the drip rate.

      (2) For cleaning:

         (a) Open the inflow tubing to continuous stream.

         (b) Continue the flow until the outflow is free of clots and sediment.

         (c) Reclamp the tubing.

11.–13. Follow the steps of the General Procedure.

Evaluation
14. Follow the General Procedure.

Documentation
15. Follow the General Procedure.

If a closed system is established after a standard Foley catheter is in place, it is necessary to use a Y-connector. One branch of the Y goes to the catheter, one to the irrigation bag, and one to the catheter. To irrigate, the drainage tubing must be clamped off. The irrigation tubing is then unclamped and fluid flows into the bladder. The irrigation tubing is reclamped, the drainage tubing is unclamped, and the fluid flows out of the bladder. This may be repeated as needed to keep the catheter patent or as ordered by the physician.

   Special Safety Note: The physician may order a specific rate of flow in milliliters per hour or may simply order that a slow continuous drip be used. The nurse is responsible for monitoring and maintaining this flow. Larger quantities of fluid can be run through as needed *to keep the catheter open and the bladder free of blood clots or debris.* To do this, simply open the clamp on the fluid and allow it to run at a rapid rate until the tubing is clear and draining freely.

   The most critical concern is that large quantities of fluid not be put into the bladder if the drainage tubing is clogged or inadvertently clamped. *This causes severe pain and could rupture the patient's bladder.* Closely watch the output of the catheter *to see that it corresponds to the amount of fluid being instilled plus any other intake.*

   Again, remember to record the amounts of all ir-

rigation solution used and to subtract it from the total amount in the collection bag. A separate record of the amount of fluid instilled can be kept to make this easier for you.

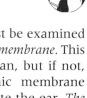

PROCEDURE FOR EAR IRRIGATION

Before an ear can be irrigated, it must be examined with an otoscope *to check the tympanic membrane.* This may have been done by the physician, but if not, you should do it. If the tympanic membrane (eardrum) is not intact, do not irrigate the ear. *The fluid could enter the middle ear and cause an infection.* You should also inspect the pinna and the external ear canal for signs of infection, open areas, the presence of cerumen, or foreign objects. An ear irrigation is most often used to remove cerumen or a foreign object in the ear.

   An ear syringe is usually used to instill the fluid, although some facilities use a water pressure device, commercially known as a Water Pik (a machine that delivers a pulsating water stream), on low pressure.

Assessment
1. Follow the General Procedure for Irrigation.

Planning
2. Use clean technique.

3. Follow the General Procedure.

4. Gather the necessary equipment.

   a. Ear syringe (usually a rubber bulb syringe) or water pressure device

   b. Emesis basin

   c. Clean towels

   d. Clean gloves

   e. Solution ordered, which is commonly saline or water. The solution is warmed to body temperature because *cold fluid striking the eardrum may cause dizziness and nausea.*

Implementation
5.–7. Follow the steps of the General Procedure.

8. Position the patient sitting or lying with the head tilted slightly forward and away from the side to be irrigated *so the ear is accessible.*

9. Place protective padding over the patient's shoulder to keep the patient dry.

10. Put on clean gloves and irrigate the ear. (If a Water Pik is used, eye protection and a gown are needed.)

   a. Place the basin under the patient's ear *to catch the solution.* The patient may be able to hold the basin in place.

   b. Fill the syringe with fluid.

   c. Straighten the ear canal as appropriate for

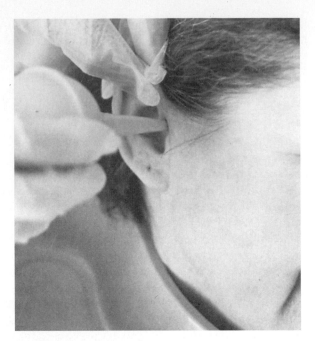

Figure 46–4. To irrigate the ear, the nurse straightens the ear canal by gently pulling the pinna upward and back, directing the flow from the bulb toward the upper part of the canal. (Courtesy Ivan Ellis).

PROCEDURE FOR EYE IRRIGATION

This is a sterile procedure, *because eyes are easily damaged by infection.* Use a sterile syringe and sterile fluid. If both eyes are to be irrigated, use separate sets for each eye *to prevent cross-contamination.* An eye irrigation is most often used to remove a foreign body or injurious fluid that has splashed into the eye. It may also be used to remove secretions caused by infection.

Assessment
1. Follow the General Procedure for Irrigation.

Planning
2. Use sterile technique. Do not touch the irrigator to the eye.
3. Follow the General Procedure.
4. Gather the necessary equipment:
   a. Sterile syringe or tubing and an IV stand if IV fluid is being used for the irrigation
   b. Sterile solution (normal saline is most common) either in a pour bottle or in a 1,000-mL intravenous bag
   c. Sterile eye shield that connects to the IV tubing if a large volume is being used (Fig. 46–5).
   d. Emesis basin
   e. Sterile cotton balls or gauze squares
   f. Sterile gloves

Implementation
5.–7. Follow the steps of the General Procedure.
8. Place the patient in the supine position. Turn the patient's head with the eye that is to be irrigated down. (The patient can be seated with the head tilted back and supported.)
9. Place padding and an emesis basin beside and below the eye. It is wise to have a large bath basin available in which *to empty the drainage basin halfway through the irrigation. This prevents it from overflowing onto the patient.*
10. Put on sterile gloves and irrigate the eye:
    a. Set up the irrigating fluid and eye shield if a large volume is being used. Pour saline into a sterile irrigation container if a smaller volume is being used.
    b. Hold the eye open with the thumb and forefinger of your nondominant hand. (Resting your hand on the patient's forehead may make this easier.)
    c. Use either syringe or continuous-flow method:
       (1) Syringe method:
           (a) Fill the syringe with 30 to 60 mL fluid.
           (b) Gently release the fluid onto the lower conjunctival sac at the inner

the patient's age. In an adult, straighten it by gently pulling the pinna upward and back. Because the ear canal in a child *is much straighter than in an adult*, gently pull it downward and back.
   d. Direct the tip of the syringe toward the top of the patient's ear canal (Fig. 46–4), so that a circular current is set up with fluid flowing in along the top and out along the bottom. With this action, *cerumen or foreign material will be irrigated out.*
      Special Safety Note: Be careful! Severe discomfort and dizziness can result from fluid directed onto the eardrum. *Cold fluid increases the chance of adverse effects.* Stop the procedure if the patient complains of severe pain.
   e. Irrigate until either the ear canal is clean or the ordered volume is used.
11. Dry the ear with a clean sponge or towel and assist the patient to a comfortable position on the affected side *to drain out excess fluid..*
12. Dispose of the used equipment and remove your gloves.
13. Follow the General Procedure.

Evaluation
14. Follow the General Procedure.

Documentation
15. Follow the General Procedure.

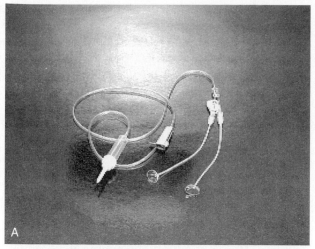

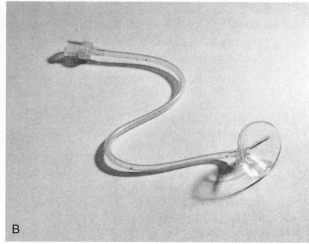

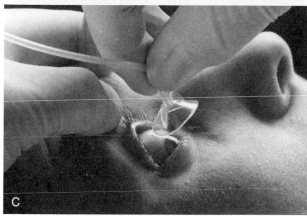

Figure 46–5. This eye irrigation system provides for continuous irrigation. **(A)** The eye shield. **(B)** Two eye shields attached to a Y-type intravenous tubing. **(C)** Placing the eye shield over the surface of the anesthetized eye for irrigation. (Courtesy MorTan Inc., Missoula, Montana)

canthus, allowing it to flow across the eye and then into the basin.

(c) Repeat as needed. Continue the procedure until the eye is clean or until the fluid ordered has been used.

(2) IV fluid method:

(a) Adjust the IV stand to its lowest height *to keep pressure low.*

(b) Attach the tubing and eye shield and hang the solution on the IV stand.

(c) Fill the tubing with fluid and eliminate the air *so it will flow evenly.*

(d) Pull back the eyelids, instill ordered topical anesthetic drops, and place the eye shield over the eyeball, allowing the lids to close over it.

(e.) Open the control valve or clamp on the IV tubing and allow the fluid to flow slowly across the eye. A continuous flow is important *for thorough cleansing, but the pressure should never cause discomfort.* The eye shield device makes it unnecessary to hold the eye open *to allow the fluid to*

flow directly onto the eye itself rather than onto the eyelid.

If an eye shield is not available, you will need to hold the eye open and hold the IV tubing, allowing the fluid to flow from the inner to the outer canthus. ***Special Safety Note:*** *Do not touch hard plastic irrigating tip of the IV line to the eye because doing so may injure the eye.* Keep the tip close to the eye *so fluid pressure is not increased by the height of the fluid container.*

If both eyes are to be irrigated, separate equipment is used for each *to prevent cross-contamination.*

11. Dry the eyelid, wiping it from the inner canthus to the outer canthus, using a sterile cotton ball or 2 × 2 gauze. Use each cotton ball or gauze only once, and discard. *This protects the opposite eye and moves any infected material away from either eye.*

12.–13. Follow the steps of the General Procedure.

Evaluation
14. Follow the General Procedure.

Documentation
15. Follow the General Procedure.

PROCEDURE FOR NASOGASTRIC TUBE IRRIGATION

The nasogastric tube is irrigated to keep it patent and functioning well.

Assessment
1. Follow the General Procedure for Irrigation.

Planning
2. Use clean technique *because the acid environment of the stomach is resistant to bacteria.* However, when there has been surgery on the stomach, sterile technique may be required.
3. Follow the General Procedure.
4. Obtain the necessary equipment, including:
   a. Prepackaged irrigation set or 60-mL syringe with an adapter, an asepto syringe, or a catheter-tip syringe along with a fluid container
   b. Solution (*normal saline is preferred because it reduces electrolyte depletion*)
   c. Emesis basin
   d. Clean gloves

Implementation
5.–7. Follow the steps of the General Procedure.
8. Position the patient so that the connection between the nasogastric tube and the suction tubing is accessible.
9. Place protective padding under the connection.
10. Put on gloves and irrigate the nasogastric tube:
    a. Turn off suction and disconnect the nasogastric tube from the connecting tubing.
    b. Fill the syringe with 30 mL fluid.
    c. Gently instill the fluid into the nasogastric tube. If the fluid will not enter the tubing, the outlet eyes may be against the mucosa. Untape the tube from the nose and move it in and out gently (not more than 1 inch either way), unless the patient has had gastric surgery and moving the tube may disrupt the operative site. *Doing this can release the end of the tube and allow you to proceed with the irrigation.* Be sure to retape the tube before you continue with the procedure *so the tube does not come out.* If the tube has an air vent, be sure that you do not instill the fluid in air vent. *Fluid in the air vent tubing prevents it from acting as safety measure to prevent excess suction on the stomach mucosa.* If the air vent tube becomes filled with gastric contents because of siphoning, you may irrigate the air vent with water and follow that with air to completely clear the air vent tubing of fluid.
    d. Aspirate the fluid back and discard it in the basin. If the fluid does not return after several attempts at aspiration, instill another 30 mL fluid. Do not continue to instill fluid after this if none is returning. *You may cause excessive distention.* Report the situation to the nurse in charge.
       In some facilities, the fluid is not aspirated. After instillation the tubing is reconnected and the suction machine aspirates the fluid. The fluid must then be added to the intake record or to a separate record of the irrigating fluid. That amount is subtracted from the suction amount when output is figured. Follow the policy of your facility.
    e. Repeat the procedure, instilling and aspirating fluid, *until the tubing is cleared of clotted material or thick mucus.*
    f. Reconnect the tubing to the suction machine. If the suction does not appear to be functioning and you have cleared the nasogastric tube, the tubing to the machine itself may be clogged. Squeeze this tubing between your fingers *to loosen the material and allow the machine to clear the tubing.* (See Module 44, Nasogastric Intubation, for the care of a patient with a nasogastric tube in place.)
11.–13. Follow the steps of the General Procedure.

Evaluation
14. Follow the General Procedure.

Documentation
15. Follow the General Procedure.

PROCEDURE FOR VAGINAL IRRIGATION (DOUCHE)

A vaginal irrigation is also called a *vaginal douche.*

Assessment
1. Follow the General Procedure for Irrigation.

Planning
2. Use clean technique *because the vagina is not sterile.*
3. Follow the General Procedure.

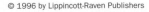

4. Gather the necessary equipment, including:
   a. Douche set with a special douche tip
   b. Solution (approximately 1,000 mL) at body temperature
   c. IV stand *(although it is possible to hold the fluid container during the procedure, you will find it is inconvenient to do so)*
   d. Waterproof pad
   e. Bedpan
   f. Tissues
   g. Clean gloves

Implementation

5.–7. Follow the steps of the General Procedure.
8. Prepare the patient:
   a. Have the patient void before beginning *because the fluid on the vulva may cause a desire to void.*
   b. Position the patient flat on her back in bed. *If the patient sits up, fluid will drain out too quickly and not contact all the tissue.*
   c. Drape the patient in the lithotomy position, with the perineal area exposed.
9. Place a waterproof pad under the patient's hips *to protect the bed* and place the patient on a bedpan to catch the fluid.
10. Put on gloves and carry out the vaginal irrigation:
   a. Wash the patient's perineal area if necessary.
   b. Fill the fluid container and connect the douche tip.
   c. Hang the container on the IV stand 18 to 24 inches above the hips *to provide appropriate pressure.*
   d. Run the fluid through the tubing *to clear the air from the tubing.*
   e. Moisten the douche tip *to lubricate it.*
   f. Run a small amount of fluid over the patient's labia *to check that the temperature of the solution is comfortable.*
   g. With the tubing clamped, insert the tip 3 to 4 inches into the vagina, at an angle toward the base of the spine, *the plane at which the vagina lies.*
   h. Unclamp the tubing and allow the fluid to flow.
   i. Rotate the tip *so the fluid contacts all vaginal tissue.*
   j. When all fluid has been used, remove the tip.
   k. Help the patient to sit on the bedpan *to allow any remaining fluid to drain out.*
11. Provide tissue *for drying the perineum.*
12.–13. Follow the steps of the General Procedure.

Evaluation

14. Follow the General Procedure.

Documentation

15. Follow the General Procedure.

PROCEDURE FOR WOUND IRRIGATION

Always use sterile technique for wound irrigations *because the body's defense created by intact skin is not present.*

Assessment

1. Follow the General Procedure for Irrigation.

Planning

2. Use sterile technique. Wound irrigations are sterile procedures *because the body's normal skin defenses against microorganisms have been breached.*
3. Wash your hands *for asepsis.*
4. Gather the necessary equipment. This will vary according to the wound, but commonly you will need the following:
   a. Irrigating set (asepto or catheter-tip syringe, solution container, receptacle for used solution). A special water pressure device may be used to irrigate seriously contaminated traumatic wounds, but this is usually done in the emergency room or in the operating room. A regular syringe may used to irrigate a small wound. A catheter may be attached to a syringe to facilitate irrigating a very deep wound.
   b. One pair of sterile gloves *if the wound is to be touched* and one pair of clean gloves, or two pairs of clean gloves *if the wound surface will not be touched.* Gown and eye protection if needed
   c. Materials for applying a new sterile dressing (including gauze squares)
   d. Solution (as ordered by the physician)
   e. Waterproof pad to protect the patient and bed
   f. Receptacle or disposable bag for soiled dressings

Implementation

5.–7. Follow the steps of the General Procedure.
8. Position the patient so that the wound is clearly exposed and the patient's body is tilted *so the solution will flow from the upper end of the wound to the lower, and then into the receptacle.*
9. Place protective padding beside and under the patient where you expect the fluid to drain.
10. Carry out the wound irrigation:
   a. Open the sterile set and pour the sterile fluid into the container.
   b. Put on clean gloves and remove the soiled dressing, using gloves *to protect yourself from body secretions.* Place soiled dressings in the receptacle along with the soiled gloves.

c. Place the receptacle to catch the fluid.

d. Put on the second pair of gloves.

e. Fill the syringe with fluid. If it is necessary to touch the wound, one sterile gloved hand is then used to touch the wound; the other gloved hand is used to manipulate the equipment and is not considered sterile after touching unsterile equipment. If clean gloves are used, remember that neither gloved hand should touch the wound surface.

f. Direct the fluid onto all parts of the wound, paying particular attention to areas with exudate or drainage.

g. Irrigate until no exudate is present, until solution returns clear, or until ordered volume has been used.

11. Use a sterile gauze square to dry the area and redress the wound, using sterile technique (see Module 35, Wound Care).

12.–13. Follow the steps of the General Procedure.

Evaluation

14. Follow the General Procedure.

Documentation

15. Follow the General Procedure.

LONG-TERM CARE

 Performing irrigations is a common procedure in the long-term care facility.

Older people may have a decrease in lacrimal or tearing ability *so that small foreign bodies such as dust particles can enter the eye or other secretions can build up.* Eye irrigations with normal saline can remove the cause of any irritation and are very soothing.

The older adult *may produce an increased amount of cerumen (earwax), which can cause pain, hearing loss, or infection.* Residents who wear canal-fitting hearing aids tend to build up more wax than those who do not wear aids *because of the close contact of the aid with the auditory canal.* This wax must be removed *so that it does not interfere with the reception of sounds.*

Because many residents have an indwelling catheter in place, the bladder or catheter irrigation is perhaps the most common irrigation needed in the long-term care facility. Any blockage of the catheter *can place the person at risk for infection secondary to retention.* Knowledge and understanding of the irrigation procedure is essential for the nurse involved in long-term care.

HOME CARE

Irrigations have long been performed in the home by either the home care nurse or a family member. For example, foreign bodies in the eye and simple ear infections require soothing irrigation. The family may have an older member residing in the home who either has a hearing deficit or wears a hearing aid. Inspection for wax buildup should take place regularly and ear irrigation performed, if appropriate, *to remove the wax.*

A common irrigation procedure done in the home is the vaginal douche. A medicated vaginal douche may be ordered to treat a vaginal infection. Vaginal douching is unnecessary for the healthy woman with normal flora of the vaginal tract, although some commercial businesses have promoted the douche as an important part of feminine hygiene. The antiseptic powders used in some commercial douche products *are irritating to some individuals* and should be used with caution. More importantly, they decrease the normal flora, making the vaginal tract more susceptible to certain infections. Client teaching may involve helping women to understand the potential harmful effects of routine douching.

CRITICAL THINKING EXERCISES

Analyze each of the three situations below to determine what assessment is needed and what you should consider in your planning. Identify two different approaches to carrying out each procedure.

• Mr. Jones had surgery for a ruptured diverticulosis of his large bowel. A partial colectomy was performed, and one area of the surgical wound is open and is to be irrigated twice daily at the time of the dressing change. The wound is then to be packed with gauze saturated with normal saline.

• Mrs. Williams has been admitted for a vaginal hysterectomy this AM. Her orders include the need for a Betadine vaginal douche before surgery.

• Mrs. Roeder brings her 12-year-old son to the emergency room. He has severe pain in his right eye from particles that blew into it when his chemistry set exploded. The physician orders an eye irrigation with 1,000 mL normal saline.

✔ PERFORMANCE CHECKLIST

General Procedure for Irrigation	Needs More Practice	Satisfactory	Comments
Assessment			
1. Verify:			
a. Type of irrigation ordered.			
b. Correct solution: amount, type, temperature, concentration.			
Planning			
2. Decide whether irrigation is clean or sterile.			
3. Wash your hands.			
4. Identify and gather the equipment needed for the specific irrigation.			
a. Solution			
b. Irrigating device			
c. Receptacle for used fluid			
d. Protective padding			
e. Clean or sterile gloves			
f. Protective eyewear or gown if needed			
Implementation			
5. Identify the patient.			
6. Explain procedure to patient.			
7. Provide privacy.			
8. Position the patient as needed.			
9. Place protective padding where needed.			
10. Put on gloves and carry out irrigation according to specific procedure below.			
11. Make sure patient is dry and comfortable.			
12. Dispose of used equipment correctly.			
13. Wash your hands.			
Evaluation			
14. Evaluate using the following criteria:			
a. Area of irrigation was thoroughly cleaned.			
b. Medication contacted desired area.			
c. Patient resting comfortably.			

(*continued*)

General Procedure for Irrigation *(Continued)*	Needs More Practice	Satisfactory	Comments
d. Amount of solution returned compared with amount instilled.			
Documentation			
15. Document the following: **a.** Type of irrigation and time performed			
b. Type, concentration, and amount of fluid used			
c. Appearance and odor of any secretions			
d. Results of procedure			
e. Patient's response			
Bladder and Catheter Irrigation: Open Technique			
Assessment			
1. Follow Checklist step 1 of the General Procedure for Irrigation (verify type of irrigation and solution amount, type, concentration, and temperature).			
Planning			
2. Use sterile technique.			
3. Wash your hands.			
4. Gather necessary equipment listed in Checklist step 4 of the General Procedure, plus: **a.** Sterile irrigation set			
b. Solution			
c. Clean gloves			
Implementation			
5–7. Follow Checklist steps 5–7 of the General Procedure (identify patient, explain procedure, provide privacy).			
8. Position patient with catheter connection accessible.			
9. Place protective padding under connection site.			
10. Put on clean gloves and carry out the bladder or catheter irrigation: **a.** Open set, using sterile technique.			

(continued)

Bladder and Catheter Irrigation: Open Technique *(Continued)*	Needs More Practice	Satisfactory	Comments
b. Pour solution from bulk container.			
c. Clean the junction of catheter and drainage tubing.			
d. Disconnect the catheter and drainage tubing and hold over receptacle.			
e. Protect the end of the drainage tubing.			
f. Instill fluid (1) For catheter irrigation: (a) Fill asepto with 30–60 mL fluid.			
(b) Insert tip of asepto into catheter and instill fluid.			
(c) Pinch catheter closed as you withdraw syringe.			
(d) Allow fluid to drain into receptacle.			
(e) Observe drainage.			
(f) Repeat as needed.			
(2) For bladder irrigation: (a) Instill the ordered fluid into the bladder.			
(b) Clamp the tubing and allow the solution to remain in the bladder for several minutes.			
(c) Unclamp the tube and allow the fluid to drain out.			
g. Reconnect catheter to drainage tubing.			
11.–13. Follow Checklist steps 11–13 of the General Procedure (make patient dry and comfortable, dispose of used equipment and gloves, and wash your hands).			
Evaluation			
14. Evaluate as Checklist step 14 of the General Procedure (area thoroughly cleansed, medication [if used] contacted desired area, patient comfortable, amount of solution returned).			

(continued)

Bladder and Catheter Irrigation: **Open Technique** *(Continued)*	Needs More Practice	Satisfactory	Comments
Documentation			
15. Document as in Checklist step 15 of the General Procedure (include type of irrigation and time performed; type, concentration, and amount of fluid used; appearance and odor of secretions; results; patient response).			
Bladder and Catheter Irrigation: Three-Way Irrigation (Continuous Drip and Cleaning)			
Assessment			
1. Follow Checklist step 1 of the General Procedure for Irrigation (verify type of irrigation and solution amount, type, concentration, and temperature).			
Planning			
2. Use sterile technique.			
3. Wash your hands.			
4. Gather necessary equipment. **a.** IV stand			
b. Solution			
c. Tubing			
d. Gloves			
Implementation			
5.–9. Follow Checklist steps 5–9 of the General Procedure (identify patient, explain procedure, provide privacy, position patient, place protective padding).			
10. Put on gloves and carry out the irrigation: **a.** Set up pole, fluid container, and tubing.			
b. Clear air from tubing by filling with fluid.			
c. Attach tubing to inflow tube on three-way catheter.			
d. Attach outflow of catheter to drainage tube and make sure outflow tube is open.			
e. Regulate flow: (1) For continuous drip, regulate drip rate.			
(2) For cleaning:			

(continued)

Bladder and Catheter Irrigation: Three-Way Irrigation (Continuous Drip and Cleaning) *(Continued)*	Needs More Practice	Satisfactory	Comments
(a) Open inflow tubing to continuous stream.			
(b) Continue flow until outflow is free of clots and sediment.			
(c) Reclamp tubing.			
11.–13. Follow Checklist steps 11–13 of the General Procedure (make patient dry and comfortable, dispose of equipment, wash your hands).			
Evaluation			
14. Evaluate as in Checklist step 14 of the General Procedure (area thoroughly cleansed, medication [if used] contacted desired area, patient comfortable, amount of solution returned).			
Documentation			
15. Document as in Checklist step 15 of the General Procedure (include type of irrigation and time performed; type, concentration, and amount of fluid used; appearance and odor of secretions; results; patient response).			
Procedure for Irrigating the Ear			
Assessment			
1. Follow Checklist step 1 of the General Procedure for Irrigation (verify type of irrigation; solution amount, type, concentration, and temperature and that the ear has been examined).			
Planning			
2. Use clean technique.			
3. Wash your hands.			
4. Gather necessary equipment. **a.** Ear syringe or water pressure device			
b. Emesis basin			
c. Clean towels			
d. Clean gloves			
e. Solution			

(continued)

Procedure for Irrigating the Ear *(Continued)*	Needs More Practice	Satisfactory	Comments
Implementation			
5.–7. Follow Checklist steps 5–7 of the General Procedure (identify patient, explain procedure, provide privacy).			
8. Position the patient with head tilted away from ear to be irrigated.			
9. Place protective padding over shoulder under ear.			
10. Put on clean gloves and irrigate the ear: **a.** Place basin under patient's ear.			
b. Fill syringe with fluid.			
c. Straighten ear canal as appropriate for age.			
d. Direct tip of syringe toward top of ear canal and instill fluid.			
e. Continue irrigating until ear is cleansed.			
11. Dry ear and position with irrigated ear down.			
12. Dispose of used equipment and remove gloves.			
13. Wash your hands.			
Evaluation			
14. Evaluate as in Checklist step 14 of the General Procedure (area thoroughly cleansed, medication [if used] contacted desired area, patient comfortable, amount of solution returned).			
Documentation			
15. Document as in Checklist step 15 of the General Procedure (include type of irrigation and time performed; type, concentration, and amount of fluid used; appearance and odor of secretions; results; patient response).			
Procedure for Eye Irrigation			
Assessment			
1. Follow Checklist step 1 of the General Procedure for Irrigation (verify type of irrigation and solution amount, type, concentration, and temperature).			

(continued)

Procedure for Eye Irrigation *(Continued)*	Needs More Practice	Satisfactory	Comments
Planning			
2. Use sterile technique. Do not touch irrigator to eye.			
3. Wash your hands.			
4. Gather necessary equipment. **a.** Sterile syringe or IV tubing and stand			
b. Sterile solution			
c. Sterile eye shield for IV tubing			
d. Emesis basin			
e. Sterile cotton balls or gauze squares			
f. Sterile gloves			
Implementation			
5.–7. Follow Checklist steps 5–7 of the General Procedure (identify patient, explain procedure, provide privacy).			
8. Position patient in supine position, with head turned toward eye to be irrigated.			
9. Place padding and emesis basin below eye.			
10. Put on sterile gloves and irrigate the eye: **a.** Set up irrigating fluid and eye shield for large volume; pour saline into sterile container for small volume.			
b. Hold eye open.			
c. Use either syringe or continuous flow (1) Syringe method: (a) Fill syringe with fluid.			
(b) Release fluid with gentle pressure, from inner to outer canthus.			
(c) Repeat as needed for cleansing.			
(2) IV fluid method: (a) Adjust IV stand to lowest height.			
(b) Attach tubing and eye shield and hang container.			
(c) Fill tubing with fluid, eliminating air.			
(d) Place eye shield over the eyeball.			
(e) Open control valve and allow fluid to flow over eye.			

(continued)

Procedure for Eye Irrigation *(Continued)*	Needs More Practice	Satisfactory	Comments
11. Dry eye from inner to outer aspect. *Note:* If both eyes are to be irrigated, treat each separately.			
12.–13. Follow Checklist steps 12–13 of the General Procedure (dispose of equipment and wash your hands).			
Evaluation			
14. Evaluate as in Checklist step 14 of the General Procedure (area thoroughly cleansed, medication [if used] contacted desired area, patient comfortable, amount of solution returned).			
Documentation			
15. Document as in Checklist step 15 of the General Procedure (include type of irrigation and time performed; type, concentration, and amount of fluid used; appearance and odor of secretions; results; patient response).			
Procedure for Nasogastric Tube Irrigation			
Assessment			
1. Follow Checklist step 1 of the General Procedure for Irrigation (verify type of irrigation and solution amount, type, concentration, and temperature).			
Planning			
2. Use clean technique. Use sterile technique if patient has had stomach surgery.			
3. Wash your hands.			
4. Obtain necessary equipment. **a.** Irrigation set or syringe			
b. Solution			
c. Emesis basin			
d. Gloves			
Implementation			
5.–7. Follow Checklist steps 5–7 of the General Procedure (identify patient, explain procedure, provide privacy).			
8. Position patient so that connection point is accessible.			

(continued)

Procedure for Nasogastric Tube Irrigation *(Continued)*	Needs More Practice	Satisfactory	Comments
9. Place padding under connection site.			
10. Put on gloves and irrigate the nasogastric tube: **a.** Turn off suction and disconnect nasogastric tube.			
b. Fill the syringe with 30 mL fluid.			
c. Gently instill fluid into the tubing.			
d. Aspirate fluid back and discard. (Alternatively, hook to suction to aspirate.)			
e. Repeat procedure as needed to clear tubing.			
f. Reconnect tubing to suction and turn on.			
11.–13. Follow Checklist steps 11–13 of the General Procedure (make patient dry and comfortable, dispose of equipment, wash your hands).			
Evaluation			
14. Evaluate as in Checklist step 14 of the General Procedure (area thoroughly cleansed, medication [if used] contacted desired area, patient comfortable, amount of solution returned).			
Documentation			
15. Document as in Checklist step 15 of the General Procedure (include type of irrigation and time performed; type, concentration, and amount of fluid used; appearance and odor of secretions; results; patient response).			
Procedure for Vaginal Irrigation (Douche)			
Assessment			
1. Follow Checklist step 1 of the General Procedure for Irrigation (verify type of irrigation and solution amount, type, concentration, and temperature).			
Planning			
2. Use clean technique.			
3. Wash your hands.			
4. Gather necessary equipment.			

(continued)

Procedure for Vaginal Irrigation (Douche) *(Continued)*	Needs More Practice	Satisfactory	Comments
a. Douche set with douche tip			
b. Solution (1,000 mL at body temperature)			
c. IV stand			
d. Waterproof pad			
e. Bedpan			
f. Tissues			
g. Clean gloves			
Implementation			
5.–7. Follow Checklist steps 5–7 of the General Procedure (identify patient, explain procedure, provide privacy).			
8. Prepare the patient **a.** Have patient void.			
b. Position patient on back in bed.			
c. Drape patient in lithotomy position.			
9. Place a waterproof pad and a bedpan under the patient.			
10. Put on gloves and carry out the vaginal irrigation. **a.** Wash the patient's perineal area.			
b. Fill fluid container and connect douche tip.			
c. Hang container on IV stand, 18–24 inches above hips.			
d. Run fluid through tubing to clear air.			
e. Moisten douche tip to lubricate it.			
f. Run small amount of fluid on labia to check for comfort.			
g. Insert tip 3–4 inches into vagina.			
h. Unclamp tubing and allow fluid to flow.			
i. Rotate tip.			
j. Remove tip when all fluid used.			
k. Help patient to sit up on bedpan.			
11. Provide tissue for drying perineum.			

(continued)

Procedure for Vaginal Irrigation (Douche) *(Continued)*	Needs More Practice	Satisfactory	Comments
12.–13. Follow Checklist steps 12–13 of the General Procedure (dispose of equipment and wash your hands).			
Evaluation			
14. Evaluate as in Checklist step 14 of the General Procedure (area thoroughly cleansed, medication [if used] contacted desired area, patient comfortable, amount of solution returned).			
Documentation			
15. Document as in Checklist step 15 of the General Procedure (include type of irrigation and time performed; type, concentration, and amount of fluid used; appearance and odor of secretions; results; patient response).			
Procedure for Wound Irrigation			
Assessment			
1. Follow Checklist step 1 of the General Procedure for Irrigation (verify type of irrigation and solution amount, type, concentration, and temperature).			
Planning			
2. Use sterile technique.			
3. Wash your hands.			
4. Gather necessary equipment. **a.** Irrigating set			
b. Two pairs of gloves and protective equipment if needed			
c. Dressing materials			
d. Solution			
e. Padding			
f. Receptacle for soiled dressing			
Implementation			
5.–7. Follow Checklist steps 5–7 of the General Procedure (identify patient, explain procedure, provide privacy).			
8. Position patient so fluid will flow appropriately.			
9. Place padding beside and under patient.			

(continued)

Procedure for Wound Irrigation *(Continued)*	Needs More Practice	Satisfactory	Comments
10. Carry out the wound irrigation: **a.** Open sterile set and pour sterile fluid into container.			
b. Put on clean gloves and remove and dispose of soiled dressing and gloves.			
c. Place receptacle to catch fluid.			
d. Put on second pair of gloves.			
e. Fill syringe with fluid, using one hand if one hand is to be used to touch wound.			
f. Direct fluid to all parts of wound.			
g. Irrigate until wound is clean or ordered volume is used.			
11. Use a sterile gauze square to dry the area and redress the wound.			
12.–13. Follow Checklist steps 12–13 of the General Procedure (dispose of equipment and wash your hands).			
Evaluation			
14. Evaluate as in Checklist step 14 of the General Procedure (area thoroughly cleansed, medication [if used] contacted desired area, patient comfortable, amount of solution returned).			
Documentation			
15. Document as in Checklist step 15 of the General Procedure (include type of irrigation and time performed; type, concentration, and amount of fluid used; appearance and odor of secretions; results; patient response).			

Short-Answer Questions

1. List two major purposes of irrigation.
   a. _cleansing_
   b. _instilling meds_

2. Mrs. Jones has had bladder surgery. An irrigation with an antibacterial medication, nitrofurantoin, has been ordered. This irrigation is probably for which of the above purposes?
   to instill medications

3. Name a type of irrigation in which sterile technique is essential.
   eye, wound, catheter, bladder

4. Name a type of irrigation in which clean technique is safe.
   vagina, ear, nasogastric tube

5. List three factors in an irrigation that can cause irritation or damage tissue.
   a. _too high temperature_
   b. _too great of pressure_
   c. _incorrect solution concentration_

6. After prostate surgery, Mr. Jefferson has a continuous three-way irrigation set up. What is the most critical safety concern with this irrigation?
   The drainage or outflow tubing Ø be blocked or clamped when fluid going in

7. Under what circumstances should an ear not be irrigated? _When the tympanic membrane is Ø intact_

8. Why is it not appropriate to administer a vaginal douche while the patient sits on a toilet?
   Fluid tends to drain out too fast and Ø come in contact c̄ all surfaces

9. Why must each eye be treated as a separate irrigation?
   To prevent spread of a microorganism from one eye to the other

10. When might a water pressure device be used to irrigate wounds? _For seriously contaminated traumatic wounds._

11. List three types of irrigations commonly performed in the long-term care facility for the older adult resident and the main reason each is done. _Eye irrigations to remove dust particles, secretions; Ear - to remove built up ear wax; catheter irrigations to keep cath patent to ↓ risk of infection_

12. Why should healthy females be cautioned in the use of vaginal douches at home?
    antiseptic powders used can cause irritation in some susceptible females

13. When are protective eyewear and a gown or apron needed for performing an irrigation?
    When any splashing might occur.

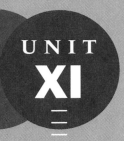

MODULE

47

ADMINISTERING MEDICATIONS: OVERVIEW

MODULE CONTENTS

PREREQUISITES

Successful completion of the following modules:[1]

VOLUME 1
Module 1 An Approach to Nursing Skills
Module 2 Basic Infection Control
Module 3 Safety
Module 5 Documentation
Module 6 Introduction to Assessment Skills

Before giving medications, you must have a satisfactory level of competence in mathematics of dosages and solutions. A math quiz follows. If you cannot answer at least 16 of the 20 problems correctly (or the number designated by your instructor), plan to complete one of the many programmed instruction units available on mathematics of dosages and solutions. Consult your instructor for guidance.

[1]For techniques related to giving medications to children, see Module 51, Administering Medications to Infants and Children. For information related to administering medications by ophthalmic, otic, nasal, skin and mucous membranes, vaginal, rectal, and inhalation routes, see Module 49, Administering Medications by Alternative Routes. For information related to parenteral medications, see Module 50, Giving Injections, Module 53, Administering Intravenous Medications and Module 58, Giving Epidural Medications.

S E L F - T E S T :   MATHEMATICS OF DOSAGES AND SOLUTIONS

Directions: *Read each problem carefully. Show your work beneath the questions, and*
place your answers in the right-hand column.

1. Pronestyl 500 mg is ordered q.i.d. for Mr. Jones. Available are 250-mg tablets of
Pronestyl. How many tablets will he receive each day?

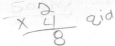

$\dfrac{500}{\times\ 4}{8}$ qid

8

2. The order reads: "Codeine phosphate gr 1/2. Tablets marked "codeine phosphate
gr 1/4" are available. How many tablets will you need for one dose?

2

3. The order for the dosage of a drug reads: "0.25 g." The only tablets available are in
milligrams. How many milligrams is 0.25 g?

0.250. g

250

4. The order reads: "Milk of magnesia 1 oz." How many milliliters will you give?

30 m

5. You are to prepare streptomycin sulfate for injection. On hand is a vial containing
1.0 g dry drug. The label reads: "Add 9.2 mL diluent to yield 10.0-mL solution."
Each milliliter will contain how many milligrams of the drug?

100 mg

6. You are to administer insulin. The vial reads: "U-100." What does this mean?

100 units/m

7. The order reads: "meperidine 75 mg IM." The meperidine available is 100 mg/mL.
How many milliliters will you give?

$\dfrac{100\,mg}{1\,ml} \times \dfrac{75\,mg}{X} = .75\,ml.$

0.75 ml

8. The order for IV fluid reads: "1,000 mL 5% glucose in water to run 10 h."
Determine the number of drops per minute the IV should run if the
administration set delivers 15 gtt/mL.

100ml hr.

9. If the centigrade temperature is 40°, what is the Fahrenheit reading?

F =

S E L F - T E S T :   MATHEMATICS OF DOSAGES AND SOLUTIONS (Continued)

10. If the adult dose of a medication is 500 mg, is the pediatric dose more likely to be 200 mg or 800 mg?

200 mg.

11. Name three factors that are commonly used to calculate pediatric dosage.

a. *weight*
b. *age*
c. *body surface area*

12. A patient is ordered to have 1,000 mL of 5% dextrose in normal saline to run over 8 h. A volume-controlled pump is to be used to deliver the IV fluid. How many milliliters per hour must you set the pump for?

$$\frac{8\,h.}{1,000\,ml} \quad \frac{1\,h.}{X\,ml}$$

$$8\overline{)1000} \quad \begin{array}{r} 125. \\ \hline 8 \\ \hline 20 \\ 16 \\ \hline 40 \end{array}$$

125 ml/h.

125 ml/h

13. How much morphine sulfate should a 6-year-old weighing 45 lb receive if the adult dosage is 10 mg?

$$\frac{45\,lb}{150\,lb.}\,X \quad \frac{X}{10\,mg} \quad 150\overline{)450}\,\frac{3}{450}$$

3 mg.

14. The usual dosage of a certain drug for a child is 20 mg/kg. The child weighs 68 lb. What would the dosage be for this child?

$$\frac{2.2\,lb.}{1\,Kg} \times \frac{68\,lb}{X} = 30.9\,Kg \quad \begin{array}{r} 30.9 \\ \times 20 \\ \hline 6180 \end{array}$$

618 mg.

15. The order reads: "Pentobarbital gr 3/4 at hs." The only drug available is marked in milligrams. How many milligrams do you need for the correct dosage?

$$\frac{60\,mg}{1\,gr.} \times \frac{X}{3/4\,gr.} = 45\,mg.$$

45 mg.

16. The order reads: "Digoxin 0.25 mg daily." The drug is available in liquid form for this patient. The label reads: "Digoxin 0.05 mg/mL." How many milliliters will you give?

$$\frac{.05\,mg}{1\,ml} \quad \frac{.25\,mg}{X} = 5\,ml.$$

5 ml

17. The order reads: "Aluminum hydroxide 1 dram as needed for indigestion." How many milliliters will you give? How many teaspoons is this?

4 or 5 ml or 1 t.

$$\frac{1}{5\,ml.}\,\frac{3}{X\,ml}$$

S E L F - T E S T :   MATHEMATICS OF DOSAGES AND SOLUTIONS (Continued)

18. The order reads: "Micro K 0.25 mg." The bottle is labeled "Micro K 250 µg/tablet." How many tablets will you give?

19. The order reads: "Metronidazole 500 mg IV q6h." You have a small IV infusion bag with a label that reads: "Metronidazole 500 mg/100 mL, give over 1 h." The equipment available delivers 15 gtts/mL. How many drops per minute should the infusion run?

20. The order reads: "Solu-Cortef 25 mg IV." The label reads: Solu-Cortef 100 mg/ 2 mL." How many milliliters will you give?

K E Y

1. 8 tablets	**12.** 125 mL/h
2. 2 tablets	**13.** 3 mg
3. 250 mg	**14.** 618 mg
4. 30 mL	**15.** 45 mg
5. 100 mg	**16.** 5 mL
6. 100 units/mL	**17.** 4 mL; 1 tsp
7. 0.75 mL	**18.** 1 tablet
8. 25 gtts/min	**19.** 25 gtts/min
9. 104°F	**20.** 0.5 mL
10. 200 mg	
11. a. age	
b. weight	
c. body surface area	

OVERALL OBJECTIVE

To understand medication administration systems, how to administer medications to patients, and how to record medication administration appropriately; to respond appropriately if a medication error occurs.

SPECIFIC LEARNING OBJECTIVES

Know Facts and Principles	Apply Facts and Principles	Demonstrate Ability	Evaluate Performance
1. Abbreviations Know meanings of abbreviations listed in Table 47–1.	Correctly interpret medication orders that include abbreviations.	Correctly use and interpret abbreviations used in preparation and administration of medications.	Evaluate own performance with instructor.
2. Equivalencies Know equivalencies listed in Table 47–2.	Given problems, work out equivalencies in apothecary, metric, and household systems.	In the clinical setting (under supervision), correctly work out problems involving equivalencies.	Evaluate own performance with instructor.
3. Administration methods Explain how medications, including narcotics, are dispensed and stored. Identify information to be found on a medication administration record.	Outline medication administration procedure used in assigned facility.	Correctly carry out medication administration procedure used in assigned facility with supervision.	Evaluate own performance with instructor using Performance Checklist and facility procedure.
4. Safety and accuracy Identify essential aspects of a complete medication order.	Analyze a medication order to determine whether it is complete.	Use three checks and six rights consistently.	Evaluate own performance with instructor.
5. Documentation Know information to be recorded regarding medications administered.	Identify documentation method used in assigned facility.	Correctly document medications administered according to method used in assigned facility.	Evaluate own performance with instructor.
6. Medication errors State nurse's responsibility when a medication error occurs.	Given a situation involving a medication error, identify appropriate nursing actions.	If a medication error occurs, carry out appropriate nursing actions.	Evaluate understanding with instructor.

LEARNING ACTIVITIES

1. Review the Specific Learning Objectives.
2. Read the section on administering medications in Ellis and Nowlis, *Nursing: A Human Needs Approach,* or comparable material in another textbook.
3. Look up the module vocabulary terms in the glossary.
4. Read through the module and mentally practice the procedure. Study as though you were planning to teach the skills to another person.
5. Study the abbreviations and equivalencies in Tables 47–1 and 47–2.
6. In the practice setting, do the following:
   a. Review the medication administration record and procedures used in your facility.
   b. Go through the procedure step by step, referring to the Performance Checklist as necessary. Use the appropriate procedures for your facility.
   c. When you know the procedure, ask your instructor to check your performance.
7. Plan with your instructor for an opportunity to administer medications in the clinical setting.

VOCABULARY

dose	route	three checks
medication administration record	six rights	unit dose
	stock drugs	

Administering Medications

Rationale for the Use of This Skill

One of the nurse's most routine and yet most critical responsibilities is the preparation and administration of medications. The responsibility extends beyond preparation and administration. The nurse must know how medicines act, the usual dosage, the desired effects, and potential side effects so that he or she can evaluate the effectiveness of the medication and recognize adverse effects promptly when they occur. You will acquire this knowledge gradually as you study pharmacology and care for patients with varying problems.[2]

▼ NURSING DIAGNOSES

The major nursing diagnosis to keep in mind when giving medications is Risk for Injury. Patients can be injured by medications given in the wrong dosage, at the wrong time, or by an incorrect route. They also can be injured by the omission of essential medications, the administration of an incorrect medication, and by incorrect documentation. Although this nursing diagnosis will not appear on the care plan, it applies to every situation in which a patient is being given medications.

Another nursing diagnosis frequently appropriate when administering medications is Knowledge Deficit. In this case the Knowledge Deficit would be related to some aspect of the medication regimen; for example, the need to be aware of drug interactions when taking antacids.

PROCEDURES RELATED TO MEDICATION ADMINISTRATION

In any healthcare facility, medications are administered according to a procedures and policies defined by that facility (Tables 47–1 and 47–2).

Storing Medications

Individual patient supplies are the most common method of storing drugs. These consist of enough medication for a single occasion, for one shift, for an entire day, or for an undefined period. These drugs are ordered by the physician, dispensed by the pharmacy labeled for the individual patient, and stored in a locked individual patient drawer or cupboard.

Drugs referred to as "scheduled" drugs (those with special control procedures mandated by federal law because of their potential for addiction or abuse) are usually kept in a locked stock supply for the unit. They are then dispensed by the nurse one dose at a time.

The *unit-dose system* consists of the provision by pharmacy personnel of prepackaged and prelabeled *individual doses* of medications for patients. Although more than one dose may be placed in the patient's medication drawer or cupboard, each dose is labeled with the drug name and dosage. Studies have shown that the unit-dose system is accurate and convenient.

Medication Administration Records

Perhaps the oldest type of record used for medication administration is that of using a card on which is recorded the patient's name and room number and the medication, dosage, and route. The nurse administering the medications checks the card against a permanent record of all medications ordered, such as a Kardex or a medication notebook. Then, using the cards as a guide, the nurse prepares and administers the medications. Documentation is

Table 47–1.	Common Abbreviations
PO	by mouth
ac	before meals
pc	after meals
q.d.	every day
q.o.d.	every other day
b.i.d.	twice a day
t.i.d.	three times a day
q.i.d.	four times a day
stat	immediately
c̄	with
s̄	without
s̄s̄	one half
hs	at bedtime
prn	as needed
qh	every hour
q2h	every 2 hours

Also see Table 47–2, Equivalencies.

[2]Note that rationale for action is emphasized throughout the module by the use of italics.

Table 47–2. Equivalencies

1. Metric doses and apothecaries equivalents

Liquid

Metric	Approximate apothecaries' equivalents
1,000 mL	1 quart
500 mL	1 pint
250 mL	8 fluidounces
30 mL	1 fluidounce
15 mL	4 fluidrams
5 mL	1 fluidram
1 mL	15 minims
0.06 mL	1 minim

Solid

130 g	1 ounce
15 g	4 drams
4 g	60 grains (1 dram)
1 g (1000 mg)	15 grains
0.5 g (500 mg)	7 ½ grains
60 mg	1 grain
30 mg	½ grain
15 mg	¼ grain
10 mg	⅙ grain
8 mg	⅛ grain
1 mg (1000 μg)	1/60 grain
0.6 mg (600 μg)	1/100 grain
0.4 mg (400 μg)	1/150 grain
0.3 mg (300 μg)	1/200 grain
0.2 mg (200 μg)	1/300 grain
0.1 mg (100 μg)	1/600 grain

2. Approximate household measures

1 teaspoonful	1 fl dr	4–5 mL
1 tablespoonful	½ fl oz	15 or 16 mL
1 jigger	1½ fl oz	45 mL
1 cup	8 fl oz	240 mL

3. Prescription abbreviations

gr	grain or grains
gtt[1]	drops
ʒ	dram
℥	ounce
aa	equal parts
ss	one half
cc[2]	cubic centimeter
g	gram
mg	milligram
μg	microgram
mL	milliliter
mEq	milliequivalent
min	minim

[1]*Gutta(e)*
[2]*Although technically not exactly equivalent, mL and cc are often used interchangeably.*

done on the patient's chart. *Because it is so easy to misplace or lose medication cards,* this system is now uncommon.

In some healthcare facilities, a large notebook or a Kardex with a page or pages containing a listing of the medications for each patient is used; this is a permanent record and a guide as the medications are prepared and administered. The notebook or Kardex is often used for documenting the administration as well.

NARCOTICS

Narcotic control is mandated by Federal legislation. Based on this legislation, individual facilities establish policies regarding access and record keeping.

Narcotics are kept in a double-locked drawer or cupboard and must be signed out by the nurse administering the drug. The record indicates how many doses remain in the supply. Signing out the narcotic documents the name of the nurse who assumed responsibility for that dose.

In most settings, narcotics are routinely counted at change of shift and anytime the supply is replenished. If the amount of medication in the drawer does not agree with the record, the situation must be reported immediately. In some settings, narcotic control is computerized, and the drug is not released from the storage container until appropriate information is entered into the computer. When this is done, routine counting is not needed.

If you need to discard part or all of a narcotic that is prepared and ready to give to a patient, you must have another nurse witness your action and co-sign the narcotic record. Follow the policy in your facility.

SAFETY AND ACCURACY

The Three Checks

Certain basic considerations always apply to medication administration. One of these considerations is the *three checks*. The name and dosage of the medication as written on the drug label are checked three times. These three times may differ somewhat depending on how the medications are stored and what the procedure is in the individual facility. Reading labels carefully three times may seem cumbersome, but medication names may be similar, dosages may differ from those ordered, and it is easy to "read" what you expect to be present if you only look one time.

Commonly, the three times for checking are as follows: 1) when choosing the medication to take out of the drawer or cupboard, 2) when the dose is in hand and can be held side-by-side with the record to compare the label and the medication administration record (MAR), and 3) one last time after all drugs have been located and before leaving the medication cart or room for the patient's bedside. (Fig. 47–1)

All drugs are kept in their individual dose package until you are at the patient's bedside. *When discussing a medication with a patient, you are then able to point out the labeled name of the drug as the patient observes its appearance. If the patient is not in the room or is unable to take the medication for some reason, you can return the medication, which is still in a labeled package, to the medication drawer for later administration because there is no chance of error in identification.* This is one of the extra safeguards that the unit-dose method provides.

The Six Rights

Additional considerations basic to the administration of medications are the *six rights*. These rights are a guide for remembering the following:

1. The right drug
2. In the right dose
3. By the right route
4. To the right patient
5. At the right time
6. With the right documentation

This is not *all* the nurse has to know, but fewer medication errors would be made if the six rights were consistently considered.

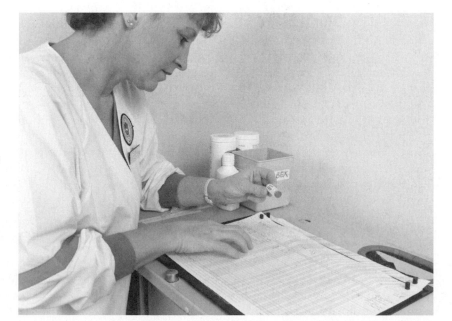

Figure 47–1. The nurse carefully checks the label against a written record.

The right drug, the right dose, the right route, and the right time are ensured by following the three checks. To ensure you have the right patient, carefully identify the patient. Some type of identification card that lists the patient's name and other identifying information, such as patient number or social security number, must be taken to the bedside *for accurate patient identification.* In systems using medication cards, the card itself is used for identifying the patient. In systems using a central medication record, you can take this record into the patient's room for identification. If you do not take the original medication record to the room, you must prepare a separate identification card. This is most easily done using the addressograph machine. Compare this card with the MAR *to ensure that it correctly identifies the patient for whom the medicine is ordered.* When you are in the patient's room, you can compare the identification card with the patient's wrist identification bracelet, or ask the patient to state or spell his or her name while you check the identification record. With confused or unconscious patients, the use of the wristband is essential. Asking the patient to state his or her name or comparing numbers eliminates the possibility that the patient may respond casually to a "yes or no" question without truly hearing what you are asking.

The patient should not be left alone until all medications have been swallowed. Although it is rare for a patient to deceive a nurse about taking medications, it does happen. It is not appropriate to leave medications at the bedside for patients to take on their own unless so ordered by the physician or unless it is a policy for certain medications on a particular unit. Medications may be inadvertently misplaced, forgotten, or mistakenly picked up by another person if they are left at the bedside. Among the medications commonly self-administered are antacids, eye medications, and inhalers. Medications that patients have been taking regularly at home, such as birth control pills, also may be their responsibility.

The nurse who prepares a given medication should administer it. Stated another way, you should administer only drugs that you prepare. *Only the person who prepared the drug knows what it is and what strength or dosage it is, unless it is still in the unit-dose packaging.*

MEDICATION ORDERS

Medications to be given in a healthcare facility must be ordered by a physician or other person with prescriptive authority in your state. Most medications are ordered for the individual patient. In some instances, a physician may establish "standing orders," which are a set of orders that they use for all of their hospitalized patients, adding individualized orders as necessary. Some also have protocols that allow nurses to use their own judgment (ie, bowel protocols).

A complete medication order should include the date, name of the drug, dosage, route of administration, frequency of administration, and signature of the prescribing person. In some facilities, the policy states that a medication is given by the oral route unless ordered differently. In those facilities, the route may not always be specified. If the order is incomplete, not clear, or does not conform to documented dosage ranges, the nurse should confer with the physician to clarify the order before giving the medication. You also may find it helpful to consult the pharmacist.

Medications that are ordered to be given on a regular basis until the order is canceled are called *routine orders.* They may be given once a day (q.d.), several times a day (b.i.d., t.i.d., q.i.d.), every other day (q.o.d.), at stated hours (q4h), or on certain days of the week only (eg, Tuesday, Thursday, and Saturday). Medications that are given when needed or requested only (a laxative for constipation, a narcotic for pain) are ordered on a *prn* (as needed) basis. *One-time only* medications are to be given on one occasion only at a specified time. Medications given prior to surgery or a diagnostic test are examples of one-time only orders. These various types of orders are transcribed onto different parts of the MAR in some facilities (Figs. 47–2 and 47–3).

Although the physician orders the medication, the facility has standard times at which medications are administered. For example, medications ordered for four times a day may be given at 9 AM, 1 PM, 5 PM, and 9 PM in some facilities but at 8 AM, 12 noon, 4 PM, and 8 PM in others. However, some medications ordered for four times a day must be given around the clock and therefore would be given at 6 AM, 12 noon, 6 PM, and 12 midnight. The nurse is responsible for identifying the appropriate times to give a medication based on its action in the body and the policy of the facility.

GENERAL PROCEDURE FOR ADMINISTERING MEDICATIONS

The general approach used to administer medications to a single patient can be modified as needed for a specific patient or for a group of patients.

(text continues on page 365)

NORTHWEST HOSPITAL MEDICATION RECORD - (ROUTINES)

Order Date	Exp. Date	Initial	ROUTINE MEDICATIONS MED - DOSE - ROUTE - FREQ	Schd Hrs	1/3/99 Init/Site	1/4 Init/Site	1/5 Init/Site	1/6 Init/Site	1/7 Init/Site	1/8 Init/Site	1/9 Init/Site
1/3/99		JE	Digoxin 0.125 mg p.o. daily	09	╳	KT PO					
				AP	╳	92					
1/4/99		KT	Lasix 40 mg. p.o. daily	09	╳	╳					
1/4/99		KT	Micro K 0.25 mg p.o. b.i.d.	09	╳	KT PO					
				21	╳	SM PO					
1/4/99		KT	Docusate Ca ÷ b.i.d.	09	╳	KT PO					
				21	╳	(SM) ✳					

DATE – TIME	1/4/99 (21)				
REFERENCE BOXES ⟶	Refused due to loose stools. SM				

SIGNATURE AND TITLE BELOW TO IDENTIFY INITIALS

JE Janice Ellis RN
KT Kay Taylor RN
SM Sue Morton RN

INJECTION SITE	CODE
DELTOID	RD/LD
ABDOMEN	RA/LA
VENTROGLUTEAL	RV/LV
GLUTEAL	RG/LG
THIGH	RT/LT

M134A REV. 1/79

Rogers, William F. M-76

09657321

Dr. J. L. Jepson

ADDRESSOGRAPH

DIAGNOSIS
Congestive heart failure

ALLERGIES
Penicillin

DIET

RECOPIED BY:

PAGE:

Figure 47–2. Medication administration record for routine medications. Note use of both initials and full signatures.

NORTHWEST HOSPITAL MEDICATION RECORD (P.R.N.'S)

(WRITE IN BELOW THE NEW P.R.N. MEDS AS ORDERED

#	Order Date	Exp. Date	Initial	MED - DOSE - ROUTE - FREQ	#	Order Date	Exp. Date	Initial	MED - DOSE - ROUTE - FREQ
1	1/3/99		JE	M. O. M. 30 cc. q.d. prn	5				
2	1/3/99		JE	Halcion 25 mg. p.o. h.s.	6				
3	1/3/99		JE	A. S. A. gr X q4h prn pain	7				
4					8				

#	Date / Time		Dose	Site	REASON	EFFECT	INIT	#	Date / Time		Dose	Site	REASON	EFFECT	INIT
2	1/3/99	2100	25 mg	p.o.	for sleep	slept	RV								
3	1/4/99	08	gr X	p o	for shoulder pain	relief	SM								
2	1/4/99	2100	25 mg	p o	sleep	slept	KT								

Order Date	INIT	STATS MED	SINGLES DOSE	PRE-OPS ROUTE	To Be Given Date	Time	INIT	(ONLY ON STATS & SINGLES) REASON	EFFECT
1/4/99	KT	Lasix 80 mg this a.m.			1/4	0900	KT	Fluid Retention	See Daily wt.

SIGNATURE AND TITLE BELOW TO IDENTIFY INITIALS			INJECTION SITE	CODE
RV Ronald Vaughn SN	JE Janice Ellis RN		DELTOID	RD/LD
SM Sue Morton RN			ABDOMEN	RA/LA
KT Kay Taylor RN			VENTROGLUTEAL	RV/LV
			GLUTEAL	RG/LG
			THIGH	RT/LT

M134A REV. 1/79

Rogers, William F. M-76

09657321

Dr. J. L. Jepson

A D D R E S S O G R A P H

DIAGNOSIS
Congestive heart failure

ALLERGIES
Penicillin

DIET
Low Na

RECOPIED BY:

PAGE:
1 of 1

Figure 47–3. Medication administration record for PRN and stat medications. Note indications of reason for administration of medications.

Assessment

1. Review the medication record used in your facility to identify whether any medications are to be given to an individual patient during your shift. Generally, medications should be given within 30 minutes of the time ordered. Exceptions to this include preoperative medications and medications given every 2 hours or more frequently. These medications must be given precisely on time.

2. Examine the MAR for accuracy and completeness as prescribed by your facility. In some facilities, the MAR is compared with the medication orders each day. In other facilities, the procedure for verifying the MAR may include a double-check system at the time the order is noted, in which case it may not be necessary to check against the order sheet. In this procedure, as in all others, follow the policy at your facility. Check the patient's name and room number, name of the medication, dosage, route of administration, and time(s) the medication is to be given. Determine whether the ordered medications have already been given or are to be held. Often that information is noted in the spot where you would indicate having given the drug.

3. Review information about the medication(s) to be administered. When you are an experienced nurse, you may have memorized this information for drugs you commonly administer. As a student, you may be expected to have written notes on each medication you are to administer. These notes should include the generic name of the drug and common trade names; the usual dosage range; the actions, side effects, and contraindications for the drug; and the nursing implications, such as the need to administer on an empty stomach, the need to take vital signs before giving, and appropriate health teaching.

   You may be permitted to use commercially prepared medication cards or a drug book. If so, you will need to individualize the information to your specific patient(s) by noting why this drug is being given to this specific patient.

4. Assess the patient *to ascertain whether the patient can take the medications as ordered* (eg, ability to swallow, level of consciousness).

5. Assess the patient *to identify a need for any prn medications ordered.*

Planning

6. Determine what equipment you will need.

7. Wash your hands *for infection control.*

8. Gather the equipment. You will need small paper cups for tablets and capsules and calibrated plastic medicine cups for liquids. In some facilities, the calibrated medicine cups are used for tablets and capsules also.

Implementation

9. Read from the record the name of the medication to be given.

10. Check the label on the medication before picking it up. (This is the first of the three checks.)

11. Pick up the medication, and check the label again, comparing it with the MAR. If the medication is in a container, do this check before you remove the medication from the container. (This is the second of the three checks.)

12. Remove the correct amount of medication for the individual dose to be given at this time.

13. Check the medication label with MAR once again. (This is the third of the three checks.) If the medication is in a unit-dose package, do this check after all medications have been identified before leaving for the patient's bedside.

14. Place the medication, still in its unit-dose package, in a container or on a tray.

15. Place a medication card or label on the prepared medication *for identification of the patient if the MAR is not to be taken into the patient room.*

16. Approach and identify the patient *to be sure you are administering medication to the correct patient.* By identifying the patient before you begin the rest of the procedure, *you avoid causing distress by mistakenly offering medication that is intended for someone else.* Although you prevent an error if you check the identification after offering the medication, the patient may feel that a mistake was almost made and may thus feel anxious. You can walk into the room and simply say, "Hello. May I check your wristband?" Another approach is to look at your identification record and say, "Hello. Would you please spell your last name for me?" or "Hello. Would you please state your full name for me?"

17. Explain what you are going to do and if appropriate, what the medication is for and how it works. The information should be presented simply, in language easily understood by the patient. Explain any specific requirements related to the drug, such as increased fluid intake. For example, you might say, "I have your Lasix for you. This is the medicine that helps to remove the extra fluid that is causing your swollen ankles." Instead, you could say, "This is the aspirin that has been ordered for your sore shoulder. It is important for you to drink a full glass of water with it. The water helps to prevent irritation of your stomach." If assessment is needed before

		DATE OF ORDER	SCHEDULED MEDICATION DOSE, ROUTE, FREQUENCY		ALLERGIES: *None*				
					DATE *1/6/99*	DATE *1/7/99*	DATE *1/8/99*	DATE *1/9/99*	DATE *1/10/99*
Ruth Brown R.N. (RB)	Elizabeth Dawson (ED)	1/5/99	Digoxin 0.25 mg p.o. q.d. 9 $\frac{00}{a.}$	N			Ⓒ		
				D	9 RB AP72	9 ED AP70			
				E					
		1/5/99	Lasix 40 mg. p.o. b.i.d. 9a – 5p	N					
				D	9 RB Ⓐ	9 ED Ⓑ			
				E	5 SM	5 SM			
Sam Morris R.N. (SM)				N					
				D					
				E					
				N					
				D					
				E					
				N					
				D					
				E					
				N					
				D					
				E					
				N					
				D					
				E					
				N					
				D					
				E					
				N					
				D					
				E					
				N					
				D					
				E					
				N					
				D					
				E					
				N					
				D					
				E					
				N					
				D					
				E					

SIGNATURE

SYMBOL KEYS: NPO - MEDICATION NOT GIVEN
PATIENT NPO
R - REFUSED MEDICATION

N - NAUSEATED
S - SEDATED
U - UNRESPONSIVE

RT - RIGHT THIGH
LT - LEFT THIGH
RD - RIGHT DELTOID
LD - LEFT DELTOID

RG - RIGHT GLUTEUS
LG - LEFT GLUTEUS
RVG - RIGHT VENTROGLUTEUS
LVG - LEFT VENTROGLUTEUS

STAMP:
Smith, John
000-92-8310
Dr. Jones

BALLARD COMMUNITY HOSPITAL
SEATTLE, WASHINGTON

Figure 47–4. Medication administration record for routine medications with special circumstances noted. **(A)** Medication given as routine. **(B)** Medication omitted. **(C)** Pulse recorded with medication administration.

you give the medication, you might say something like, "This is your blood pressure medicine. I want to take your blood pressure before you take it." If the patient expresses doubts or confusion about a medication, such as "This doesn't look the same as what I take at home" or "I've never taken *this* medication before" recheck the order before administering the drug.

18. Administer the medication as appropriate for the route used.
19. Leave the patient in a comfortable position.
20. Discard the medication container *if it is disposable*. If it is not, rinse it out and replace it on the cart for reprocessing.
21. Wash your hands.

Evaluation

22. Evaluate, using the following criteria:
    a. The *right* patient received the *right* medication in the *right* dosage by the *right* route at the *right* time, and it was documented in the *right* way.
    b. The criteria established for ascertaining the effectiveness of a specific drug were used (eg, for a given pain medication this might be "Pain relief obtained within 30 minutes").
    c. Side effects, if present, were promptly identified.

Documentation

23. Document on the medication record that the medication was given. Again, the exact method for doing this varies with the facility. Usually the name of the medication, dosage, route of administration, time, and your signature (with abbreviation indicating your position) are included. Initials are often used *to indicate that a medication has been given,* but a signature that includes at least the first initial, last name, and position (ie, RN) is usually required on the medication record at least once during each shift (see Figs. 47–2 and 47–3).

If specific assessment data are required before a medication can be given, there may be a place to document those data on the medication record. An example of such a situation is a pulse rate before a cardiac medication or a temperature before a medication to lower the temperature (Figs. 47-3 and 47-4).

If the medication is not given (eg, it may be held at the nurse's discretion or refused by the patient), indicate this on the medication record. In many facilities, this is indicated by a circle around the time that it should have been given along with an explanation in the nurses' progress notes. When the physician is notified regarding a medication not given, this also should be noted on the chart.

MEDICATION ERRORS

If a medication error occurs, it must be reported as soon as it is discovered *so that any necessary actions can be taken immediately.* In most cases, an unusual incident or quality assurance form is completed by the nurse who makes or discovers the error. The physician is notified of the error, and plans are instituted for assessing the patient for adverse effects. Check the policy in your facility regarding documentation of errors.

LONG-TERM CARE

Many long-term care facilities use a "punch card" system for dispensing oral medications. The various medications are housed in "bubbles" on cards and punched out as they are given. This system helps to prevent medication errors because the cards are a check as to whether the medications have been given.

Many individuals residing in long-term care facilities have complex medication regimens and are at high risk for adverse medication reactions based on their age and slowed body processes. Nurses in these settings must be particularly vigilant in regard to assessment.

HOME CARE

Individuals of all ages need to take medications at home. Some clients are able to manage this task on their own, and others need varying amounts of assistance. Written instructions must be individualized to the client. Home medication schedules must be worked around schedules that already exist for the client and family. For example, a medication that is to be taken three times a day could logically be given with meals if it can be taken with food and the meals are somewhat evenly spaced. Many dispensers have been designed to assist people to take the right medication in the right amount at the right time. Some of these, however, are difficult for individuals to handle. As a result, some rather ingenious devices have been designed by clients for their own use. If you are responsible for teaching clients to take medications at home, be sure to include checking for expiration dates on medication packages. In addition, teach safe and appropriate storage, especially when small children are in the environment.

CRITICAL THINKING EXERCISES

• You have checked the MAR on the two patients for whom you are caring today. The following orders are on the records:

Patient A: Digoxin 0.125 mg daily @8; hydrochlorothiazide 50 mg daily @8; KCl 40 mg b.i.d. @8, 5; multivit 1 cap. daily @8; Maalox 2 tsp. q2h prn

Patient B: Theo-Dur 100 mg b.i.d @8, 20; cefazolin 1 g IV q6h @6, 12, 18, 24; beclomethasone inhaler 2 puffs q.i.d. @8, 12, 16, 20

• Determine if these orders are complete, with all the information needed for you to give them properly. Is there any information you will need to determine whether or not to give the medications? Develop a plan for giving these medications, including the precise time you would start preparing medications and the order in which you would proceed. Explain your planning decisions.

• You are to give 9:00 AM medications to Mr. Jones. During report, you note that there are two patients on the unit with the last name of Jones. Specify the actions you can take to ensure that the correct medications are given to the correct patient.

✔ **PERFORMANCE CHECKLIST**

General Procedure for Administering Medications	Needs More Practice	Satisfactory	Comments
Assessment			
1. Review medication record for medications to be given.			
2. Examine medication administration record (MAR) for accuracy and completeness.			
3. Review information about medications to be administered.			
4. Assess patient's abilities.			
5. Assess patient's need for prn medications.			
Planning			
6. Determine equipment needed.			
7. Wash your hands.			
8. Gather equipment needed.			
Implementation			
9. Read name of medication from the record.			
10. Check the label on the medication before picking it up.			
11. Pick up medication, and compare the label again.			
12. Remove the correct amount of medication for the individual dose.			
13. Check the medication label with the MAR a third time.			
14. Place medication in its unit-dose in a container or on a tray.			
15. Place medication label on the prepared medication.			
16. Approach and identify the patient.			
17. Explain what you are going to do.			
18. Administer the medication as appropriate for the route.			
19. Leave the patient in a comfortable position.			
20. Discard disposable medication container or clean as appropriate.			

(continued)

General Procedures for Administering Medications *(Continued)*	Needs More Practice	Satisfactory	Comments
21. Wash your hands.			
Evaluation			
22. Evaluate using the following criteria: **a.** Right patient, right medication, right dosage, right route, right time, right documentation			
b. Effectiveness of drug for desired purpose			
c. Side effects			
Documentation			
23. Document that the medication was given, including name of medication, dosage, route, time, and signature.			

MODULE

ADMINISTERING ORAL MEDICATIONS

MODULE CONTENTS

PREREQUISITES

Successful completion of the following modules:

VOLUME 1
Module 1 An Approach to Nursing Skills
Module 2 Basic Infection Control
Module 3 Safety
Module 5 Documentation
Module 6 Introduction to Assessment Skills

VOLUME 2
Module 47 Administering Medications: Overview

Before giving medications, you must have a satisfactory level of proficiency in mathematics of dosages and solutions. A math quiz is presented in Module 47, Administering Medications: Overview. If you cannot answer at least 16 of the 20 problems correctly (or the number designated by your instructor), plan to complete one of the many programmed instruction units available on mathematics of dosages and solutions. Consult your instructor for guidance.

OVERALL OBJECTIVES

To understand how to administer oral medications to patients and residents with accuracy and safety, and to recognize and report adverse drug effects promptly and take corrective action.

SPECIFIC LEARNING OBJECTIVES

Know Facts and Principles	Apply Facts and Principles	Demonstrate Ability	Evaluate Performance
1. *Giving oral medications*			
Know procedure for preparation and administration of oral medication.	Adapt steps of procedures to those used in assigned facility.	Prepare and administer oral medication according to procedures in assigned facility.	Evaluate own performance with instructor.
2. *Documentation*			
Know information to be documented regarding medications administered.	Identify documentation method used in assigned facility.	Correctly document medications administered according to method used in assigned facility.	Evaluate own performance with instructor.

LEARNING ACTIVITIES

1. Review the Specific Learning Objectives.
2. Read the section on administering medications in Ellis and Nowlis, *Nursing: A Human Needs Approach,* or comparable material in another textbook. Carefully read Module 47, Administering Medications: Overview.
3. Look up the module vocabulary terms in the glossary.
4. Read through the module and mentally practice the procedure. Read as though you were preparing to teach the skills to another person.
5. In the clinical setting:
   a. Consult with your clinical instructor for an opportunity to give oral medications with supervision.
   b. Seek an opportunity to observe a nurse giving medications by the sublingual or buccal route as well as by nasogastric tube.
   c. Identify
      (1) Paper soufflé cup
      (2) Calibrated medicine container (usually made of glass or plastic but can be made of heavy waxed paper)
      (3) Mortar and pestle
      (4) Pill crusher, if available
      (5) Pill divider, if available
      (6) Medicine tray or cart
   d. Practice the explanation necessary for administration of medications to be given by the oral, sublingual, buccal, and nasogastric tube routes.

VOCABULARY

buccal	meniscus	syrup
capsule	pruritus	tablet
expectorate	sublingual	
MAR	suspension	

Administering Oral Medications

Rationale for the Use of This Skill
The majority of medications given in healthcare facilities are administered by the oral route. A patient may have a sizable number of oral medications ordered. Consequently, the nurse must be skilled in administering oral medications, incorporating sound knowledge, accuracy, and safety when providing each drug. The nurse also must be skilled in recognizing side effects.[1]

▼ NURSING DIAGNOSES

Risk for Injury is a very important nursing diagnosis to consider when administering oral medications and underscores the need to act safely when performing this procedure. Adverse effects are most likely to appear after the drug is absorbed and reaches its peak effect in the body.

Another nursing diagnosis that is specific to oral medication administration is that of Risk for Aspiration. Swallowing deficits could lead to aspirating the medication into the bronchi, *causing a life-threatening pneumonia.*

Knowledge Deficit as a nursing diagnosis requires that the nurse provide health teaching *so that the patient has basic information concerning the prescribed drug.* With this knowledge, the patient can alert the staff to any adverse reactions, such as pruritus, nausea, and others (see below).

It may be hazardous for a patient to self-administer oral medications, for a variety of reasons. For instance, a patient may have adequate knowledge of a drug, but may be unable to see the medication well or read the label or instructions clearly. A nursing diagnosis of Sensory/Perceptual Alteration: Visual may be appropriate in this situation.

Certain nursing diagnoses are associated with drug reactions. For example, a skin rash or eruption suggests a nursing diagnosis of Impaired Skin Integrity. Some medications interfere with sleep, causing Sleep Pattern Disturbance.

If a hospitalized patient consistently refuses to take a medication that is necessary for treatment, or if a person at home fails to take or renew essential prescribed medications, a nursing diagnosis of Ineffective Management of Therapeutic Regimen would be appropriate.

[1]Rationale for action is emphasized throughout the module by the use of italics.

MEASURING LIQUID MEDICATIONS

Measuring liquid medications is a special procedure. *To ensure accuracy,* read the medicine glass or cup at eye level, with the thumbnail placed at the bottom of the meniscus at the correct level on the outside of the medicine container (Fig. 48–1). The liquid should be poured from the side of the opening that is opposite the label so that the liquid does not come in contact with the label.

ASSISTING THE PERSON WITH SWALLOWING DIFFICULTIES

The nurse must consider the patient's ability to swallow when giving oral medications. Typically, it is sufficient to use a pill divider to split the solid pill into one or more pieces for easier swallowing. But sometimes it may be necessary to secure medication in liquid form or to crush pills before administering them. Crushed pills can be mixed with applesauce or ice cream *to facilitate easier swallowing.*

It is also helpful to place the patient with swallowing difficulties in high-Fowler's or a sitting position and to provide sufficient fluid for swallowing. You might also use a small plastic glass that has a section of plastic slots inside to hold the medication in a midline position near the top of the glass. As the glass is tipped, the water facilitates easy swallowing.

PROCEDURE FOR ADMINISTERING ORAL MEDICATIONS

To administer oral medications, follow the steps of the General Procedure for Administering Medications (Module 47, pages 365–366) as modified below. We have included completely the modified steps and references to the steps of the General Procedure that remain the same.

Assessment
1. Review the medication administration record (MAR) to determine the oral medications to be administered.
2. Examine the MAR for accuracy and completeness. Check the patient's name, room number, drug, dosage, and time the drug is to be given. Clarify any points about which you are unsure. See if all the medications you will need are available; if any are not, call the pharmacy so that the administration will not be delayed.

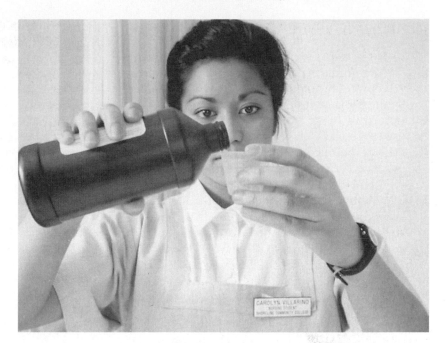

Figure 48–1. Measuring a liquid medication. The nurse holds the medicine cup at eye level, using the bottom of the concave meniscus as a guide for measurement.

3.–5. Follow steps 3 through 5 of the General Procedure: Review information about the medications to be administered; assess the patient's ability to swallow and level of consciousness; and assess the patient *to identify a need for any prn medication.*

Planning

6.–8. Follow steps 6 through 8 of the General Procedure: Determine what equipment you will need; wash your hands *for infection control*; and gather the equipment.

Implementation

9.–11. Follow steps 9 through 11 of the General Procedure: Read name of medication on the MAR; check the medication label (first check); pick up the medication and check the label again (second check).

12. Remove the correct amount of medication for the individual dose to be given at this time.
  a. For a tablet or capsule (not prepackaged):

  (1) Pour from the bottle into the bottle cap until you have the correct dosage.
  (2) Transfer to the medication cup. Generally, all pills to be given to the same patient at the same time can be placed in one container. *If the administration of a medication is contingent on a pulse or blood pressure measurement,* keep that medication separate from the others and make the measurement immediately after identifying the patient.

  b. For a liquid:
  (1) Place the bottle cap upside down on the countertop *so as not to contaminate it.*
  (2) With the medicine cup at eye level, pour the liquid to the desired level in the cup, using the bottom of the concave meniscus as your guide (see Fig. 48–1).
  (3) Pour with the label facing up *to prevent medication from running onto and distorting the label.*

Example of Nursing Progress Notes Using Narrative Format.

DATE/TIME	
5/21/99 0815	Patient admitted from acute care setting per ambulance for continuing stroke rehabilitation. Record reveals swallowing difficulties. Assessment confirms patient can only safely swallow liquids. Pharmacy informed of need to prepare medications in suspension form. ⎯⎯⎯⎯⎯⎯⎯⎯⎯⎯⎯ S. Baer, RN

    (4) Wipe the neck of the bottle with a clean paper towel before replacing the cap.

   c. For a unit-dose medication, place packages containing the correct number of tablets or capsules in the medication cup. Do not open the packages at this time.

13. Return the bottle to the shelf or drawer. Check the label again, being sure to read it carefully. (This is the third of the three checks.) For unit-dose medications, you can do this last check after all medications are prepared.

14.–17. Follow steps 14 through 17 of the General Procedure: Place medication in a container or on a tray; identify the medication with the patient's name if the MAR is not to be taken to the bedside; approach and identify the patient; explain what you are going to do and, if appropriate, provide information about the medication's actions and possible side effects.

18. Administer the medication.

   a. Give the patient a glass of fresh water. (You may have to change the water in the bedside pitcher.) If the medication has an unpleasant flavor, you can give juice with it instead of water, as long as this is not contrary to the patient's diet order or the drug manufacturer's directions. If the patient has a favorite juice, indicate it on the record *so other nurses who administer the medication will know and will not have to ask the patient again.*

   b. Watch the patient take the medication. *If you are not certain it has been swallowed, or if there seems to be a problem with swallowing,* have the patient open his or her mouth and look inside to see if the medication is still there. *If the patient cannot swallow a tablet or capsule,* give it in a vehicle, such as applesauce or jelly. It is common practice to crush tablets (except those with enteric coating) and to empty the contents from capsules to mix with the vehicle. Pills may be crushed in their unit-dose packaging or in a closed paper medication cup to avoid contaminating them with the pestle (Fig. 48–2). Pill crushers are also available (Fig. 48–3). Whole or split pills or capsules are sometimes given in a teaspoon of jelly. Unsweetened applesauce is a better vehicle for the patient with diabetes.

      Sometimes a patient will ask you to leave

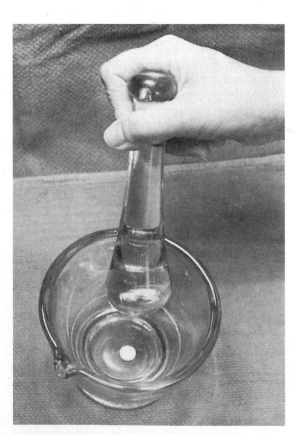

Figure 48–2. Pill being crushed with mortar and pestle. Pills may also be crushed in their unit-dose packaging to avoid contaminating them with the pestle. (Courtesy Ivan Ellis)

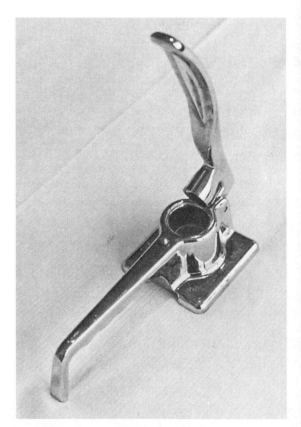

Figure 48–3. Commercially produced tablet crusher. The pill is placed in the circular area and crushed when the handle is pulled down. (Courtesy Ivan Ellis)

DATE/TIME	
11/21/99 1415	D: Patient reports continual frontal head pain. Level 3 on 0–5 scale. Has not had medication for 48 hours.
	A: Acetaminophen, p.o. administered per MAR.
	R: Patient states after one hour, "My headache is gone, I feel so much better."
	———————————————— S. Abraham, R.N.

Example of Nursing Progress Notes Using Focus Format.

a medication to be taken later. This is not appropriate *because you would not be able to document that the patient actually took the medication.* When you refuse the request, you might say, "No, I am responsible for it, so I don't want to leave it. If you can't take it now, I will come back with it later." If the medication is needed immediately, explain why it should be taken promptly. If a tablet or a capsule falls to the floor, it is considered contaminated, and you should discard it and obtain a replacement.

19.–21. Follow steps 19 through 21 of the General Procedure: Leave the patient in a comfortable position; discard the medication container; and wash your hands.

Evaluation

22. Evaluate as in step 22 of the General Procedure, using these criteria:
  a. The *right* patient received the *right* medication in the *right* dosage by the *right* route at the *right* time and it was documented in the *right* way.
  b. The criteria established for ascertaining the effectiveness of a specific drug were used.
  c. Side effects, if present, were promptly identified.

Documentation

23. Document as in step 23 of the General Procedure: Include name of medication, dosage, route, time, and signature.

SUBLINGUAL AND BUCCAL MEDICATIONS

Some medications are ordered to be given by the sublingual route (placed under the tongue) or by the buccal route (placed between the cheek and gum). These medications are absorbed through the oral mucous membranes for rapid systemic effects. In-

struct the patient not to swallow these medications, but instead to hold them in place until they dissolve completely. An alert and capable patient may place the sublingual or buccal tablet or you may place it for the patient. If you place the medication, wear clean gloves *to protect yourself from body secretions.*

ORAL MEDICATIONS ADMINISTERED AS RINSES

Some medications are used by the patient as a mouth rinse. After rinsing, some are expectorated and some swallowed. The effect of those used only as rinses is topical, with the purpose being to expose the oral mucous membrane to the drug for its local effect. After thoroughly rinsing the mouth, the patient expectorates into a basin or cup. Local anesthetic agents that are used for painful mouth lesions are examples of drugs that are used in this way.

Other medications are used first as a rinse and then swallowed for additional systemic effect. These are commonly referred to on the order form or MAR as "S&S" (swish and swallow) medications. An antifungal medication used to combat a fungal infection of the mouth is an example of a drug used in this way.

Whether the medication is a rinse or one that is rinsed and swallowed, it should be administered last if there are other medications. This provides the greatest contact with the tissues and avoids removal of the agent by any water taken with other drugs.

GIVING MEDICATIONS THROUGH A NASOGASTRIC TUBE

A patient with a nasogastric tube in place for the purpose of feeding is commonly given oral medications through the tube. The procedure is the same as for giving other oral medications, except that the medications must all be in a liquid or suspension form *so that they can be passed through the tube*. Tablets are crushed and dissolved as much as possible in water. Capsules are emptied into water. Because capsules commonly do not dissolve thoroughly, it is important to follow them with water *to flush the suspended medication completely out of the tube; otherwise the medication can occlude the tube and the patient will not receive the intended dosage*. Gel medications, such as some stool softeners, can be liquefied quickly by placing them in a plastic or paper cup and microwaving for a few minutes on a medium setting. After cooling, they can be introduced into the naso-gastric tube. Some medications can be obtained from the pharmacy as liquids or suspensions. The nurse can measure these medications in a syringe and then administer them directly from the syringe.

When giving the medications, follow the procedure in Module 29, Tube Feeding, for checking the placement of the tube and putting the medication in the tube. Do not put medications in the tube feeding itself *because it is impossible to know whether the entire dosage is administered at the appropriate time*. If a continuous feeding is being administered, stop the feeding, give the medications, flush the tubing, and resume the feeding.

LONG-TERM CARE

The resident in long-term care may have numerous medications. The nurse typically administers oral medications to several residents, making identification of each individual resident and accuracy in administration an essential responsibility. Identifying residents who may move about the facility and who may be cognitively impaired provides a challenge. To facilitate identification, some long-term care facilities place a photograph of the resident in the MAR. Nurses in long-term care typically must find ways to assist residents with swallowing difficulties or those whose coordination makes handling medications difficult.

Many residents have used large numbers of over-the-counter (OTC) medications for a time before coming to the facility. Some may be unfamiliar with the products used within the institution. Meeting the residents' needs without the use of medications is often a challenge. It is essential that the nurse in this setting provide a thorough assessment as well as health teaching regarding medications. For a variety of reasons, older adults are more susceptible to the adverse effects of medications. For instance, kidney function in the older adult may be decreased, *so dosages that are therapeutic for younger people can become toxic*. The circulatory system may be compromised, *decreasing medication distribution to the cells and metabolism*. The presence of chronic illness may also affect drug metabolism.

When administering oral medications, the nurse in long-term care has a role that is different from that of the nurse in the acute care setting. For instance, because of the number and frequency of medications to be given, the number of residents, and the kinds of physical, cognitive, and psychosocial alterations that may affect the residents (e.g., swallowing difficulties or inability to understand the medication actions or medication procedure), the nurse must give extra attention to the procedure.

HOME CARE

It is sometimes appropriate to monitor the oral medication regimen for clients living at home. As a home care nurse, you should review the medication list with the client, focusing on several aspects such as instructions, drug names and expiration dates, medication times, and OTC medications.

Some medications have instructions printed in very small type, making it difficult for some older persons to read. Suggest using a simple magnifying glass as a visual aid. Medications may have confusing brand names, so a client may unknowingly take two medications at the same time that have the same purpose. Clearly identify all medications and explain the purpose of each to the client. Instruct the client to check the expiration dates of medications; *the action of outdated drugs is less effective.*

Also, without "reminders," medication times may be completely missed, *causing inconsistent dosages.* Inexpensive plastic containers with designated times and sections for storing medications are available. One-half of an egg carton can be marked and used also for this purpose.

Assess any OTC medication the client is taking to be sure it does not conflict with prescribed medications. Instruct the client never to "lend" medications or give them to another person for whom they were not prescribed. Ensure that all medications are kept out of the reach of children. With the assistance of a home health nurse and health teaching, the client and care providers can continue administration of oral medications safely and effectively.

CRITICAL THINKING EXERCISES

- Your patient has the following oral medication orders:

  digoxin (Lanoxin) 0.125 qd
  furosemide (Lasix) 20 mg bid
  folic acid 1 mg qd
  levothyroxine sodium (L-Thyroxine) 0.05 qd
  amoxicillin 250 mg q8h
  nystatin 2 dr (S&S) tid
  docusate sodium (Doss) 250 mg qd
  triazolam (Halcion) 0.125 mg HS prn

- Formulate a general medication plan for this patient, using columns indicating the times you would be giving these medications. In the first column, note the abbreviations on the sample MAR (above) and tell why these are the appropriate times to administer each of these medications. In the second column, specify any side effects that may determine what time is most appropriate. In the third column, recommend any special health teaching that needs to be done.

- Your patient has complained of "chest pain." The physician has ordered one nitroglycerin tablet to be administered sublingually. The patient has never had this medication before. Determine what explanation you would give the patient. Describe the drug's action and the expected patient response from the drug. Explain how you would document its administration.

PERFORMANCE CHECKLIST

Procedure for Administering Oral Medications	Needs More Practice	Satisfactory	Comments
Assessment			
1. Review medication record to determine the oral medications to be administered.			
2. Examine MAR for accuracy and completeness; check that needed medications are available.			
3.–5. Follow Checklist steps 3–5 of the General Procedure for Administering Medications in Module 47 (review medication information, assess patient's ability to swallow and level of consciousness, assess need for prn medications).			
Planning			
6.–8. Follow Checklist steps 6–8 of the General Procedure (determine equipment needed, wash your hands, gather equipment).			
Implementation			
9.–11. Follow Checklist steps 9–11 of the General Procedure (read the name of the medication on the MAR, check the medication label, pick up medication and check label a second time).			
12. Remove correct amount of medication: a. Tablet or capsule (1) Pour from bottle into bottle cap until you have correct dosage.			
(2) Transfer to the medication cup unless prepackaged.			
b. Liquid (1) Remove bottle cap and place it upside down on the countertop.			
(2) Holding cup at eye level, pour liquid to desired level.			
(3) Pour with label facing up.			
(4) Wipe neck of bottle before replacing cap.			

(continued)

Procedure for Administering Oral Medications *(Continued)*	Needs More Practice	Satisfactory	Comments
c. Unit-dose medication: Place package containing medication in medication cup.			
13. Return bottle to shelf or drawer. Compare label with MAR a third time.			
14.–17. Follow steps 14–17 of the General Procedure (place medication in container or on tray, identify medication with patient's name, approach and identify patient, explain to patient).			
18. Administer the oral medication. **a.** Give patient a glass of water.			
b. Watch to be sure patient has swallowed medication.			
19.–21. Follow Checklist steps 19–21 of the General Procedure (make patient comfortable, discard medication container, wash your hands).			
Evaluation			
22. Evaluate as in Checklist step 22 of the General Procedure (six rights, desired effects, and side effects).			
Documentation			
23. Document as in Checklist step 23 of the General Procedure (name of medication, dosage, route, time, and signature).			

MODULE

ADMINISTERING MEDICATIONS BY ALTERNATIVE ROUTES

MODULE CONTENTS[1]

[1]See Module 47, Administering Medications: Overview,
for general steps using the Nursing Process.

387

PREREQUISITES

Successful completion of the following modules:

VOLUME 1
Module 1 An Approach to Nursing Skills
Module 2 Basic Infection Control
Module 3 Safety
Module 5 Documentation
Module 6 Introduction to Assessment Skills

VOLUME 2
Module 33 Sterile Technique
Module 46 Irrigations
Module 48 Administering Oral Medications

You should be able to complete satisfactorily the self-test on mathematics of dosages and solutions in Module 47, Administering Medications: Overview. If you cannot meet this level of competence, you need additional practice in mathematics of dosages and solutions. Many programmed texts are available for independent study.

Review of the anatomy and physiology of the eye, ear, nose, skin, vagina, rectum, and respiratory system.

OVERALL OBJECTIVE

To prepare and administer medications safely, using ophthalmic, otic, nasal, skin and mucous membranes, vaginal, rectal, and inhalation routes.

SPECIFIC LEARNING OBJECTIVES

Know Facts and Principles	Apply Facts and Principles	Demonstrate Ability	Evaluate Performance
1. Ophthalmic medications			
a. Technique			
State whether sterile or clean technique is used.		Use sterile technique when instilling eye medication.	Evaluate own performance with instructor.
b. Rationale			
Describe four reasons why patient might be receiving eye medication.	Given a patient situation, identify why patient might be receiving eye medication.	In the clinical setting, identify reason for eye medication.	Evaluate own performance with instructor.
c. Positioning			
Describe positioning of patient for instillation of eye medication.		In the clinical setting, correctly position patient.	Evaluate own performance with instructor.
d. Procedure			
Describe how to instill eye drops and ointments.		In the clinical setting, correctly instill eye drops and ointments.	Evaluate with instructor using Performance Checklist.
2. Otic medications			
a. Technique			
State when sterile technique is used and when clean technique is appropriate.	Given a patient situation, identify whether to use sterile or clean technique.	Use correct technique when instilling otic medication.	Evaluate own performance with instructor.
b. Positioning			
Describe positioning of adult and pediatric patients for instillation of ear drops, including position of auricle.	Given a patient situation, select appropriate positioning for patient.	In the clinical setting, correctly position adult and pediatric patients to receive ear drops.	Evaluate own performance with instructor.
c. Procedure			
Describe how to instill ear drops.		Correctly instill ear drops.	Evaluate with instructor using Performance Checklist.
State how long patient should remain on his or her side after instillation of ear drops.		Instruct patients to remain on side 5–10 minutes after instillation of ear drops.	

(continued)

SPECIFIC LEARNING OBJECTIVES (continued)

Know Facts and Principles	Apply Facts and Principles	Demonstrate Ability	Evaluate Performance
3. *Nasal medications*			
a. Technique			
State whether sterile or clean technique is used.	Given a patient situation and medication order, determine whether sterile technique is required.	In the clinical setting, use careful asepsis when instilling nasal medication.	Evaluate own performance with instructor.
b. Rationale			
Know most common reason for instilling nasal medication. State rationale for instillation of water soluble nasal medication.		In the clinical setting, check to be sure nasal medications are water soluble.	
c. Positioning			
Describe positioning of patients to receive nasal medications, including Proetz and Parkinson positions.	Given a patient situation, identify appropriate position for patient.	In the clinical setting, correctly position patient.	Evaluate own performance with instructor.
d. Procedure			
Describe how to instill nose drops and nasal sprays. State how long patient should remain in position after nose drops have been instilled.		Correctly instill nose drops and nasal sprays. In the clinical setting, instruct patients to remain as positioned for 5 minutes after instillation of nose drops.	Evaluate with instructor using Performance Checklist.
4. *Skin medications*			
a. Rationale			
State rationale for use of lotions, ointments, liniments, and powders.	Given a patient situation, state preparation that might be used.		
b. Procedure			
State how to apply medications to skin.	Given a patient situation, describe method of applying medication to skin.	Correctly apply medication to patient's skin.	Evaluate own performance with instructor.

(continued)

S P E C I F I C   L E A R N I N G   O B J E C T I V E S (continued)

Know Facts and Principles	Apply Facts and Principles	Demonstrate Ability	Evaluate Performance
5. *Mucous membrane medications*			
State where to place sublingual and buccal medications.		Correctly place medications ordered by the sublingual or buccal route.	Evaluate own performance with instructor.
		In the clinical setting, instruct patients to hold the medication in place until completely dissolved.	
6. *Vaginal medications*			
a. Positioning			
Describe positioning of patient for insertion of vaginal medications.		In the clinical setting, correctly position patient.	Evaluate own performance with instructor.
b. Procedure			
List methods of instilling vaginal medications.		Correctly administer vaginal medications.	Evaluate with instructor using Performance Checklist.
State how long patient should remain quiet after medicated douche.		Instruct patient to remain quiet for 20 minutes following douche.	
7. *Rectal medications*			
a. Positioning			
Describe positioning of patient for administration of rectal medications.		In the clinical setting, correctly position patient.	Evaluate own performance with instructor.
b. Rationale			
State rationale for administration of retention enema after bowel movement.			Evaluate with instructor using Performance Checklist.
c. Procedure			
State most common form of rectal medication.		Correctly administer rectal medication by suppository.	Evaluate own performance with instructor.
Describe how to instill rectal suppository.			
State how long patient should remain quiet after suppository insertion.		Instruct patient to remain quiet for 20 minutes following insertion of suppository.	
		Administer retention enema after patient has had bowel movement.	

(continued)

SPECIFIC LEARNING OBJECTIVES (continued)

Know Facts and Principles	Apply Facts and Principles	Demonstrate Ability	Evaluate Performance
8. Documentation State items to be included in documentation for each route discussed.	Given a patient situation, do sample recording for medication discussed.	In the clinical setting, correctly document ophthalmic, otic, nasal, skin, sublingual, buccal, vaginal, rectal, and inhaled medications.	Evaluate own performance with instructor.

LEARNING ACTIVITIES

1. Review the Specific Learning Objectives.
2. Read the section on administering drug therapy in Ellis and Nowlis, *Nursing: A Human Needs Approach,* or comparable material in another textbook.
3. Look up the module vocabulary terms in the glossary.
4. Read through the module as though you were preparing to teach the material to another person. Mentally practice the specific techniques.
5. Using a partner for a patient, in the practice setting, do the following:
   a. Simulate the instillation of eye drops. If artificial tears are available, your instructor may want you to use these or a sterile normal saline solution.
   b. Simulate the instillation of ear drops in an adult's ear. Do not use any actual drops.
   c. Simulate the instillation of nose drops and nasal sprays. Do not use any actual drops or sprays. Position your partner appropriately for the administration of a nasal spray and in the three positions described for nose drops.
   d. Using a manikin, practice the explanation and positioning for administration of a vaginal cream. Teach your "patient" self-administration.
   e. Using a manikin, practice the explanation and positioning for insertion of a rectal suppository.
   f. Practice the explanation for having patients take inhaled medications. Simulate the use of a metered-dose inhaler if one is available.
   g. Change roles with your partner and repeat steps 5a through f.
   h. Evaluate one another's performance.
6. In the clinical setting, do the following:
   a. Seek opportunities to administer medications given by alternative routes.

VOCABULARY

aspiration pneumonia	ethmoid sinus	ophthalmic	suppurating
auricle	eustachian tubes	OS	systemic
canthus	instillation	otic	topical
conjunctival sac	lacrimal system	OU	transdermal
dead air space	liniment	Parkinson's position	tympanic membrane
dermatologic	local	Proetz position	vaginal
dorsal recumbent	ocular	Sims' position	
position	OD	sphenoid sinus	
douche	ointment	suppository	

Administering Medications by Alternative Routes

Rationale for the Use of This Skill

Drugs can be administered by various routes, depending on the patient's condition, the drug, and the desired effect. The nurse must be able to prepare and administer drugs correctly using these various routes, keeping in mind the basic concepts of safe administration and those related to these special routes. The nurse's knowledge of the anatomy and physiology related to the organ being treated and of the actions, usual dosage, desired effects, and potential side effects of the drug being administered are imperative for safe practice.[2]

▼ NURSING DIAGNOSES

> The major nursing diagnosis to keep in mind when giving medications is Risk for Injury. Patients can be injured by medications given in the wrong dosage, at the wrong time, or by an incorrect route. They also can be injured by the omission of essential medications or the administration of an incorrect medication. Although this nursing diagnosis will not appear on the care plan, it applies to every situation in which a patient is being given medications.
>
> Another nursing diagnosis frequently appropriate when administering medications is Knowledge Deficit. In this situation, the knowledge deficit would be related to some aspect of the medication regimen; for example, the need for specific information related to the use of topical nitroglycerin.

PROCEDURES FOR ADMINISTERING MEDICATIONS BY ALTERNATIVE ROUTES

For each specific medication route discussed, some steps of the General Procedure for Administering Medications in Module 47 (pages 365–366) may be modified. We have included completely the modified steps and references to the steps of the General Procedure that remain the same.

[2]Note that rationale for action is emphasized throughout the module by the use of italics.

PROCEDURE FOR INSTILLING OPHTHALMIC MEDICATIONS

Ophthalmic medications are those used in the eye. They are used to soothe irritated tissue, dilate or constrict the pupil, treat eye disease, or provide anesthesia. The administration of such medications is a sterile procedure. In addition to the six rights discussed in Module 47, you must be certain you are medicating the "right" (correct) eye.

To instill ophthalmic medications, follow the General Procedure for Administering Medications (Module 47, pages 365–366) as modified below.

Assessment

1. Follow step 1 of the General Procedure for Administering Medications: Review the medication record to determine whether medications are to be administered.
2. When verifying the medication order, identify whether the medication is to be given in the right eye (OD), the left eye (OS), or both eyes (OU).
3.–5. Follow steps 3 through 5 of the General Procedure: Review medication information; assess the patient's abilities; and assess the need for prn medications.

Planning

6.–7. Follow steps 6 and 7 of the General Procedure: Determine equipment needed, and wash your hands.
8. Gather equipment needed, including a tissue, cotton ball, or gauze square *so that you can wipe away any tearing or draining of the medication out of the eye*. If the eye is suppurating, you may need gauze squares or a clean wash cloth *to clean the exterior surface of the eyelid before administering the eye medication*.

Implementation

9.–11. Follow steps 9 through 11 of the General Procedure: Read the name of the medication on the medication administration record (MAR); check the medication label; pick up the medication; and check the label a second time.
12. Be aware that eye medications are usually dispensed in dropper top bottles or from tubes of ointment. The entire bottle of eye drops is removed from the drawer. This will be taken to the bedside to administer the medication. The actual dosage must be measured directly into the eye as drops from the dropper bottle.
13.–17. Follow steps 13 through 17 of the General

Procedure: Check the medication label with the MAR a third time; place the medication in a container or on a tray; identify medication with patient's name if MAR is not to be taken to the bedside; approach and identify the patient; explain to the patient what you are going to do.

18. Administer the eye medication.
    a. Wash your hands just before administering the eye medication.
    b. Clean the eyelids and lashes if necessary. Put on gloves, and use a clean wash cloth, gauze squares, or cotton balls moistened in tap water. Move from inner canthus to outer canthus, using each cotton ball for only one wipe.
    c. Have the patient turn his or her head slightly to the side (away from the eye being medicated), and tip the head slightly backward. This can be done with the patient lying in bed or sitting in a chair.
    d. Have the patient look up.
    e. Rest your dominant hand (holding the container with dropper top or ointment tube) on the patient's forehead *to avoid inadvertently striking the patient in the eye.* Use the fingers on your other hand to pull down on the lower lid of the eye to be medicated, *exposing the lower conjunctival sac.* Exert gentle pressure with the hand resting on the patient's face. Hold a cotton ball, 2 × 2 gauze, or clean tissue *to catch any excess medication if necessary* (Fig. 49–1). Wear gloves when appropriate.

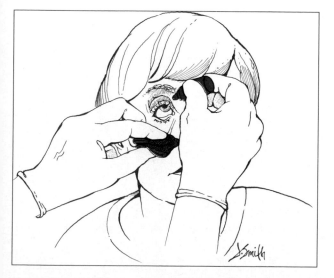

Figure 49–1. Instilling eye drops. Drop the ordered number of drops into the middle of the lowered conjunctival sac.

f. Instill medication.
    (1) Eye drops
        (a) Remove the cover of the dropper bottle.
        (b) Hold the dropper bottle tip down, close to but not touching the eye.
        (c) Squeeze the bottle to drop the ordered number of drops into the middle of the exposed conjunctival sac. Do not touch the dropper tip to the eye; *doing so will contaminate the dropper and allow microorganisms to grow and contaminate the medication. It also is uncomfortable for the patient.*
        Although most inpatient pharmacies carry only eye drops dispensed in dropper top bottles, some outpatient prescription eye drops are still dispensed in bottles in which the dropper is fastened to a separate lid. In these instances you will need to compress the bulb on the dropper, draw up the medication, and then gently squeeze the dropper to place the medication in the eye. Be sure that the tip of the dropper does not touch anything because it will be returned to the bottle.
    (2) Ointment
        (a) Squeeze out a ribbon of medication along the entire lower conjunctival sac, moving from inner canthus to outer canthus. Use the length of ointment ordered (eg, ½ in or 1 in).
        (b) Discontinue the ribbon of ointment by twisting the tube.
        (c) Wipe any excess ointment from the tube with a cotton ball, gauze, or tissue.
g. Ask the patient to close the eye gently. *If the eye is squeezed tightly shut, the ointment or drops are pushed out.* If eye drops were instilled, have the patient move the eyeball around while it is closed *to help disperse the medication.* If ointment was used, have the patient keep the eye closed a full minute following the instillation, *to allow the medication to melt.* Use tissue or gauze to wipe away excess medication.
h. *Some medications (among them atropine) have systemic effects if allowed to pass into the lacrimal system and then to be absorbed into the general circulatory system. To prevent this,* gently press the inner angle of the eye against the nose.

19. Follow step 19 of the General Procedure: Leave the patient in a comfortable position.

20. Recap the medication container, and return it to the appropriate storage location.

21. Follow step 21 of the General Procedure: Wash your hands.

Evaluation

22. Evaluate as in step 22 of the General Procedure: right patient, right medication, right dosage, right route, right time, right documentation.

Documentation

23. Document as in step 23 of the General Procedure: Note name of medication, which eye was treated, dosage, route, time, and signature.

PROCEDURE FOR INSTILLING OTIC MEDICATIONS

Medication can be introduced into the ear to soften wax, relieve pain, or treat disease. The instillation of medication to the ear is a clean procedure, *except when the tympanic membrane is not intact,* in which case sterile technique is used.

To instill otic medications, follow the General Procedure for Administering Medications (Module 47, pages 365–366) as modified below.

Assessment

1. Follow step 1 of the General Procedure for Administering Medications: Review the medication record to determine whether medications are to be administered.

2. When verifying the medication order, check whether the medication is to be given in the right ear, the left ear, or both ears.

3.–5. Follow steps 3 through 5 of the General Procedure: Review the medication information; assess the patient's abilities; and assess the need for prn medications.

Planning

6.–7. Follow steps 6 and 7 of the General Procedure: Determine equipment needed, and wash your hands.

8. Gather equipment needed, including a tissue, cotton ball, or gauze square so that you can wipe away any medication that drains out of the ear.

Implementation

9.–11. Follow steps 9 through 11 of the General Procedure: Read the name of the medication on the MAR; check the medication label; pick up the medication; and check the label a second time.

12. Obtain the medication. You will need the medication in a dropper bottle or a bottle of medica-

tion with a dropper in the lid, which will be taken to the bedside.

13.–17. Follow steps 13 through 17 of the General Procedure: Check the medication label with the MAR a third time; place the medication in a container or on a tray; identify medication with patient's name if MAR is not to be taken to the bedside; approach and identify the patient; and explain to the patient what you are going to do.

18. Administer the ear medication.

   a. Warm the medication to body temperature by holding the container in your hand for a short time or by placing the container in warm water. *Cold medication touching the eardrum may cause dizziness and may be painful.*

   b. Have the patient lie on the opposite side of the ear being medicated.

   c. Gently pull the ear auricle upward and backward (Fig. 49–2) *to straighten the canal. This allows the medication to reach all parts of the canal. In an infant or small child (younger than 3 years), the canal is almost straight,* so pull the top of the ear downward and backward.

   d. Instill the correct number of drops, directing them toward the side of the ear canal. Do not touch the dropper tip to the ear. *This will contaminate the dropper and allow microorganisms to grow and contaminate the medication.*

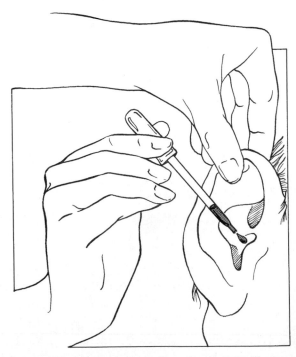

Figure 49–2. Administering ear drops to an adult. Gently pull the pinna upward and backward to straighten the canal.

e. Have the patient remain on the side for 5 to 10 minutes after the drops have been instilled *to allow maximum contact with the canal.*

f. Insert cotton loosely into the canal only if ordered. (This action is occasionally ordered *to keep the medication in contact with the canal and to prevent it from running out.*) Never pack the ear tightly.

19.–21. Follow steps 19 through 21 of the General Procedure: Leave the patient in a comfortable position; discard any disposable equipment used; and wash your hands.

Evaluation

22. Evaluate as in step 22 of the General Procedure: right patient, right medication, right dosage, right route, right time, right documentation.

Documentation

23. Document as in step 23 of the General Procedure: Note name of medication, which ear was treated, dosage, route, time, and signature.

PROCEDURE FOR INSTILLING NASAL MEDICATIONS

Nasal medication is normally ordered *to relieve nasal or sinus congestion* and is often given in the form of nose drops. Nose drops and nasal sprays are water soluble *because of the danger of aspiration pneumonia with oil-based solutions.* The administration of nasal medication is not a sterile procedure, but careful clean technique should be practiced *because of the close and direct connection between the nose and the sinuses.*

To instill nasal medications, follow the General Procedure for Administering Medications (Module 47, pages 365–366) as modified below.

Assessment

1.–5. Follow steps 1 through 5 of the General Procedure for Administering Medications: Review the medication record to determine whether medications are to be administered; examine the MAR for accuracy and completeness; review medication information; assess the patient's abilities; and assess the need for prn medications.

Planning

6.–7. Follow steps 6 and 7 of the General Procedure: Determine equipment needed, and wash your hands.

8. Gather equipment needed, including a tissue.

Implementation

9.–11. Follow steps 9 through 11 of the General Procedure: Read the name of the medication on the MAR; check the medication label; pick up the medication; and check the label a second time.

12. Obtain the medication. You will need the medication in a dropper bottle or a bottle of medication with a dropper in the lid, or nasal spray, which will be taken to the bedside.

13.–17. Follow steps 13 through 17 of the General Procedure: Check the medication label with the MAR a third time; place the medication in a container or on a tray; identify medication with patient's name if MAR is not to be taken to the bedside; approach and identify the patient; and explain to the patient what you are going to do.

18. Administer the nasal medication.

a. Have the patient clear the nasal passages, using a tissue and blowing gently.

b. Position the patient according to the area you want to medicate and the type of administration device.

   (1) Liquid drop medication: Place the patient flat on the back; this also opens the eustachian tubes.

      (a) *Ethmoidal and sphenoidal sinuses:* Place the patient in the Proetz position, with the head hanging straight back over the edge of the bed (Fig. 49–3).

      (b) *Frontal and maxillary sinuses:* Place the patient in Parkinson's position, with the head slightly over the edge of the bed and turned toward the affected side (Fig. 49–4).

   When the patient is positioned with the head hanging over the edge of the bed, you should help support the head with one hand *to prevent strain on the neck muscles.*

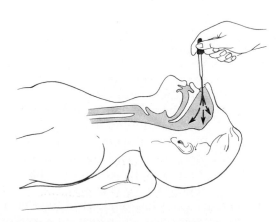

Figure 49–3. Proetz position for instilling nose drops. The patient is flat on the back with the head hanging straight back over the edge of the bed.

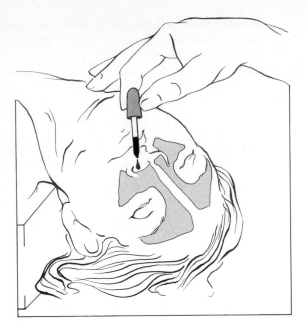

Figure 49–4. Parkinson's position for instilling nose drops. The head is slightly over the edge of the bed and turned toward the affected side.

   (2) Nasal spray: Position the patient in a chair, with the head tilted back.
 c. Instill the medication.
   (1) Dropper or dropper bottle
      (a) Draw sufficient medication for both nostrils into the dropper or simply invert the dropper bottle.
      (b) With the tip of the dropper about ⅓ in inside the nostril, instill the ordered number of drops into each side. Be careful not to touch the side of the nostrils, *which could cause the patient to sneeze.*
      (c) Have the patient remain as positioned for 5 minutes after the medication has been instilled. Caution the patient not to "sniff" the medication.
   (2) Nasal spray
      (a) Have the patient hold one nostril shut as you spray the medication into the other nostril.
      (b) Ask the patient to inhale as the spray is being administered.
      (c) Repeat on the other nostril.
      (d) Keep the patient's head back for 1 or 2 minutes. Patients often administer their own nasal sprays.
19.–21. Follow steps 19 through 21 of the General Procedure: Leave the patient in a comfortable position; dispose of used equipment; and wash your hands.

Evaluation
22. Evaluate as in step 22 of the General Procedure: right patient, right medication, right dosage, right route, right time, right documentation.

Documentation
23. Document as in step 23 of the General Procedure: Note name of medication, dosage, route, time, and signature.

PROCEDURE FOR APPLYING MEDICATIONS TO THE SKIN OR MUCOUS MEMBRANES

Medications applied to the skin for local effect are commonly in the form of lotions, ointments, or liniments and occasionally powders. *Lotions* protect, soften, soothe, and provide relief from itching. *Ointments* have an oil base, and body heat causes them to melt after application. Medications that fight infection or soothe the inflamed tissues are usually available in ointment form. *Liniments,* which are applied by rubbing, provide relief from tight aching muscles. *Powders* are applied for their soothing, drying action.
   To apply medications to the skin or mucous membranes, follow the General Procedure for Administering Medications (Module 47, pages 365–366) as modified below.

Assessment
1.–5. Follow steps 1 through 5 of the General Procedure for Administering Medications: Review the medication record to determine whether medications are to be administered; examine the MAR for accuracy and completeness; review medication information; assess the patient's abilities; and assess the need for prn medications.

Planning
6.–7. Follow steps 6 and 7 of the General Procedure: Determine equipment needed, and wash your hands.
8. Plan a method of applying the medication to the skin. Typically, application with a gloved hand is the most effective. Plan for clean gloves *to apply any topical medication that can be absorbed through the skin, like a steroid cream, to protect yourself from the medication.* You also may wish to wear gloves *to protect yourself from a medication that will stain your skin.* Sterile gloves are needed *if the skin is open.* Clean gloves are needed for mucous membranes. For small areas, cotton-tipped applicators may be adequate. Although gauze squares or cotton balls may be used, they tend to absorb large amounts of the medication, and this may in-

crease cost. Tongue blades should be avoided if possible because they are harsh to skin.

Implementation

9.–11. Follow steps 9 through 11 of the General Procedure: Read the name of the medication on the MAR; check the medication label; pick up the medication; and check the label a second time.

12. Obtain the medication. Most skin medications are in tubes that are taken to the bedside for use. If the medication is in a jar, use a sterile tongue blade to remove enough for the application. If the medication must remain sterile for application, place it in a sterile medicine cup or on a sterile gauze square. Discard any excess; do not return it to the jar.

13.–17. Follow steps 13 through 17 of the General Procedure: Check the medication label with the MAR a third time; place the medication in a container or on a tray; identify medication with patient's name if MAR is not to be taken to the bedside; approach and identify the patient; and explain to the patient what you are going to do.

18. Apply the dermal medication.

   a. Provide for the patient's privacy if necessary.

   b. Provide adequate lighting.

   c. Position the patient *so that the area to be treated is accessible.* In some cases, you may need assistance, for example, with the support of an arm or leg.

   d. Be sure the area to be treated is clean *so that the medication contacts the skin.* Skin medications are typically applied immediately after a bath or shower.

   e. Apply the medication to the area to be treated. Wear gloves when appropriate. Apply the ointments, creams, or lotions in thin, even layers unless otherwise ordered. Using gloves wastes less medication and is less irritating than using gauze. When applying the medication to the skin, take care that you do not increase discomfort through pressure or rubbing areas that are inflamed or painful. In some situations, patients can be taught to apply the medication to their own skin, especially when the area to be treated is in easy view and reach.

     To apply powder, instruct the patient to turn his or her head away *to prevent inhalation.* Spread it lightly and evenly, taking care not to let it accumulate between skin folds. Avoid shaking the powder directly over the patient. Put it in your own hand first, and then apply it to the patient.

   f. Use a light dressing to cover the area only if ordered by the physician. *Some medications should not be covered.*

19.–21. Follow steps 19 through 21 of the General Procedure: Leave the patient in a comfortable position; discard any disposable equipment; and wash your hands.

Evaluation

22. Evaluate as in step 22 of the General Procedure: right patient, right medication, right dosage, right route, right time, and right documentation.

Documentation

23. Document as in step 23 of the General Procedure: Include name of medication, dosage, route, time, signature, area treated, and appearance of the area before treatment.

Transdermal Medications

Some medications are available in a form that is readily absorbed from the skin to provide systemic effects. These are called transdermal medications. Among these are nitroglycerin, which is given for cardiac problems, and scopolamine, which is given for vertigo and nausea. The dosage of these medications must be as precise as the dosage of any other medication given for systemic effect. The correct dose may be impregnated in a small patch-type bandage. The backing is removed from the tape surface and the patch is then applied to clean skin. The medication is absorbed gradually. The patch is removed when the next dose is applied to the skin, and a new site is used for application *to avoid skin irritation from the tape or the medication.* Follow specific directions regarding such matters as showers and shampoos.

When the medication is an ointment, the order may call for a certain number of inches of ointment. A special pad of paper in which each sheet is marked in inches comes with the tube of ointment so that the nurse can carefully measure a line of ointment the diameter of the mouth of the tube and the ordered length onto the piece of paper. The paper is then placed on the skin, ointment side down, and secured around the edges with tape.

PROCEDURE FOR INSERTING VAGINAL MEDICATIONS

Creams, gels, suppositories, and douches are all used to administer vaginal medications. Vaginal medications may be needed *to treat infection, relieve discom-*

fort, or alter pH to maintain normal flora. Use clean technique when inserting vaginal medications. Be especially alert to the patient's feelings of embarrassment.

To insert vaginal medications, follow the General Procedure for Administering Medications (Module 47, pages 365–366) as modified below.

Assessment

1.–5. Follow steps 1 through 5 of the General Procedure for Administering Medications: Review the medication record to determine whether medications are to be administered; review the MAR for accuracy and completeness; review medication information; assess the patient's abilities; and assess the need for prn medication.

Planning

6.–7. Follow steps 6 and 7 of the General Procedure: Determine equipment needed, and wash your hands.

8. Read the directions on the package *to be sure that you understand how the applicator operates.* If this is the first dose, the applicator will be in the package. If previous doses have been administered, the applicator should have been washed and left in the patient's room.

Implementation

9.–11. Follow steps 9 through 11 of the General Procedure: Read the name of the medication on the MAR; check the medication label; pick up the medication; and check the label a second time.

12. Prepare the dose using the applicator as indicated in the package directions.

13.–17. Follow steps 13 through 17 of the General Procedure: Check the medication label with the MAR a third time; place the medication in a container or on a tray; identify the medication with the patient's name if MAR is not to be taken to the bedside; approach and identify the patient; and explain to the patient what you are going to do.

18. Insert the vaginal medication.
  a. Provide for the patient's privacy.
  b. Provide adequate lighting.
  c. Place the patient in the dorsal recumbent position, with knees flexed and spread as for catheterization (see Module 37, Catheterization). Sims' position also can be used.
  d. Drape the patient with the perineum exposed.
  e. Put on clean gloves.
  f. Instill the medication.

  (1) Vaginal creams: Introduce creams with a narrow, tubular applicator that has a plunger attached.
  (2) Suppositories: Introduce suppositories with a gloved and lubricated finger.
  (3) Douche
    (a) Obtain the equipment, and follow the procedure for vaginal irrigation in Module 46, Irrigations.
  g. Have the patient lie quietly for 20 minutes after the medication is inserted *to allow the medication to reach all surfaces.* In some instances a hospitalized patient can be taught to administer vaginal medications to herself.

19. Follow step 19 of the General Procedure: Leave the patient in a comfortable position.

20. Care for the equipment. *An applicator is used for the entire time the package is being used,* so wash it thoroughly with soap and water each time it is used and store it dry. Although washed, a vaginal applicator is never returned to the medication cart because of the potential for cross-contamination. It is always stored at the bedside or in the room.

21. Follow step 21 of the General Procedure: Wash your hands.

Evaluation

22. Evaluate as in step 22 of the General Procedure: right patient, right medication, right dosage, right route, right time, and right documentation.

Documentation

23. Document as in step 23 of the General Procedure: Include name of medication, dosage, route, time, and signature. In some facilities, a medicated douche is recorded on a treatment flow sheet; follow the policy in your facility.

PROCEDURE FOR ADMINISTERING RECTAL MEDICATIONS

Rectal medications are usually given for their local effect, but some (eg, aspirin suppositories) are given for systemic effect. Suppositories are most common, although creams and retention enemas also can be used. Clean technique is appropriate for all.

To administer rectal medications, follow the General Procedure for Administering Medications (Module 47, pages 365–366) as modified below.

Assessment

1.–5. Follow steps 1 through 5 of the General Procedure for Administering Medications: Review the medication record to determine whether medications are to be administered; review the MAR for accuracy and completeness; review medication information; assess the patient's abilities; and assess the need for prn medication.

Planning

6.–7. Follow steps 6 and 7 of the General Procedure: Determine equipment needed, and wash your hands.

8. Gather equipment needed, including a lubricant and a clean glove.

Implementation

9.–11. Follow steps 9 through 11 of the General Procedure: Read the name of the medication on the MAR; check the medication label; pick up the medication; and check the label a second time.

12. Prepare the medication for administration. This will include providing a lubricant and obtaining a clean glove. An applicator for a cream is treated the same way a vaginal applicator is treated.

13.–17. Follow steps 13 through 17 of the General Procedure: Check the medication label with the MAR a third time; place the medication in a container or on a tray; identify the medication with the patient's name if MAR is not to be taken to the bedside; approach and identify the patient; and explain to the patient what you are going to do.

18. Administer the rectal medication.
  a. Provide for the patient's privacy.
  b. Provide adequate lighting.
  c. Place the patient in the side-lying position. If this position is difficult for the patient, have him or her assume the dorsal recumbent position with the knees flexed.
  d. Drape the patient.
  e. Put on clean gloves.
  f. Insert the medication.
    (1) Suppository
      (a) Open the package, and lubricate the suppository if it is not prelubricated.
      (b) Using a gloved, lubricated finger, insert the suppository beyond the internal sphincter.
      (c) Ask the patient to breathe in and out through the mouth while you are inserting the suppository *to help relax the sphincter muscles*.
      (d) Have the patient lie quietly for 20 minutes after the insertion of a suppository.
    (2) Rectal cream

      (a) Introduce the cream with the special tip attached directly to the tube of cream.
      (b) Remove the tip, and clean it after each use.
    (3) Retention enema: Administer the enema after a bowel movement *for maximum absorption of the medication*. (See Module 28, Administering Enemas, for the necessary equipment and the procedure.)
  g. Clean the anal area with tissue *to remove the lubricant*.

19. Follow step 19 of the General Procedure: Leave the patient in a comfortable position.

20. Care for the equipment. An applicator is used for the entire time the package is being used, so wash it thoroughly with soap and water, and store it dry.

21. Follow step 21 of the General Procedure: Wash your hands.

Evaluation

22. Evaluate as in step 22 of the General Procedure: right patient, right medication, right dosage, right route, right time, right documentation.

Documentation

23. Document as in step 23 of the General Procedure: Include name of medication, dosage, route, time, and signature. In some facilities, a retention enema is recorded on the treatment record; follow the policy in your facility.

ADMINISTERING MEDICATIONS BY INHALATION

Medications are ordered by inhalation *for their local effect in the lungs*. They may be administered with an atomizer or nebulizer attached to oxygen or air under pressure. The medication is placed in the device, and the patient simply breathes in the mist through the device until all of the medication is gone.

Alternatively, these same medications can be administered using metered-dose inhalers, which deliver a precise amount of medication with each puff. A specific number of puffs is ordered. The patient is instructed to start inhaling as the puff is dispensed and to continue to breathe around the device, *which acts to push the mist deeper into the lungs*.

This method of administration requires considerable coordination of effort, and it is not uncommon for much of the medication to be deposited in the mouth and upper airway rather than in the lower airway where needed. Some instructions with metered-dose inhalers suggest that the patient close the lips around the device. This increases the likelihood of the medication depositing in the mouth *because no air is entering after the medication to help move it into the lungs*. The current recommendation is for the patient to place the nozzle directly in front of the open mouth and breathe deeply immediately after compressing the device.

Some nebulizers are equipped with spacer devices that facilitate delivery of the medication followed by air, again *to push the medication deeper into the lungs. Because misuse of any of these devices can result in a wrong dosage of medication or in the medication not getting into the lower respiratory tract,* you must carefully assess the patient's ability to follow the directions.

CRITICAL THINKING EXERCISES

• Mrs. Wilson, an elderly woman, has come to the clinic because of a rash on her back. The physician has prescribed a medicated cream to be used on the rash. Before leaving the clinic, Mrs. Wilson stops to ask if you will teach her husband how to apply the cream. He is in the waiting room and has not heard the physician's instructions. Determine what information you should gather before giving instructions, and identify some of the factors that you will need to consider. Then formulate two alternative approaches that you might take.

• Joel Hanson is an elderly resident of the assisted living facility where you are employed. He visited his physician today and came back with a newly prescribed inhaled bronchodilator. He brings it to you and says, "I'm not sure I understand how this works! It hardly seems that pushing down once on that thing gives you much medicine. Should I hold it down like you do for that mouth spray stuff?" Consider what you should include in your teaching. Identify what information and skills Mr. Hanson needs. Identify the potential administration errors his remarks reveal, then develop a plan for combating these misconceptions.

✔ **PERFORMANCE CHECKLIST**

Instilling Ophthalmic Medications	Needs More Practice	Satisfactory	Comments
Assessment			
1. Follow step 1 of the General Procedure for Administering Medications in Module 47: Review medication record.			
2. Examine MAR for accuracy and completeness; identify whether the medication is to be given in the right eye (OD), left eye (OS), or both eyes (OU).			
3.–5. Follow steps 3–5 of the General Procedure: Review medication information; assess patient's abilities; and assess need for prn medications.			
Planning			
6.–7. Follow steps 6 and 7 of the General Procedure: Determine equipment needed, and wash your hands.			
8. Gather equipment, including a tissue, cotton ball, or gauze square.			
Implementation			
9.–11. Follow steps 9–11 of the General Procedure: Read the name of the medication on the MAR; check medication label; pick up medication; and check label a second time.			
12. Obtain bottle of eyedrops or ointment.			
13.–17. Follow steps 13–17 of the General Procedure: Check medication label with MAR a third time; place medication in container or on tray; identify medication with patient's name; approach and identify patient; and explain to patient.			
18. Administer the eye medication. a. Wash your hands.			
b. Clean eyelids and lashes.			
c. Position patient with head slightly to affected side and tipped back.			
d. Have patient look up.			

(continued)

Instilling Ophthalmic Medications *(Continued)*	Needs More Practice	Satisfactory	Comments
e. Rest dominant hand on patient's forehead, and pull down on lower lid to open eye wide with other hand.			
f. Instill medication. (1) Eye drops (a) Remove cover of dropper bottle.			
(b) Hold tip end down.			
(c) Without touching eye, instill drops.			
(2) Ointment (a) Squeeze out medication.			
(b) Discontinue ribbon by twisting tube.			
(c) Wipe excess off tube.			
g. Ask patient to close the eye gently and move eyeball or keep eye closed as appropriate.			
h. Press inner angle of eye against nose if necessary.			
19.–21. Follow steps 19–21 of the General Procedure: Make patient comfortable; dispose of equipment; and wash your hands.			
Evaluation			
22. Evaluate as in step 22 of the General Procedure: six rights, desired effects, and side effects.			
Documentation			
23. Document as in step 23 of the General Procedure: name of medication, dosage, route, time, and signature. Add which eye was treated.			
Instilling Otic Medications			
Assessment			
1. Follow step 1 of the General Procedure for Administering Medications in Module 47: Review medication record.			
2. Examine MAR for accuracy and completeness; check whether medication is to be given in the right ear, left ear, or both ears.			

(continued)

Instilling Otic Medications *(Continued)*	Needs More Practice	Satisfactory	Comments
3.–5. Follow steps 3–5 of the General Procedure: Review medication information; assess patient's abilities; and assess need for prn medications.			
Planning			
6.–7. Follow steps 6 and 7 of the General Procedure: Determine equipment needed, and wash your hands.			
8. Gather equipment, including a tissue, cotton ball, or gauze square.			
Implementation			
9.–11. Follow steps 9–11 of the General Procedure: Read the name of the medication on MAR; check the medication label; pick up medication; and check label a second time.			
12. Obtain the medication in a dropper bottle.			
13.–17. Follow steps 13–17 of the General Procedure: Check medication label with MAR a third time; place medication in container or on tray; identify medication with patient's name; and approach and identify patient, explain to patient.			
18. Administer the ear medication. **a.** Warm medication to body temperature.			
b. Have patient lie on opposite side of ear being medicated.			
c. Pull auricle of ear to straighten canal.			
d. Instill drops.			
e. Have patient remain as positioned for 5–10 minutes.			
f. Insert cotton loosely in canal if ordered.			
19.–21. Follow steps 19–21 of the General Procedure: Make patient comfortable; dispose of equipment; and wash your hands.			

(continued)

Instilling Otic Medications *(Continued)*	Needs More Practice	Satisfactory	Comments
Evaluation			
22. Evaluate as in step 22 of the General Procedure: six rights, desired effects, and side effects. Add that correct ear was treated.			
Documentation			
23. Document as in step 23 of the General Procedure: name of medication, dosage, route, time, and signature. Add which ear was treated.			
Instilling Nasal Medications			
Assessment			
1.–5. Follow steps 1–5 of the General Procedure for Administering Medications in Module 47: Review medication record; examine MAR for accuracy and completeness; review medication information; assess patient's abilities; and assess need for prn medications.			
Planning			
6.–7. Follow steps 6 and 7 of the General Procedure: Determine equipment needed, and wash your hands.			
8. Gather equipment, including a tissue.			
Implementation			
9.–11. Follow steps 9–11 of the General Procedure: Read the name of the medication on the MAR; check the medication label; pick up medication; and check label a second time.			
12. Obtain the medication in a dropper bottle or nasal spray.			
13.–17. Follow steps 13–17 of the General Procedure: Check medication label with MAR a third time; place medication in container or on tray; identify medication with patient's name; approach and identify patient; and explain to patient.			
18. Administer the nasal medication. **a.** Have patient clear nasal passages.			
b. Position patient.			

(continued)

Instilling Nasal Medications *(Continued)*	Needs More Practice	Satisfactory	Comments
(1) Dropper: according to area you want to reach			
(2) Nasal spray: in chair with head tilted back			

c. Instill medication.
  (1) Dropper
    (a) Draw sufficient medication for both nostrils.			

(b) Insert tip and instill drops.			
(c) Have patient remain in position for 5 minutes.			
(2) Nasal spray (a) Spray medication into nostril with patient holding the other nostril closed.			
(b) Have patient inhale.			
(c) Repeat on other nostril.			
(d) Keep patient's head back for 1 or 2 minutes.			
19.–21. Follow steps 19–21 of the General Procedure: Make patient comfortable; dispose of equipment; and wash your hands.			
Evaluation			
22. Evaluate as in step 22 of the General Procedure: six rights, desired effects, and side effects.			
Documentation			
23. Document as in step 13 of the General Procedure: name of medication, dosage, route, time, and signature. Note that medication was administered nasally.			

(continued)

Applying Medications to the Skin or Mucous Membranes	Needs More Practice	Satisfactory	Comments
Assessment			
1.–5. Follow steps 1–5 of the General Procedure for Administering Medications in Module 47: Review medication record; examine MAR for accuracy and completeness; review medication information; assess patient's abilities; and assess need for prn medications.			
Planning			
6.–7. Follow steps 6 and 7 of the General Procedure: Determine equipment needed, and wash your hands.			
8. Plan a method for applying the medication using either clean or sterile gloves as appropriate, and gather appropriate equipment.			
Implementation			
9.–11. Follow steps 9–11 of the General Procedure: Read the name of the medication on the MAR; check the medication label; pick up medication; and check label a second time.			
12. Obtain the medication in a tube or jar.			
13.–17. Follow steps 13–17 of the General Procedure: Check medication label with MAR a third time; place medication in container or on tray; identify medication with patient's name; approach and identify patient; and explain to patient.			
18. Apply the dermal medication. **a.** Provide for patient's privacy.			
b. Provide adequate lighting.			
c. Position patient appropriately.			
d. Be sure area being treated is clean.			
e. Apply medication appropriately.			
f. Use light dressing if ordered.			
19.–21. Follow steps 19–21 of the General Procedure: Make patient comfortable; dispose of equipment; and wash your hands.			

(continued)

Applying Medications to the Skin or Mucous Membranes *(Continued)*	Needs More Practice	Satisfactory	Comments
Evaluation			
22. Evaluate as in step 22 of the General Procedure: six rights, desired effects, and side effects. Add correct area.			
Documentation			
23. Document as in step 23 of the General Procedure: name of medication, dosage, route, time, and signature. Include also the area treated and the appearance of the area before treatment.			
Inserting Vaginal Medications			
Assessment			
1.–5. Follow steps 1–5 of the General Procedure for Administering Medications in Module 47: Review medication record; examine MAR for accuracy and completeness; review medication information; assess patient's abilities; and assess need for prn medications.			
Planning			
6.–7. Follow steps 6 and 7 of the General Procedure: Determine equipment needed, and wash your hands.			
8. Read the package directions to understand how the applicator operates.			
Implementation			
9.–11. Follow steps 9–11 of the General Procedure: Read the name of the medication on the MAR; check the medication label; pick up medication; and check label a second time.			
12. Prepare the dose using the applicator.			
13.–17. Follow steps 13–17 of the General Procedure: Check medication label with MAR a third time; place medication in container or on tray; identify medication with patient's name; approach and identify patient; and explain to patient.			
18. Insert the vaginal medication. **a.** Provide for patient's privacy.			
b. Provide adequate lighting.			

(continued)

Inserting Vaginal Medications *(Continued)*

	Needs More Practice	Satisfactory	Comments
c. Place patient in dorsal recumbent position with knees flexed. (Sims' position also can be used.)			
d. Drape patient.			
e. Put on clean gloves.			
f. Instill medication.			
g. Have patient lie quietly for 20 minutes.			
19.–21. Follow steps 19–21 of the General Procedure: Make patient comfortable; clean or dispose of equipment; and wash your hands.			
Evaluation			
22. Evaluate as in step 22 of the General Procedure: six rights, desired effects, and side effects.			
Documentation			
23. Document as in step 23 of the General Procedure: name of medication, dosage, route, time, and signature.			
Inserting Rectal Medications			
Assessment			
1.–5. Follow steps 1–5 of the General Procedure for Administering Medications in Module 47: Review medication record; examine MAR for accuracy and completeness; review medication information; assess patient's abilities; and assess need for prn medications.			
Planning			
6.–7. Follow steps 6 and 7 of the General Procedure: Determine equipment needed, and wash your hands.			
8. Gather needed equipment, including lubricant and clean glove.			

(continued)

Inserting Rectal Medications *(Continued)*	Needs More Practice	Satisfactory	Comments
Implementation			
9.–11. Follow steps 9–11 of the General Procedure: Read the name of the medication on the MAR; check the medication label; pick up medication; and check label a second time.			
12. Prepare the medication for administration.			
13.–17. Follow steps 13–17 of the General Procedure: Check medication label with MAR a third time; place medication in container or on tray; identify medication with patient's name; approach and identify patient; and explain to patient.			
18. Administer the rectal medication. **a.** Provide for patient's privacy.			
b. Provide adequate lighting.			
c. Place patient in side-lying position.			
d. Drape patient.			
e. Put on clean gloves.			
f. Instill medication.			
g. Clean anal area.			
19.–21. Follow steps 19–21 of the General Procedure: Make patient comfortable; clean or dispose of equipment; and wash your hands.			
Evaluation			
22. Evaluate as in step 22 of the General Procedure: six rights, desired effects, and side effects.			
Documentation			
23. Document as in step 23 of the General Procedure: name of medication, dosage, route, time, and signature.			

MODULE

50

GIVING INJECTIONS

MODULE CONTENTS

(continued)

MODULE CONTENTS (continued)

Evaluation
Documentation
INTRADERMAL ADMINISTRATION
Uses
Selecting the Equipment
Selecting the Site
Procedure for Giving Intradermal
  Injections

Assessment
Planning
Implementation
Evaluation
Documentation
LONG-TERM CARE
HOME CARE
CRITICAL THINKING EXERCISES

PREREQUISITES

Successful completion of the following modules:

VOLUME 1
Module 1 An Approach to Nursing Skills
Module 2 Basic Infection Control
Module 3 Safety
Module 5 Documentation
Module 6 Introduction to Assessment Skills

VOLUME 2
Module 33 Sterile Technique
Module 47 Administering Medications: Overview

Satisfactory completion of the self-test on mathematics of dosages and solutions in Module 47, Administering Medications: Overview. If you cannot meet this level of competence, you need additional practice in the mathematics of dosages and solutions. Many programmed texts are available for independent study.

Review of anatomy as it relates to site selection for subcutaneous, intramuscular, and intradermal injections.

OVERALL OBJECTIVE

To prepare and administer subcutaneous, intramuscular, and intradermal medications safely to patients.

SPECIFIC LEARNING OBJECTIVES

Know Facts and Principles	Apply Facts and Principles	Demonstrate Ability	Evaluate Performance
1. Equipment			
a. Syringes			
Name five types of syringes available. Identify parts of syringe.	Given a patient situation, identify type of syringe appropriate for use. State which parts of syringe are kept sterile.	In the clinical setting, use correct type of syringe for injection. Handle syringe without contaminating sterile parts.	Evaluate with instructor.
b. Needles			
Identify two methods used to size needles. Identify parts of needle.	Explain system used to size gauge of needle. State which parts of needle are kept sterile for injection.	Select needle appropriate to viscosity of medication to be injected, route to be used, and size of patient. Handle needle without contaminating sterile parts.	Evaluate with instructor.
c. Medication containers			
Name two types of containers commonly used for injectable medications.	Differentiate between vial and ampule.	Correctly demonstrate removal of solution from vial and ampule.	Evaluate own performance using Performance Checklist.
2. Subcutaneous administration			
a. Advantages and disadvantages			
Name three advantages of subcutaneous medication administration over oral medication administration. Name primary disadvantage of subcutaneous medication administration.	Given a patient situation, identify advantage of giving medication subcutaneously. State implications for nurse based on disadvantage.	In the clinical setting, identify advantages of giving medication subcutaneously.	
b. Equipment selection			
State needle and syringe size most commonly used for subcutaneous injections.	Given a patient situation, select needle and syringe appropriate for subcutaneous injection.	In the clinical setting, select a needle and syringe appropriate for patient.	Evaluate own performance with instructor.

(continued)

SPECIFIC LEARNING OBJECTIVES (continued)

Know Facts and Principles	Apply Facts and Principles	Demonstrate Ability	Evaluate Performance
c. Site selection			
State angle at which needle is inserted for subcutaneous injections.	Given patient situation, identify appropriate angle for injection.	In the clinical setting, select appropriate angle for injection for patient.	Evaluate angle selection with instructor.
State three areas acceptable for subcutaneous injections.	Given a patient situation, describe which site(s) is appropriate for subcutaneous injection.	In the clinical setting, select appropriate site for injection.	Evalute site selection with instructor.
d. Injection technique			
List steps in preparation and injection of subcutaneous medications.	Adapt steps to procedures in assigned clinical facility.	Prepare and inject sterile IV saline in practice setting under supervision.	Evaluate own performance with instructor, using Performance Checklist.
		Prepare and inject medication under supervision.	
3. Intramuscular administration			
a. Advantages and disadvantages			
Describe speed of absorption of medication given intramuscularly as compared with subcutaneous administration.	Given a patient situation, select type of injection to be given in terms of absorption speed.	In the clinical setting, identify absorption speed of injection to be given.	
Name five disadvantages of intramuscular injections.	State implications for nurse based on disadvantages.		
b. Equipment selection			
State needle and syringe size most commonly used for intramuscular injections.	Given a patient situation, select needle and syringe appropriate for intramuscular injection.	In the clinical setting, select needle and syringe appropriate for patient.	Evaluate selection with instructor.
c. Site selection			
State angle at which needle is usually inserted for intramuscular injections.	Given a patient situation, identify appropriate angle for injection.	In the clinical setting, select appropriate angle for injection for patient.	Evaluate angle selection with instructor.
State four sites acceptable for intramuscular injections.	Given a patient situation, describe which site(s) is appropriate for intramuscular injection.	In the clinical setting, select appropriate site for injection.	Evaluate site selection with instructor.

(continued)

SPECIFIC LEARNING OBJECTIVES (continued)

Know Facts and Principles	Apply Facts and Principles	Demonstrate Ability	Evaluate Performance
d. Injection technique List steps in preparation and injection of medications intramuscularly, including Z-track technique.	Identify critical way in which procedure differs from subcutaneous injection.	In the practice setting, under supervision, prepare and inject sterile IV saline in one or more sites. In the clinical setting, under supervision, prepare and inject medication.	Evaluate own performance with instructor using Performance Checklist.
4. Intradermal administration			
a. Uses State two reasons for use of intradermal injection technique.	Given patient situations, identify appropriate situation for use of intradermal technique.	In the clinical setting, correctly identify situation for which intradermal injection would be used.	Evaluate with instructor.
b. Equipment selection State needle and syringe size most commonly used for intradermal injections.		In the clinical setting, select appropriate needle and syringe for intradermal injection.	Evaluate own performance with instructor.
c. Site selection State angle at which needle is inserted for intradermal injection. State two commonly used sites for intradermal injections.	Given a patient situation, select area appropriate for intradermal injection.	In the clinical setting, select site appropriate for intradermal injection.	Evaluate own performance with instructor.
d. Injection technique List steps in preparation and injection of intradermal medications.	Adapt steps to procedure in assigned clinical facility.	In the practice setting, under supervision, prepare and inject sterile IV saline intradermally. In the clinical setting, under supervision, prepare and inject intradermal medication.	Evaluate own performance with instructor using Performance Checklist.
5. Documentation Know information to be documented.	Identify documentation method used in assigned facility.	Correctly document injections given according to method used in assigned facility.	Evaluate own performance with instructor.

LEARNING ACTIVITIES

1. Review the Specific Learning Objectives.
2. Read the chapter on medication administration in Ellis and Nowlis, *Nursing: A Human Needs Approach*, or a comparable chapter in another textbook.
3. Look up the module vocabulary terms in the glossary.
4. Read through the module as though you were preparing to teach injection skills to another person. Mentally practice the specific techniques.
5. In the practice setting:
   a. Observe and become familiar with the assortment of needles and syringes available in your program and in your facility. To increase your manual dexterity before actually giving an injection, practice the sequence of movements involved: finding and cleansing the site, taking the needle cover off the needle, inserting the needle, aspirating, injecting the medication, and withdrawing the needle. You may practice these movements using a syringe and needle or simply using a pen with a cap and an alcohol swab over a table. Doing this will help you to feel comfortable handling the equipment and to remember the sequence when you are actually giving the injection. A manikin can be used to simulate an injection site.
      (1) Using a 3-mL syringe and a 1½-inch needle, draw 1 mL solution from a multiple-dose vial.
      (2) Using the same equipment, draw all the solution from an ampule containing 1 or 2 mL solution.
      (3) Demonstrate changing a needle as you would if the first one had been contaminated.
      (4) Demonstrate drawing up the equivalent of 65 units of U-100 insulin in an insulin syringe.
   b. Read the procedures.
      (1) Using the Performance Checklist as a guide, give 1 mL solution to a simulated injection site as though you were giving it subcutaneously.
      (2) Using the Performance Checklist as a guide, give 1 mL solution to a simulated injection site as though you were giving it intramuscularly.
      (3) Using the Performance Checklist as a guide, give a subcutaneous injection using either a manikin, simulation pad, or another student (if this is accepted policy), under supervision.
      (4) Using the Performance Checklist as a guide, give two intramuscular injections to a manikin, simulation pad, or another student, under supervision. Give one in the dorsogluteal site and one in the ventrogluteal site.
      (5) Using the Performance Checklist as a guide, give an intramuscular injection to a manikin, simulation pad, or another student, under supervision, using the Z-track technique.
      (6) Using the Performance Checklist as a guide, give an intradermal injection to a manikin, simulation pad, or another student under supervision.
6. In the clinical setting, when your instructor approves your practice performance, give subcutaneous, intramuscular, and intradermal injections in your facility under supervision.

VOCABULARY

ampule	intradermal	plunger	syringe
aspirate	intramuscular	prefilled cartridge	vial
barrel	Luer-Lok	(Tubex)	viscosity
bevel	lumen	reconstituted	wheal
gauge	needle	shaft	Z-track
hub	particulate matter	subcutaneous	

Giving Injections

Rationale for the Use of This Skill

The safe preparation and administration of subcutaneous, intramuscular, and intradermal medications is an important nursing responsibility that requires dexterity; sterile technique; a knowledge of the actions, usual dosage, desired effects, and potential side effects of the drug being given; and a knowledge of correct identification of site for giving the injection. Drugs given by these routes not only are absorbed more quickly than those given by mouth, but they also are irretrievable once injected. Therefore, the nurse must have a firm mathematics foundation and conscientiously use the practice of the three checks and the six rights.[1]

▼ NURSING DIAGNOSES

Risk for Injury is a priority nursing diagnosis when giving injections. Patients can be injured by injections given incorrectly or given at the wrong time, by an incorrect route, or injected into an incorrect site. Although this nursing diagnosis will not appear on the nursing care plan, it applies to every situation in which a patient is being given injections.

Knowledge Deficit is another nursing diagnosis that is commonly appropriate when administering injections. The knowledge deficit may be related to some aspect of the medication regimen; for example, the need to learn how to safely administer injections to oneself or to a family member.

Noncompliance is a nursing diagnosis that can be appropriate if the patient consistently refuses, for any reason (for example, fear of pain or a reaction), an injectable medication that is essential to treatment and that cannot be administered using another route.

EQUIPMENT

To give any injection, the nurse needs clean gloves, syringe, needle, an alcohol swab *to clean the skin*, and, of course, the medication.

Syringes

Syringes are available in various sizes, shapes, and materials. Several commercially made syringes are designed for use with specific prefilled cartridges.

Glass Syringes

Once the mainstay of every healthcare facility's syringe supply, glass syringes (Fig. 50–1) are rarely used now that plastic disposable syringes are available. Some glass syringes are still used in some settings, however, because they can be sterilized and included in surgical, obstetric, and treatment setups and because they adapt to the special tips (Luer-Lok) that are necessary for attachment to some irrigation devices.

Glass syringes are available in 2-mL, 5-mL, 10-mL, 20-mL, and 50-mL sizes. They can be secured with special control handles, which are sometimes used to administer local and regional anesthetics. The Luer-Lok is a specialized tip on the syringe that attaches the needle to the syringe by a threaded seal. This makes the connection more secure than the friction connection of a standard syringe.

Disposable Plastic Syringes

Disposable plastic syringes (Fig. 50–2) are widely used and are available in various sizes, with or without needles attached. They are usually prepackaged, either in a paper or cellophane wrapper or in a rigid plastic container.

Syringes with needles already attached are convenient and time saving if the needles are the correct size and length. The needle fits on the syringe by friction. It is designed to be secure as long as it is pushed straight on and its cover is pulled straight off. When the hub of the needle is twisted, it releases and detaches from the syringe. There are also plastic syringes that have a threaded seal to attach the needle to the syringe hub by twisting on.

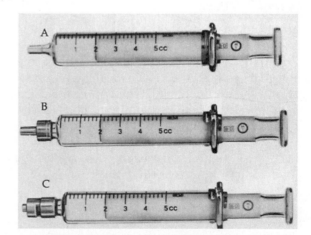

Figure 50–1. Glass syringes. **(A)** Glass Luer. **(B)** Metal Luer. **(C)** Luer-Lok. Container at eye level using the bottom of the concave meniscus as a guide for measurement. (Courtesy American Hospital Supply Corp., McGaw Park, Illinois)

[1]Rationale for action is emphasized throughout the module by the use of italics.

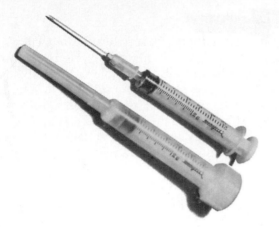

Figure 50–2. Disposable plastic syringe. This syringe is packaged in a rigid plastic container. (Courtesy Monoject Division of Sherwood Medical)

Prefilled Syringes and Cartridges

Prefilled syringes usually come with appropriate needles attached and with directions for use. Especially helpful are syringes prefilled with drugs for emergency use. Prefilled syringes are disposable.

Prefilled cartridges contain medication and have appropriate needles attached. The disposable cartridge and needle are designed to fit into a nondisposable metal or plastic cartridge holder. The cartridge must be screwed into the holder *to secure it in place*, and the plunger of the holder must be screwed into the stopper of the cartridge *so that you can aspirate* (Fig. 50–3). Although drawing up the medication is eliminated, which does make the procedure less difficult, mixing medications can be more difficult.

Insulin Syringes

Insulin syringes are marked in units specifically to measure dosages of insulin. They are available in both plastic (disposable) and glass (reusable) versions (Fig. 50–4). U-100 insulin means that there are 100 units of insulin in 1 mL. The syringe holds 1 mL and is marked directly in units. A small syringe, which holds 0.5 mL or 50 units, is also available for giving doses of less than 50 units. When given a choice, the 0.5 should be used for injecting less than 50 units *to increase accuracy*.

Tuberculin Syringes

Tuberculin syringes are usually chosen for the administration of very small amounts of medication *because they are marked in 0.01-mL increments.* They are called tuberculin syringes because they were origi-

nally used to administer small amounts of test material to check for exposure to tuberculosis. They are sometimes marked in minims as well. The accuracy of the syringe allows you to measure small quantities precisely, making these syringes ideal for infant and pediatric use. These syringes are also available in disposable plastic (Fig. 50–5) and reusable glass forms.

An insulin syringe is the safest to use when administering insulin, but insulin can also be measured accurately in a tuberculin syringe.

Needles

Needles for use with syringes come in standardized lengths (⅜–5 inches) and gauges (13–27). The needles most commonly used are ½ to 2 inches in length and 18 to 25 gauge. Both disposable and reusable versions are available. Needles currently used are disposable *to prevent the transmission of infection.*

Needles usually have a plastic hub and metal shaft. The lumen size is indicated on the hub. (Fig. 50–6 shows the parts of a needle.) The length and gauge of disposable needles are indicated on the outside of the packaging. *Sometimes color coding is used to indicate a needle's size. Because this practice is not standardized from one company to another,* you must be cautious when moving from one facility to another.

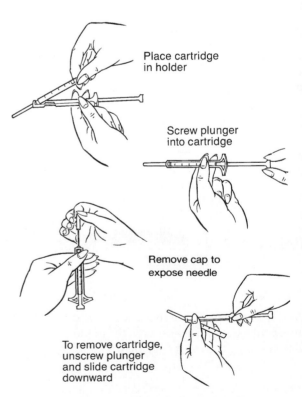

Place cartridge in holder

Screw plunger into cartridge

Remove cap to expose needle

To remove cartridge, unscrew plunger and slide cartridge downward

Figure 50–3. Prefilled cartridges and holder.

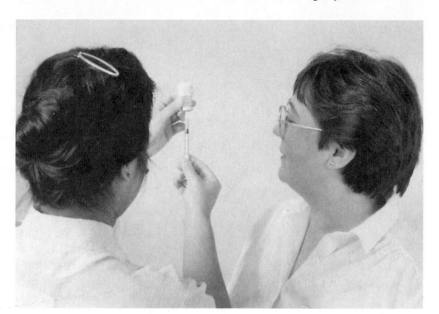

Figure 50–4. Disposable insulin syringe in use. The nurse checks the dosage of insulin with another nurse.

The larger the gauge number of a needle, the smaller the lumen. A needle with a small lumen is less painful to the patient when inserted. The choice of a needle is based on the relative viscosity or thickness of the medication. For example, most clear fluid solutions can be given intramuscularly with a 22- or 23-gauge needle. Subcutaneous injections of these kinds of fluids can be given with a 25- or 26-gauge needle. More viscous opaque medications given intramuscularly may require a 20- or 21-gauge needle. Larger needles are used primarily for blood transfusion and for injecting special intravenous fluids.

MEDICATION CONTAINERS

Two types of containers for injectable medications are the *vial* (either multiple dose or single dose) and the *ampule* (Fig. 50–7). A vial is a small, glass, round

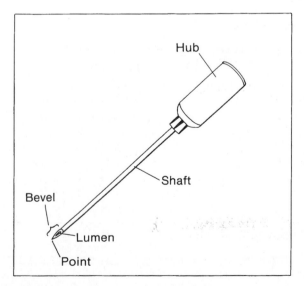

Figure 50–5. Disposable tuberculin syringe. Small amounts of medication can be measured accurately in these syringes.

Figure 50–6. The parts of a needle. Most needles currently used are disposable.

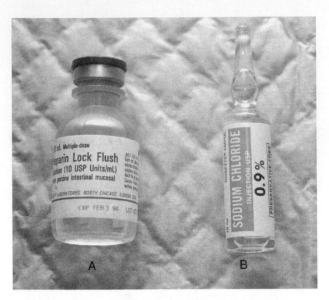

Figure 50–7. Medication containers. **(A)** Vial. **(B)** Ampule.

container with an airtight rubber stopper sealed to the glass by a metal rim. The ampule is an all-glass container that has a narrow neck. The top of the ampule must be broken off to remove the medication.

PROCEDURE FOR WITHDRAWING SOLUTIONS FROM CONTAINERS

The procedure for drawing up the medication into the syringe is the same for all types of injections. It is presented here as a separate skill that you will integrate into the overall procedure.

Vials

1. Wash your hands *for infection control.*
2. Using an alcohol or other type of antiseptic swab, clean the rubber top of the vial with a firm circular motion. Allow the alcohol to dry *to obtain maximum antibacterial action.*
3. Discard the swab.
4. Prepare the syringe and needle, selecting the

type of syringe used in your facility. Be careful to keep the needle, the syringe tip, the inside of the barrel, and the side of the plunger sterile *to prevent contamination of the medication* (Fig. 50–8).

5. Draw as much air into the syringe as the volume of solution you have calculated you will need.
6. With the vial resting on the countertop, remove the needle guard and insert the needle through the rubber top of the vial.
7. Inject the air into the vial by pushing the plunger of the syringe into the barrel. *Doing this prevents a vacuum when you withdraw the medication.*
8. Pick up the vial in your nondominant hand and hold the vial upside down at eye level. Many persons find it easier to do hold the vial between the index and middle fingers. (Practice various techniques until you feel comfortable with one.) Pull the plunger down to withdraw the necessary amount of medication. Make sure the needle tip is beneath the fluid level in the inverted vial and that you do not touch the sides of the plunger as you withdraw medication. *The sides of the plunger will touch the inside of the barrel as you manipulate to expel air and get the exact dosage. If you have touched them, they can then contaminate the inside of the barrel.*
9. Examine the medication for air bubbles and remove any that are present by keeping the syringe vertical and flicking your index finger (or a pen) against the side of the syringe over the air bubble. *The vibration will usually cause the bubble to break loose and rise to the top.* You can then push up on the plunger and expel the air into the vial. If the bubble does not rise when the syringe is tapped, you may have to push the medication back into the vial and draw up the medication again.
10. Once all air is removed from the syringe, make sure that you have the exact volume needed. *Needles and syringes are marked so that the volume in the needle and hub is considered dead space. This means that this space is full of medication when you*

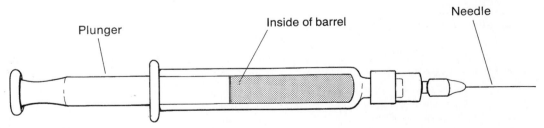

Figure 50–8. Parts of a syringe to be kept sterile. If your fingers touch the sides of the plunger, they can then contaminate the inside of the barrel.

begin to give the injection and it is still full when the injection is completed. Therefore, the exact dosage measured in the syringe is given. The practice of drawing an air bubble into the syringe to clear the medication from the needle actually creates an error in dosage by expelling the medication that is in the dead space, unless you use the air-lock technique (see pages 426–427).

11. Remove the needle from the vial.
12. Change the needle *if the medication is irritating to tissue*.
13. Replace the needle guard, being careful to touch the needle to the inside of the needle guard only. *If the needle touches the outside of the needle guard, it has been contaminated and must be replaced. To protect yourself from needle sticks*, never place the needle guard over the needle with your hand. Keep your hand that is not holding the syringe completely away from the needle guard. Some nurses simply place the needle guard in a convenient place on the counter or medicine cart and "scoop" it on. Some facilities use syringes that come housed in a case that becomes a vertical holder for the needle guard after the syringe is removed.

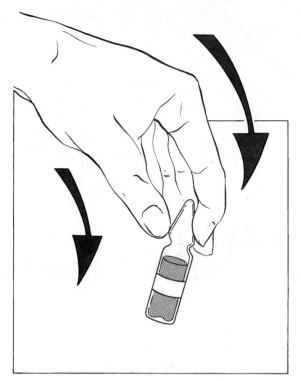

Figure 50–9. Shaking fluid to the bottom of an ampule. Grasp the ampule by the top and shake it firmly downward, as you would a thermometer.

Ampules

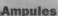

1. Wash your hands *for infection control.*
2. If the medication is in the upper part of the ampule, move it down into the lower part by flicking the tip of the ampule with your index finger. Another method is to grasp the ampule by the tip and shake it firmly downward, as you would shake down a thermometer (Fig. 50–9).
3. Using an alcohol or other type of antiseptic swab, clean the narrowest part of the ampule with a firm circular (twisting) motion.
4. Prepare the syringe and needle, using the procedure appropriate to the type of syringe used in your facility. Always use sterile technique. Many facilities provide special filter needles to withdraw medications from ampules. *The filter needle prevents the aspiration of particulate matter into the syringe.* The filter needle must not be used for injection and must be replaced with an appropriate needle after the medication has been drawn up.
5. Wrap a swab or gauze square around the neck of the ampule *to protect your hand from cuts.* Break off the top of the ampule away from yourself. To do this, hold the base of the ampule in one hand, grasp the top firmly with the other hand, and exert pressure (Fig. 50–10). Discard the top in the disposal container for "sharps."

6. Remove the needle guard.
7. Hold the ampule firmly in your nondominant hand, either resting on the counter or supported in your hand, between your index and middle fingers. Insert the needle into the open end of the ampule, being careful to touch the ampule with the needle on the inside only (Fig. 50–11).
8. Pull the plunger of the syringe back, being careful to keep the needle in the solution *to avoid drawing air into the syringe.*
9. Withdraw the needle from the ampule when you have drawn slightly more than the amount of solution needed. Most ampules are slightly overfilled *to allow sufficient medication.*
10. With the needle pointing vertically, pull back slightly to aspirate the fluid from the needle into the syringe.
11. Push the plunger gently into the barrel until 1 drop of medication appears at the point of the needle. This drop can be removed with a gentle shake of the syringe and needle over a sink or container. *Doing this prevents the medication from being on the outside of the needle and irritating the tissues as the needle is inserted.* If extra fluid must be ejected, the syringe can now be pointed downward over a sink or receptacle *so excess medication does not flow back over the needle.*

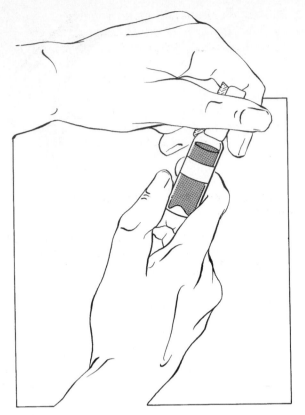

Figure 50–10. Breaking the neck of an ampule. Cover the neck of the ampule with a swab or gauze square to protect yourself from cuts. Hold the ampule away from yourself with one hand, and break the top off with the other.

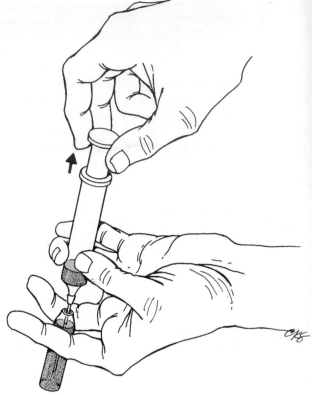

Figure 50–11. Withdrawing fluid from an ampule. Keeping the needle in the solution, pull back the plunger and withdraw the amount needed.

12. Make sure you have the exact volume needed.
13. Change the needle *if the medication is irritating to tissue or if you used a filter needle when drawing up the medication.*
14. Replace the needle guard, being careful to touch the needle to the inside of the needle guard only. *If the outside of the guard is touched, the needle has been contaminated and must be replaced.* Use a one-hand technique to replace the needle guard as previously discussed.

ENSURING ACCURATE DOSAGES

When the exact measurement of a medication is critical—for example, a dose of insulin or heparin—it is common practice to have two qualified individuals check the dosage together. The medication record and the filled syringe, still attached to the medication container if possible, are presented to the person who is doing the checking. Review the policy of the healthcare facility.

PROCEDURE FOR DRAWING UP MEDICATION WITH AN AIR LOCK

Some medications are irritating to subcutaneous tissue. These medications are given intramuscularly (IM), but they could leak back into the subcutaneous tissue. Injecting deep IM, injecting slowly so the medication can disperse, and using the Z-track technique (all of which are discussed later in this module) help to prevent leaking and irritation.

Another technique to decrease the possibility that medication will leak back into the subcutaneous tissue is the use of an *air lock*—a bubble of air which is injected after the medication and which *tends to block the needle track.* No research data support the value of using the air lock, and some researchers are concerned that errors in dosage occur if a nurse uses the air lock without understanding that there is dead space in the needle and syringe hub.

When drawing up medication with an air lock keep in mind these key concerns: having an accurate dosage of medication and giving the injection so that the air enters the tissue last. Follow these steps

1. Draw air into the syringe equal to the volume of medication needed, plus 0.4 mL.
2. When injecting air into a vial, leave 0.4 mL air in the syringe.
3. Holding the syringe vertically with the needle pointing up, draw the medication into the syringe. The air will remain at the top of the fluid. Measure the dosage by subtracting the amount of air from the total volume. Obtain the exact dosage.
4. Withdraw the syringe from the vial.
5. Still holding the syringe vertically, with the needle pointing up, expel 0.2 mL of air to clear the needle of medication. This will leave 0.2 mL of air in the syringe, and the needle will be filled with air. *The dead space in the needle is filled with air at the beginning of the injection and will be filled with air at the end, so the correct dosage will be given.* Although needles and syringes differ as to the volume of dead space, it never exceeds 0.2 mL.
6. Give the injection with the syringe in a perpendicular position *so that the air enters the tissue last.*

PROCEDURE FOR MIXING POWDERED MEDICATION FOR INJECTION

Some injectable medications come as a powder in a vial. The appropriate diluent, in the correct volume, must be injected into the vial, the contents mixed, and the medication then withdrawn. Follow these steps:

1. Read the label to determine the
   a. appropriate diluent.
   b. quantity of diluent to be used.
   c. resulting strength of the prepared medication.
2. Obtain the needed equipment:
   a. Alcohol swab
   b. Diluent
   c. Appropriate syringe
3. Cleanse the top of both the vial of diluent and the vial of powder *to decrease the potential for contamination of the needle and solution.*
4. Remove the appropriate volume of diluent from the vial, using the directions given for withdrawing solution from a container.
5. Insert the needle through the rubber stopper of the medication vial and instill the diluent toward the inside glass of the vial. *Some medications foam on direct contact with the diluent and do not mix well.*
6. Withdraw the needle and recap it, using a one-hand technique.

7. Mix the medication by gently rotating the vial between the palms of your hands. *Shaking creates bubbles, which are difficult to remove from the syringe.*
8. Draw up the appropriate dose of medication from the vial, using the directions given above.
9. If sufficient medication remains in the vial to warrant saving it and it is stable, label the vial with the date, the strength of the prepared solution, and your initials. Store it appropriately.

PROCEDURE FOR MIXING MEDICATIONS IN A SYRINGE

Commonly, physicians prescribe that injectable medications be given at the same time. It is possible to combine medications to give one injection. The important point is not to contaminate the medication in one vial with the medication from the other. Follow these steps:

1. Determine whether the two medications are compatible when mixed. This information can be found in many drug reference books or can be obtained from the pharmacy.
2. Determine the total volume of fluid that you will give if the drugs are mixed and given together. *If the volume is too large, you will need to plan for separate injections.*
3. Determine which medication you will draw up first. If one medication is in a vial and the other is in an ampule, draw up from the vial first *because it will be used again.* If both are from ampules or one-dose vials, or both are from multiple-dose vials, the order in which you draw up the medication is not important.
4. Obtain equipment:
   a. Alcohol swabs
   b. Appropriate syringe
   c. Appropriate needle
5. Clean tops of both vials or open ampules.
6. Draw up an amount of air equal to the combined volume needed if using a medication in a vial.
7. Inject the correct amount of air into each vial, first injecting air into the last medication you plan to draw up.
8. After injecting the air into the medication to be drawn up first, withdraw the exact volume of that medication needed, as described above. Be sure all air is out of the syringe.
9. Withdraw the needle from the vial.
10. Insert the needle into the second vial.
11. Turn the vial upside down and make sure that the needle is under the surface of the fluid be-

fore aspirating. *You will not be able to push bubbles out of the syringe without contaminating the first medication with the second one,* so you must be careful not to draw up air.

12. Aspirate until you have the precise volume needed for the combined medications *because the medications will mix in the syringe immediately and you cannot expel any excess without making the dosage incorrect.*

13. Withdraw the needle from the vial.

PROCEDURE FOR MIXING MEDICATIONS FROM PREFILLED SYRINGES AND CARTRIDGES

When the injectable medications ordered to be given at the same time both come in prefilled syringes or cartridges, follow these steps:

1. Determine whether the two medications are compatible when mixed.
2. Determine the total volume of fluid that you will give if the drugs are mixed and given together in the same syringe. *If the volume is too large, you will need to plan for separate injections.*
3. Measure accurate doses of medication in each of the prefilled syringes or cartridges.
4. Obtain a syringe and needle appropriate for the amount and type of medication to be given. Do not attach the needle to the syringe. If the syringe comes packaged with the needle attached, remove the needle from the syringe. Be careful not to contaminate the needle.
5. Pull back on the plunger of the syringe until there is adequate space for the total amount of medication to be given.
6. Inject the medication from each of the prefilled syringes or cartridges into the barrel of the syringe through the syringe tip.

GENERAL PROCEDURE FOR GIVING INJECTIONS

Use the General Procedure for Administering Medications (Module 47, pp. 365–366) as the basis for the General Procedure for Giving Injections, with the modifications noted below.

For each specific injection route discussed (subcutaneous, intramuscular, and intradermal), some steps of the General Procedure for Giving Injections may be modified. We have included completely the modified steps as well as references to the steps of the General Procedure that remain the same.

Assessment

1. Follow step 1 of the General Procedure for Administering Medications: Review the medication administration record (MAR) to determine whether any medications are to be administered to an individual patient.
2. Check the medications that are listed against the physician's or nurse's orders.
3. Follow step 3 of the General Procedure: Review information regarding the medication.
4. Assess the size and general build of the patient *to choose the correct size of needle for the injection.*
5. Assess whether you will need assistance to turn or protect the patient during the injection.

Planning

6. Determine the appropriate needle and syringe to be used.
7. Follow step 7 of the General Procedure: Wash your hands.
8. Gather the equipment, including the appropriate needle and syringe, alcohol swabs to use in preparing the medication and in giving the injection, and clean gloves.

Implementation

9.–10. Follow steps 9 and 10 of the General Procedure: Read the name of the medication from the record and check the label on the medication before picking it up.
11. Check the medication label a second time, then calculate the volume of medication needed. *Most medication orders are written in terms of milligrams of the drug. You will need to read the label to determine how many milligrams are found in each milliliter, to calculate how many milliliters you are to give.*
12. Draw up the correct dosage, using the techniques described for drawing up from a vial or an ampule (see pp. 000–000) or for mixing medication in a syringe (see pp. 424–426).
13. Check the label of the vial or ampule a third time and recheck your calculation of dosage.
14. Carry the syringe and alcohol swab to the bedside. When giving an injection to a child, you may wish to conceal the syringe with your hand *to avoid frightening the child as you enter the room.* In all cases, verbally prepare any child who is old enough to understand before giving the injection.
15.–16. Follow steps 15 and 16 of the General Procedure: Place MAR or identification card with the medication and identify the patient.
17. Explain the injection to the patient and identify

which site was used for the previous injection, if there was one, *to rotate to a different site and avoid excessive use of one area.*

18. Give the injection.

a. Provide privacy. Make sure there is adequate lighting and position the patient *for access to the injection site.*

b. Put on clean gloves. This step may vary with the policy of the facility and the guidelines of the nursing program. Some require clean gloves for all injections; others do not unless *there is the possibility of contact with blood.*

c. Select the appropriate injection site and clean it with a swab, using a circular motion and moving from the middle of the site outward.

d. Allow the skin to air-dry.

e. Place the swab between the third and fourth fingers of your nondominant hand. If you find this awkward, place the swab on the outer portion of the swab wrapper *to maintain cleanliness.*

f. Remove the needle guard, being careful to pull it straight off and away from the needle. Again, the needle should touch only the inside of the guard.

g. Using your nondominant hand, make the skin taut in an appropriate manner for the injection route chosen. *An injection is less painful if the skin is taut when pierced. Also, tautness allows the needle to enter the skin more easily.*

h. Hold the syringe like a dart (the barrel between the thumb and index finger of your dominant hand). The needle should be at an angle appropriate for the patient and the injection route.

i. Insert the needle through the skin with a quick dartlike thrust. Transfer your nondominant hand to the barrel of the syringe to steady it, and transfer your dominant hand to the plunger.

j. Pull back gently on the plunger (aspiration) *to be sure the needle is not in a blood vessel. Injection of a medication into a blood vessel can injure the vessel (the medication may not be appropriate for intravenous administration) and can produce a more immediate and considerably stronger effect than desired, possibly leading to serious complications.* In the remote event that blood appears in the syringe, the needle is in a blood vessel. Withdraw the needle, obtain new sterile equipment and repeat the entire procedure. You would not use the blood-tinged medication *because it is considered un-*

usable and could cause a discolored and tender area.

k. If no blood appears in the syringe, inject the medication by pushing the plunger into the barrel with slow, even pressure. *Slow infusion allows the medication to move into intracellular spaces, making room for additional fluid and reducing pain from pressure on the tissue.*

l. Using your nondominant hand, steady the tissue immediately adjacent to the puncture site and quickly remove the needle. *This prevents the skin from dragging on the needle as it is removed, which causes pain.*

m. Gently massage the injection site with the alcohol swab and discard it.

19. Follow step 19 of the General Procedure: Leave the patient in a comfortable position.

20. Discard the syringe and needle in the closest "sharps" container without replacing the needle guard. If the "sharps" container is centrally located, replace the needle guard using the one-hand technique previously discussed *to transport the needle and syringe safely.*

21. Follow step 21 of the General Procedure: Wash your hands.

Evaluation

22. Evaluate, using the following criteria:

a. The six rights were followed: right patient, right medication, right dosage, right route, right time, right documentation.

b. The correct site was used.

c. The effectiveness of the specific medication used.

d. Side effects, if present, were promptly identified.

Documentation

23. In addition to documenting the standard items (name of medication, dose, route, time, and signature), record the site of the injection. *This practice allows nurses to plan site rotation* (Fig. 50–12A and 50–12B). Also document effectiveness of medication given and presence of any side effects.

SUBCUTANEOUS ADMINISTRATION

Advantages and Disadvantages

Subcutaneous (SC or Sub-Q) injections of medication have several advantages over the oral method of administration. First, if the patient has adequate

(text continues on page 432)

DIAGNOSIS: *Left lower lobe Pneumonia* ● ● Page _1_ of _1_

ALLERGIES: *NKA*

↓ CHART ROUTINES

DRUG & STRENGTH	ROUTE & DIRECTIONS	SHIFT	DATE 1/4/99	DATE 1/5/99	DATE 1/6	DATE 1/7	DATE 1/8
1/4 Staphcillin 800 mg IM q 6 h 06 12 18 24 JE		23/07	24 Ⓐ CS 06 Ⓑ CS	24 Ⓐ CS 06 Ⓑ CS			
		07/15	12 Ⓖ PB	12 Ⓖ PB			
		15/23	18 Ⓗ EN	18 Ⓗ HW			
1/5 Heparin 10,000 U *sub cut. b.i.d.* 09 21 CS		23/07	╳				
		07/15		09 Ⓛ abd. CS			
		15/23		21 Ⓡ abd. H			
1/5 Demerol 50 mg IM *q 4 h PRN* CS		23/07	╳	╳			
		07/15		08 Ⓒ CS 12 Ⓗ CS			
		15/23		16 Ⓐ HW 20 Ⓑ HW			
		23/07					
		07/15					
		15/23					
		23/07					
		07/15					
		15/23					
		23/07					
		07/15					
		15/23					
		23/07					
		07/15					
		15/23					
		23/07					
		07/15					
		15/23					

A = RIGHT UPPER OUTER QUAD   C = RIGHT DELTOID   E = RIGHT ANTERIOR THIGH   G = RIGHT VENTROGLUTEAL
B = LEFT UPPER OUTER QUAD   D = LEFT DELTOID   F = LEFT ANTERIOR THIGH   H = LEFT VENTROGLUTEAL

Cynthia Grant F - 40
539 - 26 - 4967
Dr. John Torres

INITIAL	NAME	INITIAL	NAME	INITIAL	NAME
CS	*C. Smith, RN*	HW	*H. Williams, RN*		
PB	*P. Benitez, RN*				
EN	*E. Norton, RN*				

SWEDISH HOSPITAL MEDICAL CENTER
SEATTLE, WASHINGTON 98104

P-346 (R. 4/84) STOCK #5630

Figure 50–12. Documentation of injections. In addition to the standard items, document the site of the injection. **(A)** Standard MAR (*continued*).

This medication record and flow sheet is to be used for the documentation of all subcutaneous injections.
Label the columns with the parameters to be monitored. For example: INSULIN – Chemstrip blood glucose, lab blood glucose, type(s) of insulin. HEPARIN – Lab value (PT/PTT), heparin.

Parameters Date	Time	Injection Site	Chemstrip Blood glucose	Lab Blood glucose	Regular Insulin U-100	NPH Iletin U-100	Comments	Int.
1/4/99	0700			130				CS
	0730	E1			15 u	45 u		PB
	1130		120					PB
	1700		125					EN
	1730	E2			10 u	35 u	"hungry"	EN
	2100		210					
	2130	E3			4 u			EN
1/5/99	0710			140				CS
	0730	E4			15 u	45 u		PB

SUBCUTANEOUS INJECTION SITE CODES

C = Rt. deltoid   D = Lt. deltoid
I = Rt. abdomen   J = Lt. abdomen
E = Rt. thigh   F = Lt. thigh

This diagram shows the areas for subcutaneous injections. **For heparin the abdomen is preferred.** For insulin all sites may be used. When an injection site is used, chart the site under the Injection Site column (e.g., J4). The site may be marked off with an "X" on the diagram to facilitate the rotation plan. Each injection should be about one inch away from the other. Begin with one area and stay with that area until all the sites there have been used.

Identify Initials with Signature:			
1. PB P. Benitez, RN	4.	8.	
2. EN E. Norton, RN	5.	9.	
3. CS C. Smith, RN	6.	10.	
	7.	11.	

ADDRESSOGRAPH:

Cynthia Grant F – 40
539 – 26 – 4967
Dr. John Torres

SWEDISH HOSPITAL MEDICAL CENTER
SEATTLE, WASHINGTON

NU-32 2/90 FC/SHMC

Figure 50–12. *(continued)* **(B)** Subcutaneous injection MAR.

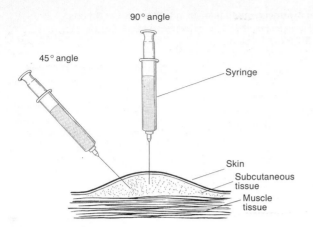

90° angle

45° angle

Syringe

Skin
Subcutaneous tissue
Muscle tissue

Figure 50–13. Subcutaneous injection. Either a 90-degree angle or a 45-degree angle may be used for subcutaneous injection if adequate subcutaneous tissue is present.

circulatory status, you can depend on rapid, almost complete absorption of the medication. Second, gastric disturbances do not affect the medication given subcutaneously. Third, the patient does not have to be conscious or rational to receive the medication.

The greatest disadvantage of subcutaneous administration is that it penetrates the body's first line of defense, the skin. Thus, it is imperative that sterile technique be used *for the patient's safety.*

Selecting the Equipment

In most instances a 25-gauge, ⅝-inch needle is used for subcutaneous injections. An extremely thin or especially obese patient may need individual variations in choice of needle or injection technique.

The maximum amount of solution that can be comfortably given subcutaneously is from 1½ to 2 mL. In many facilities, the smallest regular syringe available is 3 mL. Insulin and tuberculin syringes that hold 0.5 to 1 mL can also be used for lesser amounts.

Selecting the Site and Angle

Subcutaneous tissue lies directly below the skin. In many cases there is sufficient subcutaneous tissue present to use a 90° angle. In very thin patients you may need to use a 45° to 60° angle. The angle of insertion depends on the individual patient's size and on the needle length. In all cases, the end of the needle must lie in the subcutaneous tissue (Fig. 50–13).

The site you select will vary with individual patients and circumstances. Generally, areas are selected so that the medication is injected below the dermal layer of the skin. Avoid any areas that are tender or have signs of scarring, swelling, or inflammation. Several sites can be used, such as the upper

arms, anterior aspects of the thighs, upper back, and the abdominal wall (see Fig. 50–12**B**). It is important to rotate sites for patients who receive subcutaneous injections frequently *to decrease any local site irritation* (Fig. 50–14).

Procedure for Giving Subcutaneous Injections

To give subcutaneous injections, follow the General Procedure for Giving Injections as modified below.

Assessment
1.–3. Follow the steps of the General Procedure for Giving Injections.
4. If the patient has received other subcutaneous injections, assess the sites and note the presence of any of the reactions (described above). The properties of some medications cause more site reaction than others.
5. Follow the General Procedure.

Planning
6.–8. Follow the steps of the General Procedure.

Implementation
9.–17. Follow the steps of the General Procedure.
18. Give the subcutaneous injection.
  a.–f. Follow the steps of the General Procedure.
  g. Using your nondominant hand, gently pinch the skin at the site selected between the thumb and index finger to elevate the subcutaneous tissue. If the patient is obese, you

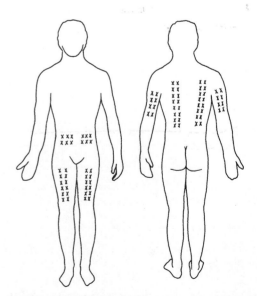

Figure 50–14. Sites used in rotating subcutaneous injections. Document the site of the injection to accurately plan site rotations.

may have to spread the skin apart firmly to make the skin taut.

    h. Use a 45° to 90° angle as selected for the individual patient (see Fig. 50–13).

    i.–m. Follow the steps of the General Procedure.

19.–21. Follow the steps of the General Procedure.

Evaluation

22. Follow the General Procedure.

Documentation

23. Document medication, dosage, route, site, time, and signature. Be sure to carefully document the site of the injection and any observations of irritation at other sites that have been used previously.

Special Concerns for Subcutaneous Injections

Heparin is a drug that is commonly given by subcutaneous injection. The preferred site was usually the abdomen. Recent research on efficacy (drug effectiveness) and bruising indicated that there were no significant differences when the drug was injected in the abdomen, thigh, or arm (Fahs and Kinney, 1991). When giving this drug, do not aspirate or massage the site afterward. *These actions might increase the capillary damage and contribute to bruising.* In addition, apply firm pressure to the injection site until all blood has stopped oozing *to help prevent bruising.* For patients who bleed or bruise easily, ice sometimes is applied to the site for 15 to 30 minutes before the injection. *Doing this causes vasoconstriction and hastens clotting.*

    Insulin and other drugs are also administered by subcutaneous injection. Some are reconstituted or mixed, so the nurse should carefully observe the directions provided by the manufacturer.

Procedure for Teaching Subcutaneous Self-Injections

As newer drugs have been developed and patients have become more knowledgeable about their treatments, there has been an increased use of subcutaneous self-injections. The nurse can teach the patient this skill. However, if the patient cannot or wishes not to perform self-injections, it may be appropriate for the nurse to teach this skill to a care provider.

    To teach subcutaneous self-injections, follow the General Procedure for Giving Injections as modified below.

Assessment

1.–2. Follow the steps of the General Procedure for Giving Injections.

3. Assess the specific drug for any guidelines on administration and the record of sites used previously.

4. Assess the knowledge base of the patient and any fears the he or she may have regarding self-injection. Also note which sites would be more appropriate for the patient or care provider.

5. Follow the General Procedure.

Planning

6. Identify the equipment needed for the injection and the items that are available for the procedure.

7.–8. Follow the steps of the General Procedure.

Implementation

9.–17. Follow the steps of the General Procedure.

18. Have the patient or care provider give the injection. Instruct the patient or the care provider to apply ice to the injection site for 1 minute before injecting. *Doing this greatly reduces any pain caused by the piercing of the skin.* Pinch skin of the injection site, inject medication at a slow and steady rate, remove needle from skin, massage gently, and discard syringe and swab.

19.–21. Follow the steps of the General Procedure.

Evaluation

22. Evaluate the skill and ease of the patient or care provider giving the injection.

Documentation

23. Teach the patient or care provider to document the date and the site that was used.

INTRAMUSCULAR ADMINISTRATION

Advantages and Disadvantages

Some of the advantages in using the intramuscular (IM) route for medications are the same as those for the subcutaneous route. For instance, the medication is almost completely absorbed, gastric disturbances do not affect the medication, and the patient does not need to be conscious or rational to receive the medication. Absorption occurs even more rapidly than with the subcutaneous route *because of the greater vascularity of muscle tissue.* Irritating drugs are commonly given intramuscularly *because very few nerve endings are in deep muscle tissue.*

    Disadvantages include the penetration of the skin, the possibility of nerve damage, pain that may linger

433

n, and the potential for abscesses.
tient teaching is necessary for the
ischarged on an IM medication.

...ng the Equipment

A 19- to 22-gauge needle is used for intramuscular injections. The choice should depend on the medication's viscosity. The needle length depends on the patient's size, but it is usually 1 to 1½ inches long. A 22-gauge, 1½-inch needle is the one most commonly used.

Syringe size varies, but generally a 3-mL syringe is used. In most facilities, no more than 3 mL medication is injected into any one intramuscular site at a time.

Selecting the Site

Dorsogluteal Site

This is perhaps the most common of the four intramuscular injection sites for adults. The injection is given in the gluteus medius muscle.

The patient should be lying prone, with the toes pointed inward. This position makes site identification easier and relaxes the muscles. For some patients, this position can be difficult or impossible. An alternative is the side-lying position. The area should be adequately exposed (that is, all clothing must be moved away) *to aid site identification*.

One of two methods may be used for locating this site. The first and most traditional is to divide the buttock into quadrants, and then give the injection in the upper outer quadrant (Fig. 50–15).

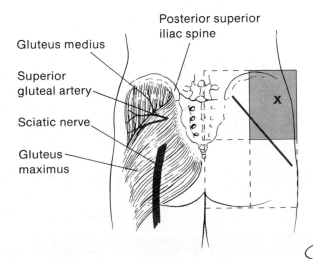

Figure 50–15. Dorsogluteal site for intramuscular injection. The quadrant outlined in solid lines surrounds the dorsogluteal site. The solid diagonal line provides another accurate way to locate this site.

Labels in figure:
Posterior superior iliac spine
Gluteus medius
Superior gluteal artery
Sciatic nerve
Gluteus maximus
X

The landmarks of the dorsogluteal site are the upper iliac crest, the inner crease of the buttocks, the outer lateral edge of the patient's body, and the lower edge of the buttock (inferior gluteal fold). These landmarks should be palpated, not merely located by sight. Errors can easily be made, particularly in the location of the iliac crest.

When you have established the location of the upper outer quadrant, give the injection 2 to 3 inches below the crest of the ilium. *Observing these precautions lessens the risk of injecting into large blood vessels or the sciatic nerve.*

The second method for locating the same site is more accurate when the patient is in the side-lying position. Draw an imaginary line between the posterior superior iliac spine and the greater trochanter of the femur (see Fig. 50–15). An injection given laterally and superiorly to this line is away from the sciatic nerve *because the line runs lateral to the nerve.*

Ventrogluteal Site

The ventrogluteal site has several advantages over the dorsogluteal site. *No large nerves or blood vessels are in the area, it is generally less fatty, and the patient on bed rest has to neither be turned nor lie directly on the injection site.* In addition, *because the gluteal muscle is not completely developed in small children,* the ventrogluteal site, rather than the dorsogluteal site, is preferred at least until a child is walking. The patient can be placed in one of several positions; prone and side-lying are preferred.

The landmarks of the ventrogluteal site are the greater trochanter, the crest of the ilium, and the anterior superior iliac spine. To identify the site, first locate these landmarks on the patient. Then place the heel of your palm on the greater trochanter. Point one finger toward the anterior superior iliac spine and an adjacent finger toward the crest of the ilium, forming a triangle with the iliac bone. (The size of your hand and the patient's bone structure may require small adjustments in hand position to form this triangle.) Use your nondominant hand to locate the site *so that your dominant hand is free to manipulate the syringe.* The injection site is near the middle of this triangle, approximately 1 inch below the iliac bone (Fig. 50–16).

When the site is located, proceed as you would for a dorsogluteal injection, except point the needle slightly toward the iliac bone as you insert it.

Vastus Lateralis Site

The lateral thigh is relatively free of major nerves and blood vessels and is accessible in the dorsal recumbent or sitting position. This site is recommend-

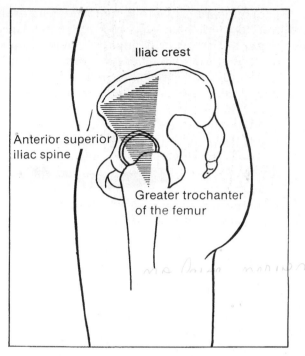

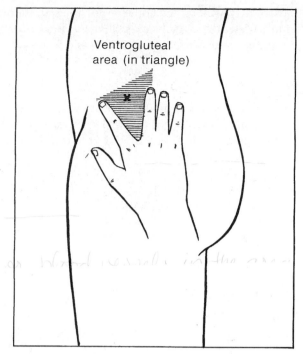

Figure 50–16. Ventrogluteal site for intramuscular injection. In this drawing, the patient is lying on the right side with the left side up. The nurse's right hand is being used to locate the site. The site can be marked with the alcohol swab and the right hand removed to handle the syringe, or the left hand can be used to give the injection while the right hand remains in place, marking the site.

ed particularly for infants and small children, *whose gluteal muscle is still undeveloped.*

In adults, the superior boundary is a hand's breadth below the greater trochanter. The inferior boundary is a hand's breadth above the knee. On the front of the leg, the midanterior thigh serves as a boundary. On the side of the leg, the midlateral thigh is the boundary. The result is a narrow band (approximately 3 inches wide) that is suitable for intramuscular injection (Fig. 50–17).

Insert the needle only to a depth of 1 inch and hold it parallel to the surface of the bed. This site is

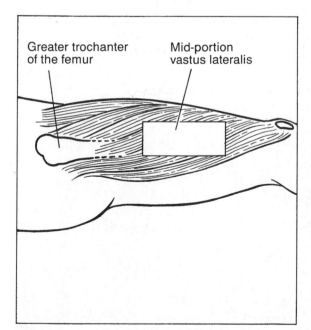

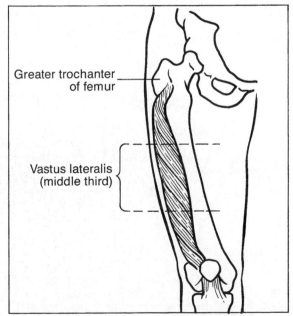

Figure 50–17. Vastus lateralis site for intramuscular injection. This site is recommended particularly for infants and small children, whose gluteal muscle is still underdeveloped.

Rectus Femoris Site

The muscle located on the anterior surface of the midlateral thigh is called the rectus femoris and can be used in the dorsal recumbent or sitting position. It is smaller than the vastus in the adult and is used only for small injections and for infants who are not yet walking and whose gluteal muscles are therefore not well developed. To concentrate the muscle mass and make the injection easier, compress the muscle tissue between your fingers. Inject straight downward into the top of the thigh to a depth that is appropriate for the age and body build of the patient (Fig. 50–18).

Deltoid Site

The deltoid muscle of the arm can also be used as a site for intramuscular injection if the muscle is well developed. Although it is easily accessible, its use is limited *because this smaller muscle is not capable of absorbing large amounts of medication*. Another, possibly more critical limitation on the use of this site *is danger of injury to the radial nerve.*

The deltoid site is rectangularly shaped. The up-

per boundary is two to three fingerbreadths down from the acromion process on the outer aspect of the arm. The lower boundary is roughly opposite the axilla. Lines parallel to the arm, one third and two thirds of the way around the outer lateral aspect of the arm, form the side boundaries (Fig. 50–19).

Although the size of the muscle varies with the size of the person, the amount of medication injected at this site should be limited to a maximum of 2 mL, preferably of nonirritating medication.

Procedure for Giving Intramuscular Injections

To give an intramuscular injection, follow the General Procedure for Giving Injections as modified below.

Assessment
1.–5. Follow the steps of the General Procedure for Giving Injections.

Planning
6.–8. Follow the steps of the General Procedure.

Implementation
9.–17. Follow the steps of the General Procedure.
18. Give the intramuscular injection.
    a.–f. Follow the steps of the General Procedure.
    g. Using your nondominant hand, spread the

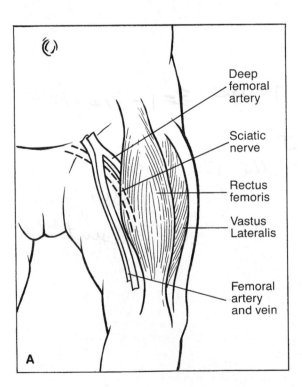
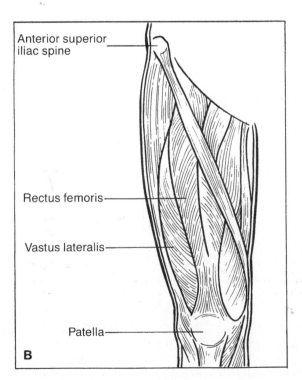

Figure 50–18. Rectus femorus site for intramuscular injection. **(A)** Infant. **(B)** Adult. This muscle is small and is therefore used only for small injections.

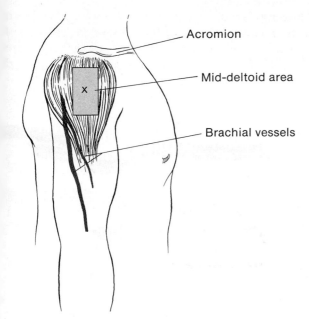

Figure 50–19. Deltoid site for intramuscular injection. The amount of medication injected at this site should be limited to a maximum of 2 mL.

Acromion

Mid-deltoid area

Brachial vessels

skin at the site selected between your thumb and index finger, making it taut. If the patient is very small or emaciated, you may have to pinch the tissue between the thumb and index finger to ensure sufficient muscle tissue.
h. Ensure that the needle is at a 90° angle.
i.–m. Follow the steps of the General Procedure.
19.–21. Follow the steps of the General Procedure.

Evaluation
22. Follow the General Procedure.

Documentation
23. Follow the General Procedure.

Procedure for Using the Z-Track Technique

The Z-track technique of intramuscular injection is used when a drug stains the tissues, such as injectable iron preparations, or is extremely irritating, such as several central nervous system drugs. *Correct use of the Z-track technique prevents a drug from leaking back up through the needle track and staining or causing irritation.* The technique may be used for any intramuscular injection *to decrease discomfort and bruising.*

The equipment used for this procedure is generally the same as for routine intramuscular injections, except that a 1½ inch needle is desirable. The dorsogluteal area is the easiest site to use for a Z-track injection.

To give a Z-track injection, follow the steps of the General Procedure for Giving Injections as modified below.

Assessment
1.–5. Follow the steps of the General Procedure.

Planning
6.–8. Follow the steps of the General Procedure.

Implementation
9.–17. Follow the steps of the General Procedure.
18. Give the Z-track injection.
   a.–f. Follow the steps of the General Procedure.
   g. Using the side of your nondominant hand, pull the skin and tissue laterally until it is taut (Fig. 50–20).
   h. Holding the syringe like a dart, insert the needle at a 90° angle.
   i. As soon as the needle is inserted, use the thumb and index finger of your nondominant hand to steady the syringe, using your dominant hand to aspirate.
   j. Do not release the tissue that has been displaced laterally.

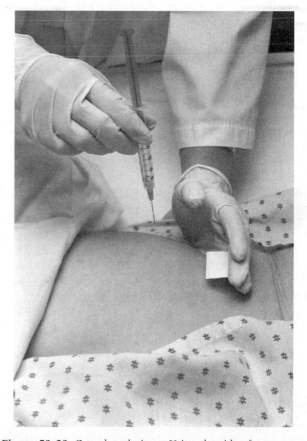

Figure 50–20. Z-track technique. Using the side of your nondominant hand, pull the skin laterally until it is taut.

k. Inject the medication slowly. Wait several seconds.

l. Remove the needle, and immediately release the skin being held taut by your nondominant hand. The skin layers will close in a Z configuration, *preventing leakage.*

m. Do not massage the injection site. The Z-track technique, when compared with standard IM injection technique, significantly decreases discomfort and the severity of postinjection irritation.

19.–21. Follow the steps of the General Procedure.

Evaluation
22. Follow the General Procedure.

Documentation
23. Follow the General Procedure.

INTRADERMAL ADMINISTRATION

Uses

The intradermal route is commonly used for diagnostic purposes, usually for diagnosing allergies and sensitivities and for administering the tuberculin test. It has the longest absorption time of all the parenteral routes.

Selecting the Equipment

Because a very small amount of drug is used, a 1-mL, or tuberculin, syringe is used, with a short (¼–⅝ inch), fine-gauge (25–27) needle.

Selecting the Site

Intradermal literally means "between the skin layers," and the injection is administered just under the epidermis. The inner surface of the forearm is the most common site, although the subscapular region of the back can be used as well.

Procedure for Giving Intradermal Injections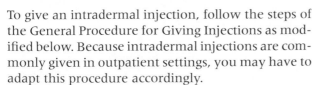

To give an intradermal injection, follow the steps of the General Procedure for Giving Injections as modified below. Because intradermal injections are commonly given in outpatient settings, you may have to adapt this procedure accordingly.

Assessment
1.–5. Follow the steps of the General Procedure.

Planning
6.–8. Follow the steps of the General Procedure.

Implementation
9.–17. Follow the steps of the General Procedure.
18. Give the intradermal injection.

a.–f. Follow the steps of the General Procedure.

g. Using your nondominant hand, stretch the skin at the selected site, making it taut.

h. Hold the syringe at a 10°–15° angle, with the bevel of the needle facing up.

i. Insert the needle just until the bevel is no longer visible (Fig. 50–21).

j. Inject the medication slowly.

k. Withdraw the needle.

l. Do not massage. A small wheal (raised area) is left at the point of injection.

m. Circle the area of injection with a skin-marking pen if the site must be assessed for reaction.

n. Assess the site at the appropriate time interval for redness and swelling.

19.–21. Follow the steps of the General Procedure.

Evaluation
22. Follow the General Procedure.

Documentation
23. Follow the General Procedure.

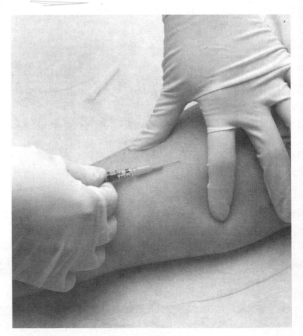

Figure 50–21. Intradermal injection technique. The syringe is held at a 10 to 15-degree angle, with the bevel of the needle facing up.

LONG-TERM CARE

Many residents in long term care settings receive medications by injection. The nurse must take into account several considerations when administering injections to elderly persons. First, these persons may be receiving multiple preparations, some orally, which may interact with the drug being injected. Second, elderly persons typically have less muscle mass than younger persons, so the technique used may have to be altered to suit the particular individual. Third, an older person's metabolism may not be as vigorous as a younger person's, so the nurse must closely monitoring drug effects. Finally, the nurse should have expertise in and understanding of pain management, because pain responses are not slowed just because a person is older.

HOME CARE

It is essential that those caring for patients in the home setting, whether professionals or lay persons, carry out the administration of injections with the same high quality of performance as that offered in any healthcare facility. An additional responsibility is the safe disposal of syringes and needles. An alternative to purchasing the type of container used in a professional setting is to use a disposable container commonly found in the home. A plastic, disposable soft drink bottle resists puncture, can be capped tightly, and does not burst under pressure. Syringes and needles can be placed there as they would be placed in the "sharps" container in the hospital. The container must be stored where children cannot reach it and must be capped before disposal.

Non-healthcare professionals who are caring for clients at home commonly need to administer medication by injection. It may be your responsibility to teach this skill to these persons. Areas for emphasis include sterile technique, accurate dosage measurement, and effective injection procedure.

CRITICAL THINKING EXERCISES

• You are to give an intramuscular injection of pain medication to a patient who has had her gallbladder removed. As you enter her room, you observe that she is lying on her back moaning. Describe your interaction with this patient and identify the site and technique that would be most appropriate.

• You are to teach a 60-year-old patient how to give a subcutaneous self-injection. Using the steps of the nursing process, create a teaching plan. Consider your interaction with the patient (or family), explanations of the equipment, technique to be used, and evaluation and documentation.

References

Centers for Disease Control. (1988). Update: Universal precautions for prevention of transmission of human immunodeficiency virus, hepatitis B virus, and other blood-borne pathogens in health care settings. *Morbidity and Mortality Weekly Report, 37,* 377–388.

Fahs, P. S., & Kinney, M. R. (1991). The abdomen, thigh and arm as sites for subcutaneous heparin injections. *Nursing Research, 40*(4), 204–207.

PERFORMANCE CHECKLIST

Procedure for Drawing Up Medication With an Air Lock	Needs More Practice	Satisfactory	Comments
1. Draw air into syringe equal to volume of medication plus 0.4 mL.			
2. Inject air into vial, leaving 0.4 mL of air in syringe.			
3. Hold syringe vertically to draw up medication. Measure dosage by subtracting the amount of air from the total volume.			
4. Withdraw syringe from vial.			
5. With syringe vertical, expel medication from needle, leaving air in the needle and 0.2 mL air in the syringe.			
6. Give injection with syringe in perpendicular position.			
Procedure for Mixing Powdered Medication for Injection			
1. Read label to determine: **a.** Diluent			
b. Quantity of diluent			
c. Resulting strength of solution			
2. Obtain equipment: **a.** Alcohol swab			
b. Diluent			
c. Syringe			
3. Clean tops of both vials.			
4. Remove appropriate volume of diluent from vial.			
5. Insert needle into vial of drug and instill diluent.			
6. Withdraw needle.			
7. Mix medication by rotating.			
8. Draw up appropriate dose.			
9. If remainder of medication is to be saved, label with date, strength, and your initials.			
Procedure for Mixing Medications in a Syringe			
1. Determine compatibility of two medications.			

(continued)

Procedure for Mixing Medications in a Syringe (Continued)	Needs More Practice	Satisfactory	Comments
2. Determine total volume of drugs to be administered.			
3. Determine medication to draw up first.			
4. Obtain equipment: a. Alcohol swabs			
b. Syringe			
c. Needle			
5. Clean tops of both vials or open ampules.			
6. Draw up amount of air equal to combined volumes.			
7. Inject air into both vials: last to be drawn up receives air first.			
8. Withdraw exact volume of medication #1. Be sure all air is removed from syringe.			
9. Withdraw needle from vial.			
10. Insert needle into vial of medication #2.			
11. Turn vial upside down and make sure that the needle is under the surface of the liquid.			
12. Draw up the exact volume of medication #2 needed.			
13. Withdraw needle from vial.			
Procedure for Mixing Medications From Prefilled Syringes and Cartridges			
1. Determine compatibility of medications.			
2. Determine total volume of drugs to be given.			
3. Measure accurate dosage of each medication to be given.			
4. Obtain an appropriate needle and syringe. If syringe has needle attached, remove it.			
5. Pull back on plunger until there is room in syringe for total amount of medication.			
6. Inject medication from each prefilled syringe or cartridge into barrel of syringe through syringe tip.			

(continued)

General Procedure for Giving Injections	Needs More Practice	Satisfactory	Comments
Assessment			
1. Follow Checklist step 1 of the General Procedure for Administering Medications in Module 47 (review medication record to identify whether any medications are to be given to an individual patient).			
2. Check medications listed against physician's or nurse's orders.			
3. Follow Checklist step 3 of the General Procedure (review medication information).			
4. Assess size and general build of patient.			
5. Assess need for assistance.			
Planning			
6. Determine appropriate needle and syringe to be used.			
7. Wash your hands.			
8. Gather equipment.			
Implementation			
9.–10. Follow Checklist steps 9 and 10 of the General Procedure (read the name of the medication from the record and check the label on the medication before picking it up).			
11. Check label again, before calculating and preparing dosage.			
12. Draw up correct dosage of medication. a. From vial (1) Wash your hands.			
(2) Clean top of vial and allow to dry.			
(3) Discard alcohol swab.			
(4) Prepare syringe and needle.			
(5) Draw air into syringe equal to amount of medication.			
(6) Insert needle into vial through rubber stopper.			
(7) Inject air into vial.			

(continued)

General Procedure for Giving Injections *(Continued)*	Needs More Practice	Satisfactory	Comments
(8) Pick up vial with nondominant hand and withdraw correct volume of medication.			
(9) Examine for air bubbles and expel them.			
(10) Recheck volume of medication for accuracy.			
(11) Remove needle from vial.			
(12) Change needle if medication is irritating.			
(13) Replace needle guard.			
b. From ampule (1) Wash your hands.			
(2) Get all medication into lower part of ampule.			
(3) Clean neck of ampule with alcohol swab.			
(4) Prepare syringe and needle.			
(5) Wrap neck of ampule and break off the top, away from yourself.			
(6) Remove needle guard.			
(7) Hold ampule in nondominant hand and insert needle into ampule.			
(8) Aspirate medication into syringe.			
(9) Withdraw needle from ampule.			
(10) Point needle vertically and pull back slightly.			
(11) Expel air from syringe.			
(12) Make sure that you have the exact volume of medication needed.			
(13) Change needle if medication is irritating.			
(14) Replace needle guard.			
13. Check label of vial or ampule and dosage.			
14. Carry syringe and swab to bedside.			

(continued)

General Procedure for Giving Injections *(Continued)*	Needs More Practice	Satisfactory	Comments
15.–16. Follow Checklist steps 15 and 16 of the General Procedure (place MAR or identification card with the medication and identify the patient).			
17. Explain to patient and identify site appropriately.			
18. Give the injection. **a.** Provide privacy.			
b. Put on clean gloves.			
c. Select the appropriate site and clean it, using a circular motion.			
d. Allow site to dry.			
e. Place swab between fingers of nondominant hand.			
f. Remove needle guard.			
g. Pinch or spread tissue as indicated.			
h. Ensure needle is at appropriate angle.			
i. Insert needle.			
j. Aspirate to be sure needle is not in blood vessel.			
k. Inject medication.			
l. Remove needle.			
m. Gently massage injection site.			
19. Follow Checklist step 19 of the General Procedure (leave patient in a comfortable position).			
20. Discard syringe and needle in "sharps" container.			
21. Follow Checklist step 21 of the General Procedure (wash your hands).			
Evaluation			
22. Evaluate using the following criteria: **a.** Six rights followed.			
b. Correct site used.			
c. Effectiveness of medication assessed.			
d. Any side effects promptly identified.			

(continued)

General Procedure for Giving Injections *(Continued)*	Needs More Practice	Satisfactory	Comments
Documentation			
23. Document medication, dosage, route, site, time, and signature. Also document effectiveness of medication given and presence of any side effects.			
Procedure for Giving Subcutaneous Injections			
Assessment			
1–3. Follow Checklist steps 1–3 of the General Procedure for Giving Injections (review medication record, check physician's order, and review medication information).			
4. Assess site if patient has had other subcutaneous injections.			
5. Follow Checklist step 5 of the General Procedure (assess need for assistance).			
Planning			
6–8. Follow Checklist steps 6–8 of the General Procedure (determine appropriate needle and syringe, wash your hands, gather equipment).			
Implementation			
9.–17. Follow Checklist steps 9–17 of the General Procedure (read the name of the medication from the record, check the label on the medication before picking it up, check label again before calculating and preparing dosage, draw up medication, check label of vial or ampule and dosage, carry syringe to bedside, place MAR or identification card with medication, identify patient, explain to patient).			
18. Give the subcutaneous injection. **a–f.** Follow Checklist steps 18 a–f of the General Procedure (provide privacy, put on clean gloves, select appropriate site and clean it, allow site to dry, place swab between fingers, remove needle guard).			
g. Pinch skin between thumb and index finger to elevate subcutaneous tissue.			
h. Use a 45°–90° angle.			

(continued)

Procedure for Giving Subcutaneous Injections (Continued)	Needs More Practice	Satisfactory	Comments
i–m. Follow Checklist steps 18 i–m of the General Procedure (insert needle, aspirate, inject medication, remove needle, massage site).			
19.–21. Follow Checklist steps 19–21 of the General Procedure (leave patient in comfortable position, discard syringe and needle in "sharps" container, wash your hands).			
Evaluation			
22. Evaluate as in Checklist step 22 of the General Procedure (six rights followed, correct site used, effectiveness of medication assessed, side effects identified).			
Documentation			
23. Document as in Checklist step 23 of the General Procedure (medication, dosage, route, site, time, signature as well as observations of irritation at other sites used previously).			
Procedure for Teaching Subcutaneous Self-Injection			
Assessment			
1.–2. Follow Checklist steps 1 and 2 of the General Procedure for Giving Injections (review medication record and check physician's order).			
3. Assess the specific drug for administration guidelines and check record of sites previously used.			
4. Assess patient's knowledge and fears; note appropriate sites.			
5. Follow Checklist step 5 of the General Procedure (assess need for assistance).			
Planning			
6. Identify equipment needed and available items.			
7.–8. Follow Checklist steps 7 and 8 of the General Procedure (wash your hands and gather equipment).			

(*continued*)

Procedure for Teaching Subcutaneous Self-Injection *(Continued)*	Needs More Practice	Satisfactory	Comments
Implementation			
9.–17. Follow Checklist steps 9–17 of the General Procedure (read the name of the medication from the record, check the label on the medication before picking it up, check label again before calculating and preparing dosage, draw up medication, check label of vial or ampule and dosage, carry syringe to bedside, place MAR or identification card with medication, identify patient, explain to patient).			
18. Have the patient give the injection.			
19.–21. Follow Checklist steps 19–21 of the General Procedure (leave patient in comfortable position, discard syringe and needle in "sharps" container, wash your hands).			
Evaluation			
22. Evaluate as in Checklist step 22 of the General Procedure (six rights followed, correct site used, effectiveness of medication assessed, side effects identified).			
Documentation			
23. Teach patient to document date and site used.			
Procedure for Giving Intramuscular Injections			
Assessment			
1–5. Follow Checklist steps 1–5 of the General Procedure for Giving Injections (review medication record, check physician's order, review medication information, assess patient's size and build, assess need for assistance).			
Planning			
6–8. Follow Checklist steps 6–8 of the General Procedure (determine appropriate needle and syringe, wash your hands, gather equipment).			

(continued)

Procedure for Giving Intramuscular injections *(Continued)*	Needs More Practice	Satisfactory	Comments
Implementation			
9–17. Follow Checklist steps 9–17 of the General Procedure (read the name of the medication from the record, check the label on the medication before picking it up, check label again before calculating and preparing dosage, draw up medication, check label of vial or ampule and dosage, carry syringe to bedside, place MAR or identification card with medication, identify patient, explain to patient).			
18. Give the intramuscular injection. **a.–f.** Follow Checklist steps 18 a–f of the General Procedure (provide privacy, put on clean gloves, select appropriate site and clean it, allow site to dry, place swab between fingers, remove needle guard).			
g. Spread skin with thumb and index finger.			
h. Ensure that needle is at 90° angle.			
i.–m. Follow Checklist steps 18 i–m of the General Procedure (insert needle, aspirate, inject medication, remove needle, massage site).			
19.–21. Follow Checklist steps 19–21 of the General Procedure (leave patient in comfortable position, discard syringe and needle in "sharps" container, wash your hands).			
Evaluation			
22. Evaluate as in Checklist step 22 of the General Procedure (six rights followed, correct site used, effectiveness of medication assessed, side effects identified).			
Documentation			
23. Document as in Checklist step 23 of the General Procedure (medication, dosage, route, site, time, and signature).			

(continued)

Procedure for Using the Z-Track Technique	Needs More Practice	Satisfactory	Comments
Assessment			
1.–5. Follow Checklist steps 1–5 of the General Procedure for Giving Injections (review medication record, check physician's order, review medication information, assess patient's size and build, assess need for assistance).			
Planning			
6.–8. Follow Checklist steps 6–8 of the General Procedure (determine appropriate needle and syringe, wash your hands, gather equipment).			
Implementation			
9.–17. Follow Checklist steps 9–17 of the General Procedure (read the name of the medication from the record, check the label on the medication before picking it up, check label again before calculating and preparing dosage, draw up medication, check label of vial or ampule and dosage, carry syringe to bedside, place MAR or identification card with medication, identify patient, explain to patient).			
18. Give the Z-track injection. **a.–f.** Follow Checklist steps 18 a–f of the General Procedure (provide privacy, put on clean gloves, select appropriate site and clean it, allow site to dry, place swab between fingers, remove needle guard).			
g. Pull skin and tissue laterally until taut.			
h. Hold syringe like a dart and insert needle at 90° angle.			
i. Aspirate.			
j. Do not release laterally displaced tissue.			
k. Inject medication slowly.			
l. Remove needle and immediately release skin.			
m. Do not massage injection site.			

(continued)

Procedure for Using the Z-Track Technique *(Continued)*	Needs More Practice	Satisfactory	Comments
19.–21. Follow Checklist steps 19–21 of the General Procedure (leave patient in comfortable position, discard syringe and needle in "sharps" container, wash your hands).			
Evaluation			
22. Evaluate as in Checklist step 22 of the General Procedure (six rights followed, correct site used, effectiveness of medication assessed, side effects identified).			
Documentation			
23. Document as in Checklist step 23 of the General Procedure (medication, dosage, route, site, time, and signature).			
Procedure for Giving Intradermal Injections			
Assessment			
1–5. Follow Checklist steps 1–5 of the General Procedure for Giving Injections (review medication record, check physician's order, review medication information, assess patient's size and build, assess need for assistance).			
Planning			
6–8. Follow Checklist steps 6–8 of the General Procedure (determine appropriate needle and syringe, wash your hands, gather equipment).			
Implementation			
9–17. Follow Checklist steps 9–17 of the General Procedure (read the name of the medication from the record, check the label on the medication before picking it up, check label again before calculating and preparing dosage, draw up medication, check label of vial or ampule and dosage, carry syringe to bedside, place MAR or identification card with medication, identify patient, explain to patient).			

(continued)

Procedure for Giving Intradermal Injections *(Continued)*	Needs More Practice	Satisfactory	Comments
18. Give the intradermal injection. **a.–f.** Follow Checklist steps 18 a–f of the General Procedure (provide privacy, put on clean gloves, select appropriate site and clean it, allow site to dry, place swab between fingers, remove needle guard).			
g. Stretch skin at selected site.			
h. Hold syringe at 10°–15° angle, with needle bevel facing up.			
i. Insert needle just until bevel is no longer visible.			
j. Inject medication slowly.			
k. Withdraw needle.			
l. Do not massage.			
m. Circle site with marking pen.			
n. Assess site for reaction at appropriate time.			
19.–21. Follow Checklist steps 19–21 of the General Procedure (leave patient in comfortable position, discard syringe and needle in "sharps" container, wash your hands).			
Evaluation			
22. Evaluate as in Checklist step 22 of the General Procedure (six rights followed, correct site used, effectiveness of medication assessed, side effects identified).			
Documentation			
23. Document as in Checklist step 23 of the General Procedure (medication, dosage, route, site, time, and signature).			

MODULE

51

ADMINISTERING MEDICATIONS TO INFANTS AND CHILDREN

MODULE CONTENTS

PREREQUISITES

Successful completion of the following modules:

(continued)

P R E R E Q U I S I T E S (c o n t i n u e d)

If you are giving medications by routes other than the oral route, you will need to complete the appropriate additional module.

Module 49   Administering Medications by Alternative Routes
Module 50   Giving Injections
Module 53   Administering Intravenous Medications

Proficiency in mathematics of dosages and solutions is also essential to safe medication administration. This is especially critical with regard to medications for children. Because dosages are small, even minimal numerical errors can have serious consequences. Additionally, children are typically more sensitive to adverse effects of medication because of their immature metabolic systems. See Module 48, Administering Oral Medications, for a self-test on the mathematics of dosages and solutions.

OVERALL OBJECTIVE

To adapt medication administration procedures to the special needs of infants and children.

SPECIFIC LEARNING OBJECTIVES

Know Facts and Principles	Apply Facts and Principles	Demonstrate Ability	Evaluate Performance
1. Safety and accuracy State the nurse's responsibility for safe dosage.	Given a situation, identify safety hazards.	Maintain safety and accuracy when administering medications to infants and children.	Evaluate safety with instructor.
2. Calculating pediatric dosages State the formula for obtaining a safe child's dose when the reference provides a dose per kilogram. State the formula for obtaining a safe child's dose when an adult dose is given and the child's weight is known. State the formula for obtaining a safe child's dose when an adult dose is given and a chart is available for determining child's body surface area.	Select correct formula to calculate a safe child's dosage, using the information available.	Calculate safe child's dosage when the reference provides a dosage per kilogram. Calculate a safe child's dosage when the child's weight is known. Calculate a safe child's dosage when both weight and height are known.	Check accuracy of calculation with instructor.
3. Dosage forms for children State the age at which a child can usually swallow tablets and capsules.			
4. Parent involvement Discuss appropriate ways parents may be involved in giving medications.	Give an example of how you might involve a parent in giving an oral medication.	Include parents when giving medication to a child.	Evaluate interaction with instructor.
5. Vehicles for the administration of oral medications List five vehicles commonly used to administer oral medications. State four factors to be considered when deciding which vehicle to use for mixing with a medication.	Given a specific situation, identify an appropriate vehicle to administer a medication.	Use an appropriate vehicle to administer a medication to a child.	Evaluate choice with instructor.

(continued)

S P E C I F I C   L E A R N I N G   O B J E C T I V E S (c o n t i n u e d)

Know Facts and Principles	Apply Facts and Principles	Demonstrate Ability	Evaluate Performance
6. *Measuring pediatric dosages*			
Identify which tablets can be divided.	Given a situation, choose a method of measuring a liquid medication.	Measure a liquid medication in a syringe.	Evaluate choice with instructor.
List methods of measuring liquids for children.			
7. *General approaches to giving medications to children*			
Identify seven general approaches to giving medications to children.	Give an example of how each approach might affect nursing action.	In the clinical setting, choose an approach to be used for a specific child.	Evaluate choice with instructor.
8. *Techniques for gaining the child's cooperation*			
List three techniques for gaining a child's cooperation.	Give examples of situations in which each technique might be used.	In the clinical setting, choose a technique for gaining a child's cooperation.	Evaluate choice with instructor.
9. *Restraining children for injections*			
Describe three methods of restraining an infant or child.	Give examples of situations in which each method of restraining an infant or child for an injection might be used.	In the clinical setting, choose a method for restraining a specific child for an injection.	Evaluate choice with instructor.
10. *Procedure for administering pediatric medications*			
List additional steps that must be taken when assessing a child for medication administration.	Adapt steps to individual patient situation.	Under supervision, give medication to a child or infant.	Evaluate own performance with instructor.
List the various factors that affect planning of medication administration to children.			
11. *Documentation*			
Know information to be documented.	Identify documentation method used in assigned facility.	Correctly document medication given to child.	Evaluate own performance with instructor.

LEARNING ACTIVITIES

1. Review the Specific Learning Objectives.
2. Read through the module as though you were preparing to teach these concepts and skills to another person. Mentally practice the techniques.
3. For the list of medications below, calculate the safe dosage for the child described. (Answers appear at the end of Learning Activities.)
   a. Meperidine (Demerol), adult dose 50 mg, child's weight 44 lb
   b. Penicillin G, adult dose 600,000 units, child's height 4 feet 1 inch and child's weight 68 lb. Find body surface area and calculate safe dosage.
   c. Tetracycline, child's dosage 25 to 50 mg/kg/day divided into four doses. What is the safe individual dose for a 20-kg child?

Answers for Practice Problems:
   a. 14.67 mg
   b. 352,941 units
   c. 250-mg dose (1000 mg/day)

4. In the practice setting:
   a. Examine various scored tablets. Practice breaking a scored tablet.
   b. Examine a 3-mL, a 5-mL, and a 1-mL (tuberculin) syringe. Compare the accuracy with which you could draw up 0.2 mL in each.
   c. Examine various liquid medications. Practice drawing up a correct dosage of oral medication in a syringe.
   d. Practice positioning a child for topical medications.
   e. Practice different methods of restraining a child for an injection.
5. In the clinical setting, arrange with your instructor to give medications to a child. Include an oral medication, an injection, and a topical medication.

Administering Medications to Infants and Children

Rationale for the Use of This Skill
When children require medications, it is often necessary to use special techniques to administer the medication(s) safely and successfully. Knowledge of physical growth and development is essential to enable you to make informed decisions regarding the necessary technique.[1]

▼ NURSING DIAGNOSIS

The major nursing diagnosis to keep in mind when giving medications to children is Risk for Injury. Children can be injured by medications given in the wrong dosage, at the wrong time, or by an incorrect route. They can also be injured by the omission of essential medications, the administration of an incorrect medication, or by inaccurate documentation. Although this nursing diagnosis will not appear on the nursing care plan, it applies to every situation in which a child is being given medications.

SAFETY AND ACCURACY

Safety and accuracy take on special meaning when you are giving medications to infants and children. Besides observing the three checks and the six rights, you must pay special attention when computing dosage. Although the physician computes the dosage when ordering the medication, the nurse should also compute the dosages *as a double check for safety.* If the nurse's computation indicates that the ordered dosage exceeds the safe dose level, it is the nurse's responsibility to consult with the physician, pharmacist, or nursing supervisor *to clarify the correct dosage before proceeding.*

Safety enters into each action taken. *Children are dependent on the adults around them for protection from the hazards of modern healthcare.* The nurse's judgment and discretion are crucial. Safety must be considered when deciding how to administer the medication, whether to restrain the child, how to restrain the child, and in every aspect of care.

[1]Rationale for action is emphasized throughout the module by the use of italics.

CALCULATING PEDIATRIC DOSAGE

Many standard references provide the recommended dosage for children as a dosage *per kilogram of body weight.* When this is the case, the correct dosage is easily figured, using this formula:

If the scales available do not weigh in kilograms, you can first compute the weight in kilograms by dividing the weight in pounds by 2.2.

$$\begin{array}{c}\text{Recommended} \\ \text{dosage} \\ \text{per kilogram}\end{array} \times \begin{array}{c}\text{Child's} \\ \text{weight in} \\ \text{kilograms}\end{array} = \begin{array}{c}\text{Safe} \\ \text{child's} \\ \text{dosage}\end{array}$$

Other commonly used formulas for calculating a safe pediatric dosage are based on weight and body surface area. The formula based on body surface area is considered the most accurate *because it reflects several parameters related to metabolism and size.* The body surface area is found by plotting weight and height on a nomogram such as that found in Fig. 51–1.

To find body surface area:

1. Locate the child's height on the scale to the left.
2. Locate the child's weight on the scale to the right.
3. Draw a straight line between the two and read the surface area in square meters from the scale labeled SA.

The line on the chart shows that for a child 116 cm tall and weighing 19 kg the body surface area is 0.78 m². In the center of the chart is a simple scale for using weight only for the child of normal height and weight.

$$\frac{\begin{array}{c}\text{Body surface area of} \\ \text{child in square meters}\end{array}}{\begin{array}{c}1.7 \\ \text{(Average adult body} \\ \text{surface in} \\ \text{square meters)}\end{array}} \times \begin{array}{c}\text{Average} \\ \text{adult} \\ \text{dose}\end{array} = \begin{array}{c}\text{Safe} \\ \text{child's} \\ \text{dose}\end{array}$$

The formula based on weight is commonly used, *because it is not necessary to have a nomogram available.* This formula is considered to have a fair degree of accuracy and is called *Clark's Rule.*

$$\frac{\begin{array}{c}\text{Weight of child} \\ \text{in pounds}\end{array}}{\begin{array}{c}150 \\ \text{(Average adult weight} \\ \text{in pounds)}\end{array}} \times \begin{array}{c}\text{Average} \\ \text{adult} \\ \text{dose}\end{array} = \begin{array}{c}\text{Safe} \\ \text{child's} \\ \text{dose}\end{array}$$

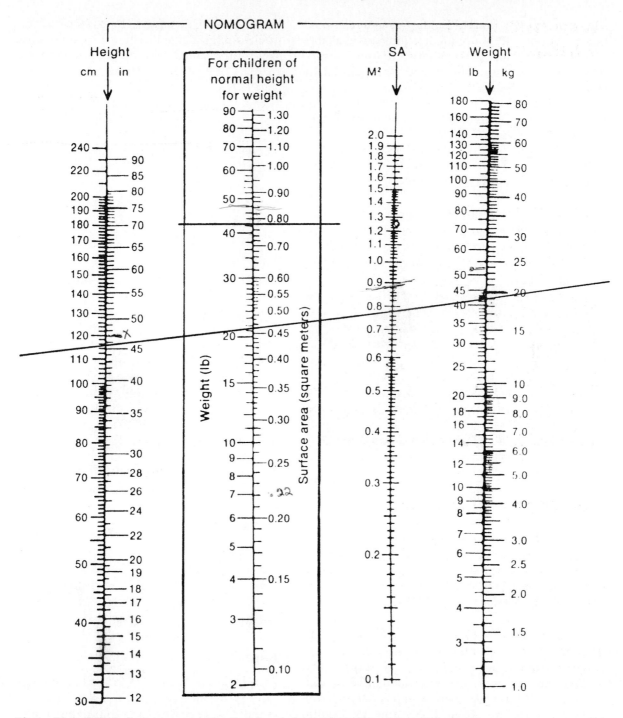

Figure 51–1. Body surface nomogram. Use the left scale for height and the right scale for weight to locate the surface area on the scale labeled SA. Use the scale in the rectangle to determine surface area using weight only for the child of normal height and weight. (From Behrman, R. E., (Ed) (1992), *Nelson's textbook of pediatrics*, 14th ed. Philadelphia: W. B. Saunders, p. 1827)

No formula for determining pediatric dosage is totally correct *because children respond to drugs differently than adults.* When an ordered dosage is larger than that identified as safe through calculation, consult with the pharmacist and the physician. The dosage may be appropriate based on the individual drug action, but an error in dosage is possible and must be investigated.

DOSAGE FORMS FOR CHILDREN

Most children can easily learn to swallow tablets and capsules by ages 4 or 5 years. Some children may be taught to take tablets as early as age 2, but this is unusual. Other children still cannot swallow tablets at ages 6 or 7. Knowing the abilities of the individual child is important. Many medications are available in a liquid form that is suitable for children. It is always appropriate to consult with the pharmacist with regard to whether a liquid form is available. Sometimes tablets may be crushed and mixed with a soft food, such as applesauce or ice cream, *to facilitate the child's taking them.*

PARENT PARTICIPATION

In many hospitals, parents and other family members are encouraged to spend as much time as possible with the child. When giving medications to a child whose parent is present, include the parent as well as the child in your planning.

Explain to the parent what the medicine is. If the medicine causes any special care needs, such as a need for increased fluid intake, share that information *so the parent can participate effectively in the child's care.*

Typically, a child will take an oral medication with minimal distress if it is given by the parent. This procedure is perfectly acceptable *as long as you stay to see that the medication is swallowed.* If you are giving an injection that is painful, do not ask the parent to restrain the child unless no other options are available. *This way the parent maintains the role of comforter and protector and is not associated with causing pain.* It is usually most helpful to the child if the parent stays and offers reassurance that the procedure will soon be over *so the child does not feel abandoned.*

VEHICLES FOR ADMINISTRATION OF ORAL MEDICATIONS

Some foods and fluids are used *to make oral medications more palatable.* Honey, syrup, jelly, custard, applesauce, and other fruits may be mixed with crushed tablets *to make them easier for the child to swallow.* A puréed food or viscous liquid, such as syrup, holds particles in suspension. The medication should be mixed with the smallest amount of food possible *so the child is more likely to take the entire amount.* Liquid medication may be mixed with juice or soda. Again, a small amount is used. The vehicle chosen is determined by the child's preferences, the taste of the medication (a strong taste is more effectively masked by a food with a distinct flavor), the diet prescribed for the child, and the nature of the medications. For example, one would not choose a sugared food for a diabetic child. Or if the medica-

tion cannot be given with foods containing calcium, one would not give it with ice cream or custard.

It is unwise to mix a medication with the child's regular food or bottle for two reasons. *First, if the child fails to eat all the food or finish the bottle, he or she has not received the complete dose, yet it is impossible to tell exactly what amount has been omitted. Second, the child may transfer dislike of the medication to dislike of the food, and this may interfere with adequate nutrition.*

MEASURING PEDIATRIC DOSAGES

Tablets

Whole tablets are used when possible *because this makes dosage more accurate.* Tablets are broken only if they are scored by the manufacturer. *Scoring allows for a fairly clean break and accurate dosage. It is almost impossible to break an unscored tablet accurately.* Sometimes a tablet can be dissolved in a carefully measured amount of water, and then the correct portion of the solution given. This method is accurate if the medication dissolves completely.

One effective way of crushing a tablet to mix with a vehicle is by using a mortar and pestle (see Fig. 48–2). On some units a commercial pill crusher (see Fig. 48–3) may be available. If neither of these is available, the tablet may be crushed between two spoons (Fig. 51–2A). Whichever method you choose, leave the tablet in the unit-dose package while it is being crushed, if possible (Fig. 51–2B). *The packaging keeps the medication clean and keeps the full amount contained so no part of the dose is lost.* If the tablet does not come in a unit-dose package, you can place it inside a paper medicine cup before crushing.

Liquids

Liquids can be measured in a medicine cup. *For accuracy,* a syringe (without a needle) should be used to measure very small amounts of liquid medication (Fig. 51–3A). *The smallest syringe that will measure the correct amount will give the most accurate dosage.* The medication can then be administered using the syringe (Fig. 51–3B).

Some liquid medicine comes with a medicine dropper, with measuring gradations marked on the dropper. The dropper is used to measure the medication but not to give the medication orally *because the dropper must be kept clean so it can be returned to the bottle.* A dropper without calibrations will not pro-

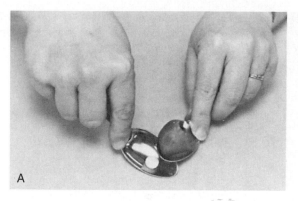
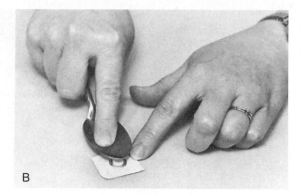

Figure 51–2. **(A)** Crushing a tablet between two spoons. **(B)** Crushing a tablet in a unit-dose package. (Courtesy Ivan Ellis)

vide an accurate drug measurement. Avoid transferring a liquid medication among containers unnecessarily *because some of the medication will cling to the container each time it is transferred, and an inaccurate dose may result.* Calibrated spoons, syringes, and droppers are available in several sizes (for example, 0.5 tsp, 1 tsp, 2 tsp, 3 tsp) and can be purchased at most pharmacies (Fig. 51–4A). Parents can be advised to use these devices when administering medications at home (Fig. 51–4B).

GENERAL APPROACHES TO ADMINISTERING MEDICATIONS TO A CHILD

1. Be honest and direct with both the child and the parents. It is important to establish and maintain trust with children. If trust is established, *the child will cooperate more effectively in care.*
2. Acknowledge the child's feelings and behavior.

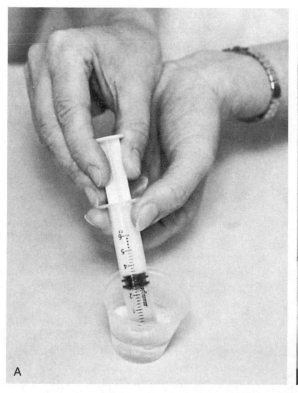
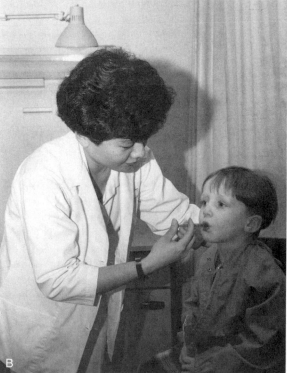

Figure 51–3. **(A)** Measuring an oral liquid in a syringe. **(B)** Nurse using a syringe to administer liquid medication to a toddler.

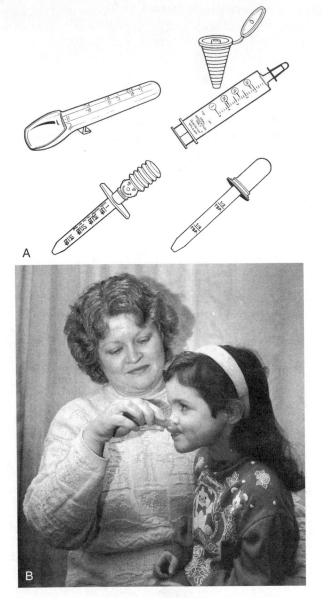

Figure 51–4. (A) Calibrated spoons, syringes, and droppers are available in several sizes (for example, 0.5 tsp., 1 tsp., 2 tsp., 3 tsp.) and can be purchased at most pharmacies. (Courtesy Apothecary Products, Inc., Burnsville, Minnesota) **(B)** Mother using calibrated spoon to give medication.

The child may be angry or upset. Telling the child that he or she should feel positive or cooperative is setting an unrealistic expectation. *Acceptance of the child's feelings enhances the child's feelings of self-worth.* If the child rejects you because you have caused discomfort, continue to be warm and positive toward the child, but do not press for a positive response.

3. Praise the child freely. *Praise is an effective reinforcer* and should be used at every opportunity. *The child who receives a lot of praise feels good about himself or herself and is better able to withstand adverse events.*

4. Offer only appropriate choices. *Whenever a choice is offered to a child, either alternative must be acceptable.* If no alternative is acceptable, do not offer one. Do not say, "Do you want to take your medicine now?" "No" is an unacceptable alternative. Instead, say, "It is time for your medicine. Do you want to take it with orange juice or grape juice?"

5. Be quick and positive in your actions. *If you hesitate or delay the process, you offer more opportunity for the child to respond negatively. The child will perceive your hesitancy and become more anxious and reluctant.*

6. Offer all explanations in terms appropriate for the child's age. For a toddler, this may mean you say only, "Okay, take this." For a 5-year-old, you might say, "Here is some medicine to help you feel better." For a 10-year-old, you could say, "This medicine is to help your throat infection." *A child's need for information is directly related to the ability to understand that information.*

7. Expect cooperation, but be prepared for noncooperation. *Expectations are transmitted to the child in various ways. In most instances the child will respond to your expectations.* If you expect cooperation, the child will cooperate. If you expect the child to resist, he or she often will. *Some children will not cooperate whatever the situation,* and you should be prepared for this. For instance, if you are giving an injection, have everything ready and arrange ahead of time for others to help restrain the child. Those assisting should be unobtrusively present and should be called on to help the child "hold still" until the procedure is finished. Restraining should be regarded as a safety measure and not as punishment.

GAINING THE CHILD'S COOPERATION

Diverting the young child's or infant's attention with a toy or a game may *decrease concern about the medication.* This is not to imply that you sneak up on a child or lie, but simply give the child another interest on which to focus.

Role playing is sometimes successful in gaining a child's cooperation. The child first gives "pretend" medication to a doll or stuffed toy, and then the nurse gives the medication to the child. In the case of an injection it is more appropriate to give the medication to the child first, and then let the child pretend to give an injection.

For a toddler, making a game of taking medications, such as pretending a spoon is an airplane heading for the "hangar" (the open mouth), *can encourage participation by a reluctant child and make the process almost enjoyable.* In turning medicine time into a fun time, be careful not to give the impression that medicine is not really being given (honesty) or that not taking the medication is a choice. Do not pretend the medicine is candy *because this presents an unsafe situation. A child may seek to have additional "candy" when at home and may take medication inappropriately.*

Forcing a child to take oral medication is not wise. *A child who is crying and upset may aspirate a medication. Medication forced into a child's mouth may be spit out. A child who is very upset may even vomit the medication.*

TECHNIQUES FOR ADMINISTERING MEDICATIONS TO CHILDREN

Take care to prevent aspiration when administering liquid medications to infants. Elevate the infant's head and use your thumb to depress the infant's chin to open the mouth. Then, using the dropper included with the medication or the plastic syringe in which the medication was measured, slowly drop the medication onto the middle of the tongue. If you are using a syringe, remember to remove the plastic syringe cap before injecting into the infant's mouth *to prevent aspiration of the syringe cap by the infant.* The nurse can also insert a disposable dropper or syringe into the side of the mouth parallel to the nipple while the infant is being fed, or put the medication into an empty nipple for the infant to suck. Remember that medications are never added to a bottle of formula *because of the danger that the infant will not drink all of the formula, leaving the amount of medication taken in doubt.*

To help older children who have difficulty swallowing tablets or pills, have them place the pill near the back of their tongue and then drink liquid to wash it down. Some facilities have special glasses that have a shelf that holds the pill. As the child drinks the liquid in the glass, the pill is carried to the back of the throat and swallowed. These cups may be purchased at a pharmacy for home use.

RESTRAINING CHILDREN FOR INJECTIONS

When an injection is ordered, you will need to plan ahead for restraining a child who is younger than school age. For a child aged 5 to 10 years, you may still need another person to help the child "hold still." When choosing a restraining technique, you must first identify the injection site you intend to use (see Module 50, Giving Injections). Discuss the intended site with the person who will assist you in restraining the child. *The goal of restraining a child for an injection is to keep the body still, so the needle does not cause tissue damage.* Also make sure the child's hands cannot reach the syringe and that both hands and arms are positioned so they cannot strike the hands of the person giving the injection.

You may be able to restrain an infant effectively while you give the injection by using your dominant arm to stabilize the baby's body and your other hand to hold the leg firmly (Fig. 51–5). Holding a child on his or her side, with head and arms tucked under one arm and legs tucked under the other, works well when restraining a child while someone else gives an injection (Fig. 51–6).

For a small child who does not resist, you may be able to do this yourself, using the arms to hold the child and having your hands free to give the injection. If the child resists, it is safer to have a second person devote all his or her attention to restraining while you devote your attention to giving the injection.

On occasion, a larger child will resist injections. When this happens and the injection is essential (such as a preoperative sedation), it may be necessary to have two adults to help restrain—one restraining the upper body and arms and one restraining the legs (Fig. 51–7).

Restraining a small child for nose drops or ear drops can usually be done by the person giving the medication. If you place the child across the crib, bed, or lap, with the head toward you extended over the edge, you can hold the head still as you give the drops (Fig. 51–8).

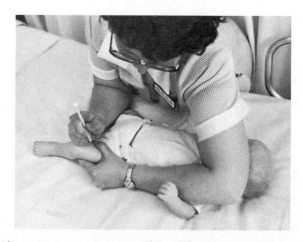

Figure 51–5. Restraining an infant while giving an injection.

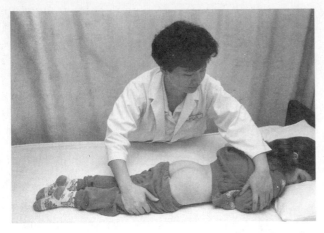

Figure 51–6. Restraining a child for someone else to give an injection.

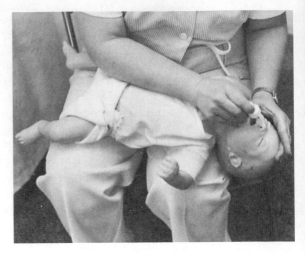

Figure 51–8. Holding a young child to give nose drops. (Courtesy Ivan Ellis)

GENERAL PROCEDURE FOR PEDIATRIC MEDICATION ADMINISTRATION

Assessment

1. Review the medication record used in your facility *to identify whether any medications are to be given to an individual child on your shift.*
2. Examine the medication administration record (MAR) for accuracy and completeness. Check the child's name and room number, the name of the medication, the dosage, the route of administration, and the time(s) the medication is to be given. In addition, be sure to check whether the ordered medications have already been given or if they are to be held. If a vehicle is needed to administer the medication, you may also find information about the child's preference on the MAR.
3. Review information about the medication(s) to be administered. In addition to the generic name of the drug and the common trade names, you will need to know the usual dosage range. If a specific safe child's dose is not given, compute a safe dose using one of the formulas given. If there is any discrepancy, consult with the physician or pharmacist before proceeding. Also review the actions, side effects, and contraindications for the drug as well as information regarding the absorption, detoxification, and excretion of the drug as they relate to the maturity of the child. Finally, you need to be aware of any nursing implications as well as the reason(s) *this* child is receiving *this* medication.
4. Identify the child's physical growth and development level, with special concern for swallowing ability, and the need for additional personnel if the child will need to be restrained. In addition, plan an approach to the child that is appropriate to his or her developmental level.
5. Assess the child *to identify a need for any as-needed (prn) medications ordered.* The child may not be able to request a needed medication, or may not wish to *because, for example, he or she dislikes the taste or does not wish to receive an injection.* To assess a need for pain medication, you may find that using a pain rating scale such as the one pictured is helpful (Fig. 51–9).

Planning

6. Determine what equipment you will need. Consider whether vital signs need to be measured before giving any of the medications, whether a syringe or calibrated spoon is needed to measure small liquid doses accurately, and whether you will need a vehicle to make the medication more acceptable.

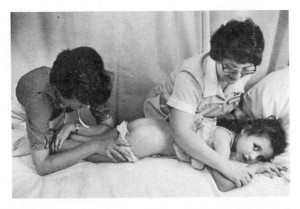

Figure 51–7. Two persons restraining a child for an injection.

Wong-Baker Faces Pain Rating Scale

| 0 | 1 | 2 | 3 | 4 | 5 |

Figure 51–9. The Wong-Baker Faces Pain Rating Scale. Child is told that each face is for a person who feels happy because he or she has no pain (hurt) or sad because there is some or a lot of pain. **FACE 0** is very happy because there is no hurt at all. **FACE 1** hurts just a little bit. **FACE 2** hurts a little more. **FACE 3** hurts even more. **FACE 4** hurts a whole lot. **FACE 5** hurts as much as you can imagine, although you don't have to be crying to feel this bad. The child is asked to choose the face that best describes how he or she is feeling. This chart is recommended for persons aged 3 years and older. (From Wong, D., 1993, *Whaley & Wong's essentials of pediatric nursing.* 4th ed. St. Louis: Mosby, p. 597.)

7. Wash your hands *for infection control.*
8. Assemble all of the equipment you will need. *Delays related to trips out of the room for forgotten items increase any anxiety already present in the child.*

Implementation

9. Read the name of the medication to be given from the record.
10. Check the label on the medication before picking it up (first check).
11. Pick up the medication and check the label again, comparing it with the MAR (second check). If the medication is in a container, do this check before you remove the medication from the container.
12. Remove the exact amount of medication for the child's dose to be given at this time. Use your planned method for measuring accurate dosage. The facility may have a policy requiring that a second nurse verify dosage on some medications, such as insulin.
13. Check the medication label with the MAR once again (third check).
14. Place the medication in a container or on a tray. If the medication is in a unit dose package, leave it in the package until you reach the bedside and determine that it will actually be given.
15. Place a medication card or label on the prepared medication *for identification of the child if the MAR is not to be taken to the patient room.*
16. Approach and identify the patient *to be sure you are administering medication to the correct patient.* Always check the identification band. You may also verify with a parent that you have the right child in addition to checking the name band.
17. Explain what you are going to do and, if appro-

priate, what the medication is for and how it works. The explanation should be appropriate to the child's age and developmental level.
18. Give the medication as appropriate for the route planned, adding planned actions related to:
    a. Making the medication acceptable to the child
    b. Approaching the child
    c. Restraining as needed
19. Watch the child take the medication. If you are not certain it has been swallowed, or if there seems to be a problem with swallowing, have the child open the mouth and look inside to see if the medication is still there.
20. Leave the child in a comfortable position.
21. Discard the medication container if it is disposable. If it is not, rinse it out and place it in the appropriate place for reprocessing.
22. Wash your hands.

Evaluation

23. Evaluate, using the following criteria:
    a. Right child, right medication, right dosage, right route, right time, right documentation.
    b. The criteria established for determining the effectiveness of a specific drug were used and documented.
    c. Side effects, if present, were promptly identified.

Documentation

24. Document on the medication record that the medication was given. Include:
    a. Name of medication
    b. Dosage
    c. Route

d. Time of administration
e. Initials
f. Signature with abbreviation indicating your designation
g. Any specific assessment data required before medication administration

25. Successful methods of administering medications to a child should be added to the Nursing Care Plan.

HOME CARE

When parents must give medications to children at home, they are faced with the same problems and concerns that nurses encounter in the hospital. The major concern is safety, and a secondary concern is the technique for medication administration.

Nurses should counsel parents to safely store medications out of reach of children. The importance of clearly differentiating medicine from food or candy should be emphasized because children may enjoy the taste of flavored medications and try to take more as they would a desired snack food. Teaching parents to read labels carefully is critical to medication safety. Some medications must be scheduled with meals and others given on an empty stomach. These scheduling details are important for medication effectiveness. Sometimes the nurse can offer parents hints for ways to remember medication administration times. For instance, scheduling medications in relationship to a meal, naptime, bedtime, or some other regular activity may help. A chart for checking off dosages may also be of assistance. It is essential to individualize teaching and planning to the situation in each home.

Measuring doses accurately is another important aspect of safety. Household spoons vary in size and are not reliable for administering most children's medications. Many children's medications come with measuring droppers, which should be used when preparing medications. Most pharmacies carry calibrated measuring spoons and droppers designed to be used with infants and children. These devices provide accurate measurement and can help prevent spilling (see Fig. 51–4**A**) when giving a liquid to a child.

Families may also need help with techniques of administering medications to children. Any of the techniques presented in this module might be useful in specific home situations. You might demonstrate how to give a medication while the child is in the hospital or clinic and, if possible, offer the parent an opportunity to give it with you there as support before being expected to manage this task at home. When this is not possible, describe techniques and answer questions raised by the parents.

CRITICAL THINKING EXERCISES

You are caring for a 7-year-old boy whose medication orders include an intramuscular injection. He received this medication the day before, but there is no note on the MAR or his chart regarding his response. Before preparing the medication, you sit down with the boy and his mother and explain that, although he may make noise during the procedure, he must "hold still." Your final question of him is, "Do you think you will be able to hold still by yourself, or should I get someone to help you?" After a thoughtful silence he replies, "You'd better get help." Unit staff members are extremely busy. The boy's mother is there. Will you ask her to assist in restraining the boy? Discuss and give rationale for your decision.

✔ PERFORMANCE CHECKLIST

General Procedure for Administering Medications to Infants and Children	Needs More Practice	Satisfactory	Comments
Assessment			
1. Review the medication record to identify whether any medication(s) are to be given to a child on your shift.			
2. Examine the MAR for accuracy and completeness. Check the child's name and room number, the name of the medication, the dosage, the route of administration, and the time(s) the medication is to be given.			
3. Review information about the medication(s) to be administered. Check reference for a safe child's dose or compute a safe dosage.			
4. Identify the child's physical growth and development level, including swallowing ability, and need for additional personnel if child will need to be restrained.			
5. Assess child's need for any prn medications ordered.			
Planning			
6. Determine what equipment you will need.			
7. Wash your hands.			
8. Assemble equipment.			
Implementation			
9. Read the name of the medication to be given from the record.			
10. Check the label on the medication before picking it up.			
11. Pick up medication and check the label again, comparing it with the MAR.			
12. Remove exact amount of medication for the child's dosage.			
13. Check the medication label with the MAR again.			
14. Place the medication in a container or on a tray.			

(continued)

General Procedure for Administering Medications to Infants and Children (Continued)	Needs More Practice	Satisfactory	Comments
15. Place medication card or label on the prepared medication if MAR will not be taken into room.			
16. Approach and identify patient.			
17. Explain what you are going to do.			
18. Give medication, adding planned actions related to: a. Making the medication acceptable to the child			
b. Approaching the child			
c. Restraining as needed			
19. Watch the child take the medication.			
20. Leave the child in a comfortable position.			
21. Discard the medication container.			
22. Wash your hands.			
Evaluation			
23. Evaluate, using the following criteria: a. Six rights maintained.			
b. Effects were documented.			
c. Side effects were identified.			
Documentation			
24. Document accurately. Include: a. Name of medication			
b. Dosage			
c. Route			
d. Time of administration			
e. Initials			
f. Signature with designation			
g. Any specific assessment data required			
25. Add successful methods of administering medications to the nursing care plan.			

MODULE

52

PREPARING AND MAINTAINING INTRAVENOUS INFUSIONS

MODULE CONTENTS

PREREQUISITES

Successful completion of the following modules:

(continued)

P R E R E Q U I S I T E S   (c o n t i n u e d)

VOLUME 2
Module 33 Sterile Technique
Module 47 Administering Medications: Overview

Satisfactory completion of the self-test on mathematics of dosages and solutions in Module 47, Administering Medications: Overview. If you cannot meet this level of proficiency, you need additional practice in the mathematics of dosages and solutions. Many programmed texts are available for independent study.

Review of the anatomy and physiology of the vascular system.

OVERALL OBJECTIVE

To prepare and maintain intravenous infusions accurately, with comfort and safety for patients.

SPECIFIC LEARNING OBJECTIVES

Know Facts and Principles	Apply Facts and Principles	Demonstrate Ability	Evaluate Performance
1. Equipment			
a. Fluid containers			
Describe two types of fluid containers.		In the clinical setting, select correct fluid container and check for clarity and sterility.	Verify selection with instructor.
State rationale for checking fluid for clarity and sterility.			
b. Administration sets			
State purpose of each type of administration set.	Given a patient situation, identify type of administration set needed.	In the clinical setting, select correct administration set.	Verify selection with instructor.
2. Monitoring and maintaining an infusion			
Describe phlebitis.	Given a patient situation, differentiate between phlebitis and infiltration.	In the clinical setting, make complete assessment of IV.	Verify adequacy of assessment with instructor.
Describe infiltration.			
List causes of obstruction of flow.	Given a patient situation, identify problem that exists with IV.	In the clinical setting, determine correct action for problems identified.	Verify decision with instructor.
List appropriate checks to be made when assessing IV.		Document assessment.	
3. Regulating the flow			
State two methods for calculating correct drip rate.	Given a patient situation, identify whether IV must be regulated.	Calculate drip rate correctly.	Verify calculation with instructor.
		Regulate IV correctly.	
4. Removing and replacing a gown			
Describe method for removing and replacing gown with IV in place.		In the practice or clinical setting, remove and replace gown with IV in place.	Check IV to be sure it is infusing properly when finished.
5. Changing fluid containers and tubing			
State frequency for changing fluid container and tubing.		In the practice setting, change IV tubing, fluid container, and dressing correctly.	Evaluate own performance using Performance Checklist.
State appropriate procedure for dressing IV site.			

(*continued*)

SPECIFIC LEARNING OBJECTIVES (continued)

Know Facts and Principles	Apply Facts and Principles	Demonstrate Ability	Evaluate Performance
6. Discontinuing intravenous infusion			
Describe procedure for discontinuing IV.		In the clinical setting, discontinue IV.	Check site for bleeding and inflammation. Evaluate performance with instructor.
7. Documentation			
State what should be documented regarding IV.		In the clinical setting, document information related to IVs correctly.	Use Performance Checklist to check documentation.

LEARNING ACTIVITIES

1. Review the Specific Learning Objectives.
2. Read the section on intravenous fluid in Ellis and Nowlis, *Nursing: A Human Needs Approach,* or comparable material in another textbook.
3. Look up the module vocabulary terms in the glossary.
4. Read through the module as though you were preparing to teach the concepts and skills to another person. Mentally practice the skills.
5. In the practice setting:
   a. Examine the IV equipment. Identify each of the following:
      (1) Microdrip (pediatric sets) and macrodrip venosets. Differentiate between the two.
      (2) Secondary administration sets (piggybacks)
      (3) Safety needles and needleless devices
      (4) Extension tubing
      (5) In-line filters
      (6) Controlled-volume sets (Peditrol, Soluset, Volutrol)
      (7) IV poles
      (8) Fluid containers (bottles, plastic bags)
      (9) Any infusion control devices available
      (10) Armboards
   b. Read the directions on the package regarding how to set up the brand of equipment you will be using.
   c. Set up an IV line as if it were to be started. Pay particular attention to maintaining sterility.
   d. Attach the end of the IV line to another fluid container, so the fluid will run from the first container to the second. This will simulate an ongoing IV line.
   e. Regulate the drip rate by manual control or using an ICD.
      (1) To 32 drops/minute
      (2) To whatever rate would be needed to deliver the fluid remaining in the container in 4 hours. You will have to figure the drip rate. Consult the equipment container to identify the drops per milliliter delivered by the tubing.
   f. Change the fluid container only.
   g. Change the fluid container and IV tubing and redress.
   h. Using a manikin, remove and replace a gown with the IV in place.[1]
   i. Remove the IV from the manikin's arm as if you were discontinuing the IV.
6. Practice documentation for the following situations:
   a. You have hung an IV, 1000 mL D_5W, to be given over 8 hours from 4:00 PM to 12:00 midnight.
   b. You are maintaining an IV, and it is the end of your shift. On the previous shift, 1000 mL D_5W was started. When your shift began, 100 mL had been given; 50 mL fluid remained. (Simulate any observation data that would be needed.)
   c. You are carrying out an order to discontinue an IV. The entire amount, 500 mL normal saline, has been given.

VOCABULARY

bolus	fluid overload	intravenous
cannula	infiltration	phlebitis
embolus	infusion	thrombophlebitis

[1] If you do not have a manikin, consult with your instructor on improvising a substitute.

Preparing and Maintaining Intravenous Infusions

Rationale for the Use of This Skill

Intravenous infusions are used when patients need fluids, electrolytes, or nutritional supplements that cannot be taken orally. Such infusions are also used when continuous administration of intravenous medications is necessary.

Because the infusion provides direct access to the bloodstream, it involves many hazards: it provides an optimum entry for infectious organisms; it can allow foreign material, including air, to be introduced and to act as emboli; it can cause bleeding; and both the equipment and the solution can irritate the tissue. The nurse is responsible to protect the patient from these dangers.

In addition, ensuring that the infusion flows at the correct rate is a critical nursing responsibility. Too rapid a flow can create a fluid overload of the circulatory system, potentially resulting in death if not corrected. A flow that is too slow may deprive the patient of needed fluid, electrolytes, or medication. The nurse must monitor and maintain the correct infusion rate.

The nurse also is responsible to ensure that the correct fluid is administered, using the appropriate equipment.[2]

▼ NURSING DIAGNOSES

The major nursing diagnosis to keep in mind when preparing and maintaining intravenous infusions is Risk for Injury. Patients can be injured by an intravenous infusion given at an incorrect rate. They can also be injured by the omission of an additive or by the administration of an incorrect infusion or additive in the infusion.

Patients are also at risk for injuries related to tissue irritation from the equipment or the solution. Although this nursing diagnosis will usually not appear on the nursing care plan, it applies to every situation in which a patient is receiving an intravenous infusion.

A second nursing diagnosis related to preparing and maintaining intravenous infusions is Risk for Infection. Patients are at risk for infection related to the disruption of skin integrity inherent in the presence of an intravenous infusion.

Fluid Volume Excess, a third possibility, is usually related to too much fluid over a brief period or perhaps related to an incorrect infusion rate or equipment malfunction.

[2]Rationale for action is emphasized throughout the module by the use of italics.

EQUIPMENT

Fluid Containers

Fluid containers are available in 50-mL and 100-mL sizes partially filled and in 150-, 250-, 500-, and 1000-mL sizes. The most common size is 1000 mL. *Fluid in containers, regardless of size, is comparable in cost,* so it is not a great saving to the patient to supply fluid from a small-volume container as an interim if a larger container is ordered but has not arrived on the unit.

Some fluid containers are glass bottles. *For the fluid to flow out of the bottle, there must be some kind of mechanism to allow air to enter the bottle.* This can be a vent incorporated into the bottle (Fig. 52–1).

If no air vent is in the bottle, there must be an air vent in the administration set. The air vent usually has a filter *that removes contaminants from the air entering the bottle.*

Most IV fluids are now supplied in plastic containers (Fig. 52–2). *Because the plastic container collapses as fluid is removed, no air vent is needed. This prevents nonsterile air from coming in contact with the IV fluid.*

Plastic containers have a characteristic that is of special concern to nurses. They can absorb some types of ink and transport the ink to the fluid. For this reason it is appropriate to do all marking on tapes that can be adhered to the container and not to use any type of ink marker on the plastic. It is also advisable not to use felt-tip pens, *both because the ink may penetrate the surface of the plastic container and because it may become illegible if it comes into contact with moisture. To minimize the potential for infection and possible complications,* the

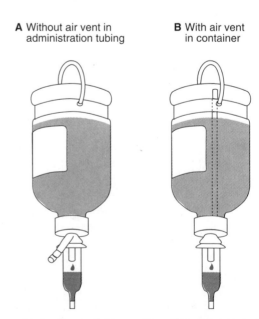

A Without air vent in administration tubing   **B** With air vent in container

Figure 52–1. Glass IV fluid containers. If no air vent is in the bottle, there must be an air vent in the administration set.

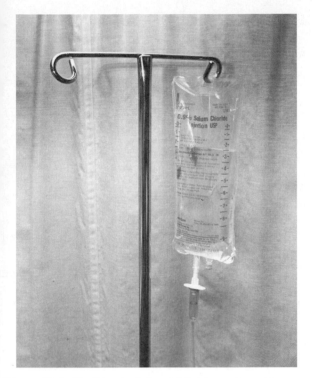

Figure 52–2. Flexible plastic bag IV fluid container. (Courtesy Ivan Ellis)

nurse should closely inspect all containers before administration. Check for leaks, cracks, damaged caps, particulate material, and expiration date.

Another concern is the fact that some medications or additives in IV solutions adhere to the inner surface of a plastic container, *so the patient does not receive an accurate amount of the additive.* For this reason, IV solutions with these additives are prepared by the pharmacy in glass bottles.

Administration Sets

The conventional administration set consists of plastic tubing with a plastic spike that is inserted into the fluid container. The spike must be kept sterile. Below the spike is a drip chamber, *which allows the rate of fluid administration to be monitored by counting the drops falling into the chamber.* If an infusion control device (ICD) is in use, the drop rate within the drip chamber may be monitored by a sensor. The pump cartridge serves as a volumeter, so that the device delivers a programmed volume or rate within a specified period (see the section on ICDs, which follows).

Intravenous tubing with an integral air vent is shown in Fig. 52–3.

Nonvented tubing to be used with a plastic or glass container that has an airway looks much the same, except there is no air vent on the side of the drip chamber. Vented tubing may be used on a contain-er that has an airway or on a plastic container. The fluid will still flow, although the plastic container may not collapse evenly *because of the air in the container.* A ventless glass bottle will not empty if non-vented tubing is used. Special tubing, some with an additional cartridgelike chamber, is used with volume-controlled infusion devices. Review the procedure for the type(s) used in your facility.

If the flow rate is not monitored by an ICD, it is usually controlled by a roller clamp. A screw clamp is also found on some types of tubing, but its primary purpose is to turn the flow on or off. *It does not provide an accurate way to control a flow rate manually.*

The syringe tip (male adapter end of the tubing) fits into the hub of the needle in the vein. Most sets have one or more soft rubber entry ports that reseal after puncture by a needle. These ports are used to inject medications into the IV line. *If any other part of the plastic is punctured with a needle, a leak will result.*

Administration sets are constructed so the orifice in the drip chamber delivers a predictable number of drops for each milliliter of fluid. The most common sets are called *macrodrip sets.* These deliver 10 to 20 drops/mL (cc)[3] (see Fig. 52–3). The drop factor for an individual set is usually given on the box supplied with the product. Sets vary, so consult the manufacturer's package for a correct figure for the delivery rate. Remember that this figure is correct for regular, water-type fluids. *When viscous fluids such as those containing amino acids and fats are given, the number of drops can vary. Because of this, most facilities use an infusion control device to deliver these solutions.*

Most manufacturers also supply *microdrip sets* (Fig. 52–4). These sets deliver 60 drops/mL and can be identified by the fine metal orifice in the drip chamber.

Blood administration sets are characterized by a larger lumen, which delivers fewer drops per milliliter, and a large built-in filter in the drip chamber, which removes any clots or precipitates in the blood (see Module 56, Administering Blood and Blood Products).

Secondary Sets

These sets are designed to allow more than one fluid container to be hung at the same time, in one of three ways. Using a *tandem setup,* the second container is attached to the first by the secondary set. The fluid container on the secondary set (farthest from the patient) empties first, *because this is where the air enters and because it is higher.*

[3]See Table 47–2, Equivalencies, in Module 47, Administering Medications: Overview.

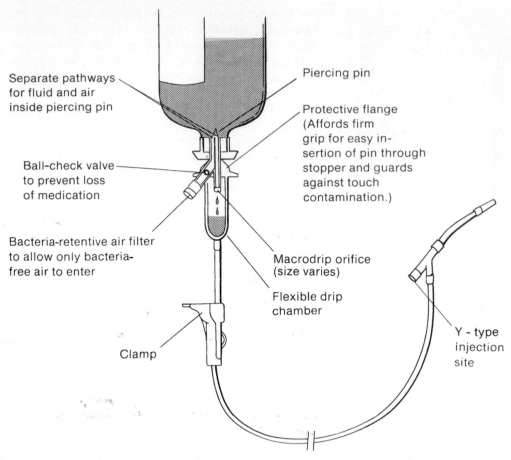

Separate pathways
for fluid and air
inside piercing pin

Piercing pin

Protective flange
(Affords firm
grip for easy in-
sertion of pin through
stopper and guards
against touch
contamination.)

Ball-check valve
to prevent loss
of medication

Bacteria-retentive air filter
to allow only bacteria-
free air to enter

Macrodrip orifice
(size varies)

Flexible drip
chamber

Y - type
injection
site

Clamp

Figure 52–3. Regular (macrodrip) IV administration set. Note that the airway is in the set. (Courtesy Abbott Laboratories, Chicago, Illinois)

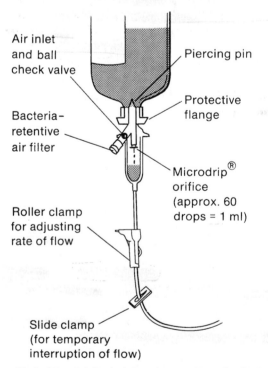

Air inlet
and ball
check valve

Piercing pin

Protective
flange

Bacteria-
retentive
air filter

Microdrip®
orifice
(approx. 60
drops = 1 ml)

Roller clamp
for adjusting
rate of flow

Slide clamp
(for temporary
interruption of flow)

Figure 52–4. Microdrip® administration set. Note the fine metal orifice in the drip chamber. (Courtesy Abbott Laboratories, Chicago, Illinois)

The second method is the *piggyback setup.* The secondary set is used to attach the second bottle to the primary set's tubing. Using the piggyback setup, either bottle can be made to run by shutting off the tubing to one container above the junction and keeping the tubing to the other container open (Fig. 52–5).

The piggyback setup is most commonly used to deliver small volumes of fluid containing medications. In this situation, both lines are left open and the piggyback container is hung higher than the original container. The higher container runs in first. When that container is empty, a special valve at the piggyback entry port allows the lower container to start running.

Two containers can also be hung at the same time by using a *Y-type administration set* (Fig. 52–6). When both arms of the Y are open, the container with the fluid at a higher level empties first, and then the other container empties. The Y set can also be used to alternate solutions.

If the tubing does not contain a special stop valve for the container that empties first, the infusion must be closely monitored. The branch to the container emptying

A variety of "needleless" systems are also available. Some use plastic cannulas that puncture a specially designed IV lock device, and others use a unit with a mechanical valve recessed in a plastic covering. Any male Luer connector can then be used to access this system (Fig. 52–8).

Extension Tubing

Extension tubing is a length of IV tubing with a male adapter on one end and a female adapter on the other, so it can be attached to the main set to create longer tubing. Some extension tubing has a clamp. Extension tubing is commonly added *to allow a patient greater mobility* (Fig. 52–9).

In-Line Filters

In-line filters (Fig. 52–10) are sometimes used *to guard against particulate matter and bacteria entering IV fluids. They also trap small air bubbles.* These filters are typically an integral part of the tubing and are positioned near the end that connects the tubing and the needle. They look like they contain white cotton. When flushing the IV tubing, always thoroughly saturate the filter with solution *to obtain a steady flow of fluid.*

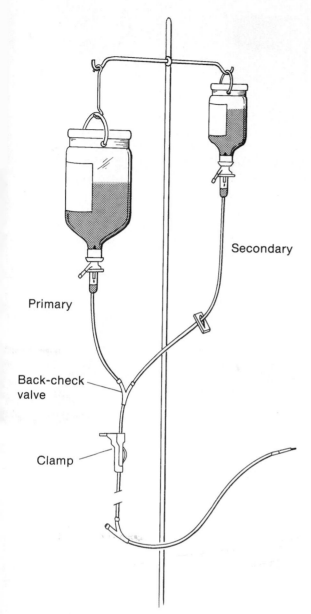

Figure 52–5. Secondary piggyback set. When the piggyback container is empty, a special valve at the piggyback entry port allows the lower container to start running again. (Courtesy Abbott Laboratories, Chicago, Illinois)

first must be turned off while fluid remains in the tube. *If air is allowed to enter one arm of the Y, it will be pulled into the fluid stream coming from the second bottle and could cause a significant air embolus.*

Safety Needles and Needleless Devices

Special needles that protect the staff from accidental sticks ("needle-lock" devices) are available for use when attaching secondary lines. The needle is surrounded with rigid clear plastic that slides over the injection port, guides the needle into the injection port, and secures the needle in place (Fig. 52–7).

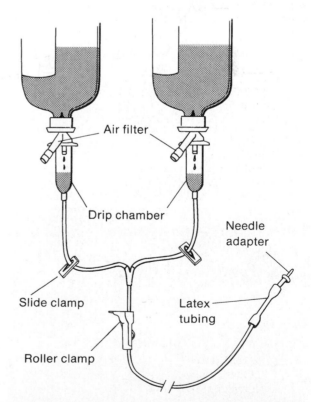

Figure 52–6. Y-type administration set. When both arms of the Y are open, the container with the fluid at a higher level empties first. (Courtesy Abbott Laboratories, Chicago, Illinois)

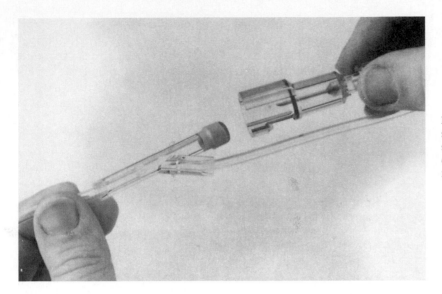

Figure 52–7. Safety needles. The needle is surrounded with rigid clear plastic, which slides over the injection port, guides the needle into the injection port, and secures the needle in place.

Controlled-Volume Sets

Controlled-volume administration sets (Fig. 52–11) have a 100- to 250-mL chamber, which is attached just below the fluid container. The drip chamber is below this chamber. These sets usually deliver a microdrip, or 60 drops/mL. Some controlled-volume

administration sets deliver a macrodrip, or regular drip, at 15 drops/mL. Check the package to make sure you know the correct drop factor. Controlled-volume sets are used when medication must be added to a limited fluid volume or when there is high risk from fluid overload as for the pediatric patient. Another device, primarily for pediatric use, is

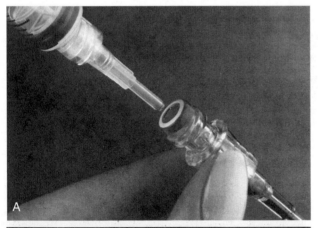

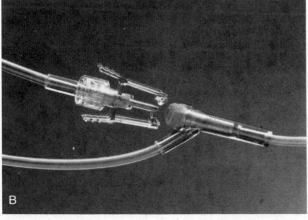

Figure 52–8. Selected components of a "needleless" system. **(A)** Blunt plastic cannula prepared to enter pre-slit injection site. **(B)** Secondary injection set with blunt plastic cannula prepared to enter pre-slit injection port on primary IV set. Note Lever Lock clamps designed to hold the secondary injection set securely in place. (Courtesy Baxter Healthcare Corporation, Round Lake, Illinois)

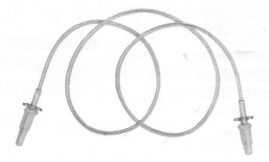

Figure 52–9. Extension tubing. Extension tubing is often added to allow patients greater mobility.

the Benzing retrograde set, which delivers a measured dosage of drug and at the same time displaces an equal amount of maintenance solution from the IV line. More common brands of controlled-volume sets are Peditrol, Soluset, and Volutrol.

IV Poles

IV poles or stands can be attached to a bed, placed on casters on the floor, or suspended from the ceiling with chains or hooks (Fig. 52–12). *The height of the fluid container affects the flow rate. The higher the fluid container, the greater the pressure and the faster the rate.*

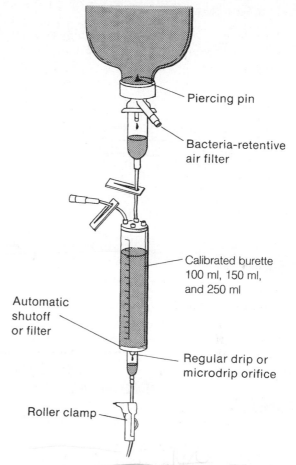

Piercing pin

Bacteria-retentive air filter

Calibrated burette 100 ml, 150 ml, and 250 ml

Automatic shutoff or filter

Regular drip or microdrip orifice

Roller clamp

Figure 52–11. Controlled-volume administration set. These sets are often used when medication must be added to a limited fluid volume or for administering fluids to children. (Courtesy Abbott Laboratories, Chicago, Illinois)

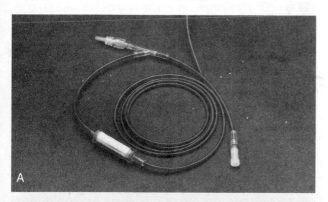

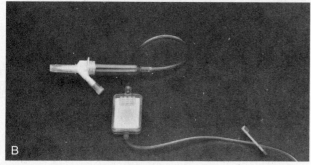

Figure 52–10. In-line filters. **(A)** Distal in-line filter. **(B)** Proximal in-line filter located near drip chamber. (Courtesy Abbott Laboratories, Abbott Park, Illinois)

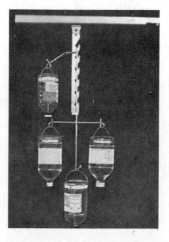

Figure 52–12. IV stands. IV poles and stands can be attached to a bed, placed on casters on the floor, or suspended from the ceiling with chains or hooks. (Courtesy American Hospital Supply Corp., McGaw Park, Illinois)

Extension Hangers

Various metal wires or plastic hooks may be used to hang one bottle on an IV pole lower than the other. The higher bottle then flows in first (see Fig. 52–5).

Armboards

An armboard is a rigid plastic or cardboard device used to immobilize a hand or arm to assure that an IV site is not disrupted. Commercially produced armboards often consist of a padded flat or molded board. Disposable armboards of heavy cardboard material are also available (Fig. 52–13). Reusable armboards should be disinfected between uses.

Armboards are used infrequently *because they interfere with the motion of the wrist or elbow joint, or both. Also, hand veins are preferred for the site of IV needles. The veins in the antecubital fossa are reserved for drawing blood and other essential tests.* Occasionally, however, *when a patient has hand veins that cannot be used or is extremely restless or confused,* an armboard is used to immobilize the needle site. Although armboards come in various lengths, use the shortest board to accomplish the task *so that maximum mobility can be maintained.* If the need for an armboard arises and none is available, improvise with cardboard padded with towels.

Infusion Control Devices

Healthcare facilities are increasing their use of infusion control devices (ICDs) because these devices provide safer intravenous therapy for patients and save valuable staff time. Because more than two dozen manufacturers are producing ICDs, you will need to investigate the types used in your facility and follow the specific instructions for their use. For purposes of this module, we discuss these devices in general terms.

An ICD is most commonly used when the IV fluid contains a medication and a precise rate of administration is necessary to maintain a therapeutic blood level; when the fluid contains an additive that might have adverse effects if given too rapidly (such as a high concentration of glucose or amino acids); or when the patient is unable to tolerate any excess fluid volume.

Two types of devices are available to regulate the flow rate of an intravenous infusion—controllers and pumps. Regardless of which is used, it is essential for the nurse to know that when the tubing is released from the machine, it must be manually regulated by using the clamp unless the device in use provides "free flow protection"—that is, includes a mechanical or electronic safety mechanism that prevents free flow. Without free flow protection, the roller clamp is totally open when the machine is operating, and if it is not adjusted when the tubing is released, *the patient receives a bolus of solution.* You need to become familiar with the devices in use where you practice.

Both controllers and pumps can be either volumetric or nonvolumetric. Volumetric devices deliver a specific desired volume over a long period. An example is the administration of total parenteral nutrition (TPN). Devices that are nonvolumetric are designed to deliver a constant drop rate over a short period. One example is the administration of medications to patients with heart irregularities or seriously low blood pressure. Nonvolumetric devices are less accurate than volumetric ones *because the drop size of different solutions can vary,* depending on the viscosity of the fluid.

Controllers

The least complex type of controller is one that regulates the rate in drops per minute. This type of device has a drop counter and a mechanism for applying pressure to the tubing. It is set for the desired number of drops per minute (nonvolumetric device). Controllers such as these are being replaced by models in which flow rates can be set in milliliters per hour (volumetric devices).

In the controller, gravity is responsible for the pressure in the tubing. Changing the height of the fluid container changes the pressure and thus the flow. If the IV infiltrates, the flow will eventually stop *because the pressure of gravity is less than the tissue pressure that will build up as the IV infiltrates.* This feature makes the controller the preferred device when the fluid contains a medication that could cause tissue damage if infiltration occurred.

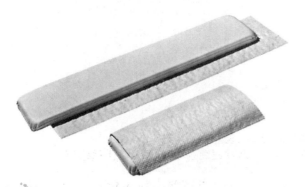

Figure 52–13. Armboards. It is best if you use the shortest board available to accomplish the task, so that maximum mobility can be maintained. (Courtesy American Hospital Supply Corp., McGaw Park, Illinois)

The controller can deliver a constant rate of flow but will not necessarily deliver a precise volume of flow, because variations in IV tubing and fluid viscosity affect the size of the drop. This feature makes it appropriate for situations where rate of flow is important for titrating medication dosage but the exact volume of fluid delivered is not critical.

Pumps

There are three types of pumps: syringe, peristaltic, and cassette. *Syringe pumps* are designed to deliver measured doses of medications and are discussed in Module 53, Administering Intravenous Medications. *Peristaltic pumps* deliver IV solutions by a squeezing action on the tubing. *Cassette pumps* collect a small, specified amount of solution in a reservoir and then deliver that volume. *Cassette pumps require special tubing,* which makes them more expensive to use than controllers. Pumps are set for milliliters per hour, and the fluid is then delivered at that rate. *Because of their high degree of accuracy in volume administered,* these devices are best suited to situations in which the volume administered is critical, such as in the infant or for TPN.

Pumps do not depend on gravity to maintain a rate of flow. Pressure is provided by a mechanism within the system. This positive pressure allows the fluid to be administered into an arterial line, where pressure is needed to overcome the arterial blood pressure. The same pressure is a disadvantage when infiltration occurs. *The machine can continue to pump fluid into the tissue, causing an extensive infiltration if the patient is not assessed frequently.*

All pumps have multiple alarm systems that notify you when the infusion is occluded, when air is in the system, or when the desired infusion volume has been reached. Alarms may alert you to other problems, too, depending on the type of device(s) in use in your facility. Multiple electronic infusion control devices may be in use when the patient is an acutely ill individual receiving a variety of fluids and medications.

Check the manufacturer's directions for specific information on operating the pumps in your facility (Fig. 52–14).

Newer infusion control devices include a combination pump and controller (the user chooses the function desired) and a pump that delivers infusions through two separate channels with separate controls for each line. A new ambulatory pump, controlled by a microprocessor, weighs less than 1 pound and is the size of a small portable radio.

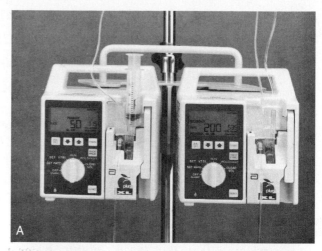

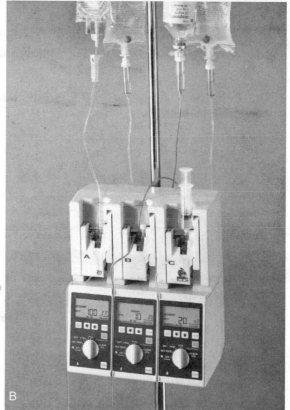

Figure 52–14. Volumetric infusion systems offer dual channel drug delivery which can deliver fluids from bags, bottles, syringes, and vials. **(A)** Two pumps are mounted to a tandem carrier. **(B)** A single pump with 3 separate channels and 3 individual lines to the patient. (Courtesy Abbott Laboratories, Abbott Park, Illinois)

MONITORING AND MAINTAINING AN INFUSION

An important nursing responsibility is to monitor an IV infusion and to maintain its flow. Monitoring involves looking for signs and symptoms of phlebitis (or thrombophlebitis), infiltration, and obstruction

DATE/TIME	
2/3/99	IV site inflammation:
1430	S "When I move it, my hand hurts where the tube goes in."
	O IV site slightly reddened. IV patent and infusing last 150 ml of ordered solution.
	A Potential phlebitis at IV site.
	P Observe IV site q h until completion of infusion.
	D. Myers, NS

Example of Nursing Progress Notes Using SOAP Format.

of flow. Maintaining the infusion includes taking actions to assure patency, adjusting the rate, changing the site dressing, and changing the fluid container and tubing.

Phlebitis—inflammation of the vein—can be present with or without a clot in the vein. When there is a clot, the condition is technically thrombophlebitis. In actual practice the two terms are used interchangeably. Phlebitis is characterized by redness, warmth, pain, and swelling at the IV site. It seems to occur more rapidly when electrolytes (especially potassium) are in the solution and when antibiotics are being administered through the IV, and results from direct irritation of the vessel.

When phlebitis occurs, the course of action is determined by the *degree* of the problem. Table 52–1 shows one method of scaling degrees of phlebitis along with appropriate interventions.

Infiltration is the leaking of IV fluid into the surrounding tissue. Pallor, swelling, coolness, pain at the site, and usually a diminished IV flow rate are all indications of infiltration. Infiltration is caused most often by a cannula that has become dislodged and penetrated a vein wall. The term "cannula" refers to both metal needles and various plastic intravenous access devices. It can also occur around a plastic cannula that has been in place for an extended period. An infiltrated IV must be discontinued. Degrees of infiltration can also be scaled. Table 52–2 shows a method of scaling infiltration along with corresponding interventions.

Decreased flow rate or cessation of fluid flow are indications of occlusion. Occlusion may be caused by a clot forming over the cannula lumen, by particulate matter clogging the filters, by the lumen of the cannula being positioned against the wall of the vein, by kinking or pressure on the tubing, or by a position of the arm that occludes the vessel proximal to the IV site. The nurse should locate the source of the obstruction and correct it (Table 52–3).

The entire infusion should be checked systematically each time the nurse is at the patient's bedside. In addition, IVs should be routinely checked every 4 hours for rate of flow and level of fluid. Insertion

---

Table 52–1.   Evaluation and Treatment of IV Phlebitis

Assessment Grading Criteria	Interventions
1+ Pain at site*	1. Assess severity of phlebitis.
2+ Pain at site or along vein Mild erythema localized at site	2. Discontinue IV catheter.*
	3. Apply warm pack to site assessed 3+ or greater.
3+ Pain at site or along vein Erythematous at site and streaking along vein	4. Determine if drug/fluid is causative factor of phlebitis. Arrange for drug dilution or rate change, if appropriate.
	5. 3+ and 4+; Initiate QA[1] Problem Record
4+ Pain and severe erythematous streak along vein Palpable cord or induration of vein area	6. 4+; Report problem to physician; obtain order for K-Pad® treatment. Notify unit RN if they are to be involved in treatment plan.

*1+Phlebitis—Intervention steps 3 and 4 may be initiated first to determine if mild pain relieved without removing IV catheter; reassess site in 1–2 h.
[1] Quality assurance
Courtesy Swedish Hospital Medical Center.

Table 52–2. Evaluation and Treatment of IV Infiltration

Assessment Criteria	Interventions

1+ Small area of swelling at or above IV site
2+ Area of swelling areound IV site > 1″ and < 2″
3+ Area of swelling > 2″; involves one surface or extremity
    Skin cool over swollen area
4+ Gross infiltrate involving circumference of extremity
    Skin very tight and cold to touch
	1. Determine if infiltrated fluid/medication is a vesicant; refer to tx of extravasation.
	2. Assess severity of infiltrate; discontinue IV catheter
	3. Grade 3+ and 4+; Elevate extremity on two pillows.
	4. Grade 4+: Notify unit RN and initiate QA[1] Problem Record.

[1] *Quality assurance*
Courtesy Swedish Hospital Medical Center

sites should be routinely checked every 8 hours for redness, swelling, temperature changes, and patient comfort (Centers for Disease Control, 1983).

PROCEDURE FOR MONITORING AND MAINTAINING AN INFUSION

Assessment

1. Review the form used to monitor IVs in your facility to identify whether an individual patient has intravenous fluids infusing.
2. Examine the IV record for accuracy and completeness as prescribed by your facility, noting the
   a. Number of the IV infusing
   b. Ordered contents of the fluid container
   c. Time the IV was hung
   d. Time the IV is to be completed. Note also if another IV is to follow the one currently infusing.
3. Review information about the IV fluid infusing, if you are not familiar with it.
4. Identify the patient *to be sure you are performing the procedure for the correct patient.*

5. Explain that you are monitoring the intravenous infusion.
6. Review the entire system for obvious problems.
7. Check the IV container.
   a. Note the date and time.
   b. Verify that the correct solution is infusing.
   c. Verify that the number of the fluid container is correct.
   d. Note the fluid level in the container. Verify that at the current rate, the fluid will be infused at the designated time.
8. Inspect the drip chamber.
   a. Check that the drip chamber is filled to an appropriate level. There is usually a mark on the drip chamber indicating the level to which it should be filled.
   b. Check that it is dripping.
   c. Check that the rate is correct.
9. Check the tubing over its entire length for kinks or obstructions.
10. Examine the IV site for signs of phlebitis or infiltration:
    a. Skin color and temperature
    b. Pain
    c. Swelling

DATE/TIME	
7/20/98 1900	D: C/O pain at left hand IV site. Area around IV site swollen and cool. IV not infusing. A: IV discontinued with cannula intact. Warm moist pack applied to IV site and left arm elevated on two pillows. IV nurse notified for restart. R: States "The pain is almost gone." <div align="right">C. Abbott, R.N.</div>

Example of Nursing Progress Notes Using Focus Format.

Table 52–3. Troubleshooting IV Problems

Problem	Action	Rationale
1. IV off schedule	**a.** Calculate rate to finish IV over remaining time If new rate is over 3mL/min for adult or drastically changed (more than 20% increase), consider patient's condition and consult with physician before increasing rate. **b.** Reset flow	**a.** Fluid is absorbed and used over time. Too rapid infusion will simply result in high urine output. If a patient's cardiovascular system is inadequate, fluid overload may occur. **b.** If fluid is behind schedule, infusing at original rate will result in inadequate fluid intake for 24-h period. **c.** Calculating new rate provides adequate fluids in an evenly distributed pattern. **d.** Exact rate may be critical to patient and should be determined by physician.
2. Incorrect solution	**a.** Slow rate to minimum. **b.** Initiate change to correct solution. **c.** Assess patient. **d.** Follow incident procedure for facility. **e.** Notify physician.	You may want to minimize amount of incorrect solution given without losing access to the vein. In some instances the type of solution is critical, and laboratory tests may be necessary to determine action.
3. Tubing kinked	Straighten tubing and check flow rate again.	Kinked tubing slows flow rate. When kink is removed, rate may increase significantly.
4. Flow stopped	Take the following steps to reestablish flow: **a.** Look for obstruction of tubing and correct if present. **b.** Open regulator completely, move to new position, and regulate again if flow begins. **c.** Reposition arm. **d.** Place bottle lower than needle to see if blood flows back, indicating cannula and tubing are patent. **e.** Gently raise cannula hub. If this starts flow, support hub with cotton ball or gauze 2 × 2. **f.** Note height of fluid container and adjust if it is not at least 3 feet above IV site. **g.** Pinch off tubing close to arm above soft rubber section of tube. Then squeeze soft rubber firmly. **h.** Obtain sterile needle and syringe. Insert into injection port closest to IV site. Pinch off tubing above syringe and aspirate. Then open flow.	**a.** Pressure of arm, side rails, and other equipment can obstruct IV tubing. **b.** Changes in position or "fatigue" of plastic may alter flow rate. **c.** Flexing or twisting the forearm can obstruct vein proximaly to IV site, stopping flow. **d.** Pressure in vein causes blood backflow when pressure in tubing is reduced. **e.** Cannula tip may be against wall of vein or a valve, obstructing flow. **f.** The force of gravity may not be adequate to overcome the pressure of the blood in the vein. **g.** Slight pressure may force wall of vein away from needle. It may also release small clot. (A clot small enough to be dislodged in this manner is small enough not to be of danger as an embolus.) **h.** Aspiration can remove clot or clogged fluid. (Clot or clog moves into syringe and is removed, so it is not hazardous to patient.)

(continued)

Table 52–3. Troubleshooting IV Problems (Continued)

Problem	Action	Rationale
5. Bubbles in tubing	**a.** For a few small bubbles high in tubing: (1) Turn off flow. (2) Stretch tubing taut downward. (3) Flick tubing with fingernail. Bubbles will flow up to drip chamber. (4) Start flow and regulate. **b.** For large amounts of air high in tubing: (1) Turn off flow. (2) Insert sterile open needle into injection port close to air. (3) Open flow slowly. When air reaches needle it will bubble out. (4) Start flow and regulate. **c.** For air low in tubing, below last port: (1) Turn off flow. (2) Obtain sterile needle and syringe. (3) Insert into port closest to IV site. (4) Pinch tubing distal to port and close it off. (5) Aspirate air into syringe. Blood will return into tubing. (6) Start flow rapidly to flush out blood. (7) Regulate flow.	**a.** Air is lighter than fluid and therefore rises. **b.** Because air is lighter than fluid, when it reaches opening it rises out of tubing. **c.** Aspiration creates suction, pulling contents of tubing—including air—into syringe.
6. Drip chamber full of fluid, so drip is not visible	For flexible drip chamber: **a.** Pinch off tubing. **b.** Invert container **c.** Squeeze fluid back into container. **d.** Hang up bottle. **e.** Release tubing.	With drip chamber full, it is not possible to monitor fluid rate. When fluid is squeezed into container, air at top of bottle can enter drip chamber.
7. Solution falls below drip chamber and fluid container is empty	**a.** If tubing is scheduled to be changed: (1) Slow drip rate. (2) Follow directions for changing fluid container and tubing. **b.** If tubing does not need to be changed: (1) Obtain next fluid container, syringe and needles. (2) Connect tubing in use to new container. (3) Fill drip chamber. (4) Aspirate column of air through port on tubing. (5) Regulate flow rate.	**a.** Prevent IV from clotting off. **b.** Aspiration creates suction, pulling contents of tubing—including air—into syringe.

11. If an armboard is being used, remove it periodically to move the arm or leg or *to examine for skin irritation and circulatory impairment*. Then replace the armboard.

12. Identify the specific problem present.

Planning
13. Using the chart on troubleshooting IV problems, plan an appropriate course of action.

Implementation
14. Carry out the action planned.

Evaluation
15. Evaluate, using the following criteria:
   a. Any problem present is identified and corrected.
   b. The correct intravenous infusion is infusing at the correct rate.

Documentation
16. On the flow sheet, note that the correct IV is running, the rate at which it is running, and the appearance of the site.

17. If any problems were identified and corrected,

note those on the nurses' notes or on the flow sheet, as prescribed by your facility.

REGULATING THE INTRAVENOUS INFUSION

The intravenous drip rate must be regulated in drops per minute to provide the ordered quantity of fluid over the ordered period. Many manufacturers provide tables that give this information, but the nurse should know how to compute the rate when tables are not available. Below we give two methods of calculation. Try both and determine which is easier for you.

To calculate the rate using either method, you need three pieces of information:

1. Volume of fluid to be infused
2. Length of time this volume of fluid is to run
3. "Drop factor" (number of drops per milliliter) for the administration set, which is commonly found on the package. (Most administration sets provide 10 gtt/mL, 15 gtt/mL, or 20 gtt/mL. Microdrip sets and most controlled-volume sets provide 60 gtt/mL.)

Method 1

Use the following formula:

$$\frac{\text{volume (in ml)} \times \text{drop factor}}{\text{time in minutes (hours} \times 60)} = \frac{\text{gtt}}{\text{min}}$$

Method 2

1. Divide the total volume by the number of hours to obtain the *milliliters per hour*.

$$\frac{\text{volume}}{\text{hours}} = \text{ml/hr}$$

2. Divide the milliliters per hour by 60 to obtain the *milliliters per minute*.

$$\frac{\text{ml/h}}{60} = \text{ml/min}$$

3. Multiply the milliliters per minute by the drop factor to obtain the *drops per minute*.

$$\text{ml/min} \times \text{drop factor} = \text{gtt/min}$$

Note: The drop rate of microdrip sets, which deliver 60 drops/mL, is always equal to the number of milliliters per hour. Try a few examples using the methods above to check this.

If you are regulating an infusion that is being con-

trolled with an ICD, consult the instructions for the specific device. Most ICDs have to be programmed in the reset mode. Then turn to "operate." If you are using an ICD set in milliliters per hour, use step 1 of method 2 above to calculate the rate.

PROCEDURES FOR CHANGING THE FLUID CONTAINER, TUBING, AND DRESSING

Assessment

1. Review the physician's orders. Pay particular attention to the type of fluid and solution concentration and to the infusion rate. Many abbreviations are used; three of the most common are for concentrations of dextrose or saline.

5% dextrose in water $= D_5W$ or 5% D/W

5% dextrose in normal saline $= D_5N/S$ or 5% D/NS

half-strength normal saline $= \frac{1}{2}N/S$

If you do not understand the orders, be sure to ask.

2. Verify when the tubing and dressing were last changed. *The Centers for Disease Control and Prevention (1983) currently recommend that all IV tubings be changed at least every 72 hours, to decrease the incidence of phlebitis at the site* (see Monitoring and Maintaining an Infusion, earlier in this module). The CDC further recommends that IV dressings be changed every 48 to 72 hours. *Fluid containers are changed every 24 hours.*

Planning

3. Determine what equipment you will need.
4. Wash your hands *for infection control.*
5. Select the equipment.
   a. Obtain the correct fluid, using the three checks.
   b. Select an infusion set. Consider the amount of fluid to be administered and the rate. *If a very slow rate is needed, a microdrip set will provide more accurate regulation. If medications are to be given, a set with multiple injection ports may be needed. For an infant or child, the use of a controlled-volume set is usually routine.*
   c. Note that extension tubing may be needed *to give the patient more mobility.*
   d. Be aware that tape will be needed *to tape the line in place.*
   e. Obtain gloves *to protect yourself from exposure to blood.*
   f. If you will be changing the dressing, gather the items you will need to redress the site according to your facility's procedure.

Implementation

6. Set up the equipment.

a. Examine the fluid container against a light *to check for cracks (if glass), cloudiness, particulate matter, or other evidence of contamination.* If in doubt, do not use the fluid. Select another container and save the potentially contaminated container to be returned to the pharmacy or the central processing department. Check a plastic container for leakage by squeezing. Dampness on the outside of plastic bags is condensation from the sterilization procedure and is expected.

b. Open the package containing the tubing. Be sure to maintain the sterility of the connectors. If the connectors are covered with plastic caps, leave the plastic caps in place until you are ready to connect the tubing. Check the drop factor of the tubing.

c. Open the entry area of the fluid container according to the manufacturer's directions. There should be evidence that the container was sealed, which certifies sterility. Be careful not to contaminate the entry port.

d. Follow the manufacturer's directions about cleaning the entry port with an alcohol swab. Most fluid containers are sealed, so the entry area is sterile and does not need to be cleaned if not touched.

e. Close the regulator on the tubing *so you do not inadvertently fill the tubing with air and spill fluid on the floor.*

f. Insert the spike into the fluid container through the correct entry port.

g. Invert the fluid container with the tubing hanging down. It is convenient to be able to hang the container on a hook or IV pole at this time.

h. For a flexible-plastic drip chamber, squeeze the chamber to fill it half full with fluid. A rigid drip chamber usually fills when the container is inverted.

i. Hold the end of the tubing over a basin or a waste container. Open the regulator gradually and allow the tubing to fill. If the end of the tubing is tightly capped, the cap must be carefully removed *to allow the tubing to fill.* Allow a small amount of fluid to flow out of the line *to clear any particulate matter in the tubing.* Replace the cap when the tubing is full. Be sure all large bubbles are eliminated. *Very tiny bubbles that together do not constitute a large bubble cannot cause an embolus that is dangerous,* so there is no need for alarm if a small bubble is inadvertently administered. However, it is not wise practice to knowingly administer *any* air.

7. Identify the patient *to be sure you are performing the procedure for the correct patient.* Place a towel under the arm *to protect the linen.*

8. Explain what you plan to do.

9. Hang the new fluid container on the IV pole beside the current container.

10. Remove the tape and dressing on the IV site to expose the hub of the cannula. Be gentle and careful. Do not pull at the cannula *or you may dislodge it.*

11. Examine the IV site for signs of swelling or inflammation.

12. Put on gloves *to protect yourself from exposure to blood.*

13. When the hub is exposed, shut off the IV flow.

14. Hold the hub of the cannula firmly and remove the tubing with a twisting motion.

15. Continue holding the hub of the cannula with one hand while you remove the cap of the new tubing and insert it firmly into the hub with the other.

16. Immediately start the new IV infusion at a slow drip rate.

17. Redress the site according to your facility's procedure. If your facility has no procedure, use the following:

a. Clean the site. Povidone-iodine swabs (acudyne, Betadine) are commonly used. However, a recent study indicated that products containing chlorhexidine gluconate were more effective than other agents at reducing bacterial growth (Larson, 1994).

b. Apply a small amount of water-soluble iodine ointment to the needle site. In some facilities an antibiotic ointment, such as Neosporin, is used.

c. If it is the policy of your facility, place a folded 2 × 2 gauze square *under* the cannula *so the site can be observed. This also protects the skin from the cannula and stabilizes it at the correct angle.*

d. Remove gloves.

e. Make an occlusive, or airtight, seal over the dressing with tape or a transparent dressing. The transparent dressing is applied so the cannula hub is outside the dressing and does not have to be removed to change the tubing or examine the site.

f. Write the date, time dressed, and your initials directly on the tape *to facilitate record keeping.* The date and time of *starting* the IV may also be recorded on the tape each time the dressing is changed. In some facilities a special adhesive label is used for this purpose.

18. Regulate the IV to the ordered infusion rate.
19. Mark the container at the beginning level of the fluid with the time the IV was started. Note the time the fluid is to be completed at the bottom of the container. Mark appropriate intervals (such as the fluid level at 2-hour intervals). *This information facilitates monitoring the rate of the IV.* You may mark directly on glass bottles with a large marking pen. You may also place a piece of tape the length of the bottle and mark on that. Commercial tapes are made for this purpose. With a plastic container, remember that you must mark only on a tape *to prevent absorption of ink into the fluid.* This step may be completed when you first obtain the container.
20. Dispose of the used equipment.
21. Wash your hands.

Evaluation

22. Evaluate, using the following criteria:
    a. Tubing and fluid container are changed with no contamination.
    b. IV site is observed and dressing is replaced and dated.
    c. The correct intravenous fluid is running at the correct rate.

Documentation

23. For documentation purposes, IVs can be treated the same as for three other categories: 1) medications, 2) fluids, and 3) assessment.
    a. As for medications, include the exact time the IV was started and stopped and the exact contents in detail.
    b. As for fluids, carefully document quantities of fluid intake (commonly on the intake and output worksheet) to facilitate assessing the patient's fluid balance.
    c. As for assessment, note the patient's response, especially when the fluid infusing might be expected to cause a local reaction. Some charts contain a separate sheet on which IVs are recorded (Fig. 52–15), but the fluid quantities are still entered on the intake and output sheet. Another option for healthcare facilities is a parenteral therapy record (Fig. 52–16). On other charts, IVs are recorded with medications and treatments. Most facilities number each bottle sequentially *to facilitate accuracy in administration and record keeping.*

    When complete tubing is changed or when the IV site is redressed, a notation is made on

IV FLOW RECORD

I V S T A R T	START : SITE	℞ Hand			
	TIME / # ATTEMPTS	1100 / 1	/		/
	GAUGE / LENGTH	18 / 1½"	/		/
	TYPE	Angiocath			
D C	D/C : TIME / SITE EVAL.	/	/		/
	CATHETER INTACT				
	CONVERTED TO HEP LOCK : TIME				
A B G	SITE / ALLENS TEST	/	/		/
	ECCHYMOSIS / HEMATOMA	/	/		/
	INITIALS	JL			

		2300 - 0700	0700 - 1500	1500 - 2300
I V	SITE EVALUATION TIME / CONDITION			1600 OK
	HOURLY BOTTLE CHECK	00-01-02-03 04-05-06-07	08-09-10-11 12-13-14-15	16-17-18-19 20-21-22-23
	DRESSING △ / TUBING △	/	Ø / Ø	Ø / Ø
	INFUSION DEVICE:		Ø	Ø
	SITE EVALUATION TIME / CONDITION			
	HOURLY BOTTLE CHECK	00-01-02-03 04-05-06-07	08-09-10-11 12-13-14-15	16-17-18-19 20-21-22-23
	DRESSING △ / TUBING △		/	/
	INFUSION DEVICE:			
	INITIALS		JL	EK

DATE	IV #	AMOUNT AND SOLUTION	ADDITIVES	INITL'S	TIME IV HUNG	TIME IV COMPLT	FLOW RATE CC/HR	INFU- SION DEVICE	SHIFT CHANGE STATUS TIME	IV #	#CC LEFT TO CNT
6/23/99	1	1000 ml LR		JL	1100	2100	100	Ø			
	2	1000 ml D₅NS		EK	2100		100	Ø	22	2	900

Figure 52–15. IV Flow Record portion of 24-hour Flow Sheet. Space for nurse's signature is on another part of form.

PARENTERAL ACCESS*	08	09	10	11	12	13	14	15	⑯	17	18	19	20	21	22	23	24	01	02	03	04	05	06	07

location, type, use
(1) _LW_ / _P_ / _C_   0800 WNL
(2) _____ / _____ / _____   1600 Site slightly reddened. No swelling or % tenderness
(3) _____ / _____ / _____   2400 WNL
WNL = patent, dressing intact, no redness, tenderness, swelling
☐ NONE

SITE LOCATION CODES:
R = right   FT = foot
L = left   J   = jugular
W = wrist   SC = subclavian
FA = forearm   FM = femoral
AC = antecubital   ABD = abdominal
UA = upper arm   SP = spinal

CATHETER TYPES:
P = peripheral venous catheters
CV = central venous catheters
H-art = hepatic artery catheter
epi = epidural catheter
subq = subcutaneous catheter
intrap = intraperitoneal catheter

USE CODES:
C = Continuous infusion
I = Intermittent

Figure 52–16. Parenteral Access Site Assessment portion of Physical Assessment Flow Sheet. Note criteria for WNL at left of form. Space for nurse's signature is on another part of form.

a separate flow sheet, on the IV sheet, or on the nurses' notes.

PROCEDURE FOR CHANGING THE CONTAINER ONLY

Assessment

1. Review the physician's orders to determine type of fluid.
2. Verify when the tubing and dressing were last changed *to be certain that there is no need for a tubing or dressing change at this time.*

Planning

3. Wash your hands *for infection control.*
4. Obtain the correct container of fluid, using the three checks.

Implementation

5. Take the new fluid container to the bedside.
6. Identify the patient *to be sure you are performing the procedure for the correct patient.*
7. Explain what you are going to do, if appropriate. There may be no need to awaken the patient if he or she is asleep *because you can change the container without disturbing the patient.*
8. Remove the cover from the entry port and place the container on the bedside stand.
9. Turn off the IV flow.
10. Invert the old fluid container.
11. Remove the tubing connector. Be careful not to touch the tubing end.

12. Insert the tubing into the new container.
13. Invert the new container and hang it on the IV pole.
14. Turn on the flow and regulate the rate.
15. Dispose of the old container.
16. Wash your hands.

Evaluation

17. Evaluate, using the following criteria:
    a. Fluid container is changed with no contamination.
    b. IV site and dressing are assessed for any problems.
    c. The correct intravenous fluid is infusing at the correct rate.

Documentation

18. Document:
    a. Time of fluid container change and exact contents of new container
    b. Amount of fluid infused from old container
    c. Assessment of IV site and dressing as facility policy requires.

PROCEDURE FOR CHANGING A GOWN OVER AN IV

In some facilities, gowns with shoulder seams that open and close with snap fasteners are available for patients with IVs. If such gowns are not available, use the following procedure:

DATE/TIME	
1/10/99 8:15 AM	Tubing and dressing changed on IV site. Site Clear. S. Storm, NS

Example of Nursing Progress Notes Using Narrative Format.

To Remove

1. Remove the gown from the free arm and chest.
2. Gather the sleeve on the IV arm until it forms a compact circle of fabric. Hold this circle firmly.
3. Move the sleeve down over the arm, being particularly careful as you pass over the IV site. The sleeve should now be around the tubing, not around the arm.
4. Move the gown up the tubing toward the fluid container.
5. Remove the fluid container from the standard.
6. Slip the gown over the fluid container.
7. Rehang the container.

To Replace

Proceed in the opposite direction.
1. Gather the appropriate sleeve of the gown into a firm circle.
2. Remove the fluid container from the IV stand.
3. Slip the gown over the fluid container (Fig. 52–17).
4. Rehang the fluid container.
5. Carefully move the gown over the tubing and onto the arm.
6. Adjust the gown on the IV arm.
7. Place the patient's other arm in the gown and fasten the gown.

PROCEDURE FOR DISCONTINUING AN IV

Assessment

1. Check the orders carefully. *It is painful as well as expensive for patients to have an IV restarted after it has been discontinued by mistake.*

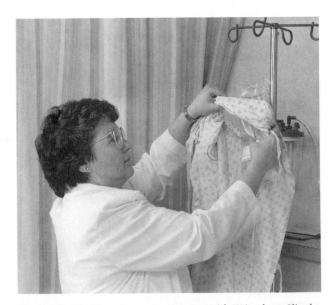

Figure 52–17. Changing patient's gown with IV in place. Slip the gown over the fluid container before moving the gown over the tubing and onto the arm.

Planning

2. Determine what equipment you will need.
3. Wash your hands *for infection control.*
4. Select the necessary equipment.
   a. Sterile cotton ball or an alcohol swab (safe but uncomfortable) or a 2 × 2 sterile gauze square.
   b. Adhesive bandage (such as a Band-Aid)
   c. Clean gloves

Implementation

5. Identify the patient *to be sure you are performing the procedure for the correct patient.*
6. Explain to the patient what you plan to do.
7. Shut off the IV flow.
8. Carefully remove the tape and dressing.
9. Put on clean gloves *to protect yourself from exposure to blood.*
10. Hold the cotton ball, gauze square, or alcohol swab (according to your facility's policy) above the entry site. Be ready to exert pressure as soon as the needle is out, but do not exert pressure on the site while pulling the cannula out. *The pressure compresses the vein wall between the needle and the swab and can damage the vein.*
11. Remove the cannula by pulling straight out in line with the vein. Check the cannula *to make sure no part of it has broken off and remains in the patient.*
12. Immediately put pressure on the site *to control bleeding.*
13. Elevate the patient's arm for about 1 minute. Keep pressure on the site until any bleeding is controlled.
14. Remove gloves.
15. Put the adhesive bandage over the site.
16. Remove all the equipment. Be sure to note the volume of fluid remaining in the container, *to record intake accurately.*
17. Wash your hands.

Evaluation

18. Evaluate, using the following criteria:
   a. Intravenous infusion is discontinued.
   b. Any bleeding is controlled.
   c. Cannula is intact.

Documentation

19. Document appropriately.
   a. On the flow sheet or nurses' notes, document that the IV was discontinued with cannula intact, your assessment of the site, and the time.
   b. On the intake and output sheet, document the intake from the IV that has occurred on your shift. To do this accurately, you will

DATE/TIME	
12/19/99 2038	All fluid infused. IV DC'd with catheter intact. Catheter site without signs of infiltration or infection. —————— S. Juarez, NS

Example of Nursing Progress Notes Using Narrative Format.

have to check whether any fluid was administered on the previous shift and subtract that amount from the total amount of fluid administered from the container.

LONG-TERM CARE

Because an increased number of patients are being admitted to long-term care facilities for rehabilitation or transitional care before returning home, IV infusions and electronic infusion control devices are being seen with greater frequency in these settings. Although the procedures themselves vary little from those used in acute care settings, fragile elderly residents need especially careful monitoring. Increased susceptibility to peripheral infections, fragility of veins, and risk for fluid overload demand more frequent and meticulous inspection of IV sites and schedules.

HOME CARE

Home infusion therapy has become quite common and is related to early discharge from hospitals as well as the need for IV therapy or medications in the treatment of many chronic conditions. In addition, the recognition that hospitalization can be a stressful and disruptive event for patients, especially children, has led hospitals, home health agencies, and private enterprises to set up programs for home infusion therapy.

If you are employed in an acute or chronic care facility and are aware that the individual for whom you are caring will be going home on IV fluids, you will need to coordinate your teaching with that of the agency responsible for overseeing this aspect of care. Generally, the focus of the teaching program is to prepare patients, family members, or other caregivers to administer the required IV therapy safely and independently, using the equipment required.

Teaching requires a careful assessment of caregiver ability, equipment, and home setting. Limited intellectual capacity or manual dexterity as well as fear, distance of the home from the supervising agency, inability to speak English, and risky therapy are among the challenges that may be encountered (Sudela, Newsom, Fox, Summers, & Patel, 1993). Effective and thorough communication is one of the most critical factors that influence the success of a home infusion therapy program.

CRITICAL THINKING EXERCISES

• It is the beginning of your shift and you are doing a routine assessment of all IVs for which you are responsible. When you inspect Mrs. Callihan's IV container, you discover that the solution infusing is not the one ordered. Determine how you will proceed. Plan how you will explain your actions to Mrs. Callihan.

• Home infusion therapy has been ordered for Juanita Gomez, age 5. The pediatric hospital where you are employed has a home care program through which the therapy will be supervised. Juanita's mother works part-time outside the Gomez home. In addition, you know that although Juanita speaks fluent English, her mother's English is quite limited. Evaluate the challenges in this situation and devise ways in which they might be addressed.

References

Centers for Disease Control. (1983). *Guidelines for prevention of intravascular infections.* Washington, DC: US Department of Health and Human Services.

Larson, E. (1994). Does antiseptic make a difference in intravascular device-related complications? *Heart & Lung, 23*(1), 90–92.

Sudela, K., Newsom, T., Fox, L., Summers, P., & Patel, B. (1993). Pediatric home infusion therapy: Obstacles and opportunities. *Journal of Home Health Care Practice, 6*(1), 40–52.

✔ PERFORMANCE CHECKLIST

Procedure for Monitoring and Maintaining an Infusion	Needs More Practice	Satisfactory	Comments
Assessment			
1. Identify whether patient has IV fluids running.			
2. Examine IV record for accuracy and completeness. a. Number of IV infusing			
b. Ordered contents of fluid container			
c. Time IV was hung			
d. Time IV is to be completed			
3. Review information about IV infusing if not familiar with it.			
4. Identify patient.			
5. Explain that you are monitoring the IV infusion.			
6. Review entire system for obvious problems.			
7. Check IV container. a. Date and time			
b. Correct solution infusing			
c. Number of IV container is correct			
d. Fluid level in container and designated time of completion			
8. Inspect drip chamber. a. Filled to appropriate level			
b. Dripping			
c. Rate correct			
9. Check tubing for kinks or obstructions.			
10. Examine IV site for phlebitis or infiltration. a. Skin color and temperature			
b. Pain			
c. Swelling			
11. If armboard in use: Remove, examine for skin irritation and circulatory impairment, and replace.			
12. Identify specific problem present.			

(continued)

Procedure for Monitoring and Maintaining an Infusion (Continued)	Needs More Practice	Satisfactory	Comments
Planning			
13. Using the chart on troubleshooting IV problems, plan appropriate course of action.			
Implementation			
14. Carry out action planned.			
Evaluation			
15. Evaluate, using the following criteria: 　a. Any problem present identified and corrected			
b. Correct intravenous infusion running at correct rate			
Documentation			
16. On flow sheet, note that correct IV is running, the rate, and appearance of site.			
17. If problems identified and corrected, note on nurses' notes or flow sheet.			
Procedures for Changing the Fluid Container, Tubing, and Dressing			
Assessment			
1. Review physician's order for type of fluid and infusion rate.			
2. Check date of last tubing and dressing change.			
Planning			
3. Determine equipment you will need.			
4. Wash your hands.			
5. Select correct fluid container and correct tubing and obtain tape and gloves.			
6. Select the equipment. 　a. Correct fluid			
b. Appropriate infusion set			
c. Extension tubing			
d. Tape			
e. Gloves			
f. Dressing materials if needed.			

(continued)

Procedures for Changing the Fluid Container, Tubing, and Dressing *(Continued)*	Needs More Practice	Satisfactory	Comments
Implementation			
7. Set up equipment. **a.** Examine fluid container.			
b. Open package containing tubing and check drop factor of tubing.			
c. Open entry area of fluid container.			
d. Clean entry port if necessary.			
e. Close regulator on tubing.			
f. Insert spike of tubing into container.			
g. Invert container and hang it up.			
h. Fill drip chamber.			
i. Hold end of tubing over basin or waste container and fill tubing with fluid, expelling all air.			
8. Identify patient and protect linen.			
9. Explain what you plan to do.			
10. Hang new container on stand beside current container.			
11. Remove tape and dressing from IV site.			
12. Examine site.			
13. Put on gloves.			
14. Shut off flow of old IV tubing.			
15. Hold cannula hub while removing old tubing.			
16. While holding hub, remove cap of new tubing and insert it into cannula hub.			
17. Start new infusion at a slow rate.			
18. Redress site. **a.** Clean site with povidone-iodine swab.			
b. Apply ointment to site.			
c. Place sterile 2 × 2 gauze under needle at the entry site.			
d. Remove gloves.			
e. Use tape to make an airtight seal around the dressing.			

(continued)

Procedures for Changing the Fluid Container, Tubing, and Dressing *(Continued)*	Needs More Practice	Satisfactory	Comments
f. Write date and time of dressing change on tape.			
19. Regulate IV to ordered rate.			
20. Mark container with the times of beginning and ending and with intermediate times, to facilitate monitoring.			
21. Dispose of used equipment.			
22. Wash your hands.			
Evaluation			
23. Evaluate, using the following criteria: **a.** Tubing and fluid container changed with no contamination.			
b. IV site observed and dressing replaced and dated.			
c. Correct intravenous infusion running at correct rate.			
Documentation			
24. Record information in correct location for your facility.			
a. Time started and stopped and exact contents of IV.			
b. Fluid intake from discontinued container.			
c. Assessment of IV line and site and patient's response.			
Procedure for Changing the Container Only			
Assessment			
1. Check physician's order for type of fluid.			
2. Verify when tubing and dressing were last changed.			
Planning			
3. Wash your hands.			
4. Select correct fluid container.			
Implementation			
5. Take new fluid container to bedside.			
6. Identify the patient.			

(continued)

Procedure for Changing the Container Only *(Continued)*

	Needs More Practice	Satisfactory	Comments
7. Explain what you are going to do.			
8. Remove cover from entry port of new container.			
9. Turn off IV flow.			
10. Invert old fluid container.			
11. Remove tubing without contamination.			
12. Insert tubing into new container.			
13. Invert and hang new container.			
14. Start and regulate flow rate.			
15. Dispose of old container.			
16. Wash your hands.			
Evaluation			
17. Evaluate, using the following criteria: **a.** Fluid container changed without contamination			
b. IV site and dressing assessed			
c. Correct intravenous fluid infusing at correct rate			
Documentation			
18. Document: **a.** Time of fluid container change and exact contents of new container			
b. Amount of fluid infused from old container			
c. Assessment of IV site and dressing			
Procedure for Removing Patient's Gown			
1. Remove gown from free arm and chest.			
2. Gather sleeve into circle.			
3. Move sleeve down over arm.			
4. Move gown up tubing, toward container.			
5. Remove fluid container from stand.			
6. Slip gown over container.			
7. Rehang container.			

(continued)

Procedure for Replacing Patient's Gown	Needs More Practice	Satisfactory	Comments
1. Gather sleeve into circle.			
2. Remove fluid container from stand.			
3. Slip gown over container.			
4. Rehang container.			
5. Move gown over tubing and onto arm.			
6. Adjust gown on arm.			
7. Put gown on free arm and fasten.			
Procedure for Discontinuing an IV			
Assessment			
1. Check orders.			
Planning			
2. Determine equipment you will need.			
3. Wash your hands.			
4. Select necessary equipment. 　a. Sterile cotton ball, alcohol swab, or 2 × 2 gauze square			
b. Adhesive bandage			
c. Clean gloves			
Implementation			
5. Identify patient.			
6. Explain procedure to patient.			
7. Shut off IV flow.			
8. Remove tape and dressing.			
9. Put on gloves.			
10. Hold swab above entry site.			
11. Remove cannula by pulling straight out.			
12. Put pressure on site.			
13. Elevate patient's arm for 1 minute, keeping pressure on site until bleeding is controlled.			
14. Remove gloves.			
15. Put adhesive bandage over site.			
16. Remove all equipment.			

(*continued*)

Procedure for Discontinuing an IV *(Continued)*	Needs More Practice	Satisfactory	Comments
17. Wash your hands.			
Evaluation			
18. Evaluate, using the following criteria:			
a. Intravenous infusion is discontinued.			
b. Any bleeding is controlled.			
c. Cannula is intact.			
Documentation			
19. Document appropriately.			
a. Document that IV was discontinued with cannula intact, assessment of site, time.			
b. Document intake from IV occurring on your shift.			
Troubleshooting Problems			
1. IV off schedule			
a. Calculate rate.			
b. Reset flow.			
2. Incorrect solution			
a. Slow rate.			
b. Change to correct solution.			
c. Assess patient.			
d. Follow incident procedure.			
e. Notify physician.			
3. Tubing kinked			
a. Straighten tubing.			
b. Check flow rate.			
4. Flow stopped			
a. Look for obstruction and correct.			
b. Open regulator completely, move to new position, regulate again if flow begins.			
c. Reposition arm.			
d. Place bottle lower than needle.			
e. Gently raise cannula hub.			
f. Note height of fluid container and adjust if it is not at least 3 feet above IV site.			

(continued)

Troubleshooting Problems *(Continued)*	Needs More Practice	Satisfactory	Comments
g. Pinch off tubing close to arm above soft rubber section of tube and squeeze soft rubber firmly.			
h. Obtain sterile needle and syringe, insert needle into injection port closest to IV site, pinch off tubing above syringe and aspirate. Open flow.			
5. Bubbles in tubing **a.** For a few small bubbles: Turn off flow, stretch tubing downward, flick tubing with fingernail, start flow and regulate.			
b. For large amounts of air high in tubing: Turn off flow, insert sterile needle into injection port close to air, open flow slowly so when air reaches needle it bubbles out, start flow, and regulate.			
c. For air low in tubing: Turn off flow, obtain sterile needle and syringe, insert into port closest to IV site, pinch tubing distal to port, aspirate air into syringe (blood will return into tubing), start flow rapidly to flush out blood, regulate flow.			
6. Drip chamber full of fluid **a.** Pinch off tubing.			
b. Invert container.			
c. Squeeze fluid back into container.			
d. Hang up bottle.			
e. Release tubing.			
7. Solution falls below drip chamber with fluid container empty **a.** If tubing scheduled to be changed: Slow drip rate, obtain new fluid container and tubing, insert new tubing into needle hub, regulate flow rate.			
b. If tubing does not need to be changed: Obtain next fluid container, connect tubing to new container, fill drip chamber, aspirate column of air, regulate flow rate.			

MODULE

53

ADMINISTERING INTRAVENOUS MEDICATIONS

MODULE CONTENTS

PREREQUISITES

Successful completion of the following modules:

VOLUME 1

Module 1 An Approach to Nursing Skills
Module 2 Basic Infection Control
Module 3 Safety
Module 5 Documentation
Module 6 Introduction to Assessment Skills

VOLUME 2

Module 33 Sterile Technique
Module 47 Administering Medications: Overview
Module 50 Giving Injections
Module 52 Preparing and Maintaining Intravenous Infusions

Satisfactory completion of the self-test on mathematics of dosages and solutions in Module 47, Administering Medications: Overview. If you cannot meet this level of proficiency, you need additional practice in the mathematics of dosages and solutions. Many programmed texts are available for independent study.

Review of the anatomy and physiology of the vascular system.

OVERALL OBJECTIVE

To prepare and administer intravenous (IV) medications using an IV access that is in place and one of the following methods: a controlled-volume administration set, a small-volume container, a syringe infusion pump, a patient-controlled analgesia infuser, an intermittent infusion adapter (IV lock or heparin lock), or a controller.

SPECIFIC LEARNING OBJECTIVES

Know Facts and Principles	Apply Facts and Principles	Demonstrate Ability	Evaluate Performance
1. Hazards			
State signs and symptoms that can indicate adverse reaction to IV medication.		In the clinical setting, evaluate patient's response to IV medication.	Verify own evaluation with instructor.
2. Equipment			
List various types of equipment available and purpose of each.	Given a specific situation, identify equipment needed.	In the clinical setting, choose correct equipment.	Validate choice with instructor.
3. IV medication and administration			
Know where to find information on preparation of IV medication.	Given a specific IV medication order, take appropriate steps to seek information needed.	In the clinical setting, locate and use appropriate information when preparing IV medication.	Double-check preparation, and recheck with instructor.
a. Preparing the medication			
Explain compatibility of IV fluids.	Given a specific IV medication order, check for compatibility.	In the clinical setting, prepare IV medication correctly.	
b. Adding medications to IV fluid			
State reason for injecting only at injection ports.	Identify entry port on fluid container into which medication should be injected.	Add medication to IV fluid container maintaining sterility.	Evaluate own performance using Performance Checklist.
c. Using a controlled volume administration set			
Identify purpose of controlled-volume set. State amount of fluid to be used for diluting medication when using controlled-volume set.	Identify situations in which controlled-volume set is necessary.	Give medication using controlled-volume administration set.	Evaluate own performance using Performance Checklist.
d. Using a small-volume container and secondary administration set			
Identify purpose of small-volume container.	Identify situations in which small-volume container and secondary administration set could be used.	Give medications correctly, using small-volume container and secondary administration set.	Evaluate own performance using Performance Checklist.

(continued)

S P E C I F I C   L E A R N I N G   O B J E C T I V E S (c o n t i n u e d)

Know Facts and Principles	Apply Facts and Principles	Demonstrate Ability	Evaluate Performance
e. Using a syringe infusion pump			
Explain purpose of syringe infusion pump.	Identify appropriate situations for using a syringe infusion pump.	Give medications correctly using syringe infusion pump.	Evaluate own performance using Performance Checklist.
f. Using a patient-controlled analgesia (PCA) infuser			
Identify purpose of a PCA infuser.	Identify appropriate situations for using a PCA infuser.	Teach patients how to use the PCA effectively. Give medications safely and correctly, using the PCA.	Evaluate own performance using Performance Checklist.
g. Using an intermittent infusion adapter (IV lock or heparin lock)			
List reasons for using an IV lock. Explain purpose of heparin or saline solution in lock.	Identify situations in which IV lock would be useful.	Give medication into IV lock. Add heparin or saline solution to lock to maintain patency of IV lock.	Evaluate own performance using Performance Checklist.
h. Using an infusion controller			
Explain purpose of infusion controller.	Identify appropriate situations for using an infusion controller.	Give medications correctly using infusion controller.	Evaluate own performance using Performance Checklist.
i. IV push			
Explain reasons for differences in rate of injection. Explain how to decrease discomfort of IV push medications.	Identify entry port on IV tubing to be used for injection.	Maintain sterile technique while injecting medication at correct rate.	Evaluate own performance using Performance Checklist.

LEARNING ACTIVITIES

1. Review the Specific Learning Objectives.
2. Read the section on IV infusions in Ellis and Nowlis, *Nursing: A Human Needs Approach,* or comparable material in another textbook.
3. Look up the module vocabulary terms in the glossary.
4. Read through the module as though you were preparing to teach the contents to another person. Mentally practice the skills.
5. In the practice setting, do the following:
   a. Draw up medication as you would for an intramuscular injection, using a 21- or 22-gauge needle.
      (1) Inject the medication into an IV fluid container through the correct port, using sterile technique.
      (2) Invert the bottle, observe, and withdraw the needle.
   b. Draw up second dose of medication.
      (1) Inject this into the air vent of the IV bottle.
      (2) Withdraw the needle, invert the bottle, and observe the result.
   c. Draw up medication.
      (1) Set up a controlled-volume administration set (Peditrol, Soluset, Volutrol).
      (2) Fill the controlled-volume reservoir with 100 mL fluid.
      (3) Add the medication.
      (4) Start the flow rate.
      (5) Close both the airway and inlet to the reservoir. Observe the effect.
      (6) Close the airway, and open the inlet to the reservoir. Observe the effect.
      (7) Close the exit to the reservoir, and open the airway and inlet. Observe the effect.
   (8) Regulate the flow to administer medication in 30 minutes. (Calculate the correct rate.)
   d. Draw up the medication using a small-gauge (25 or 26) needle. On an existing IV line, choose an entry port.
      (1) Inject the medication directly into the IV line.
      (2) Watch for air bubbles forced into the line.
      (3) Consider the speed with which the medication can be given.
   e. Draw up the medication using a large-gauge needle. On an existing IV line, choose an entry port. Repeat steps (1) through (3) in step d above. Note the difference in effect of the large- and small-gauge needles.
   f. Draw up medication and heparinized saline or normal saline solution in separate syringes. Inject into the IV lock.
   g. Set up a small-volume container, adding medication in the same way you added medication to the fluid container. Attach the secondary set to an ongoing IV, and regulate the rate.
6. In the clinical setting, do the following:
   a. Inquire about what equipment is available in your clinical facility for administering medications by the IV route.
   b. Arrange with your instructor to observe and carry out (with supervision) IV medication administration using an IV access already in place, a controlled-volume administration set, a small-volume container, a syringe infusion pump, a patient-controlled analgesia infuser, or an intermittent infusion adapter (IV lock).

VOCABULARY

additive	compatible	intermittent infusion	piggyback
anticoagulant	diluent	adapter	thrombophlebitis
bolus	IV lock or heparin lock	laminar airflow hood	venipuncture

Administering Intravenous Medications

Rationale for the Use of This Skill

Intravenous (IV) medications are being used with increasing frequency when rapid effect is necessary, when medications are too irritating to be given by another route, or when the discomfort of frequent intramuscular injections is to be avoided. IV medications also are commonly used for critically ill patients and when a constant blood level of a drug must be maintained.

The nurse must be aware of the potential hazards of IV medications. Sterile technique must be faultless to prevent infection, and all aspects of the procedure must be done correctly. Of course, careful attention to the three checks and six rights is always necessary for safety.[1]

▼ NURSING DIAGNOSIS

The major nursing diagnosis to keep in mind when giving IV medications is Risk for Injury. Patients can be injured by IV medications given in the wrong dose, at the wrong time, or at an incorrect rate of speed. They also can be injured by the omission of essential medications, the administration of an incorrect medication, or inaccurate documentation.

Patients also are at high risk for injuries related to tissue irritation from the equipment or the medication being administered. Although this nursing diagnosis will not appear on the nursing care plan, it applies to every situation in which a patient is receiving an IV medication.

HAZARDS OF ADMINISTERING INTRAVENOUS MEDICATION

Because an IV medication is immediately available to body tissue, any severe reaction to a medication may happen immediately. The major danger is from reactions that interfere with respiratory, circulatory, or neurologic function. Whenever a medication is given IV, observe for noisy respirations, changes in pulse rate, chills, nausea, or headache. *These can be early signs of severe reaction.* If any of these occur, discontinue the medication, and carefully assess the patient. Notify the physician.

[1]Note that rationale for action is emphasized throughout the module by the use of italics.

In addition to these general symptoms, be aware of the possible adverse reactions specific to the medication being given and of possible incompatibilities of different drugs that affect only certain people.

Many IV medications are irritating to the vein and can cause local pain, redness, and swelling, a condition known as *thrombophlebitis.* This may involve the formation of a clot.

Drug incompatibilities can alter or negate the effects of drug(s) or more seriously, cause the patient to experience untoward reactions. Factors that can affect incompatibility are concentration of the drug, length of time in contact, ionic or electrolyte strength, and pH level. Drug incompatibilities can be visual or chemical. A visual incompatibility may be evidenced by precipitation, color change, cloudiness, or the formation of gas bubbles. Chemical incompatibilities can cause the drugs to become inactive or toxic. For example, antibiotics often become unstable when the pH of a solution is very high or very low. *One of the most important ways to prevent incompatibilities is to become knowledgeable about the classifications of drugs that are likely to cause this problem.*

The literature accompanying the medication is one of the best sources of information about incompatibilities and about the appropriate diluent, amount of diluent, and how slowly or rapidly to give the medication. (A rate of 1 mL/min is considered slow.) *The speed of instillation can be related to the desired effect of the medication.* For example, if the patient has suddenly become seriously ill, the physician may order a drug to be given as rapidly as possible. The rate of instillation also can affect the degree of irritation to the vein, *which can cause patient discomfort.* Giving the medication slowly *allows the drug to become diluted by the flow of blood in the vein, which makes it less irritating and less painful.* Again, you should carefully read the literature provided by the manufacturer. If it does not answer your questions, consult a reference book, or contact the pharmacist for assistance.

EQUIPMENT

Bolus or Push IV Medications

IV medications are sometimes ordered to be given as a *bolus* or *push,* which means that a measured amount of medication, diluted or undiluted, is manually instilled through some type of IV device or directly into the vein by venipuncture. When this is the case, the basic equipment is the same as for an intramuscular injection. To begin, select the size of syringe appropriate for the quantity of medication. A small-gauge needle (one with a high gauge number, 25 or 26) injects the medication more slowly; a large-gauge needle (one with a low gauge number, 19 or 20) injects medication rapidly. *The size selected depends on how fast the medication must be given in relation to its viscosity.*

Additive IV Medications

The fluid container has a special entry port for adding medications. In some facilities, medications are added to IV fluids only in the pharmacy, *where an area of minimal contamination from microorganisms is maintained through the use of a laminar airflow hood.* If IV additives are added on the nursing unit, the nurse is responsible to add the medication to the container in an area that is as free from potential contamination as possible.

When adding medications to IV fluids, take precautions *to ensure that the medication and the fluid are thoroughly mixed.* If a medication is lighter or heavier than the solution, it tends either to float or to fall to the bottom of the container, *which means that the patient receives a concentrated dosage of the added medication rather than the desired mixture. To prevent this,* thoroughly agitate the IV bag or bottle before administering. If the added medication has a lipid or oil base, shake the container every 15 to 30 minutes during the infusion. Use a long needle when adding medications through the port of a container *so the medication does not become trapped in the area around the port.*

A small-volume container (minibottle or partial-fill bag) holds 50 to 100 mL of solution. It is used to administer a small volume of medication that must be diluted. The medication is added to the container in the pharmacy or on the nursing unit, and the container is then hung as a secondary administration set.

A controlled-volume administration set (Peditrol, Soluset, Volutrol) is attached to a regular, large IV fluid container. *This set allows a measured volume of fluid to be withdrawn from the large container. The medication can then be added to the controlled-volume reservoir and given at the appropriate rate.* (For a complete discussion of the various types of infusion control devices, see Module 52, Preparing and Maintaining Intravenous Infusions.)

An intermittent infusion adapter, also called an IV lock or heparin lock, is *designed to provide ready access to a vein without having an IV infusing continuously.* A cannula (which may be either a needle or a catheter) is placed in the vein. Attached to the cannula hub is a very short tubing with one or two IV entry ports at the end or a straight male adapter with a rubber cap. A dilute heparinized saline or normal saline solution is injected through the port into the needle and tubing to fill them. *This solution prevents blood from coagulating and blocking the needle.* Whenever the lock is used, it must be refilled with fresh heparinized saline or normal saline solution. If heparinized saline is used, most facilities use a solution containing 10 U of heparin in 1 mL of saline. (Prefilled cartridges are available for this purpose.)

Some facilities have a policy to flush peripheral intermittent infusion adapters with normal saline only (Peterson & Kirchhoff, 1991; Kleiber, Hanrahan, Fagan, & Zittergruen, 1993). These investigators have found that heparin and saline were equally effective in maintaining the patency of the IV lock, but the incidence of pain was greater with the heparin flush solution (Kleiber, et al., 1993). When saline only is used, there is no need for concern regarding giving IV drugs incompatible with heparin or about the effect of heparin on systemic coagulation. Because agencies have varying policies and procedures, in this chapter, these devices are called IV locks.

"Needle-lock" and "needleless" devices that protect the staff from accidental needle sticks are available for use when injecting medications into IV access devices. The needle-lock device is designed to secure an IV connection so that it does not become dislodged. It is composed of a needle surrounded with rigid clear plastic that slides over the injection port, guides the needle into the injection port, and secures the needle into place.

A variety of needleless systems are available. Some use plastic cannulas that puncture a specially designed IV lock device, while others use a unit with a mechanical valve recessed in a plastic covering. Any male Luer connector can then be used to access this system. These systems are costly, but the number of needle stick injuries has been significantly reduced where they are in use (Dugger, 1992; Prince, Summers, & Knight, 1994). A potential disadvantage is that in some cases, there are many component parts to the system, not all necessarily compatible with standard IV locks and tubing. In this module, we assume that conventional needles are in use and specify "needle" in situations in which a needle is the device commonly used. We refer to needle, needle-lock, or needleless connector when all are commonly used. If needleless devices are used in your facility, you will need to become familiar with the directions for their use.

An alcohol swab is needed *for cleaning* whenever a surface is punctured by a needle. Tape may be needed *to reinforce the point of attachment.* Because the sticky residue left by tape may attract microorganisms, devices with Luer-Loks or needle-locks at the points of attachment are preferred.

ADMINISTERING INTRAVENOUS MEDICATIONS

Use the General Procedure for Administering Medications (Module 47, pages 365-366) as the basis for the General Procedure for Administering Intravenous Medications, with the modifications noted below.

For each specific procedure for administering IV medications discussed (Adding to a New Fluid Container, Adding to an Existing Fluid Container, Using a Controlled-Volume Administration Set, Using a Small-Volume Parenteral, Using a Syringe Infusion Pump, Using a Patient-Controlled Analgesia Infuser, Giving Medication by IV Push into an Existing IV, and Giving Medication into an Intermittent Infusion Adapter [IV Lock]), some steps of the General Procedure for Administering IV Medications may be modified. We have included completely the modified steps and references to the steps of the General Procedure that remain the same.

GENERAL PROCEDURE FOR ADMINISTERING INTRAVENOUS MEDICATIONS

Assessment

1. Validate the physician's orders for the medication.
2. Examine the medication administration record (MAR) for accuracy and completeness as prescribed by your facility. Check the patient's name and room number, the name of the medication, the dosage, and the time(s) the medication is to be given. Check for any medication allergies. Note especially whether the ordered medication(s) has already been given or is to be held.
3. Assemble information on the drug, including its effects, the dilution, the rate of administration, and any potential for incompatibility with other IV fluids or medications being given. Each IV medication has specific properties. It is essential that you know a medication's expected actions and potential adverse reactions when you administer IV medication. *Because the system is affected so rapidly,* observe the patient closely for side effects or reactions while the medication is being given and immediately after it is given. Be prepared to act promptly should an emergency occur.
4. Assess the patient to see what type of IV access is present—that is, whether an existing IV infusion is running, whether an IV lock is in place, or whether a venipuncture must be done to administer the medication.

5. Follow step 5 of the General Procedure for Administering Medications: Assess the patient *to identify a need for any prn medications ordered.*

Planning

6. Determine the equipment you will need. If the patient has been receiving IV medications, there may be some equipment in the room.
7. Follow step 7 of the General Procedure: Wash your hands *for infection control.*
8. Select the appropriate equipment based on the necessary method of administration. Often the physician's orders specify the method of IV administration. If an access to the vein is not present, the medication must be given by a nurse skilled in venipuncture. *When multiple IV push medications are needed,* the nurse may request an order for an IV lock from the physician.

"Add to the IV" indicates that the medication should be placed in the large-volume container and will be administered for the time designated for the fluid. Medications given this way must be stable in solution for the length of time the infusion is to run.

Many medications are administered intermittently. These are diluted and mixed in small volumes of solution and are usually prepared in the pharmacy and sent to the units clearly labeled for individual patients. If the medication comes in a small bottle or bag, it is hung piggyback, using a secondary administration set attached to an injection port of the primary IV.

Ready-to-mix IV drug systems also are in use. These systems use minibags filled with a diluent solution, along with vials containing commonly used drugs in powder form. The nurse attaches the vial containing the ordered medication to a port with a break-away seal on the minibag. Next, the nurse squeezes solution into the vial and squeezes and releases the bag to transfer the solution and dissolve and mix the medication. This system allows reconstitution as needed on the clinical unit. The system does not use any exposed spikes or needles (Fig. 53–1).

A second method for delivering small-volume medications is with a syringe infusion pump (Fig. 53–2). This is a small battery-run device that can be carried by an ambulatory patient, hung on a stand, or placed on the bedside table. The medication-filled syringe, prepared either in the pharmacy or by a nurse on the unit, is attached to small-diameter tubing and placed in the pump. The tubing is attached to the IV access. *An alarm on the device alerts the nurse when all the medication has been infused.*

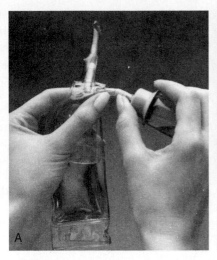 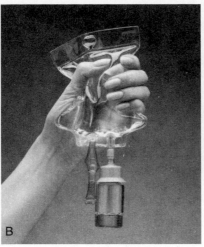 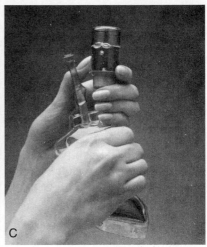

Figure 53–1. Ready-to-mix intravenous drug system. **(A)** After making sure there are no leaks, the nurse creates a fluid pathway by snapping the breakaway seal. **(B)** The nurse then holds the bag with the medication vial beneath it and squeezes solution from the minibag to half fill the vial. **(C)** Next, the nurse inverts and shakes the vial to suspend the medication in the diluent, then squeezes and releases the bag to transfer the solution and dissolve and mix the medication. (Courtesy Baxter Healthcare Corporation, Round Lake, Illinois)

Both of these small-volume methods cost less than other methods, *because tubing can be used for 48 to 72 hours with compatible medications.* Some facilities have extended the use of tubing to 72 to 96 hours based on their own incidence of complications. Follow the policy in your facility.

The nurse must always use a sterile needle when starting medications through an existing line—that is, one within the 48- to 72-hour limit—and the delivery needle must be replaced with another sterile needle at the completion of the instillation. *A contaminated needle could spread*

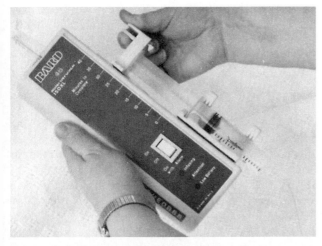

Figure 53–2. Syringe infusion pump. The syringe is placed into the pump so that the upper ridge on the syringe rests on the flange of the pump.

microorganisms to the tubing. The cost of changing needles is minimal, and the procedure greatly reduces the chance of infection at the site.

Implementation

9.–11. Follow steps 9 through 11 of the General Procedure: Read the name of the medication to be given from the record; check the label on the medication before picking it up (first check); and pick up the medication and check the label again, comparing it with the MAR (second check).

12. Determine whether the ordered medication has already been given or is to be held. This is particularly important with medications being administered by the IV route.

13. Follow step 13 of the General Procedure: Check the medication label with the MAR once again (third check).

14. Prepare the medication, using sterile technique. *If the medication is incompatible with the solution already in the line,* prepare a syringe of 5 mL sterile normal saline, half of which will be used to flush the IV line before administering the medication, and the remaining half is used after giving the medication. If you cannot find any information that tells you whether the medications are compatible, it is safer to proceed as if they are not.

15.–17. Follow steps 15 through 17 of the General Procedure: Place a medication card or label on the prepared medication *for identification of the patient if the MAR is not to be taken into the patient's room.* Approach and identify the patient *to be sure you are administering the medication to the correct patient.* Explain what you are going to do and if appropriate, what the medication is for, how it works, and what the patient will experience.

18. Administer the medication in the appropriate manner. See the next sections for specific procedures. Flush the line before and after giving the medication if necessary. Observe the patient carefully while you are giving the medication *to identify any complications immediately.*

19. Follow step 19 of the General Procedure: Leave the patient in a comfortable position.

20. Dispose of the equipment correctly.

21. Follow step 21 of the General Procedure: Wash your hands.

Evaluation

22. Evaluate, using the following criteria:
    a. Six rights were followed: The right patient received the right medication in the right dosage by the right route at the right time, and it was documented in the right way.
    b. The medication was given over the correct time.
    c. The criteria established for ascertaining the effectiveness of a specific drug were used. For example, for a given pain medication, this might be "Pain relief obtained within 10 minutes."
    d. Side effects, if present, were promptly identified.

Documentation

23. Indicate on the medication record that the medication was given. Record the name of medication, dosage, IV route used, the time, and your initials.

24. If 50 or 100 mL fluid is given, add this amount to the intake record if this is the policy. *The cumulative volume of fluid over 24 hours could be significant for the patient on measured intake and output.*

Adding to a New Fluid Container

Medications, vitamins, and electrolytes may be added to the main IV fluid container to be administered over many hours. *Medications given this way provide for a stable blood level. Vitamins and electrolytes given in this manner are available to the body as they are needed.*

To add medications, vitamins, or electrolytes to a new fluid container, follow the steps of the General Procedure for Administering IV Medications as modified below.

Assessment

1. Review the medication record *to determine if any medications, vitamins, or electrolytes are to be added to the main IV fluid container.*

2. Examine the MAR or IV record for accuracy and completeness as prescribed by your facility. Verify the patient's name and room number, the name of the additive, the dosage, and the time over which the fluid is to run.

3. Review information about the medication, vitamin, or electrolyte to be added. Validate that the additive is compatible with the fluid in the main IV container.

4.–5. Follow the steps of the General Procedure for Administering IV Medications.

Planning

6.–7. Follow the steps of the General Procedure.

8. Select the appropriate equipment.
    a. Obtain a large-volume fluid container that has the ordered IV fluid. Be careful when checking this fluid *because all medications are not compatible with all IV fluids.* Your facility may stock 1,000-mL bags of certain IV fluids with potassium chloride 20 mEq or 40 mEq already added *for convenience and safety.*
    b. Use a syringe and needle to draw up the medication or additive to add it to the IV fluid. You also will need an alcohol swab *to prepare the injection site.*

Implementation

9.–17. Follow the steps of the General Procedure.

18. Inject the additive into the new fluid container.
    a. Open the top of the new fluid container, and identify the injection port. This may be designated by the word *Add* or by a triangle on the rubber top. On a plastic bag, the injection port usually appears as a conventional soft rubber injection port, which is self-sealing. If you inserted a needle through the plastic, *you would cause a leak.*
    b. Clean the port with an alcohol swab *for infection control.*
    c. Inject the medication. If the container has an air vent, be sure you do not inadvertently inject into it.
    d. Tilt the container back and forth *to mix the additive thoroughly.*
    e. Hang the new infusion container following the steps in Module 52, Preparing and Maintaining Intravenous Infusions. (Spike entry port of container with tubing, close roller clamp, invert container, and squeeze to fill drip chamber.)
    f. Regulate the flow.

(1) If you are using an infusion control device, thread the tubing through the device according to manufacturer's instructions, and set controls to desired milliliters per hour.

(2) If you are not using an infusion control device, slowly open the roller clamp, and time flow to desired rate.

g. Label the new fluid container with the name and amount of additive, the date and time, and your initials.

19.–21. Follow the steps of the General Procedure.

Evaluation
22. Follow the General Procedure.

Documentation
23.–24. Follow the steps of the General Procedure.

Adding to an Existing Fluid Container

Occasionally it will be necessary to add a medication, vitamin, or electrolyte to an existing fluid container. Be sure to verify precisely the amount of fluid left in the fluid container *to ensure accurate calculation of administration rate.*

To add medications, vitamins, or electrolytes to an existing fluid container, follow the steps of the General Procedure for Administering IV Medications as modified below.

Assessment
1. Review the orders *to verify that a medication, vitamin, or electrolyte is to be added to an existing fluid container.*
2. Examine the MAR or IV record for accuracy and completeness as prescribed by your facility. Verify the patient's name and room number, the name of the additive, the dosage, and time over which the remainder of the fluid is to run.
3. Review information about the medication, vitamin, or electrolyte to be added. Validate that the additive is compatible with the fluid in the existing fluid container.
4.–5. Follow the steps of the General Procedure for Administering IV Medications.

Planning
6.–7. Follow the steps of the General Procedure.
8. Select the necessary equipment:
   a. Needle and syringe of the appropriate size to draw up the medication
   b. Alcohol swab to prepare the injection site

Implementation
9.–17. Follow the steps of the General Procedure.
18. Inject the medication, vitamin, or electrolyte to the existing fluid container.

a. Turn off the IV flow.
b. Invert the fluid container.
c. Clean the medication port with an alcohol swab.
d. Inject the medication into the appropriate medication port on the container.
e. Tilt the container back and forth *to mix the additive thoroughly.*
f. Label the container appropriately.
g. Rehang the IV container.
h. Regulate the flow rate as ordered.

19.–21. Follow the steps of the General Procedure.

Evaluation
22. Follow the General Procedure.

Documentation
23.–24. Follow the steps of the General Procedure.

Using a Controlled-Volume Administration Set

Controlled-volume administration sets are most commonly used in pediatric settings and in situations in which the patient can tolerate only small amounts of fluid. These also are used instead of small-volume parenterals to dilute medication and deliver it intravenously over short periods of time, usually 30 minutes to one hour.

To administer medication using a controlled-volume administration set, follow the steps of the General Procedure for Administering IV Medications as modified below.

Assessment
1. Review the medication record and the IV infusion record *to verify that a medication is to be administered intravenously and to validate that the medication to be administered and the IV fluid being infused are compatible.*
2. Examine the MAR for accuracy and completeness as prescribed by your facility. Verify the patient's room number, the name and dosage of the medication, the amount of the compatible diluent to be used, and the time over which the fluid and medication are to be administered.
3.–5. Follow the steps of the General Procedure for Administering IV Medications.

Planning
6.–7. Follow the steps of the General Procedure.
8. Select the appropriate equipment:
   a. A controlled-volume administration set to attach to the existing fluid container (if this is a new order)
   b. Syringe and needle of the appropriate size to

draw up the medication and an alcohol swab to prepare the injection site

Implementation

9.–17. Follow the steps of the General Procedure.

18. Administer the medication using the controlled-volume administration set.

a. Open the inlet to the controlled-volume chamber. Fill with 50 to 100 mL, depending on the dilution suggested by the drug manufacturer. (Usually 100 mL is used unless the patient has a fluid restriction.)

b. Tightly close the inlet to the chamber.

c. Check the chamber. If it is hard plastic, make sure the air vent is open.

d. Turn on the drip from the chamber to check that the system is functioning correctly before adding medication.

   (1) *If the system does not work, the filters may be clogged,* and you will need to replace the set.

   (2) If the system is functioning, turn off the drip again.

e. Clean the entry port of the fluid chamber with an alcohol swab.

f. Insert the needle through the entry port, and inject the medication.

g. Calculate the drip rate, and regulate the flow. Remember that the controlled-volume set usually has a microdrip orifice. In all sets that deliver 60 drops/mL, the drip rate is the same as the number of milliliters per hour. This needs to be monitored closely to 1) add more fluid to the chamber when the medication finishes (for cautious IV fluid therapy) or 2) open the clamp to restart the flow from the IV container.

h. Label the chamber with the name and amount of medication, date, time, and your initials.

19.–21. Follow the steps of the General Procedure.

Evaluation

22. Follow the General Procedure.

Documentation

23.–24. Follow the steps of the General Procedure.

Using a Small-Volume Parenteral

This method of administration is known as a partial-fill, a piggyback, a minibottle, or a small-volume parenteral. To administer medication using a small-volume parenteral, follow the steps of the General Procedure for Administering IV Medications as modified below.

Assessment

1.–5. Follow the steps of the General Procedure for Administering IV Medications.

Planning

6.–7. Follow the steps of the General Procedure.

8. Select the correct equipment.

a. For an IV lock (intermittent infusion adapter), you will need regular long IV tubing *to give the patient enough line to move about comfortably.* You also will need a needle, needle-lock device, or needleless access device to fasten to the end of the line and insert in the IV lock. The needle should be 1 in long. *A longer needle cannot enter the port completely, which means that the exposed portion could become contaminated with microorganisms. A longer needle can damage the lock itself or the catheter within the vein.* A 19-, 20-, or 21-gauge needle is preferred. *Larger needles put such large holes in the soft rubber cap that the lock may begin to leak. Smaller needles restrict the flow and make it difficult to administer a very viscous solution in the appropriate length of time.* You also will need an alcohol swab and tape *to fasten the tubing to the arm.*

b. For attaching to an existing infusion, you will need a secondary administration set. These sets usually come with a needle enclosed to allow you to insert the secondary set into the primary set. Most manufacturers include an extension hanger in the secondary set package. If the package you are using does not contain an extension hanger, check to find where one can be obtained on your unit. You also will need an alcohol swab and tape *to fasten the secondary set onto the primary set or the needle to the IV lock* if the access device is not a needle-lock or a needleless device or if it does not have a Luer Lok.

c. For attaching a new container to an existing secondary or conventional line, you will need a new sterile needle. Although the needle on the line was sterile and was stored in a cover, *it is impossible for you to know if the needle has become contaminated in any way. Because needles are inexpensive,* it is a prudent practice to change them. You also will need an alcohol swab and tape *to secure the line.*

Implementation

9.–17. Follow the steps of the General Procedure.

18. Administer the medication using a small-volume parenteral.

a. If the container did not come from the pharmacy as a labeled, mixed medication, follow the directions given above for adding to a fluid container, and label the container with the medication, dosage, time, and your initials.

b. If you are using a new tubing set, do the following:

(1) Close the regulator on the tubing.

(2) Clean the top of the small container.

(3) Attach the administration set to the container.

(4) Place the needle or connector on the end of the tubing.

(5) Hang the small container (or hold it up), and fill the drip chamber half full of fluid.

(6) Remove the needle cover, and open the regulator *to allow the tubing to fill with fluid and the air to be expelled;* then recover the needle or connector.

(7) Hang the small container on the IV pole.

(8) Place the main IV container on an extension hanger, *so it is lower than the small container. This allows the liquid in the small container to be instilled first.*

(9) Clean the entry port near the top of the administration set.

(10) Insert the needle from the secondary set into the high port.

(11) Open the regulator on the secondary set.

(12) Use the regulator on the primary line to set the drip rate. When the small container has emptied, the main IV will begin to drip again at the rate set for the small container. At that time, you may need to return to the room to regulate the main IV.

(13) Tape the connection where a needle without a Luer Lok enters the port. It is wise to tape the needle cover at the connection point also. *This way it is readily available to cover the needle when the secondary set must be removed. Covering a needle for removal from the secondary line is a safety precaution for the staff.* Anytime you place a needle cover on a needle, use the one-hand technique discussed in Module 50, Giving Injections.

c. If you are using an existing line, do the following:

(1) Identify the correct used small container and tubing. If multiple medications are being given by secondary set and the drugs are incompatible, a different tubing is used for each. The tubings are changed every 48 to 72 hours, as are all IV tubings, *to guard against the possibility of infection from a contaminated line.*

(2) Clean the top of the new small container.

(3) Make sure the regulator is turned off.

(4) Remove the old small container from the IV pole, and detach the tubing.

(5) Insert the spike of the used tubing into the new small container.

(6) Hang the small container on the IV pole.

(7) Hang the main IV container on the extension hanger.

(8) If the needle for the secondary set is still attached to the primary set, you do not need to take the needle out of the port. If the needle was not attached but was hanging loose or in a used needle cover, change it *for sterility.* Then cleanse the port and reinsert the new needle.

(9) Remove air in the secondary line by "back-filling." To do this, hold the small container lower than the main IV. Then open the regulator on the secondary line. Fluid will begin to flow from the main IV line into the secondary line. Allow the fluid to flow until the fluid has filled the drip chamber halfway.

(10) When the fluid is at the appropriate level in the drip chamber, hang the small container on the IV pole.

(11) Set the correct drip rate for the medication by using the regulator on the main IV. When the medication has finished running, the main IV will begin to drip at the same rate set for the small container. You may need to return to the room to regulate the IV to its previous rate.

(12) Tape the connection, with the needle cover present, as discussed previously.

19.–21. Follow the steps of the General Procedure.

Evaluation

22. Follow the General Procedure.

Documentation

23.–24. Follow the steps of the General Procedure.

Using a Syringe Infusion Pump

The infusion pump is used for small volumes of medication, usually 50 mL or less. In many facilities, syringes containing the medication in a predetermined level of solution are prepared in the pharmacy. When the pump is activated, the medication is delivered at the correct rate (see Fig. 53–2).

To administer medication using a syringe infusion pump, follow the steps of the General Procedure for Administering IV Medications as modified below.

Assessment

1.–2. Follow the steps of the General Procedure for Administering IV Medications.

3. Review information about the medication(s) to be administered. If more than one medication is being administered using the syringe infusion pump, you will need to know if the same tubing can be used for both medications, that is, whether or not they are compatible.

4. and 5. Follow the steps of the General Procedure.

Planning

6.–7. Follow the steps of the General Procedure.

8. Select the appropriate equipment.
  a. Infusion pump, which is usually requisitioned from the central processing department and charged to the patient
  b. Special thin IV tubing designed for these pumps
  c. Sterile 1-in needle, needle-lock device, or needleless access device; syringe; an alcohol swab; and tape

Implementation

9.–13. Follow the steps of the General Procedure.

14. Check the syringe from the pharmacy to make sure you have the right medication for the right patient in the right dosage at the right time, or draw up the medication in the predetermined amount of solution. When the medication is prepared in the pharmacy, it may come with a small air bubble in the syringe. This allows all of the medication to be infused *because the air bubble fills the hub when the syringe is emptied.*

15.–17. Follow the steps of the General Procedure.

18. Administer the medication using the syringe infusion pump.
  a. If you are setting up the syringe infusion pump:
    (1) Attach the end of the tubing that has small "butterfly wings" to the syringe.
    (2) Attach the other end of the tubing to the needle.
    (3) Attach a label to the tubing indicating the date and time.
    (4) Remove the needle cover, and manually flush the tubing and needle with solution. Be careful not to allow medication to get into the air or onto your hands *because of the potential for resistant organism development if antibiotics are sprayed or dribbled into the environment.* Replace the needle cover using the one-

hand technique discussed in Module 50, Giving Injections.
    (5) Using the clips on the pump, place the syringe into the pump so that the upper ridge on the syringe rests on the flange of the pump. Secure the syringe into the pump by lowering the sliding clamp. *This clamp determines the rate of flow.*
    (6) Clean the port to be used, and insert the needle.
    (7) Hang the pump on the IV pole, or place it on the table.
    (8) Turn the rocker switch of the pump on, with or without alarm as desired. When the pump is working properly, a green light will flash on and off.
    (9) Tape the hub of the needle in place.
    (10) When the medication has been infused, the pumping action will stop; solution will remain in the tubing. Remove the needle, and replace it with a covered sterile needle, which should be taped to the pump or IV pole.
  b. If you are using an existing infusion pump, do the following:
    (1) Check the tubing *to be sure it has not been in use for more than 48 to 72 hours.* IV tubing should be replaced every 48 to 72 hours *to decrease the chances of infection* (Centers for Disease Control, 1983). If you are giving the same medication or one that is compatible, you can use the same tubing.
    (2) Remove the used syringe, and discard it.
    (3) Attach the tubing to the new syringe.
    (4) Replace the existing needle with a 1-in sterile needle or connector.
    (5) Place the syringe in the pump.
    (6) Insert the needle or connector into the port as before, and turn on the pump.

19.–21. Follow the steps of the General Procedure.

Evaluation

22. Follow the General Procedure.

Documentation

23.–24. Follow the steps of the General Procedure.

USING A PATIENT-CONTROLLED ANALGESIA INFUSER

Patient-controlled analgesia (PCA) is a system for administering IV pain medications. The patient is able to activate the system when the need for medication arises. PCA is available in two major types—electronic and mechanical.

The electronic version of PCA delivers pain medication through a computer-controlled infusion pump. The unit can be programmed to deliver a continuous infusion, an adjustable patient-controlled dose (sometimes called a *bolus*), or both. A lockout interval also may be specified. During that time, the machine will not deliver another dose. In addition, a 4-hour limit may be set. The nurse programs the infuser according to the physician's orders.

The continuous infusion is ordered to provide the patient with a baseline amount of medication continuously *to prevent deep troughs in serum drug levels.* The patient-controlled dose is the number of milliliters of fluid that is to be given for each individual dose. The physician orders the number of milligrams of drug in each milliliter, or the pharmacy may provide a standardized solution. Morphine sulfate with 1 mg/mL and meperidine with 10 mg/mL are common solutions. The individual injection dose is then calculated to match the physician's prescription. The lockout interval is ordered *to prevent the patient from getting too much medication.* It can be adjusted to specify a period from several minutes to several hours. The *4-hour limit* is set *to limit the total volume to be infused over any consecutive 4-hour period.*

The pump holds a syringe inside a locked case. This syringe is attached to a port on the patient's IV line by a microbore (small-diameter) tubing that has an antireflux valve *to prevent reverse pressure into the syringe.* The medication in the syringe is administered when the patient pushes a control button attached to the machine (Fig. 53–3).

The computer contains a clock and a rechargeable battery *so that the device can be unplugged for transport or ambulation.* The computer records each attempt by the patient to receive medication and each dosage of medication given. By keying in a code on the machine, it is possible to get a complete history of the use of the pain medication, including the total number of milliliters used from the current syringe, the number of attempts and the number of injections given during each hour, and the dose and interval programmed into the machine.

The mechanical PCA is disposable and uses gravity rather than electricity to deliver the medication. Although this device is much less expensive than the electronic version, it does have some limitations. The delivery rate is set at either 2 or 5 mL/h. The patient-controlled dose volume is 0.5 mL and cannot be adjusted. Lockout times are preset at 6 or 15 minutes. This means the strength of the medication solution must be adjusted accordingly. Because the de-

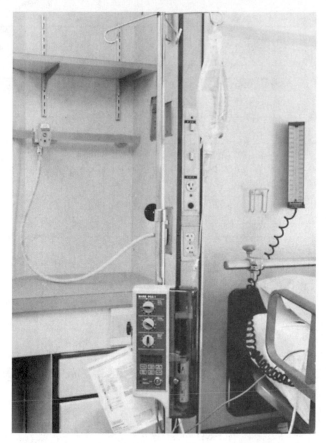

Figure 53–3. PCA infuser. The medication is administered when the patient pushes a control button attached to the machine.

vice cannot be reset, if the patient should need a change in medication dosage, the patient will need a new infuser.

Because patients on either type of PCA are receiving IV narcotics, careful assessment of respiratory status, sedation level, and analgesic effect is essential. Figure 53–4 gives an example of a flow sheet used to record the monitoring of a patient on a PCA.

For the PCA to be effective, the patient must be alert and oriented. Careful teaching is needed *for the patient to use the PCA effectively.* It is important to emphasize that the administration is safe *because the machine is programmed to give only the prescribed dose and cannot give the patient too much medication or too many injections.* It is also important to encourage the patient to use the medication *to maintain comfort* and not to wait a specified time to seek more medication. Even small children can be taught to use PCA effectively.

In evaluating the effectiveness of PCA, the nurse should consider whether the patient is frequently attempting to get injections unsuccessfully. This may indicate that the patient is not feeling adequate pain relief. Excessive sedation or respiratory depres-

Start new record daily at 2400.

DATE   *6-12-99*

PCA

MEDICATION *morphine sulfate*			CONCENTRATION (mg/ml) *1 mg/ml.*							
TIME	*0015*	*0200*								
BOLUS DOSE (ml)	*1 ml.*	*Ø*	*Ø*	*Ø*	*Ø*	*Ø*	*Ø*	*Ø*	*Ø*	*Ø*
PCA DOSE (ml)	*.5 ml.*	→	→	→	→	→	→	→	→	→
INTERVAL (min.)	*10 min.*	→	→	→	→	→	→	→	→	→

EPIDURAL

TIME										
PF MORPHINE										
FENTANYL										

CONTINUOUS INFUSION

MEDICATION			CONCENTRATION (mg/ml)							
INITIALS										

CONTINUOUS INFUSION / EPIDURAL / PCA (Please circle)					INITIAL	SIGNATURE
SHIFT	2200 0600	0600 1400	1400 2200	24 HR TOTAL	*ML*	*M. Lewis RN*
TOTAL ATTEMPTS	*40*	*36*	*30*		*DB*	*D. Baker RN*
TOTAL INJECTIONS	*40*	*36*	*30*		*MK*	*M. Keithly RN*
TOTAL ml USED	*20*	*18*	*15*			
TIME SYRINGE CHANGE	*Ø*	*Ø*	*2100*			
ml DISCARDED	*Ø*	*Ø*	*4 ml*			
INITIALS	*ML*	*DB*	*MK*			

PATIENT CARD IMPRINT

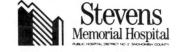

Stevens
Memorial Hospital
PUBLIC HOSPITAL DISTRICT NO 2 SNOHOMISH COUNTY

PAIN MANAGEMENT FLOW SHEET

SMH NUR 041 (REV. 10/91)

Figure 53–4. Flow sheet for administering IV medications.

sion may indicate that the individual dose is too large for the patient or that the interval between injections is too short.

To set up a PCA unit, refer to the specific directions for the brand used in your facility. Also refer to your facility's policy book for guidelines on managing the narcotics used in the machine and monitoring the patient.

Giving Medication by IV Push Into an Existing IV

To give medication by IV push into an existing IV, follow the steps of the General Procedure for Administering IV Medications as modified below.

Assessment
1.–2. Follow the steps of the General Procedure for Administering IV Medications.
3. Review information about the medication(s) to be given. Especially note the recommended speed of injection and the dilution and diluent, if appropriate.
4.–5. Follow the steps of the General Procedure.

Planning
6.–7. Follow the steps of the General Procedure.
8. Select the appropriate equipment.
  a. Syringe large enough to accommodate the medication and the correct amount of diluent, if any is needed
  b. Needle appropriate to the viscosity of the medication and to the recommended speed of injection
  c. Alcohol swab

Implementation
9.–17. Follow the steps of the General Procedure.
18. Administer the medication by IV push into the existing IV infusion.
  a. Identify the injection port closest to the patient. (*An injection port must be used because it is self-sealing. Puncturing the plastic tubing will create a leak.*)
  b. Clean the port with an alcohol swab.
  c. Insert the needle firmly into the port.
  d. Pinch off the IV line between the port and the end of the bottle *to close it off. Doing this prevents the medication from going up into the bottle.*
  e. Inject the medication at the correct rate, taking into account the amount of tubing between the injection port and the IV insertion site. If the amount of medication to be injected is small and the distance to the IV insertion site large, you will need to recalculate the IV rate of flow *to ensure that the medication does not enter the patient's body at a rate too rapid to be safe.* Alternatively, you can flush the IV

tubing with an amount of normal saline equal to the amount of fluid in the tubing between the injection port and the IV insertion site. If the normal saline is injected at the appropriate rate, the medication will enter the patient's circulation at the correct rate.
  f. Observe the patient for any immediate effects or side effects.
  g. Release the tubing when the injection is completed.
  h. Withdraw the needle.
19.–21. Follow the steps of the General Procedure.

Evaluation
22. Follow the General Procedure.

Documentation
23.–24. Follow the steps of the General Procedure.

Giving Medication Into an Intermittent Infusion Adapter (IV Lock)

This is a variation of giving an IV push medication. To give medication into an intermittent infusion adapter (IV lock), follow the steps of the General Procedure for Administering IV Medications as modified below.

Assessment
1.–2. Follow the steps of the General Procedure for Administering IV Medications.
3. Review information about the medication(s) to be given. Especially note the recommended speed of injection and the dilution and diluent, if appropriate.
4.–5. Follow the steps of the General Procedure.

Planning
6.–7. Follow the steps of the General Procedure.
  8. Select appropriate equipment.
  a. Syringe large enough for medication and diluent, if needed
  b. Needle appropriate to viscosity of medication and speed of injection
  c. Separate syringe for the heparinized or normal saline solution. If more than one medication is to be given, prepare enough heparinized or normal saline for the number of flushes you will need to do.
  d. Enough alcohol swabs for the number of medications and flushes to be administered

Implementation
9.–13. Follow the steps of the General Procedure.
14. Prepare the medication and the heparinized or normal saline solution in separate syringes.
15.–17. Follow the steps of the General Procedure.
18. Administer the medication using an intermittent infusion adapter (IV lock).

a. Locate the IV lock. It is usually on the forearm or the back of the hand.
b. Inspect the site. Look for signs of phlebitis, and check that the cannula has not dislodged.
c. Clean the port of the IV lock with an alcohol swab.
   (1) If normal saline is being used in the lock or if heparinized saline is being used in the lock and the medication is compatible with heparin, proceed to step d.
   (2) If heparinized saline is being used in the lock and the medication is *not* compatible with heparin, flush the lock with 2 to 2.5 mL normal saline before and after the injection of the medication.
d. Insert the needle of the syringe with medication or the needle on an infusion pump tubing firmly through the soft rubber while stabilizing the lock with your nondominant hand.
e. Aspirate gently to see if blood returns *to verify the lock's position in the vein*. In some facilities, it is no longer policy to aspirate, because blood may not return *if the vein collapses*.
f. If blood returns, inject the medication at the recommended rate.
g. If blood does not return, *the cannula may be against the wall of the vein, or it may be dislodged.* Inject a small amount of medication while feeling the tissue over the site with your fingertips.
   (1) *If the medication is being injected into the tissue,* you can feel a small swelling. Also, ask the patient whether he or she feels discomfort. *The heparinized saline solution usually produces burning when injected into the subcutaneous tissue.* If evidence indicates that the medication is going into the subcutaneous tissue, remove the lock and replace it.
   (2) If there is no evidence that medication is moving into the tissue, inject a bit more medication, continuing to check for burning and swelling. Continue to give the medication in this manner.
h. Withdraw the needle after all medication is given.
i. Clean the injection port again.
j. Insert the needle of the heparinized or normal saline-filled syringe.
   (1) If normal saline is being used in the lock or if heparinized saline is being used in the lock and the medication is compatible with heparin, proceed to step k.
   (2) If heparinized saline is being used in the lock and the medication is *not* compati-

ble with heparin, flush with 2 to 2.5 mI normal saline before injecting the heparinized saline.
k. Inject the solution slowly, no faster than 1 mL/min.
l. Remove the syringe and needle from the port.
19.–21. Follow the steps of the General Procedure.

Evaluation
22. Follow the General Procedure.

Documentation
23.–24. Follow the steps of the General Procedure.

LONG-TERM CARE

Many residents in long-term care facilities need IV medications, especially those who are recovering from stays in acute care facilities and those who are terminally ill. Although the equipment may differ, the procedures will not vary significantly from those used in acute care facilities.

HOME CARE

IV medications are increasingly used in home care settings to treat clients with a variety of chronic or acute conditions. Caring for clients at home requires careful choices regarding equipment and appropriate teaching and supervision. Whether the client needs IV antibiotics, chemotherapy, pain management, or more than one of these, easily operated pumps are available to permit maximum freedom of movement and minimum manipulation of equipment.

Some infusion systems can deliver up to four drugs with one system. Others are automated and can be programmed by the pharmacist to deliver medications at a set rate or intermittently at set intervals. Some have a lock-out system, ensuring that the patient or caregiver will not change the rate or amount of drug delivered once it is set by the pharmacist. Continuing improvements in equipment and teaching aids are making home infusion therapy an increasingly safe and cost-effective alternative for adults and children with a wide variety of diagnoses.

CRITICAL THINKING EXERCISES

• You are caring for a patient who is to receive two medications intravenously at 0800. One is to be given "IV push" into an IV lock, and the other is to be delivered using a syringe infusion pump and the same IV lock. How will you organize these tasks? Identify what you will need to consider as you assess and plan.

• A patient has been receiving IV antibiotics for 24 hours. The next dose is due in 1 hour. When you examine the IV site, you note that the area around the cannula is reddened. Determine what further data you should collect. What are your concerns at this time? Identify at least two alternative approaches to this problem.

References

Centers for Disease Control (1983). *Guidelines for control of nosocomial infection.* Washington, DC: US Department of Health and Human Services.

Dugger, B. (1992). Introducing products to prevent needlesticks. *Nursing Management, 23*(10), 62–66.

Kleiber, C., Hanrahan, K., Fagan, G., & Zittergruen, M. (1993). Heparin vs. saline for peripheral IV lines in children. *Pediatric Nursing, 19*(4), 405–409.

Peterson, F., & Kirchhoff, K. (1991). Analysis of the research about heparinized versus nonheparinized lines. *Heart & Lung, 20*(6), 631–42.

Prince, K., Summers, L., & Knight, M. (1994). Needleless IV therapy: Comparing three systems for safety. *Nursing Management, 25*(3), 80N, 80P.

✔ PERFORMANCE CHECKLIST

General Procedure for Administering Intravenous Medications	Needs More Practice	Satisfactory	Comments
Assessment			
1. Validate the orders.			
2. Examine the medication administration record (MAR) for accuracy and completeness.			
3. Assemble information on the drug, including effects, dilution, rate of administration, and potential for incompatibility with other fluids or medications being given.			
4. Assess patient to see what type of intravenous (IV) access is present.			
5. Follow step 5 of the Performance Checklist: General Procedure for Administering Medications in Module 47: Assess patient to identify need for any prn medications ordered.			
Planning			
6. Determine equipment needed.			
7. Follow step 7 of the General Procedure: Wash your hands.			
8. Select appropriate equipment.			
Implementation			
9. –11. Follow steps 9 through 11 of the General Procedure: Read name of medication from record; check label on medication; and pick up medication and check label again, comparing it with MAR.			
12. Determine whether medication has been given or is to be held.			
13. Follow step 13 of the General Procedure: Check medication label with MAR again.			
14. Prepare the medication, using sterile technique.			

(continued)

General Procedures for Administering Intravenous Medications *(Continued)*	Needs More Practice	Satisfactory	Comments
15.–17. Follow steps 15 through 17 of the General Procedure: Place label on prepared medication to identify patient if MAR is not to be taken to bedside; approach and identify patient; explain what you are going to do.			
18. Administer the medication appropriately.			
19. Follow step 19 of the General Procedure: Leave patient in comfortable position.			
20. Dispose of equipment correctly.			
21. Follow step 21 of the General Procedure: Wash your hands.			
Evaluation			
22. Evaluate using the following criteria: **a.** Six rights followed (right patient, right medication, right dosage, right route, right time, right documentation).			
b. Medication given for correct time.			
c. Criteria established for determining medication's effectiveness used.			
d. Side effects promptly identified.			
Documentation			
23. Indicate on the medication record that the medication was given, including name of medication, dosage, IV route used, time, and your initials.			
24. If 50 or 100 mL fluid was given, add amount to intake record.			
Adding to a New Fluid Container			
Assessment			
1. Review medication record to determine if any medications, vitamins, or electrolytes are to be added.			
2. Examine MAR or IV record for accuracy and completeness.			
3. Review information about the medication, vitamin, or electrolyte to be added.			

(continued)

Adding to a New Fluid Container *(Continued)*	Needs More Practice	Satisfactory	Comments
4.–5. Follow steps 4 and 5 of the Performance Checklist: General Procedure for Administering Intravenous Medications: assess patient to see what type of IV access is present and to identify need for any prn medications ordered.			
Planning			
6.–7. Follow steps 6 and 7 of the General Procedure: Determine equipment needed, and wash your hands.			
8. Select appropriate equipment **a.** Large-volume fluid container with ordered IV fluid			
b. Syringe, needle, and alcohol swab			
Implementation			
9.–17. Follow steps 9 through 17 of the General Procedure (read name of medication from record; check label on medication; pick up medication, and check label again, comparing it with MAR; determine whether medication has been given or is to be held; check medication label with MAR again; prepare medication, using sterile technique; place label on prepared medication to identify patient if MAR is not to be taken to bedside; approach and identify patient; and explain what you are going to do.			
18. Inject additive into new fluid container. **a.** Open top of new fluid container, and identify injection port.			
b. Clean port with alcohol swab.			
c. Inject medication.			
d. Tilt container back and forth to mix additive.			
e. Hang new infusion container.			
f. Regulate the flow.			
g. Label new fluid container with name, amount of additive, date, time, your initials.			

(continued)

Adding to a New Fluid Container *(Continued)*	Needs More Practice	Satisfactory	Comments
19.–21. Follow steps 19 through 21 of the General Procedure: Leave patient in a comfortable position; dispose of equipment correctly, and wash your hands.			
Evaluation			
22. Evaluate as in step 22 of the General Procedure: Six rights followed, medication given over correct time, criteria established for determining medication's effectiveness used, and side effects promptly identified.			
Documentation			
23.–24. Document as in steps 23 and 24 of the General Procedure: Indicate on medication record that medication was given, including name of medication, dosage, IV route used, time, and your initials; if 50 or 100 mL fluid was given, add amount to intake record.			
Adding to an Existing Fluid Container			
Assessment			
1. Review orders to verify that an additive is to be added to an existing fluid container.			
2. Examine the MAR for accuracy and completeness.			
3. Review information about the additive.			
4.–5. Follow steps 4 and 5 of the Performance Checklist: General Procedure for Administering Intravenous Medications: Assess patient to see what type of IV access is present and to identify need for any prn medications ordered.			
Planning			
6.–7. Follow steps 6 and 7 of the General Procedure: Determine equipment needed, and wash your hands.			
8. Select appropriate equipment **a.** Needle and syringe to draw up medication			
b. Alcohol swab			

(continued)

Adding to an Existing Fluid Container *(Continued)*	Needs More Practice	Satisfactory	Comments
Implementation			
9.–17. Follow steps 9 through 17 of the General Procedure: Read name of medication from record; check label on medication; pick up medication, and check label again, comparing it with MAR; determine whether medication has been given or is to be held; check medication label with MAR again; prepare medication, using sterile technique; place label on prepared medication to identify patient if MAR is not to be taken to bedside; approach and identify patient; and explain what you are going to do.			
18. Inject additive into existing fluid container. **a.** Turn off the IV flow.			
b. Invert fluid container.			
c. Clean medication port with alcohol swab.			
d. Inject medication into appropriate medication port.			
e. Tilt container back and forth to mix additive.			
f. Label container appropriately.			
g. Rehang IV container.			
h. Regulate the flow rate.			
19.–21. Follow steps 19 through 21 of the General Procedure: Leave patient in a comfortable position; dispose of equipment correctly, and wash your hands.			
Evaluation			
22. Evaluate as in step 22 of the General Procedure: Six rights followed, medication given over correct time, criteria established for determining medication's effectiveness used, and side effects promptly identified.			

(continued)

Adding to an Existing Fluid Container *(Continued)*	Needs More Practice	Satisfactory	Comments
Documentation			
23.–24. Document as in steps 23 and 24 of the General Procedure: Indicate on medication record that medication was given, including name of medication, dosage, IV route used, time, and your initials; if 50 or 100 mL fluid was given, add amount to intake record.			
Using a Controlled-Volume Administration Set			
Assessment			
1. Review MAR and IV infusion record to verify that a medication is to be given IV and to validate that the medication and the IV fluid infusing are compatible.			
2. Examine MAR for accuracy and completeness.			
3.–5. Follow steps 3 through 5 of the General Procedure for Administering Intravenous Medications: Assemble information on the drug; assess patient to see what type of IV access is present and to identify need for any prn medications ordered.			
Planning			
6.–7. Follow steps 6 and 7 of the General Procedure: Determine equipment needed, and wash your hands.			
8. Select appropriate equipment **a.** Controlled volume set			
b. Syringe, needle, and alcohol swab			

(continued)

Using a Controlled-Volume Administration Set *(Continued)*	Needs More Practice	Satisfactory	Comments
Implementation			
9.–17. Follow steps 9 through 17 of the General Procedure: Read name of medication from record; check label on medication; pick up medication, and check label again, comparing it with MAR; determine whether medication has been given or is to be held; check medication label with MAR again; prepare medication, using sterile technique; place label on prepared medication to identify patient if MAR is not to be taken to bedside; approach and identify patient; and explain what you are going to do.			
18. Administer the medication using the controlled volume administration set. **a.** Open the inlet to the controlled-volume chamber, and fill with 50–100 mL fluid from large-volume fluid container.			
b. Tightly close the inlet to the chamber.			
c. Check the chamber. If hard plastic, be sure air vent is open.			
d. Turn on drip from chamber to determine that system is functioning. Turn off drip again.			
e. Clean entry port with alcohol swab.			
f. Insert needle through entry port, and inject medication.			
g. Regulate the flow.			
h. Label chamber with name and amount of medication, date, time, and your initials.			
19.–21. Follow steps 19 through 21 of the General Procedure: Leave patient in a comfortable position; dispose of equipment correctly, and wash your hands.			

(continued)

Using a Controlled-Volume Administration Set (Continued)	Needs More Practice	Satisfactory	Comments
Evaluation			
22. Evaluate as in step 22 of the General Procedure: Six rights followed, medication given over correct time, criteria established for determining medication's effectiveness used, and side effects promptly identified.			
Documentation			
23.–24. Document as in steps 23 and 24 of the General Procedure: Indicate on medication record that medication was given, including name of medication, dosage, intravenous route used, time, and your initials; if 50 or 100 mL fluid was given, add amount to intake record.			
Using a Small-Volume Parenteral			
Assessment			
1.–5. Follow steps 1 through 5 of the Performance Checklist: General Procedure for Administering Intravenous Medications: Validate the orders; examine MAR for accuracy and completeness; assemble information on the drug; and assess patient to see what type of IV access is present and to identify need for any prn medications ordered.			
Planning			
6.–7. Follow steps 6 and 7 of the General Procedure: Determine equipment needed, and wash your hands.			
8. Select appropriate equipment			
a. For IV lock: regular long IV tubing; needle, needle-lock device, or needleless access device; alcohol swab; and tape			
b. For attaching to existing infusion: secondary administration set, extension hanger, alcohol swab, and tape			
c. For attaching a new container to an existing secondary or conventional line: new sterile needle, alcohol swab, and tape			

(continued)

Using a Small-Volume Parenteral *(Continued)*	Needs More Practice	Satisfactory	Comments
Implementation			
9.–17. Follow steps 9 through 17 of the General Procedure: Read name of medication from record; check label on medication; pick up medication, and check label again, comparing it with MAR; determine whether medication has been given or is to be held; check medication label with MAR again; prepare medication, using sterile technique; place label on prepared medication to identify patient if MAR is not to be taken to bedside; approach and identify patient; and explain what you are going to do			
18. Administer the medication using a small-volume parenteral **a.** If container did not come from pharmacy, follow previous directions for adding to a fluid container, and label the container with medication, dosage, time, and your initials.			
b. If using a new tubing set (1) Close regulator on tubing.			
(2) Clean top of small container.			
(3) Attach administration set to small container.			
(4) Place needle or connector on end of tubing.			
(5) Hang small container, and fill drip chamber half full.			
(6) Remove needle or connector cover; open regulator; fill tubing with fluid; and replace cover.			
(7) Hang small container on IV pole.			
(8) Place main IV bottle on extension hanger.			
(9) Clean entry port near top of administration set.			
(10) Connect secondary set to high port.			

(continued)

Using a Small-Volume Parenteral *(Continued)*	Needs More Practice	Satisfactory	Comments
(11) Open regulator on secondary set.			
(12) Regulate rate for secondary container using regulator on main set.			
(13) Tape connection, including needle or connector cover.			
c. If using an existing secondary line (1) Identify correct used small container and tubing.			
(2) Clean top of new small container.			
(3) Make sure regulator is turned off.			
(4) Remove old small container from IV pole, and detach tubing.			
(5) Insert spike of used tubing into new small container.			
(6) Hang small container on IV pole.			
(7) Hang main IV container on extension hanger.			
(8) If needle or connector is not attached to primary set, change it, clean port, and connect.			
(9) Remove air in secondary line by back-filling.			
(10) When fluid is at appropriate level in drip chamber, hang small container on IV pole.			
(11) Set correct drip rate, using regulator on main IV.			
(12) Tape the connection, including connector cover.			
19.–21. Follow steps 19 through 21 of the General Procedure: Leave patient in a comfortable position; dispose of equipment correctly; and wash your hands.			
Evaluation			
22. Evaluate as in step 22 of the General Procedure: Six rights followed, medication given over correct time, criteria established for determining medication's effectiveness used, and side effects promptly identified.			

(continued)

Using a Small-Volume Parenteral *(Continued)*	Needs More Practice	Satisfactory	Comments
Documentation			
23.–24. Document as in steps 23 and 24 of the General Procedure: Indicate on medication record that medication was given, including name of medication, dosage, intravenous route used, time, and your initials; if 50 or 100 mL fluid was given, add amount to intake record.			
Using a Syringe Infusion Pump			
Assessment			
1.–2. Follow steps 1 and 2 of the Performance Checklist: General Procedure for Administering Intravenous Medications: Validate the orders, and examine the MAR for accuracy and completeness.			
3. Review information about medications to be administered, especially regarding compatibility with other medications being given using the syringe infusion pump.			
4.–5. Follow steps 4 and 5 of the General Procedure: Assess patient to see what type of IV access is present and to identify need for any prn medications ordered.			
Planning			
6.–7. Follow steps 6 and 7 of the General Procedure: Determine equipment needed, and wash your hands.			
8. Select appropriate equipment **a.** Syringe infusion pump			
b. Special thin tubing			
c. Syringe, needle, or other connector; alcohol swab; and tape			

(continued)

Using a Syringe Infusion Pump *(Continued)*	Needs More Practice	Satisfactory	Comments
Implementation			
9.–13. Follow steps 9 through 13 of the General Procedure: Read name of medication from record; check label on medication; pick up medication, and check label again, comparing it with MAR; determine whether medication has been given or is to be held; and check medication label with MAR again.			
14. Check syringe from pharmacy to make sure it is the right medication for the right patient in the right dosage at the right time, or draw up the medication in the predetermined amount of solution.			
15.–17. Follow steps 15 through 17 of the General Procedure: Place label on prepared medication to identify patient if MAR is not to be taken to bedside; approach and identify patient; and explain what you are going to do.			
18. Administer the medication using the syringe infusion pump. **a.** If you are setting up the syringe infusion pump (1) Attach proper end of tubing to syringe.			
(2) Attach other end of tubing to needle or connector.			
(3) Attach label to tubing, indicating date and time.			
(4) Remove needle or connector cover, and flush tubing. Replace cover using one-hand technique.			
(5) Place syringe into pump.			
(6) Clean port, and attach needle or connector.			
(7) Hang pump on IV pole, or place on table.			

(continued)

Using a Syringe Infusion Pump *(Continued)*	Needs More Practice	Satisfactory	Comments
(8) Turn on pump, with or without alarm.			
(9) Tape hub of needle in place.			
(10) When infusion is completed, replace used needle or connector with sterile one, and tape to pump or IV pole.			
b. If you are using an existing infusion pump			
(1) Check tubing to be sure it is not older than 48–72 hours.			
(2) Remove used syringe and discard.			
(3) Attach tubing to new syringe.			
(4) Replace existing needle or connector with sterile needle or connector.			
(5) Place syringe in pump.			
(6) Insert needle or connector as before, and turn on pump.			
19.–21. Follow steps 19 through 21 of the General Procedure: Leave patient in a comfortable position; dispose of equipment correctly; and wash your hands.			
Evaluation			
22. Evaluate as in step 22 of the General Procedure: Six rights followed, medication given over correct time, criteria established for determining medication's effectiveness used, and side effects promptly identified.			
Documentation			
23.–24. Document as in steps 23 and 24 of the General Procedure: Indicate on medication record that medication was given, including name of medication, dosage, intravenous route used, time, and your initials; if 50 or 100 mL fluid was given, add amount to intake record.			

(continued)

Giving Medication by IV Push into an Existing IV	Needs More Practice	Satisfactory	Comments
Assessment			
1.–2. Follow steps 1 and 2 of the Performance Checklist: General Procedure for Administering Intravenous Medications: Validate the orders, and examine MAR for accuracy and completeness.			
3. Review information about medication(s) to be given, especially noting recommended speed of injection and dilution and diluent, if needed.			
4.–5. Follow steps 4 and 5 of the General Procedure: Assess patient to see what type of IV access is present and to identify need for any prn medications ordered.			
Planning			
6.–7. Follow steps 6 and 7 of the General Procedure: Determine equipment needed, and wash your hands.			
8. Select appropriate equipment. **a.** Syringe large enough for medication and diluent, if needed			
b. Needle appropriate to viscosity of medication and speed of injection			
c. Alcohol swab			
Implementation			
9.–17. Follow steps 9 through 17 of the General Procedure: Read name of medication from record; check label on medication; pick up medication, and check label again, comparing it with MAR; determine whether medication has been given or is to be held; check medication label with MAR again; prepare medication, using sterile technique; place label on prepared medication to identify patient if MAR is not to be taken to bedside; approach and identify patient; and explain what you are going to do.			

(*continued*)

Giving Medication by IV Push into an Existing IV (Continued)	Needs More Practice	Satisfactory	Comments
18. Administer medication by IV push into existing IV infusion. a. Identify injection port closest to patient.			
b. Clean port with alcohol swab.			
c. Insert needle into port.			
d. Pinch off tubing above port.			
e. Inject medication at correct rate.			
f. Observe patient.			
g. Release tubing when injection is completed.			
h. Withdraw needle.			
19.–21. Follow steps 19 through 21 of the General Procedure: Leave patient in a comfortable position; dispose of equipment correctly; and wash your hands.			
Evaluation			
22. Evaluate as in step 22 of the General Procedure: Six rights followed, medication given over correct time, criteria established for determining medication's effectiveness used, and side effects promptly identified.			
Documentation			
23.–24. Document as in steps 23 and 24 of the General Procedure: Indicate on medication record that medication was given, including name of medication, dosage, intravenous route used, time, and your initials; if 50 or 100 mL fluid was given, add amount to intake record.			
Giving Medication into an Intermittent Infusion Adapter (IV Lock)			
Assessment			
1.–2. Follow steps 1 and 2 of the Performance Checklist: General Procedure for Administering Intravenous Medications: Validate the orders, and examine MAR for accuracy and completeness.			

(*continued*)

Giving Medication into an Intermittent Infusion Adapter (IV Lock) *(Continued)*	Needs More Practice	Satisfactory	Comments
3. Review information about medication(s) to be given, especially noting recommended speed of injection and dilution and diluent, if needed.			
4.–5. Follow steps 4 and 5 of the General Procedure: Assess patient to see what type of IV access is present and to identify need for any prn medications ordered.			
Planning			
6.–7. Follow steps 6 and 7 of the General Procedure: Determine equipment needed, and wash your hands.			
8. Select appropriate equipment. **a.** Syringe large enough for medication and diluent, if needed			
b. Needle appropriate to viscosity of medication and speed of injection			
c. Separate syringe and needle for heparinized or normal saline solution			
d. Enough alcohol swabs for number of medications and flushes to be administered.			
Implementation			
9.–13. Follow steps 9 through 13 of the General Procedure. Read name of medication from record; check label on medication; pick up medication, and check label again, comparing it with MAR; determine whether medication has been given or is to be held; and check medication label with MAR again.			
14. Prepare the medication and heparinized or normal saline solution in separate syringes.			
15.–17. Follow steps 15 through 17 of the General Procedure: Place label on prepared medication to identify patient if MAR is not to be taken to bedside; approach and identify patient; and explain what you are going to do.			

(continued)

Giving Medication into an Intermittent Infusion Adapter (IV Lock) *(Continued)*	Needs More Practice	Satisfactory	Comments
18. Administer the medication using an intermittent infusion adapter (IV lock). **a.** Locate IV lock.			
b. Inspect site.			
c. Clean port with alcohol swab. (1) If normal saline is being used in the lock or if heparinized saline is being used in the lock and the medication is compatible with heparin, proceed to step d.			
(2) If heparinized saline is being used in the lock and the medication is *not* compatible with heparin, flush lock with 2.5 mL normal saline before and after injection of the medication.			
d. Insert needle or connector of syringe with medication or on infusion pump tubing into IV lock.			
e. Aspirate.			
f. If blood returns, inject at recommended rate.			
g. If blood does not return, inject small amount while checking for swelling and discomfort. (1) If medication is going into subcutaneous tissue, remove lock and replace.			
(2) If medication does not appear to be going into tissue, continue to inject slowly, checking for burning and swelling.			
h. Withdraw needle.			
i. Clean injection port again.			
j. Insert needle or connector of heparinized or normal saline-filled syringe. (1) If normal saline is being used in lock or if heparinized saline is being used in lock and medication is compatible with heparin, proceed to step k.			
(2) If heparinized saline is being used in lock and medication is *not* compatible with heparin, flush with 2.5 mL normal saline before injecting heparinized saline.			

(continued)

Giving Medication into an Intermittent Infusion Adapter (IV Lock) *(Continued)*	Needs More Practice	Satisfactory	Comments
k. Inject solution slowly.			
l. Remove syringe and needle or connector from port.			
19.–21. Follow steps 19 through 21 of the General Procedure: Leave patient in a comfortable position; dispose of equipment correctly; and wash your hands.			
Evaluation			
22. Evaluate as in step 22 of the General Procedure: Six rights followed, medication given over correct time, criteria established for determining medication's effectiveness used, and side effects promptly identified.			
Documentation			
23.–24. Document as in steps 23 and 24 of the General Procedure: Indicate on medication record that medication was given, including name of medication, dosage, intravenous route used, time, and your initials; if 50 or 100 mL fluid was given, add amount to intake record.			

? QUIZ

Short-Answer Questions

1. Why is a needle inserted into an IV line only at an injection port?

_____

2. If there is no designated speed of injection for an IV push medication, how fast should it be injected and why? _____

_____

3. When adding medications to a small- or large-volume container, why should you agitate the solution to mix it thoroughly? _____

_____

4. What are two effects of drug incompatibilities? _____

_____

5. What are two resources for determining the actions and possible incompatibilities of drugs?

_____

6. What is the purpose of an intermittent infusion adapter? _____

_____

7. Why must the premeasured syringe of medication be accurately placed in the infusion pump?

_____

8. Why is normal or heparinized saline solution left in the IV lock? _____

_____

9. How many milliliters of fluid are usually used to dilute the medication in a controlled-volume administration set? _____

_____

MODULE

54

CARING FOR CENTRAL INTRAVENOUS CATHETERS

MODULE CONTENTS

547

M O D U L E   C O N T E N T S (c o n t i n u e d)

Implementation
Evaluation
Documentation
PROCEDURE FOR ACCESSING A
 SUBCUTANEOUS CATHETER PORT
Assessment
Planning

Implementation
Evaluation
Documentation
LONG-TERM CARE
HOME CARE EXERCISES
CRITICAL THINKING EXERCISES

P R E R E Q U I S I T E S

Successful completion of the following modules:

VOLUME 1
Module 1 An Approach to Nursing Skills
Module 2 Basic Infection Control
Module 3 Safety
Module 5 Documentation
Module 6 Introduction to Assessment Skills

VOLUME 2
Module 33 Sterile Technique
Module 35 Wound Care
Module 47 Administering Medications: Overview
Module 52 Preparing and Maintaining Intravenous Infusions
Module 53 Administering Intravenous Medications

Review the anatomy and physiology of the large central veins in the neck and chest and of the right atrium.

OVERALL OBJECTIVE

To care for a patient with any of the various types of central venous infusion catheters by assisting with insertion, changing dressings, providing intravenous (IV) therapy and drawing blood.

SPECIFIC LEARNING OBJECTIVES

Know Facts and Principles	Apply Facts and Principles	Demonstrate Ability	Evaluate Performance
1. General information			
a. Purposes			
State two common reasons for using a central intravenous (IV) line.	When given an example of a patient with a central IV line, identify the purpose of the line.	In the clinical setting, identify the reason a specific patient has a central IV line.	Evaluate with your instructor.
b. Complications			
State two major complications associated with central IV lines.	Given a patient situation with a complication of a central IV line occuring, identify the complication.	In the clinical setting, make appropriate observations to identify complications.	Evaluate with your instructor.
2. Standard central venous line			
List common sites for insertion of the standard central venous line. Describe the procedure used for inserting a central IV line.	Given a patient situation, identify the rationale for the site chosen.	In the practice or clinical setting, select correct equipment for inserting a central IV line.	Evaluate selection with your instructor.
3. Changing the central IV dressing			
State four purposes of changing the central IV dressing. List the supplies used in your facility for changing a central IV dressing. Explain the rationale for using various antiseptic agents for cleansing the skin when inserting a subclavian line or changing a subclavian dressing. Describe the procedure for changing the central IV dressing.	Select appropriate materials for central IV dressing.	In the practice setting, change a central IV dressing.	Evaluate your own performance using the Performance Checklist and consulting with instructor.

(continued)

SPECIFIC LEARNING OBJECTIVES (continued)

Know Facts and Principles	Apply Facts and Principles	Demonstrate Ability	Evaluate Performance
4. *Changing the fluid container and the tubing*			
State the special concern when changing the tubing on the central IV line. Describe the procedure for changing the fluid container and the tubing.	Given a patient situation, identify appropriate actions when changing the fluid container and tubing on a central line.	In the practice setting, change the fluid container and tubing on a central IV line safely.	Evaluate own performance using the Performance Checklist and consultation with your instructor.
5. *Peripherally inserted central catheter (PICC)*			
Identify the special problems associated with a PICC.	Outline actions that can prevent the development of problems related to the PICC.	In the practice setting, care for patient with PICC.	Evaluate own performance in consultation with instructor.
6. *Surgically implanted central IV catheter*			
Describe the Hickman, the Broviac, double-lumen Hickman catheters, and subcutaneous catheter ports, pointing out similarities and differences. List the uses of these catheters.			
a. Changing the exit site dressing			
List supplies needed for changing the exit site dressing.		In the practice setting, change an exit site dressing.	Evaluate own performance with instructor using the Performance Checklist.
b. Establishing an intermittent line with a heparin lock			
List supplies needed to establish an intermittent line with a heparin lock. Describe the procedure for establishing the intermittent line.		In the practice setting, set up a central line as an intermittent line with a heparin lock.	Evaluate own performance with instructor using the Performance Checklist.
c. Irrigating a central IV catheter			
List supplies and equip-needed to irrigate the line. Describe the procedure for irrigating a central IV line.		In the practice setting, irrigate a central line.	Evaluate own performance with instructor using the Performance Checklist.

(*continued*)

SPECIFIC LEARNING OBJECTIVES (continued)

Know Facts and Principles	Apply Facts and Principles	Demonstrate Ability	Evaluate Performance
d. Giving a medication through an intermittent central IV catheter			
List supplies and equipment needed to give a medication through the catheter. Describe the procedure for giving a medication through the central IV line.		In the practice setting, give a medication through the central line.	Evaluate own performance with instructor using the Performance Checklist.
e. Drawing blood through a central IV catheter			
List supplies needed for drawing blood through a central IV catheter.		In the practice setting, go through the procedure for drawing blood from a central IV catheter.	Evaluate own performance with instructor using the Performance Checklist.
f. Accessing a subcutaneous catheter port			
List supplies and equipment needed to access a port.	Given a patient situation, identify what problem in accessing the port might be present and what nursing action is appropriate.	In the practice setting, access a subcutaneous catheter port.	Evaluate own performance with instructor using the Performance Checklist.

LEARNING ACTIVITIES

1. Review the Specific Learning Objectives.
2. Look up the module vocabulary terms in the glossary.
3. Read through the module as though you were preparing to teach the contents to another person. Mentally practice the skills.
4. Examine the various central IV catheters used in the facility in which you practice.
5. Review the following procedures in the procedure book for your facility:
   a. Central IV dressing change
   b. Central IV catheter care
   c. Hickman catheter care
   d. Broviac catheter care
   e. Subcutaneous catheter port (Port-a-cath, Infus-a-port) care
6. Arrange for time to practice handling central IV catheters.
7. In the practice setting, do the following:
   a. Practice the procedures outlined in the Performance Checklist.
   b. When you have mastered these procedures, select another student, and critique one another's performance using the Performance Checklist.
   c. Arrange for your instructor to evaluate your performance.
8. In the clinical setting, do the following:
   a. Identify patients with central IV catheters in place.
   b. Arrange an opportunity to observe care for these patients.
   c. Ask your instructor for an opportunity to carry out the specific care needed by the patient.

VOCABULARY

air embolism
Broviac catheter
cardiac output
cephalic vein
Groshong catheter
Hickman catheter
inferior vena cava
Infus-a-port
Intrasil catheter
noncoring needle
Port-a-cath
right atrium
sclerose
septicemia
subclavian vein
subcutaneous catheter port
superior vena cava
Trendelenburg's position

Caring for Central Intravenous Catheters

Rationale for the Use of This Skill

In modern healthcare settings, many patients are receiving intravenous (IV) medications and nutritional solutions. Many of these products are irritating to small veins but are tolerated without local irritation in large vessels that have a high-volume blood flow, allowing for rapid dilution of the product. Because of the increased use of all IV products, in many patients all available small vessels have been used repeatedly and have subsequently become irritated or sclerosed or in other ways are unusable. For these patients, the central IV catheter (or central venous line as it is also called) offers an effective route for the administration of needed therapy. Because of the direct access to the central circulation, the special dynamics of blood flow in the large central veins, and the difficulty in replacing central IV catheters, specialized care techniques are required.[1]

▼ NURSING DIAGNOSES

Risk for Infection is a major nursing diagnosis for patients with central lines. First, the solution is flowing directly into the central circulation. *Any bacteria introduced with the fluid circulate freely, and generalized septicemia may result.* Second, *the catheter enters through the skin and provides a direct path that microbes may follow from the surface, along the outside of the catheter, and into the central circulation. Also, septicemia may easily result. Many of the steps in the procedures for care are designed to guard the patient against this high infection risk.* The nurse must carefully observe the entry site for redness, swelling, or exudate *to identify local infection.* The nurse also must assess for elevated temperature, malaise, and chills *to identify systemic infection.*

Potential Complication: *Air embolism* is another special risk for the patient with a central IV catheter. *As a result of the dynamics of fluid flow and pressure changes within the thoracic cavity, negative pressure develops in the large central veins, facilitating their filling and returning blood to the heart and thus maintaining adequate cardiac output.* When a catheter is placed in one of these large veins, negative pressure occurs at the tip of the catheter, facilitating the movement of fluid from the catheter into the vein. *If the catheter is not filled with fluid and is open to the air,*

the negative pressure at the tip draws air into the catheter, creating an air embolism. Of course, *the amount of air that actually enters the catheter depends on the amount of negative pressure and the length of time negative pressure is exerted against an open catheter.* The amount of air needed to create an air embolus large enough to be symptomatic is not known. Some authorities believe that 50 mL of air may cause a fatal air embolus. No data substantiate this. *Because an air embolus can interfere with effective emptying of the ventricles and diminish cardiac output even when not great enough to cause death*, it is wise to eliminate air entirely by careful technique. Care should be taken not to frighten the patient by overzealous behavior, because inadvertently allowing a single small air bubble to enter the line will certainly not cause problems for the patient. Symptoms that may indicate air embolus include shortness of breath, irregularities in the apical heartbeat, and chest discomfort. If the patient is being monitored, arrhythmias may be observed.

To prevent air embolism, many central venous catheters are produced with a clamp located near the external end that can be closed whenever the catheter is being opened to the air. If the catheter does not have a clamp, a 6-in extension tubing with a clamp may be attached for the same purpose.

TYPES OF CENTRAL INTRAVENOUS CATHETERS

Several types of central IV infusion catheters are in use. The various standard central IV lines, the surgically inserted central IV line, and the central IV line with a peripheral exit site are discussed briefly. Other types of central IV lines may be used in your facility. By analyzing the type of line in use, you should be able to adapt these procedures to your situation as necessary.

Standard Central Intravenous Catheters

The standard central venous line is inserted by a physician or specially trained nurse using a sterile procedure. The catheter may be sutured to the skin at the exit site and may be short or long. The most common insertion site is the right or left subclavian vein, but the right cephalic vein or the right or left internal jugular vein also may be used (Fig. 54–1). Care for all is the same.

[1]Note that rationale for action is emphasized throughout the module by the use of italics.

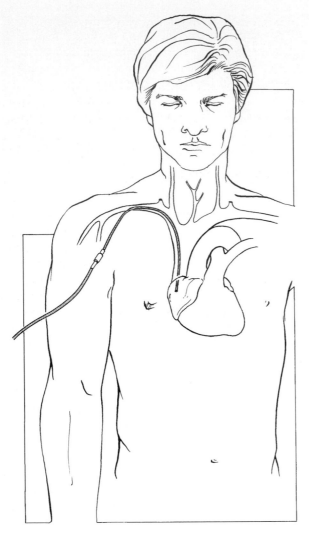

Figure 54–1. Subclavian IV line in place. Note the entry point and the position of the tip of the catheter in the right atrium.

A variety of short catheters designed for insertion through the internal jugular vein, including the Arrow and Hon brand catheters, are available. These are short catheters, approximately 1 in long, that are inserted in the same way that a standard Angiocath IV is inserted. Internal jugular catheters are often inserted in surgery by an anesthesiologist. In some facilities, nurses are certified to insert internal jugular catheters.

Internal jugular catheters may be single, double, or triple lumen in construction. The multiple-lumen catheter has separate color-coded ports, each going to a different lumen. Each lumen exits separately from the other lumens. *It is therefore possible to designate each for a separate purpose. For example, the triple-lumen catheter can have one lumen designated for nutritional solutions, another for drawing blood, and the third for intermittent medications.* Any one, any two, or all

three may be capped and filled with heparinized saline or saline solution *for intermittent use.*

The long catheter is inserted in a more complex procedure and has the potential for more side effects. It is threaded farther into the vein until the tip rests in the superior vena cava outside the right atrium. These catheters must be inserted by a physician, most often by a surgeon. The following procedure describes assisting with the insertion of these catheters.

Peripherally Inserted Central Intravenous Catheters

The peripherally inserted central catheter is referred to as a PICC or a central catheter with a peripheral exit site. This is a long central IV catheter that is inserted into a vein in the arm through an intracath needle. The catheter is then threaded from a spool through the needle into the subclavian vein until its tip rests outside the superior vena cava. In some facilities, PICC catheters are inserted by specially certified registered nurses. The catheter volume is 0.4 mL.

This catheter facilitates the administration of fluids and medications that can be infused only into the large central veins without the use of the more complex procedure necessary to insert a conventional central IV line or the surgical procedure to implant a catheter. This type of line also may be used to measure central venous pressure and to draw blood (Fig. 54–2). Fluoroscopy is used to verify its position. PICC lines may be left in place for a prolonged period of time and can be used to infuse substances that cannot be placed into peripheral veins.

In most facilities, care is identical to that given for the standard central IV line. In some facilities, the care is the same as that given for other peripheral IVs unless nutrient solutions are being administered. Be sure to check the policy in your facility.

Clear lines of communication must be established *so that members of the healthcare team are aware that this is not a peripheral IV line.* In addition to recording this information in the permanent medical record and on the Kardex, it is wise to note the type of line being used by writing directly on the dressing or on a piece of tape placed over the dressing. Then, *even if someone has not thoroughly read the patient record, the information will be immediately apparent when the line is used or given care.*

Surgically Inserted Central Intravenous Catheters

Central lines that are used for patients being treated for cancer or other major illnesses must be resistant to displacement and infection to be useful for a pro-

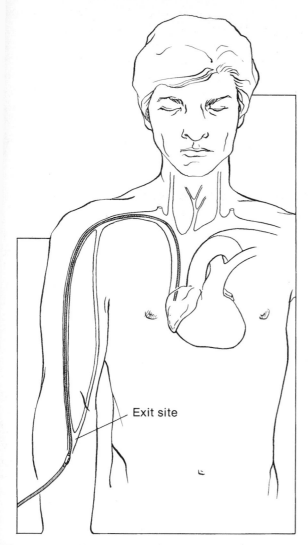

Figure 54–2. The peripherally inserted central IV catheter (sometimes called a PICC).

longed time. Therefore, surgically inserted catheters are commonly used for these patients. These types of catheters may stay in place for months or sometimes years.

Subcutaneous Catheter Ports

The subcutaneous catheter port (Port-a-cath, Infus-a-port, or Hickman port) is a surgically inserted central IV line that does not have an external exit site. The catheter ends in a reservoir that has a rubber diaphragm for a top and is implanted under the skin. To access it, the nurse uses a special needle inserted through the skin (see page 573). The subcutaneous port can be filled with heparinized saline and used intermittently or connected to IV fluids and medications. *Because it has no exit site, the potential for infection is decreased,* but a needle puncture is needed

each time it is used. It is cared for as if it were a standard central IV line, except that a larger volume of heparinized saline (5 mL) is needed to fill it (Fig. 54–3).

These devices appear to be more susceptible than other central lines to clotting closed when used for drawing blood. Therefore, the nurse must thoroughly flush it after all blood drawing.

Hickman and Broviac Catheters

The *Hickman catheter* is a right atrial catheter that is surgically inserted into the chest and into a central vein. As shown in Figure 54–4, it is tunneled under the chest tissue after it exits from the vein so that the exit site at the skin is a distance from the exit from the vein. In the subcutaneous tunnel, the catheter is surrounded by a Dacron cuff, which *allows tissue to grow into the material, forming a seal against microbes. It takes approximately 3 weeks for the catheter to thoroughly heal into place. The time varies depending on the patient's health and healing ability.*

The internal diameter of the Hickman catheter is 1.6 mm. This is large enough to allow withdrawal of blood and infusion of fluid into the vein. This type of catheter may be kept open with a continuous infusion or may be capped and filled with heparinized saline to be used as an intermittent access to the vein. The Hickman catheter may have one, two, or three lumens.

The *Broviac catheter* is a similar single-lumen catheter that is inserted in the same way as the Hickman catheter. The major difference between the two is that the Broviac catheter has an internal diameter of 1 mm, so it cannot be used for drawing blood. It is used only for infusing fluids.

The double-lumen Hickman catheter is actually a fusion of two Hickman catheters or of a Broviac catheter and a single-lumen Hickman catheter (Fig. 54–5).

The double-lumen catheter is used principally to allow adequate nutrients to be infused without interruption, while allowing medications to be given and blood to be drawn intermittently. A continuous infusion of a nutritional solution is administered through the smaller-lumen Broviac, while the larger-lumen Hickman is used for drawing blood samples (with the Broviac temporarily clamped) and for infusing medications (may be done simultaneously with the infusion of the nutrient solution). When both lumens are the same size (Hickman diameter), either lumen may be used for all purposes.

Care is the same for all three catheters. The insertion site is dressed as any surgical site until it has healed (see Module 35, Wound Care). The exit site

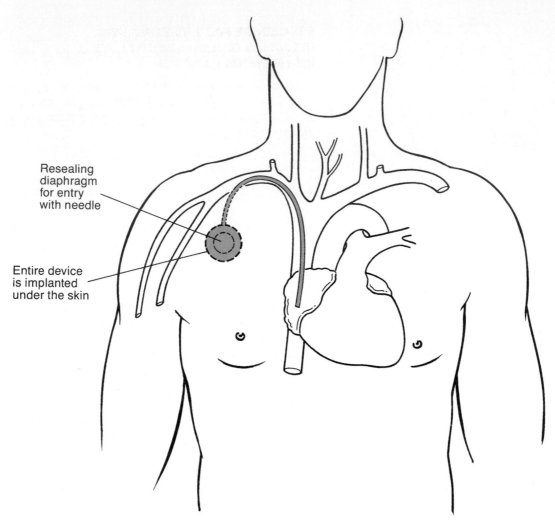

Resealing
diaphragm
for entry
with needle

Entire device
is implanted
under the skin

Figure 54–3. The implanted central IV port. The IV catheter is threaded into the right atrium. The catheter exits the vein and attaches to the metal reservoir, which has a resealable rubber diaphragm on the top.

must be cared for and dressed, and a special technique is necessary for drawing blood from the Hickman line. When the line is used intermittently, it must be filled with heparinized saline *to prevent coagulation at the tip, which would occlude the line. Because these lines are intended for long-term use,* the patient and the family must be taught to carry out the care at home. A clamp is kept on the catheter whenever fluid is not being infused *to guard against inadvertent separation of the cap and line, with the resulting risk of air embolism.* Plastic clamps are in place on most central catheters. When one is not already present, a bull dog clamp is placed on the line over a piece of tape. *The tape protects the tubing from possible damage from the metal clamp.*

Groshong Catheters

The Groshong catheter is a surgically implanted central venous catheter made of silicone rubber. It is inserted through a tunnel in a manner similar to a Hickman catheter. It has a specially designed tip that allows the pressure of fluid being instilled to open the tip and administer fluid. The tip also can be opened by the negative pressure created by a syringe and therefore can be used for drawing blood. However, the tip will not open from the blood pressure in the central vein, *so no blood can get into the catheter and form a clot.* In addition, the patient is protected from air embolism *because the tip does not allow the negative pressure in the chest to be transmitted to the catheter*

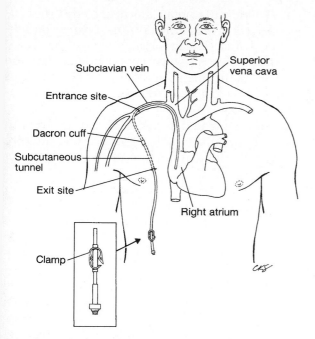

Figure 54–4. A surgically inserted central intravenous catheter shown with a built-in clamp. This is a Hickman catheter.

lumen. This catheter is filled with normal saline when not in use. *Because no heparin is administered to keep it open,* it is safer for the patient who should not receive heparin. However, some facilities do use heparin solution in Groshong catheters. You will need to follow the procedure in your facility.

PROCEDURE FOR ASSISTING WITH INSERTION OF A STANDARD CENTRAL INTRAVENOUS CATHETER

This procedure is based on the General Procedure for Assisting With Diagnostic and Therapeutic Procedures in Module 12, Assisting With Diagnostic and Therapeutic Procedures, pp. 252–253. The nurse's role is assisting with the catheter insertion at the bedside. It is a sterile procedure.

Assessment

1. Check the order for insertion of a central IV line.
2. Determine whether your facility requires a signed permission form for this procedure. If so, ensure that this form is obtained before proceeding.
3. Assess the patient's ability to participate in and tolerate the procedure.
   a. Assess whether the patient can be positioned flat or in Trendelenburg's position.
   b. Assess the patient's ability to hold breath on command. *Some physicians may ask that patients hold their breath during insertion.*
   c. Assess the patient's ability to understand and follow directions in regard to the position of the head and remaining still.

Planning

4. Wash your hands *for infection control.*
5. Obtain the necessary equipment and supplies. In many facilities, a standard disposable set is used

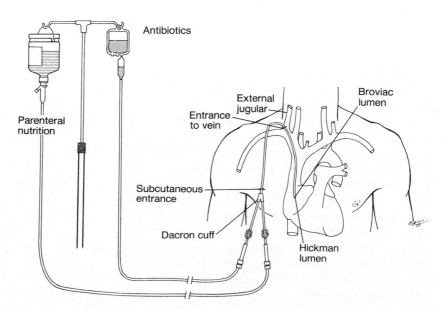

Figure 54–5. The double-lumen Hickman catheter.

for inserting central IV lines. If such a set is used, be sure to check the contents, *so you know which other items you will need.* The following supplies are commonly used:

a. Masks for all those assisting with the procedure *to reduce the possibility of contamination from microbes from the nose and mouth.* In some facilities, the procedure specifies that the patient also be masked. *Because this often creates anxiety,* in most facilities the patient is positioned with the face away from the insertion site, and the drapes are positioned to provide a screen between the patient's nose and mouth and the insertion site.

b. Sterile gown for the physician inserting the catheter. In some facilities, a sterile gown is not required, but a clean gown is used to cover the physician's clothes *to protect against contamination of the site and to protect the physician.*

c. Two pairs of sterile gloves of the appropriate size for the physician.

d. Skin preparation materials. Procedure in some facilities includes the use of acetone to defat the skin. *Evidence has shown, however, that removing the normal protective coat increases skin irritation and local inflammation and does not lower the infection rate,* so it is not recommended.

Povidone-iodine swabs or solution and sterile gauze swabs are an excellent skin antiseptic, but a potential for skin reaction exists. A large area is prepared and the solution allowed to dry. *This process liberates free iodine and is the basis for the effectiveness of this solution in lowering the bacterial count.*

Tincture of iodine may be used as an antiseptic agent, but because it often causes skin reactions, it is removed with 70% alcohol after it has dried. *This lessens the incidence of skin reaction and preserves the antiseptic effect.*

Also, 70% alcohol alone may be used as a skin antiseptic.

e. Scissors to clip hair if necessary

f. 1% lidocaine for use as a topical anesthetic

g. Sterile drapes *to drape the site.* A fenestrated drape (one with a hole in the center) is commonly used, or four plain drapes may be used *to surround the area.* Towel clips to hold the plain drapes in place are useful but not essential.

h. Suitable catheter and a syringe. A 16-gauge, 20-cm catheter is a common size. The catheter may be either polyethylene or silicone rubber.

i. Suturing materials. 000 silk sutures with atraumatic needles attached are commonly used. A needle holder, a hemostat, and scissors are needed.

j. IV fluid with tubing attached, ready to be connected to the catheter. A 6-in extension tubing with a clamp is often used on central lines. This is treated as a part of the primary line and allows the line to be clamped when tubing is being changed or other procedures are performed.

k. Dressing materials *to dress the exit site.* Various techniques can be used for dressing the central IV site, each requiring slightly different materials.

(1) Transparent, moisture- and vapor-permeable dressing material (OpSite, Tegaderm) is gaining favor as a dressing material. *It allows for easy inspection of the site; stays moist but does not allow excess moisture to accumulate beneath the dressing due to its moisture- and vapor-permeable nature; and forms an effective barrier to microbes. Because nurses can observe the site without removing the dressing,* this type of dressing is changed less frequently than others—in some facilities only once a week. Some recent research indicates the insertion site infection rate may be higher under transparent dressings than under gauze dressings. Encourage your facility to examine its policies in light of its own infection rate and appropriate research.

(2) Large adhesive bandages with water-repellent backing are included in many prepackaged kits. There is adhesive on all four edges of the bandage's gauze pad *so the dressing may be securely adhered to form an occlusive seal.*

(3) Plastic adhesive material may be used *to cover a gauze dressing* placed directly over the site. Two 3 × 3 gauze squares are used for the underneath dressing. Tape also may be used *to fasten the edges of this type of dressing more securely.*

(4) 3 × 3 gauze squares and impermeable plastic tape may be used *to form an occlusive dressing over the site. If the patient's skin is sensitive to this kind of tape,* use hypoallergenic paper tape instead.

(5) Povidone-iodine ointment is used *to seal the opening through which the catheter passes into the body, regardless of the type of dressing used. This seal helps prevent microbes from entering.* Studies indicate that *using an antiseptic or antimicrobial ointment at an IV insertion site lessens the incidence of local infection.* In some facilities, an antibiotic ointment is used. *Povidone-iodine ointment is more effec-*

tive in preventing fungal infections and also prevents bacterial infections. Antibiotic ointment is more effective against bacterial infections but allows fungal infections to develop. Either type of ointment may cause skin irritation.

l. Sterile towel *to provide a sterile field.* If a prepackaged set is used, the wrapper may serve as the sterile field.

Implementation

6. Check the patient's identification *to be sure you are performing the procedure for the correct patient.*

7. Explain the procedure to the patient. The patient who is alert needs a careful, nonthreatening explanation of the procedure *to reduce anxiety.* The explanation should focus on what the patient will experience. Briefly explain the advantage of this method of access to the vein: Both arms may be free for movement, and the arms may be spared further discomfort from IV lines. You also should point out that special care procedures will be used that were not used for the peripheral IV lines, such as a more elaborate procedure for the dressing change. Emphasize that these procedures are added safety measures. During the procedure, the area will be anesthetized, *so the insertion will not be painful.* A sedative may be ordered by the physician. Explain that lying still is important *to facilitate the physician's task* and that the patient may be asked to inhale and then bear down briefly while the tubing is attached. (This is a Valsalva maneuver.) Doing this prevents air embolus, although you may not wish to explain this in detail because it might frighten the patient unnecessarily.

If the patient cannot understand the explanations, you will need to make brief statements throughout the procedure *to reduce anxiety.* Emphasize that you are there to help the patient. Extra assistants may be needed *if the patient must be restrained to maintain immobility.*

8. Prepare the unit.

a. Provide for privacy.

b. Ensure a clean table is available on which to set up a sterile field for all the supplies. If an overbed table is used, it is prudent to clean the surface thoroughly with a germicidal agent, such as 70% alcohol, or a phenol disinfectant, *because overbed tables may have been used to hold urinals, bedpans, or other contaminated items.*

c. Set up the equipment on the table. Using sterile technique, arrange a sterile towel or the wrapper of the package to form a sterile field. Then carefully place all sterile equipment within the field.

9. Place the patient in a supine position. If this is not possible for the entire procedure, be prepared to place the patient in a flat position for the time needed. A slight Trendelenburg's position is desirable when the vein is entered and when the tubing is being connected. *With the patient in Trendelenburg's position, slight positive pressure occurs in the central veins and protects against air embolism. This positioning also causes the vessels to dilate, facilitating insertion.* If the bed cannot easily be adjusted from flat to Trendelenburg's, the patient may have to be placed in a slight Trendelenburg's position for the entire procedure. If the patient cannot tolerate this position, he or she remains lying flat during all parts of the procedure, and connections are made quickly *to lessen the opportunity for air to enter the catheter.* Place a rolled towel under the shoulder on the side being used for the insertion *to provide better access to the vein.*

10. Assist with the procedure by supporting the patient psychologically and assisting the physician as needed. An experienced nurse may be able to accomplish both tasks simultaneously. As a beginner, you may find it easier if two nurses are present, *so one can focus on the patient, and the other can take care of procedural needs.*

a. Maintain touch with the patient. Often this takes the form of holding the patient's hand.

b. Help the patient maintain the proper position by supporting the head if necessary.

c. Give positive reinforcement to the patient for cooperative efforts.

d. Provide feedback to the patient *to reassure that the procedure is progressing satisfactorily.*

e. If difficulties are encountered, try to reassure the patient *so anxiety does not increase.*

f. If necessary, remind others in the environment that the patient is alert even though the face is covered. Discourage inappropriate comments by staff.

g. Open equipment or supply packages *so the contents are accessible to the physician without risking contamination of the sterile gloves.*

h. If asked, hold the vial of anesthetic while the physician withdraws the medication.

i. When asked, connect the heparin lock to the catheter and prepare the tape for stabilizing the catheter on the skin.

j. Complete the dressing, if asked.

11. After the line has been inserted, do the following:
    a. Remove the drapes, and position the patient comfortably.
    b. Ensure that an x-ray to verify correct placement is done before IV fluids are started. Begin providing the prescribed fluid as soon as the x-ray report is available *so the patient is receiving all the fluid required at a rate that allows for appropriate use.*
    c. Remove all used supplies and packaging materials. Most will be disposable. Care for nondisposable items according to your facility's procedure.
    d. Wash your hands *for infection control.*

Evaluation

12. Evaluate using the following criteria:
    a. Patient comfortable.
    b. The IV line—*all connections securely fastened. You will find a variety of IV connection securing devices for this purpose. If there is not a connection securing device, the connection is taped. A connecting device is preferred because tape attracts microbes.*
    c. The dressing—*secure.*
    d. The fluid after it is started—flow not obstructed and rate correctly set.

Documentation

13. Document on the patient's chart:
    a. Time the central IV line was inserted
    b. Type and size of the catheter
    c. Site used
    d. Solution started and the rate of administration. In some facilities, this information may be recorded on an IV flow sheet. If it is recorded on the narrative, the same information is included.
    e. Patient's response
    f. Time you received the report of the x-ray taken to verify the position of the catheter and what was reported. If the catheter is not properly placed in the vein, you will need to notify the physician immediately and ensure that no IV fluids are started.

PROCEDURE FOR CHANGING THE STANDARD CENTRAL INTRAVENOUS DRESSING

The same procedure may be used for changing dressings over all types of central lines when they are newly inserted.

The frequency with which these dressings are changed is not standardized. In some facilities where standard gauze and tape dressings are used, the dressings are changed daily or every other day. In other facilities, such dressings are changed three times weekly on a prescribed schedule. In some facilities where transparent, moisture-permeable dressings (OpSite and Tegaderm) are used, dressings are left in place until they begin to loosen or for 1 week, whichever comes first. This method saves nursing time. No specific recommendation is forthcoming from the Centers for Disease Control and Prevention at this writing. It would be appropriate to watch the literature closely for research results and specific recommendations. Meanwhile, continue to follow the procedure designated in your facility. In addition to regularly scheduled changes, the dressing is changed if it pulls loose or becomes wet, *because this situation increases the potential for contamination of the entry site.*

The dressing change permits careful assessment of the insertion site, thorough cleansing of the area and removal of any debris that might foster microbial growth, application of antiseptic or antimicrobial agents to decrease future growth of microbes, and application of new sterile dressing materials to replace those that may have become contaminated.

Assessment

1. Check the date and time of the last dressing change.
2. Review the facility procedure *to identify the appropriate dressing materials to use.*

Planning

3. Wash your hands *for infection control.*
4. Obtain the necessary supplies, including:
    a. Mask for the nurse *to prevent contamination of the sterile field from microorganisms of the mouth*

DATE/TIME	
12/28/99 11:00 AM	No. 16, 20 cm single-lumen subclavian intravenous catheter inserted by Dr. M. Sanchez at 10 AM. Position verified by x-ray. 1,000 mL D₅W with 40 mEq KCl started at 30 mL/h. Pt. resting comfortably with all vitals stable. See graphic record. —— R. Nichols, RN

Example of Nursing Progress Notes Using Narrative Format.

nose, and throat. In some facilities, a mask is used for both patient and nurse, and in others no masks are used. Follow the policy in your facility.

b. Disinfectant or germicidal cleansing agent *to prepare a clean surface to use as a base for the sterile field*

c. Sterile gloves *to maintain the dressing's sterility and protect the patient from infection*

d. Cleansing materials. These vary from facility to facility, but most commonly used are hydrogen peroxide applied with cotton-tipped applicators *to cleanse any exudate from the site or to remove crusts around the catheter* and povidone-iodine solution and gauze squares or povidone-iodine swabs *to cleanse and disinfect the skin.* When swabs are used, you do not need sterile gloves, because the hands are separated from contact with the wound. Some facilities use acetone, but this is not recommended, as discussed previously. Tincture of iodine may be used and then followed with 70% alcohol to remove the iodine *to decrease the incidence of skin reaction to the tincture of iodine. For patients with sensitivity to iodine,* 70% alcohol alone may be used.

e. Dressing supplies for the site vary, as discussed previously. Select those used in your facility.

f. Antiseptic or antimicrobial ointment *to decrease microorganisms at the insertion site*

g. Clean gloves to remove the soiled dressing

Implementation

5. Check the patient's identification *to be sure you are performing the procedure for the correct patient.*

6. Explain the procedure to the patient.

7. Clean the overbed table with disinfectant and allow it to dry, or cover it completely because the table is frequently soiled by urinals, bedpans, and used tissues.

8. Place the patient in the supine position, with the head turned away from the insertion site.

9. Put on a mask if your facility procedure requires its use.

10. Set up your materials on the overbed table. Open sterile packages so the contents are accessible but remain protected. If a prepackaged set is used, open it so the outer wrap is a sterile field.

11. Put on clean gloves, remove the old dressing, and discard it into a paper bag or appropriate receptacle. *Clean gloves protect your hands from possible contact with drainage from the wound.*

12. Take off the gloves, and wash your hands.

13. Inspect the site carefully, especially noting any redness, swelling, or drainage, *to assess for infection and reaction to the materials used in cleansing. If irritation is noted without signs of infection,* it is appropriate to change to an alternate cleansing material or to use only hydrogen peroxide.

14. Put on the sterile gloves.

15. Cleanse the area around the catheter.

a. Use the hydrogen peroxide *to remove secretions, crusts, or exudate.*

b. Use the antiseptic solution *to cleanse the entire site and surrounding area.* Cleanse in a circular manner, starting at the catheter and moving outward in concentric circles. Do not go back over areas previously cleansed. Cleanse an area 3 in from the site in all directions *to provide a wide area of antiseptic protection.*

c. Allow the antiseptic solution to dry. *This provides good contact with the antiseptic activity of the agent.* If you used tincture of iodine, you then use 70% alcohol to remove the iodine and allow the alcohol to dry. *This provides maximum antiseptic action.*

16. Obtain a small amount of antiseptic or antibiotic ointment on an applicator, and apply it to the insertion site, completely filling the space and occluding it. *This provides a mechanical and a chemical barrier to microbes.*

17. Apply the new dressing.

a. If using gauze squares and tape, place one gauze square under the catheter and one over the insertion site. Arrange the catheter so the connection end is outside the dressing. *This allows the tubing to be changed without disturbing the dressing.* Remove the sterile gloves, and tape the dressing down on all sides. To seal the edge under the catheter completely, cut a small slit in the tape, and slide this onto each side of the catheter *to secure the dressing* (Fig. 54–6).

b. If using a plastic adhesive drape material, place one gauze square under the catheter and one over the insertion site. Remove the gloves, and pull the backing off the plastic. Place it over the gauze, and begin pressing it down from one side to the other. When securing it at the catheter, mold the plastic around the catheter to form a seal (Fig. 54–7).

c. If using a transparent, moisture- and vapor-permeable dressing (OpSite or Tegaderm), do not use gauze squares. *Skin moisture will gradually escape through the dressing material.* Remove your gloves before handling the materials. Peel off the backing gradually as you apply the material to the skin *so it goes on*

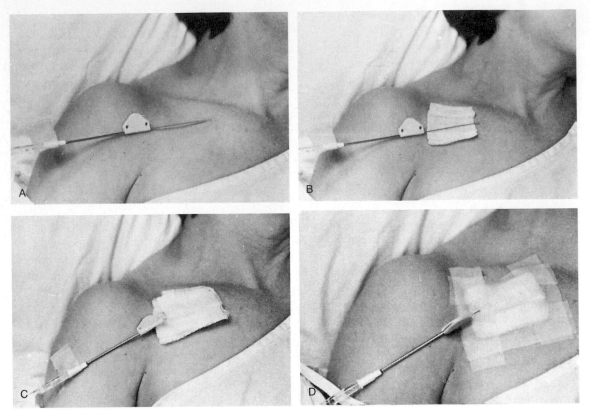

Figure 54–6. Using gauze squares as a dressing for a subclavian IV line. **(A)** Catheter and insertion site. **(B)** The first gauze square is placed under the catheter. **(C)** The second gauze square is placed over the catheter exit site. **(D)** The edges are taped down to form a seal on all sides. Note how the tape is placed around the catheter. (Courtesy Ivan Ellis)

smoothly. Allow enough slack *so you can mold the dressing material around the catheter, forming a seal* (Fig. 54–8).

Commercially produced transparent dressings also are designed for use with central lines (Fig. 54–9).

18. If there is not a connector device, change the tape over the connection between the catheter and the IV tubing. *Replacing the tape lessens the accumulation of microbes.* Make tabs on each end of the tape *so it can be removed easily,* and then apply the tape around the connection securely (Fig. 54–10).

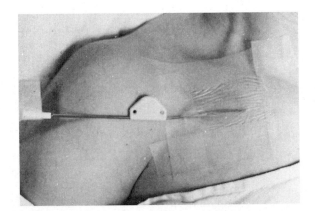

Figure 54–7. Using a clear plastic adhesive drape over the subclavian dressing. (Courtesy Ivan Ellis)

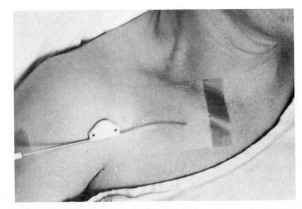

Figure 54–8. Dressing the subclavian IV line with transparent, moisture-permeable dressing (OpSite). (Courtesy Ivan Ellis)

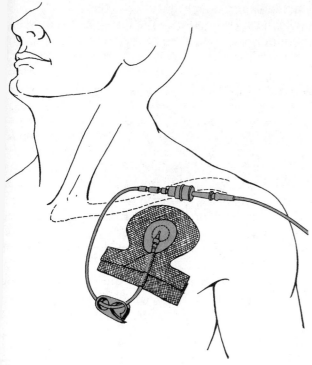

Figure 54–9. Commercial dressing for a central line. The line is connected to the IV tubing with a screw connection. Note the plastic clamp on the line.

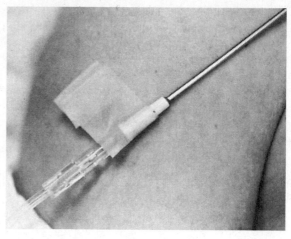

Figure 54–10. Taping the connection between the catheter and the IV tubing. (Courtesy Ivan Ellis)

    b. The IV line—*flow not obstructed, rate correctly set, and all connections secure.*
    c. The dressing—*secure.*

Documentation

25. Document the dressing change according to the procedure in your facility, either on a flow sheet or on the progress notes. Be sure a description of the site is included.

19. Label the dressing with date and time of changing by writing on the dressing itself or by writing on a piece of tape placed on the dressing. Use a pen with ink that will not rub off.
20. Reposition the patient *for comfort.*
21. Dispose of all packages and materials used.
22. Wash your hands.
23. Remove and discard your mask, if you are wearing one.

Evaluation

24. Evaluate using the following criteria:
    a. Patient comfortable.

PROCEDURE FOR CHANGING THE EXIT SITE DRESSING ON A SURGICALLY INSERTED LINE

The exit site on a surgically implanted catheter is distant from the entrance into the bloodstream, and the Dacron cuff provides a barrier to ascending infection on the outside of the catheter. Therefore, the procedure requires sterile technique but is usually less extensive than for the standard central IV catheter.

    If the dressing over the exit site is gauze, it may be changed daily for the first 3 weeks after surgical insertion. If the dressing is transparent, it may be left

DATE/TIME	
12/30/99 9:30 AM	D: *Subclavian site clean and dry with no drainage, redness, or swelling; sutures remain intact.* A: *Subclavian site dressing changed.* R: *Patient states no pain or discomfort at site.* M. Washington, NS

Example of Nursing Progress Notes Using Focus Format.

in place for several days before it is changed. In some facilities, the dressing is changed only when soiled or loose or at specified intervals, such as three times a week. When the exit site is thoroughly healed, the procedure is usually different. A common practice is to leave the exit site open without a dressing after it is fully healed. After healing, the exit site is cleaned as necessary with hydrogen peroxide. *To prevent pulling,* the tubing is clamped to the patient's underclothing, or a small gauze square is taped over the site and the catheter clamped to the dressing.

Assessment

1. Check the date and time of the last dressing change.
2. Review the facility procedure *to identify the appropriate dressing material to use.*

Planning

3. Wash your hands *for infection control.*
4. Gather the necessary supplies.
   a. Hydrogen peroxide and sterile cotton-tipped applicators
   b. Povidone-iodine swabsticks or povidone-iodine solution and additional sterile cotton-tipped applicators. In some facilities, you also need an alcohol wipe.
   c. Povidone-iodine ointment or triple antibiotic ointment
   d. Sterile 2 × 2 gauze squares
   e. Paper tape
   f. Clean gloves
   g. Sterile gloves and mask are not needed. *Because the exit site is a distance from the entry into the vein, the infection danger is considerably lessened.* Sterile equipment is used, and the sterility of all items that touch the exit site is maintained. *This has been demonstrated to provide adequate protection against infection.*

Implementation

5. Identify the patient *to be sure you are performing the procedure on the correct patient.*

6. Explain the procedure to the patient.
7. Put on clean gloves to remove the old dressing and inspect the site for redness, exudate, and swelling, *which might indicate infection.* Use clean gloves for handling the soiled dressing *to protect yourself from infection.* Check also for skin reaction to the iodine products.
8. Using the sterile cotton-tipped applicators, cleanse the exit site with hydrogen peroxide. Remove any crusts that have formed. Use a new sterile applicator each time it is necessary to dip into the container of peroxide *so you do not contaminate the supply.* Cleanse outward for 3 inches in all directions from the catheter, using a spiral that starts at the catheter and progresses outward *so microbes are moved away from the exit site.*
9. Cleanse the same area in the same way using the povidone-iodine swabsticks or cotton-tipped applicators dipped in povidone-iodine solution.
10. Allow the iodine solution to dry on the skin for 2 or 3 minutes. *This frees the iodine and leaves an antiseptic film on the skin.* In some facilities, the iodine cleansing is done first, and the iodine is allowed to dry, then the peroxide cleansing is done. Doing this does not leave the antiseptic film on the skin, but *removing the iodine may lessen the chance of skin reaction.* Follow the procedure established in your facility.
11. Squeeze antiseptic ointment directly onto the exit site, completely occluding the opening around the catheter. *Doing this provides a mechanical and a chemical barrier against microbes.*
12. Lift the catheter up, and use a povidone-iodine swabstick to cleanse it from the exit site to the connector. *Doing this decreases the number of bacteria present and moves them away from the exit site.* In some facilities, this step is done with an alcohol wipe.
13. Place one 2 × 2 gauze square under the catheter and one over the exit site *to provide an absorbent*

DATE/TIME	
7/28/99	S States Hickman site has no soreness or discomfort.
1000 AM	O Hickman entry site is clean, dry, and without redness or swelling.
	A Site healing well.
	P Continue with standard nursing care protocol.
	J. Swisher RN

Example of Nursing Progress Notes Using SOAP Format.

surface between the plastic of the catheter and the skin and to act as a barrier between outside contaminants and the exit site.

14. Tape the dressing in place *to secure it.*
15. Loop the catheter, and tape it to the body. *Looping prevents direct pull on the catheter and lessens the chance of disturbing it. Taping the catheter down prevents it from twisting and being caught on clothing.*
16. Write the date and time of the change on the dressing itself. *This provides immediate reference for those caring for the patient.*
17. Dispose of used equipment and packaging materials.
18. Wash your hands.

Evaluation

19. Evaluate using the following criteria:
    a. Patient comfortable.
    b. Dressing secure.
    c. Catheter not under tension.

Documentation

20. Document the dressing change as appropriate in your facility, either on a flow sheet or on the progress record. Include the appearance of the site.

PROCEDURE FOR CHANGING THE FLUID CONTAINER AND THE TUBING

When changing an IV fluid container connected to a central line, use the same technique as for changing a container on a conventional IV line.

When changing the tubing, *take special precautions to protect the patient against air embolism caused by the negative pressure at the catheter's tip.* This procedure is based on the Procedure for Changing the Fluid Container, Tubing, and Dressing in Module 52, Preparing and Maintaining IV Infusions, pp. 490–492.

Assessment

1.–2. Follow steps 1 and 2 of the Procedure for Changing the Fluid Container, Tubing, and Dressing in Module 52: Check the chart for the physician's order for type of fluid, and verify when the tubing and dressing were last changed.

Planning

3.–5. Follow steps 3 through 5 of the Procedure for Changing the Fluid Container, Tubing, and Dressing in Module 52: Determine the equipment you will need. Wash your hands *for infection control.* Select the correct IV fluid and equipment based on whether a regular tub-

ing, microdrip tubing, or infusion control device tubing is needed.

Implementation

6.–13. Follow steps 6 through 13 of the Procedure for Changing the Fluid Container, Tubing, and Dressing in Module 52: Set up equipment, identify the patient, and explain what you plan to do. Hang the new container on the IV pole. Remove tape and dressing from old tubing, examine site, put on gloves, and shut off IV flow.
14. Remove the tape, if any is present, from the connection between the catheter and the tubing.
15. Cleanse the junction between the catheter and the tubing with an alcohol swab, and allow it to dry *to decrease the number of microbes in the area.*
16. Clamp the line if there is a clamp on the tubing *to prevent air embolism. Most central venous catheters have a plastic clamp as an integral part of the equipment. In those that do not, a special clamp without teeth that remains closed (a bulldog clamp) is usually kept on a piece of tape attached to the tubing so that it is available.*

    If there is no clamp, you must do one of three things to increase intrathoracic pressure and prevent air embolism: Pinch or fold the tubing; place the patient in Trendelenburg's position, which will slow the flow in the vein, *thus increasing venous pressure;* or have the patient take a deep breath and hold it while you change the tubing *to increase intrathoracic pressure.* This last method is called the Valsalva maneuver and should be done just at the time of the tubing change.
17. Loosen the old tubing from the connection by twisting it, but do not disconnect it.
18. Remove cap from new tubing.
19. Remove the old tubing from the connector, and insert the new tubing immediately (Fig. 54–11).
20. Start the new fluid at a slow rate.
21. Tape the connection as previously described or secure the connector firmly.

Evaluation

22. Evaluate using the following criteria:
    a. Patient comfortable.
    b. Line patent, flow rate correct, and connections secure.
    c. Dressing secure and intact.

Documentation

23. Document as follows:
    a. IV flow sheet: time, fluid container discontinued, fluid container added, tubing change
    b. Intake and output record

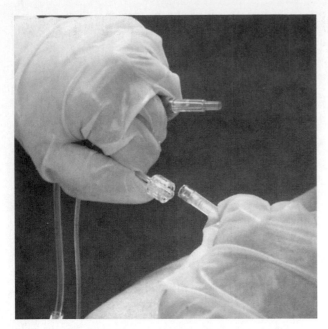

Figure 54–11. Hold the new IV line carefully to prevent its contamination while you separate the used tubing from the catheter.

PROCEDURE FOR ESTABLISHING A HEPARIN LOCK ON A CENTRAL INTRAVENOUS CATHETER

When a Hickman line or central IV catheter is being used for intermittent infusion and drawing of blood, it must be capped with a special type of injection cap that screws onto the line like a jar lid. This cap is used *to make sure the cap does not become dislodged accidentally, providing an opportunity for air to enter.* As in the regular IV lock, the catheter must be filled with a heparinized saline solution *to prevent clots from forming at the tip of the catheter and occluding it.* A solution of 10 to 100 U heparin per milliliter of normal saline is the most common mixture. The heparin solution is injected at least twice a day *to maintain patency of the catheter.* Some facilities are experimenting with using a stronger heparin solution (100–500 U/mL) and allowing longer intervals between additions of new solution. Check the policy in your facility.

As another precaution against accidental opening of the central IV line, an integral clamp is usually in place. The surgically inserted catheter may not have an integral clamp; instead, a clamp without teeth, such as a shunt clamp (sometimes called a Scribner clamp, cannula clamp, or bulldog clamp) is used. Even though the clamp has no teeth, *to prevent damage to the catheter,* the clamp is placed over a piece of tape on the line. *Remember that a Hickman line may be in place for months and that repairs and replacement are problems.* Thus, careful handling is essential.

When the line is being used, the clamp is kept attached to the dressing or a tape for safe keeping.

Assessment
1. Check the order for discontinuing IV fluids and establishing a heparin lock on a central line.
2. Check the facility procedure for the type of solution to be used.
3. Check the type of central IV line in place and the number of milliliters of fluid necessary to fill it.

Planning
4. Wash your hands *for infection control.*
5. Gather the necessary equipment.
   a. Sterile screw-type cap. Some types of central IV lines do not use a screw cap. For these lines, a regular male adapter for an IV line is used. A cap that is accessed with needle or one of the needleless devices may be used.
   b. Syringe with heparinized saline and a 1-in needle or special tip for accessing the needleless device. *The Hickman catheter has an internal volume of 2 mL. An extra 0.5 mL (2.5 mL total) is usually added to make sure the tip of the catheter is free of clots. The 1-in needle is used because it is less likely to penetrate beyond the tip and damage the reservoir wall.* A 20-gauge or smaller needle is used *because repeated punctures with large needles can lead to leaks in the rubber diaphragm.* Surgically implanted ports hold 5 mL of solution. Some facilities use a larger volume to irrigate the catheter or port. Follow the procedure in your facility.
   c. Tape. Plastic tape is commonly used *because it is thick and protects the catheter from the clamp better than other tape does. Also, it does not usually leave adhesive residue when removed.*
   d. Appropriate clamp if one is not already in use on the line. It is common practice to attach a clamp to the dressing of a Hickman line even when a continuous infusion is being administered. *This makes the clamp accessible during tubing changes and blood drawing.* An extension tubing within an integral clamp is commonly placed on a conventional central line.
   e. Alcohol swab
   f. Clean gloves

Implementation
6. Identify the patient *to be sure you are performing the procedure for the correct patient.*
7. Explain the procedure to the patient.
8. Place the tape over the catheter, if needed. Make folded-over pull-tabs at each end of the tape *so it will be easy to remove for replacement.* Tape is not needed if there is an integral plastic clamp.

Table 54–1.	Example of Flow Sheet for Documenting Starting a Heparin Lock						
Date	**IV #**	**Content**	**Start**	**Stop**	**Amount**	**Signature**
9/12/99	5	5%D/NS	1600	2210	500 mL	N. McGill, SN
9/12/99	Heparin lock to IV		2210			N. McGill, SN

9. Turn off the IV infusion.

0. Put on gloves *to protect yourself from the possibility of any blood returning through the catheter,* although this is not likely.

1. Place the clamp on the catheter (over the tape for bulldog clamp).

2. Cleanse the junction of the catheter and the tubing with an alcohol swab *to decrease the number of microbes in the immediate area when the tubing is opened.* Allow the solution to dry before proceeding.

3. Open the package containing the sterile cap. Hold the cap carefully by the outside rim of the rubber injection cap. *To preserve sterility,* do not touch the end that will be placed in the central IV line.

4. Loosen the IV tubing connector by twisting it.

5. Remove the IV tubing, and insert the injection cap, being careful to maintain sterility of the ends of the catheter and the cap. Screw the cap in securely by hand. Do not use excessive force *because this will make the cap difficult to remove.* The IV tubing may be capped with a sterile needle or needleless connector and used at a later time or may be discarded depending on the patient's needs.

6. Insert the needle or needleless connnector of the filled syringe into the cap. A needle is placed in the center *where the rubber is thinnest.* Follow the instructions for the specific needleless connector being used.

7. Release the clamp.

8. Inject 2.5 mL heparinized saline into the catheter. In some facilities, the following alternative is used.
   a. Inject 2 mL heparinized saline.
   b. Inject the remaining 0.5 mL heparinized saline as you are clamping the catheter. *This is done to provide a slight positive pressure in the tubing, thereby preventing backflow into the tip of the catheter.* No research data demonstrate that this step is necessary. Follow the procedure in your facility.

9. Replace the clamp on the catheter.

0. Remove the needle and syringe from the cap.

Evaluation
21. Evaluate using the following criteria:
   a. Patient comfortable.
   b. Catheter not caught in clothing.
   c. Catheter clamp secure.

Documentation
22. Discontinuing the continuous infusion and placing a heparin lock on the central line are typically noted on the IV flow sheet. If this is not the case in your facility, make a brief note on the progress record (Table 54–1).

PROCEDURE FOR IRRIGATING AN INTERMITTENT CENTRAL INTRAVENOUS CATHETER

If the catheter is being used for intermittent administration of drugs and for drawing blood, carefully maintain the patency of the catheter by periodically irrigating it with a heparinized saline solution. Use the schedule stipulated in the policy of your facility.

Assessment
1. Determine when medications are being administered or blood is being drawn. *If these two procedures are done regularly, the heparin injected after each procedure is adequate irrigation to maintain patency. If the catheter is not being used regularly,* develop a schedule for irrigation. Follow the policy in your facility (every 12 hours is common).

2. Check your facility's policy on the strength of heparinized saline and the amount to be used. The two most common strengths and amounts are 2.5 mL of 10 U/mL and 2.5 mL of 100 U/mL. Some facilities flush with saline before using the heparin solution *to ensure that the line is patent.*

Planning
3. Wash your hands *for infection control.*

4. Gather the necessary equipment.
   a. Syringe with 2.5 mL heparinized saline, with a 1-in needle or needleless connector
   b. Povidone-iodine or alcohol wipe.
   c. Clean gloves

Medication	12/23/99	12/24/99	12/25/99
Ampicillin 500 mg IV 6-12-18-24	6KD 12RS 18MN 24KD	6KD	
Heparin Flush 10 U/mL 2.5 mL 6-12-18-24	6KD 12RS 18MN 24KD	6KD	

Table 54–2. Example of Flow Sheet for Documenting Heparin Irrigation of a Central Line as a Separate Entry

d. Normal saline solution—2.5 mL in a syringe with a 1-in needle or connector as indicated by your facility procedure

Implementation

5. Identify the patient *to be sure you are performing the procedure for the correct patient.*
6. Explain the procedure to the patient.
7. Put on gloves *to protect yourself from the possibility of accidental separation of the tubing and blood return that would contaminate your hands.*
8. Cleanse the cap by scrubbing for 1 minute with the antiseptic swab. *This provides mechanical cleansing and antiseptic action. For maximum antiseptic effect, allow the solution to dry.*
9. Insert the needle or connector into the cap.
10. Remove the clamp from the catheter.
11. Inject 2.5 mL heparinized saline. If resistance is felt, and the solution cannot be injected or the injection causes pain, pause and have the patient turn. Try again. *If the catheter was resting against the wall of the vein or against a valve, turning will cause the catheter to move and the solution can then be injected with ease. If you still cannot inject the solution with ease, notify the physician. The catheter may be occluded.*
12. Optional steps:
    a. Inject the first 2 mL heparinized saline.
    b. Clamp the catheter while injecting the remaining 0.5 mL of solution.
13. Reclamp the catheter if not done as part of step 10.
14. Remove the needle (or connector) and syringe from the cap and remove gloves.

Evaluation

15. Evaluate using the following criteria:
    a. Patient comfortable.
    b. Catheter clamp secure.
    c. Catheter not caught in clothing.

Documentation

16. Usually the nurse will document the heparin flush on the medication record. In some facili-

ties, all procedures related to the central line are recorded on a special flow sheet (Table 54–2).

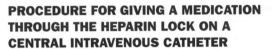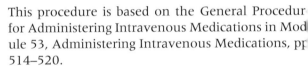

PROCEDURE FOR GIVING A MEDICATION THROUGH THE HEPARIN LOCK ON A CENTRAL INTRAVENOUS CATHETER

This procedure is based on the General Procedure for Administering Intravenous Medications in Module 53, Administering Intravenous Medications, pp 514–520.

Assessment

1. Validate the orders.
2. Examine the MAR for accuracy and completeness.
3. Review information about the medication, especially noting recommended speed of injection, dilution and diluent, and compatibility with heparinized saline. The pharmacist may be consulted if the information is not available in your unit references. *If the medication is not compatible with the heparinized saline,* incorporate the optional steps listed in the module.
4. Check your unit procedure for the strength of heparin solution to use.
5. Assess the patient to identify the need for any prn IV medications ordered.

Planning

6. Determine the equipment you will need.
7. Wash your hands *for infection control.*
8. Obtain the necessary supplies.
    a. Medication in a syringe with a 1-in needle or connector or in a small-volume parenteral container with tubing and a 1-in needle or connector attached. (See Module 53, Administering Intravenous Medications, for preparation instructions.)
    b. Povidone-iodine or alcohol swab

c. Syringe containing 2.5 mL heparinized saline, with a 1-in needle or connector

d. Clean gloves

e. Optional: Syringe with 5 mL plain saline solution or two syringes with 2.5 mL saline in each if the medication is incompatible with the heparin. Check the policy in your facility.

Implementation

9. Read the name of the medication on the MAR.

10. Check the label on the medication, and pick it up (first check).

11. Check the label again, comparing it with the MAR (second check).

12. Prepare the medication.

13. Check the medication label with the MAR again (third check).

14. Place a label on the prepared medication to identify the patient if the MAR is not to be taken into the room.

15. Prepare and label the heparinized saline solution and plain saline if needed.

16. Identify the patient *to be sure you are performing the procedure for the correct patient.*

17. Explain the procedure to the patient.

18. Administer the medication by IV push or piggyback set.

   a. Put on gloves *to protect yourself from the possibility of accidental separation of the tubing and blood return that would contaminate your hands.*

   b. Cleanse the cap by scrubbing for 1 minute with the antiseptic swab *for mechanical cleansing and antiseptic action.* Allow the solution to dry.

   c. Optional steps *if medication is not compatible with heparin:*

     (1) Insert needle or connector of syringe with plain saline in the cap.

     (2) Release the clamp.

     (3) Inject 2.5 mL saline to flush the heparin from the line.

     (4) Reclamp the line.

     (5) Remove the saline syringe.

   d. Insert the needle or connector for the medication into the cap.

   e. Release the clamp.

   f. Inject the medication at the rate ordered or as recommended by the manufacturer. If an infusion set is used, regulate the infusion set to the correct rate to deliver the medication as ordered or recommended by the manufacturer (Fig. 54–12).

   g. When all the medication has been injected or infused, clamp the catheter over the tape.

   h. Remove the needle or connector from the cap.

   i. Scrub the cap again for 1 minute *if the medication has been infusing over an extended period. If the medication was injected over 5 minutes or less,* it is not necessary to rescrub the cap.

   j. Optional steps if the medication is not compatible with heparin: Follow steps 19.c.(1) through 19.c.(5) above *to flush the medication out before the heparin is instilled.*

   k. Instill the heparinized saline using steps 19.c.(1) through 19.c.(5) for flushing the line with saline.

19. Optional steps followed in some facilities when heparinizing central lines:

     (1) Inject the first 2 mL heparinized saline into the catheter.

     (2) Clamp the catheter while injecting the

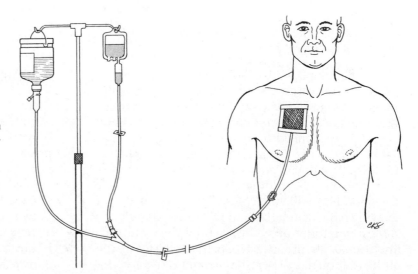

Figure 54–12. Administering medication through the Hickman catheter using a piggyback administration set.

Table 54–3. Example of Flow Sheet for Documenting An Intravenous Medication and Heparin Flush In One Entry

			12/23	12/24
12/23/99	Ampicillin	6	KD	KD
	500 mg IV	12	RS	
	followed by			
	2.5 mL	6	MN	
	heparin	12	KD	
	flush · q6h,			
	6-12-6-12			

remaining 0.5 mL of heparin so the syringe is not emptied.

20. Leave the patient in a comfortable position.

21. Dispose of the used equipment and gloves.

22. Wash your hands *for infection control.*

Evaluation

23. Evaluate using the following criteria:

   a. Six rights followed: Right patient, right medication, right dosage, right route, right time, right documentation.

   b. Medication given over correct time period.

   c. Catheter clamp secure.

   d. Catheter not caught in clothing.

   e. Criteria established for determining effectiveness of medication were used.

   f. Side effects promptly identified.

Documentation

24. Document the medication on the medication record. The heparin flush is usually noted with the medication and charted at the same time (Table 54–3).

PROCEDURE FOR DRAWING BLOOD THROUGH A CENTRAL INTRAVENOUS CATHETER

Some central catheters may be used for drawing blood and for administering fluids and medications. The criteria for determining suitability are usually the internal diameter of the catheter and the material of which it is made. Larger diameter catheters are less likely to clot with blood and become unusable. Silicone rubber catheters are more flexible and are smoother, which decreases the likelihood that drawing blood through them will cause clotting.

Most surgically implanted central lines are routinely used for drawing blood. With many of the multiple-lumen catheters, one lumen is reserved for drawing blood. There is a great advantage to the patient in having all blood drawn through an existing line rather than having multiple needle sticks on already difficult veins. Follow the policy of your facility regarding which central catheters may be used for drawing blood and who is permitted to draw blood.

The procedure presented here is for drawing blood through a Hickman line. The only difference for other catheters is that they may be shorter and need less solution to clear them. If a multiple-lumen catheter is in use, shut off the other lines temporarily while drawing the blood *to prevent erroneous laboratory test results based on large amounts of solution in the blood.*

Assessment

1. Determine the suitability of the central IV catheter for drawing blood. The policy or procedure book for your facility is usually the best resource for this information.

2. Determine which ordered laboratory tests require blood specimens.

3. Consult the laboratory or a reference *to identify the amount of blood needed and the type of laboratory specimen tube (eg, heparinized, plain) that should be used to obtain blood for the planned tests.* These are often designated by the color of the test tube's rubber stopper (eg, red top, green top, lavender top).

Planning

4. Wash your hands *for infection control.*

5. Gather the necessary equipment.

   a. One empty 5-mL syringe without a needle or an extra 5 mL test tube for the blood collection device.

   b. One syringe large enough to aspirate the amount of blood required for the laboratory test ordered or a blood collection device that holds blood sample tubes and appropriate connector

   c. One syringe with 20 mL saline *to flush blood from the line.* In some facilities two 10-mL syringes are used.

   d. One syringe with 2.5 mL heparinized saline *to reheparinize the line and prevent clotting*

   e. Sterile 2 × 2 gauze squares *to hold the cap* or a sterile needle in its cover *to place on the end of an IV tubing*

   f. Povidone-iodine or alcohol swab *to cleanse the cap*

   g. Test tubes appropriate for the type of specimen needed. It is wise to mark each tube *so you know the amount of blood needed for that particular test.*

   h. Tape *to secure all connections*

   i. Clean gloves *to protect your hands from possible contamination*

j. Eye protection *to protect your eyes from the possibility of blood splashing from an accident with the syringe or the blood tube.* Face shields and goggles are the best eye protection *because they completely shield the eyes from all directions.* Regular eyeglasses may be considered adequate eye protection in some instances, but they do not protect from the side. Check the policy in your facility as to whether or not eyeglasses may be used for eye protection.

Implementation

6. Identify the patient *to be sure you are performing the procedure for the correct patient.*
7. Explain the procedure to the patient.
8. Remove the protective tape holding the cap or line firmly in place.
9. Put on clean gloves and eye protection.
10. Cleanse the junction of the catheter and the cap with the antiseptic swab for 1 minute, and allow it to dry. *This decreases the number of microbes in the immediate area.*
11. Open the package of sterile 2 × 2 gauze squares.
12. Check to make sure the catheter is firmly clamped over the tape.
13. Remove the cap or line from the catheter, and place the cap between two sterile 2 × 2 gauze squares. Put a sterile capped needle on the IV line if one is in use. Hold the end of the catheter in your fingers *so it does not touch anything.* The cap is removed when blood is being drawn *so it does not become damaged from the large-diameter needles that are necessary to draw blood. The damaged cap will begin to leak and admit microbes. It must be discarded and replaced. If a needleless connector system is being used, this is not a concern.* Some facilities keep a supply of sterile caps, and a fresh cap is placed on the line each time the cap is removed.
14. Connect an empty 5-mL syringe or collection device to the catheter.
15. Release the clamp on the catheter.
16. Aspirate 5 mL fluid from the catheter, or engage extra test tube into collection device. *This will completely remove the heparinized saline or IV fluid from the catheter, and the catheter will be filled with undiluted blood.* If the syringe will not aspirate with ease, have the patient turn. *Turning will move the tip of the catheter in the vein* and if it was against the wall of the vein or a valve, will allow it to move away. Gently aspirate again. If you still cannot aspirate, stop the procedure, and notify the physician.
17. Reclamp the catheter. Remember, the catheter must always be clamped when the syringe is being attached or removed *so the patient is protected from air embolism.*
18. Remove the first syringe from the catheter or test tube from the collection device and discard it, along with its contents. *This blood has heparinized saline mixed in it and therefore would provide erroneous results on laboratory tests.*
19. Attach the empty syringe or next test tube *to draw blood from the catheter.*
20. Unclamp the catheter.
21. Aspirate the amount of blood needed for the tests into the syringe (Fig. 54–13), or engage test tubes one at a time into the blood collection device.
22. Reclamp the catheter after aspirating or each time a test tube is removed or inserted into the collection device *to guard against air entering.*
23. Remove the syringe of blood from the catheter. The blood should not be allowed to remain in the syringe because it may clot. At this point, you may wish to ask another person to assist you by putting the correct amount of blood into the correct test tubes while you are finishing with the catheter. As you become more experienced, the next steps will be done rapidly, and there will be no problem with the blood remaining in the syringe while you finish. If using a blood collection device that holds the blood sample tubes, this is not a concern because *the blood will be aspirated directly into the tube.*
24. Attach the syringe with 20 mL saline.
25. Unclamp the catheter.
26. Inject the saline. *This flushes all blood from the catheter.* Some facilities use less than 20 mL of saline. The important point is to flush thoroughly *so no blood residue remains in the tubing to occlude it.*
27. Clamp the catheter.
28. Remove the empty syringe.
29. Attach the syringe with the heparinized saline solution to the catheter. *The heparin will prevent clotting in the catheter.*
30. Unclamp the catheter.
31. Inject 2.5 mL heparinized saline solution. Optional step: Inject the last 0.5 mL while clamping the catheter.
32. Clamp the catheter.
33. Remove the empty syringe.
34. Replace the cap or IV line on the catheter, being careful to maintain sterility of the catheter and of the cap or IV line.
35. Inject the blood into the proper laboratory test tubes if not using a blood collection device.
36. Tape the cap to the catheter *for extra security* if indicated. Be sure to make tabs at the ends of the tape *so that removal is easier.*

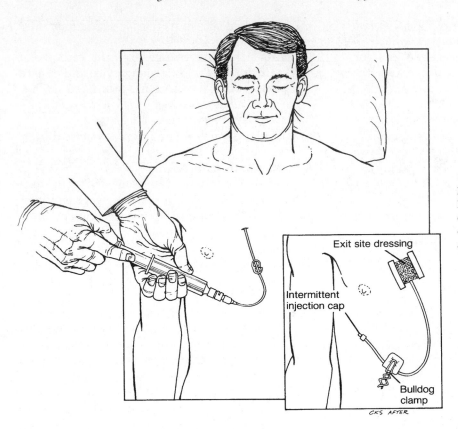

Figure 54–13. Drawing blood from a Hickman catheter. An integral clamp is on the catheter. The inset shows a catheter without an integral clamp with a bulldog clamp in place over tape.

37. Discard used equipment and gloves.
38. Wash your hands.
39. Send the blood to the laboratory with the correct requisition forms and labeling. The laboratory specimens are usually enclosed in a plastic bag *for safe handling during transport.*

Evaluation
40. Evaluate using the following criteria:
   a. Catheter clamp secure.
   b. Catheter not caught in clothing.
   c. Appropriate blood sample obtained.

Documentation
41. Document on a flow sheet or on a progress record that blood was drawn from the central line and sent to the laboratory.

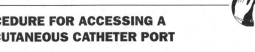

PROCEDURE FOR ACCESSING A SUBCUTANEOUS CATHETER PORT

To administer IV fluids or medications or to heparinize an implanted infusion port, you must first access it. This means that you need to insert a special noncoring needle into the port. A noncoring needle has a tip constructed so that it opens a slit into the rubber diaphragm and does not create a hole from a segment "cored" out. The access needle can be a straight needle attached to a syringe to administer medication or draw blood or may be right-angle needle (sometimes called a Huber needle) that is used to connect to an IV line. Noncoring needles are shown in Figure 54–14.

Assessment
1. Check the physician's order to determine whether an ongoing access or simply temporary access is needed and medications that need to be given.
2. Identify the type and location of the patient's subcutaneous port.

Planning
3. Wash your hands *for infection control.*
4. Obtain the equipment you will need.
   a. Three povidone-iodine swabs
   b. Dry cotton swab or 2 × 2 gauze
   c. Sterile gloves
   d. Alcohol swabs in addition to the povidone-iodine swabs if used in your facility
   e. An empty syringe with an extension tubing that has a clamp attached to a noncoring needle
   f. One of the following groups of supplies
   For temporary access:
   (1) Materials to draw blood or give medication
   (2) Syringe with heparinized saline in the dilution

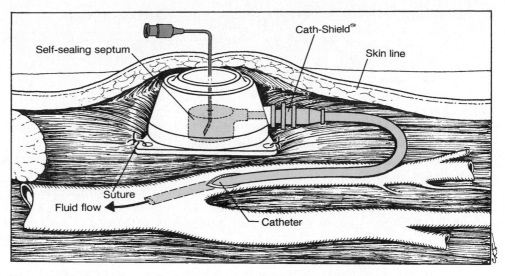

Figure 54–14. Noncoring needles leave only a smooth slit in the rubber diaphragm.

prescribed by your facility (frequently 100 U/mL) to reheparinize the line when you have finished. If you are only reheparinizing a port that is not being used, you may use a straight noncoring needle attached directly to the syringe of heparinized saline. If you must change syringes, you will need to use a right-angle needle attached to extension tubing as listed previously *to clamp the line closed while you are changing syringes.*

(3) Medication ordered. Remember to use the six rights and three checks when preparing any medication.

For ongoing access:

(1) IV fluid with tubing set up and ready to attach (see Module 52, Preparing and Maintaining Intravenous Infusions)

g. In some facilities, ethyl chloride spray is used *to decrease discomfort* caused by the needle entry. If used in your facility, obtain spray.

Implementation

5. Check the patient's identification *for safety.*

6. Explain the procedure to the patient *to alleviate anxiety and elicit the patient's cooperation.*

7. Provide for patient privacy.

8. Prepare a clean surface to set up your equipment *so that your materials will not become contaminated and so that they are convenient.*

9. Place the patient in a supine or semi-Fowler's position and expose the port site. *This makes the area easier to access.*

10. Put on a mask *to reduce the chance of microorganisms from your mouth and nose contaminating the site.* In some facilities, this is not part of the pro-

cedure. In others, both patient and nurse wear a mask. There is no evidence to support one method over another. Follow the policy in your facility.

11. Set up your equipment on the table in the order you will use it. *This helps you to remember what you must do next and makes the procedure go more quickly.* Open sterile packages to have the contents ready to use.

12. Put on clean gloves *to protect your hands from disinfectants.*

13. Palpate the area over the port *to determine exactly where the port is located.*

14. Prepare the skin *to lessen the chance of infection at the site.*

   a. Swab the area with povidone-iodine in concentric circles starting at the center and moving out to form a circle approximately 3 to 4 in in diameter. Do this three times with separate swabs.

   b. Allow the solution to remain on the skin for 1 full minute.

   c. If your facility procedure calls for cleaning the iodine solution off with alcohol, do it at this time.

   d. Use a dry sterile swab to dry the skin site.

   e. If your facility procedure calls for ethyl chloride spray, use it at this time. Spray the site until it appears frosted.

15. Take off and discard the clean gloves, and put on sterile gloves. *Using sterile gloves makes sure that organisms are not introduced by your hands.*

16. Attach the extension tubing and syringe to the needle. (Some manufacturers make noncoring needles with tubing attached.) Leave the clamp on the tubing open at this time *so that you will be* *able to aspirate the syringe after you have accessed the port.*

17. Palpate the site with your nondominant hand *to determine the site of the diaphragm*, and hold the edges of the port firmly in place *to prevent its shifting as you access it*.

18. Using your dominant hand, insert the needle firmly straight into the center of the diaphragm until you feel it touch the needle stop in the bottom.

19. Hold the needle firmly in place while you aspirate. *A blood return indicates that the port is functioning*. If blood does not return immediately, having the patient turn to either side, cough slightly, and take deep breaths *may move the catheter in the vessel enough that blood will return*. If you cannot get blood to return, *the catheter may be plugged (the most likely cause) or the end may have migrated out of the vessel*. In this case, remove the needle, and notify the physician.

20. If the port is functioning, proceed to draw blood, administer medications, attach fluid set, or flush and heparinize the line as planned. Use the procedures previously outlined.

21. Complete the procedure.
    a. For intermittent access, remove the needle after flushing and heparinizing.
    b. For ongoing access, tape connections and apply dressing as described previously.

Evaluation

22. Evaluate using the following criteria:
    a. Catheter dressing and tapes intact.
    b. Site clean and free of signs of infection.
    c. Correct medication given or correct blood sample obtained.

Documentation

23. Document that implanted port was accessed, including date and time, on the IV flow sheet or the progress notes.

24. Document any heparin or medication given on the medication record.

LONG-TERM CARE

Traditionally, individuals with central lines did not receive care in long-term care settings. However, as the healthcare system changes, this practice also is changing. Some long-term care settings now admit people who have long-term central IV lines. The care of these residents is the same as for patients in an acute care setting.

HOME CARE

Increasing numbers of individuals who need long-term IV therapy, including those who need long-term antibiotic therapy for cardiac infections, parenteral nutrition on an ongoing basis, or pain medication or other ongoing therapies, and their home caregivers are being taught to care for central IV catheters. In some instances, the client maintains the catheter at home but receives therapy on an inpatient basis. In other instances, the client administers therapy at home as well. When the client is not able to manage this care, a family member or friend may be the primary home caregiver.

To enable clients to assume this highly technical care, the nurse must carefully plan an instructional program. Instruction begins while the individual is still in the hospital. A home care nurse provides follow-up care for ongoing assessment and to help with problem-solving in the home environment.

CRITICAL THINKING EXERCISES

• Jeff Madison has had Crohn's disease for many years. Because his recent exacerbation was particularly severe, a central venous catheter for total parenteral nutrition is to be inserted. The procedure will be done tomorrow morning. As you plan for Jeff's care, determine what concerns he might have about this procedure and how the procedure is carried out. Specify what teaching will be needed and about what he will need to talk. Describe what you will need to do to assist with such a procedure in your setting. Identify your immediate concerns for the patient after the procedure; how will you address these concerns in your planning?

• Margaret Sand, age 83, was admitted with severe pneumonia. Because her veins were so poor, the physician decided that a PICC line should be inserted to provide IV access for fluids and antibiotics. The certified IV nurse has just inserted the PICC line. Specify what concerns you will have and what monitoring you should do. When can the PICC line be used to start the ordered fluids and antibiotics? What care guidelines should you establish? Explain whether Mrs. Sand's age has any influence on your care planning.

✔ **PERFORMANCE CHECKLIST**

Procedure for Assisting With the Insertion of the Standard Central Intravenous Catheter	Needs More Practice	Satisfactory	Comments
Assessment			
1. Check order.			
2. Obtain signed permission, if needed.			
3. Assess patient's ability to participate in and tolerate the procedure. **a.** Position flat or in Trendelenburg's?			
b. Able to hold breath?			
c. Able to understand and follow directions?			
Planning			
4. Wash your hands.			
5. Obtain necessary equipment and supplies. **a.** Masks			
b. Sterile gown for physician			
c. Two pairs of sterile gloves			
d. Skin preparation materials			
e. Scissors to clip hair			
f. Topical anesthetic agent			
g. Sterile drapes			
h. Suitable catheter and syringe			
i. Suturing materials			
j. Intravenous (IV) fluid with tubing attached			
k. Dressing materials			
l. Sterile towel			
Implementation			
6. Check patient's identification.			
7. Explain procedure to patient.			
8. Prepare the unit.			
9. Place patient in a supine position.			
10. Support patient, and assist with procedure. **a.** Maintain touch.			
b. Help patient maintain position.			

(continued)

Procedure for Assisting With the Insertion of the Standard Central Intravenous Catheter *(Continued)*	Needs More Practice	Satisfactory	Comments
c. Give positive reinforcement to patient.			
d. Provide feedback to alleviate anxiety.			
e. Reassure patient.			
f. Remind others that patient is alert, if necessary.			
g. Open equipment and supplies.			
h. Hold anesthetic vial.			
i. Connect IV lock.			
j. Complete dressing.			
11. When completed line has been inserted: **a.** Remove drapes, and position patient comfortably.			
b. Order X-ray.			
c. Remove used supplies and packages.			
d. Wash your hands.			
Evaluation			
12. Evaluate the following: **a.** Patient comfort			
b. IV line for secure connections			
c. Dressing secure			
d. Fluid, after started, for line patency and rate			
Documentation			
13. Document on patient's chart: **a.** Time the central IV line was inserted			
b. Type and size of catheter			
c. Site used			
d. Solution and rate of administration			
e. Patient's response			
f. Time X-ray report received			

(continued)

Changing the Standard Central Intravenous Dressing	Needs More Practice	Satisfactory	Comments
Assessment			
1. Check date and time of last dressing change.			
2. Review facility procedure to identify appropriate dressing materials.			
Planning			
3. Wash your hands.			
4. Obtain necessary supplies.			
a. Masks, as directed by facility policy			
b. Disinfectant cleansing agent for table			
c. Sterile gloves			
d. Cleansing materials			
e. Dressing supplies			
f. Antiseptic ointment			
g. Clean gloves			
Implementation			
5. Check patient's identification.			
6. Explain procedure to patient.			
7. Clean overbed table, and allow to dry.			
8. Place patient in supine position, with head turned away from site.			
9. Put on mask.			
10. Set up materials on overbed table.			
11. Put on clean gloves and remove old dressing, and discard it.			
12. Remove gloves, and wash your hands.			
13. Inspect site carefully.			
14. Put on sterile gloves.			
15. Cleanse area.			
a. Use hydrogen peroxide, moving in a spiral pattern beginning at the exit site.			
b. Cleanse area with antiseptic solution in a similar pattern for 2 minutes.			
c. Allow antiseptic solution to dry.			

(*continued*)

Changing the Standard Central Intravenous Dressing *(Continued)*	Needs More Practice	Satisfactory	Comments
16. Apply antiseptic ointment to exit site with cotton-tipped applicator.			
17. Apply new dressing.			
18. Change tape over connection between catheter and IV tubing if necessary.			
19. Label dressing with date and time.			
20. Reposition patient for comfort.			
21. Dispose of packages and materials.			
22. Wash your hands.			
23. Remove mask.			
Evaluation			
24. Evaluate, using the following criteria: **a.** Patient comfortable.			
b. IV line for patency and correct flow, connections secure.			
c. Dressing secure.			
Documentation			
25. Document on flow sheet or on narrative record.			
Changing the Exit Site Dressing			
Assessment			
1. Check date and time of last dressing change.			
2. Review facility procedure to identify appropriate dressing materials.			
Planning			
3. Wash your hands.			
4. Gather necessary supplies. **a.** Hydrogen peroxide and sterile cotton-tipped applicators.			
b. Povidone-iodine swabsticks or solution and applicators (in some facilities you also need an alcohol wipe)			
c. Antibacterial ointment			
d. Sterile 2 × 2 gauze squares			

(continued)

Changing the Exit Site Dressing *(Continued)*	Needs More Practice	Satisfactory	Comments
e. Paper tape			
f. Clean gloves			
Implementation			
5. Identify patient.			
6. Explain procedure to patient.			
7. Put on clean gloves to remove old dressing and inspect site.			
8. Cleanse with hydrogen peroxide and applicators in a spiral fashion outward for 3 in, removing any crusts.			
9. Cleanse with povidone-iodine swabs in the same way.			
10. Allow iodine solution to dry on skin.			
11. Apply antibacterial ointment to exit site.			
12. Cleanse catheter from exit site outward, using povidone-iodine or alcohol wipe.			
13. Place one gauze square under catheter and one over exit site, touching only outside of gauze.			
14. Tape dressing in place.			
15. Loop catheter, and tape it to body.			
16. Write date and time on dressing.			
17. Dispose of used materials and packages.			
18. Wash your hands.			
Evaluation			
19. Evaluate using the following criteria: **a.** Patient comfortable.			
b. Dressing secure.			
c. Catheter not under tension.			
Documentation			
20. Document on a flow sheet or on the narrative record.			

(continued)

Changing the Fluid Container and the Tubing	Needs More Practice	Satisfactory	Comments
Assessment			
1.–2. Follow steps 1 and 2 of the procedure for Changing the Fluid Container, Tubing, and Dressing in Module 52, Preparing and Maintaining Intravenous Infusions: Check physician's order and date of last tubing change.			
Planning			
3.–5. Follow steps 3 through 5 of Changing the Fluid Container, Tubing, and Dressing: Determine needed equipment, wash your hands, and select the correct tubing.			
Implementation			
6.–13. Follow steps 6 through 13 of Changing the Fluid Container, Tubing, and Dressing: Set up equipment, identify the patient, explain what you plan to do, hang the new container, remove old tape and dressing, examine site, put on gloves, and shut off IV.			
14. Remove tape from connection.			
15. Cleanse junction between catheter and tubing.			
16. Clamp line or plan for method to prevent air from entering catheter.			
17. Loosen old tubing by twisting it and leave connected.			
18. Remove cap from new tubing.			
19. Remove old tubing from connector, and insert new tubing.			
20. Start new fluid at a slow rate.			
21. Tape connection.			

(continued)

Changing the Fluid Container and the Tubing *(Continued)*	Needs More Practice	Satisfactory	Comments
Evaluation			
22. Evaluate the following: **a.** Patient comfort			
b. Patency, correct flow, and secure connections			
c. Dressing secure			
Documentation			
23. Document as follows: **a.** IV flow sheet: time, fluid discontinued, fluid added, tubing change			
b. Intake and output record			
Establishing a Heparin Lock on a Central Intravenous Catheter			
Assessment			
1. Check order.			
2. Check facility procedure for type of solution used.			
3. Check type of line in place and number of milliliters necessary to fill it.			
Planning			
4. Wash your hands.			
5. Gather necessary equipment. **a.** Sterile screw-type injection cap			
b. Syringe with 1-in needle or connector and heparinized saline			
c. Tape			
d. Clamp for line			
e. Alcohol swab			
f. Clean gloves			
Implementation			
6. Identify patient.			
7. Explain procedure to patient			
8. Place tape over catheter, making folded tabs at ends.			
9. Turn off IV infusion.			

(continued)

Establishing a Heparin Lock on a Central Intravenous Catheter *(Continued)*	Needs More Practice	Satisfactory	Comments
10. Put on gloves.			
11. Place clamp on catheter (over tape if a bull-dog clamp).			
12. Cleanse junction of catheter and tubing.			
13. Open package containing sterile cap.			
14. Loosen IV tubing by twisting it.			
15. Remove IV tubing, and insert injection cap.			
16. Insert needle of syringe into center of cap.			
17. Release clamp.			
18. Inject the heparinized saline. Alternative: Inject remaining 0.5 mL of solution while clamping catheter.			
19. Replace clamp.			
20. Remove needle and syringe and gloves.			
Evaluation			
21. Evaluate using the following criteria: a. Patient comfortable.			
b. Catheter clamp secure.			
c. Catheter not caught in clothing.			
Documentation			
22. Document on the intravenous flow sheet or on the narrative record.			
Irrigating an Intermittent Central Intravenous Catheter			
Assessment			
1. Determine when medications are being administered or blood is being drawn.			
2. Check facility policy regarding strength and amount of heparinized saline to be used.			
Planning			
3. Wash your hands.			
4. Gather necessary equipment. a. Syringe with heparinized saline and 1-in needle or needleless connector.			
b. Povidone-iodine or alcohol swab			

(continued)

Irrigating an Intermittent Central Intravenous Catheter *(Continued)*	Needs More Practice	Satisfactory	Comments
c. Clean gloves			
d. Normal saline solution			
Implementation			
5. Identify patient.			
6. Explain procedure to patient.			
7. Put on gloves.			
8. Cleanse cap by scrubbing for 1 minute.			
9. Insert needle or connector into cap.			
10. Remove clamp from catheter.			
11. Inject heparinized saline into line. Optional steps: a. Inject first 2 mL into line.			
b. Inject remaining 0.5 mL while clamping line.			
12. Reclamp catheter.			
13. Remove needle and syringe from cap and remove gloves.			
Evaluation			
14. Evaluate using the following criteria: a. Patient comfortable.			
b. Catheter clamp secure.			
c. Catheter not caught in clothing.			
Documentation			
15. Document heparin flush on medication record or on special flow sheet for Hickman catheter.			
Giving a Medication Through the Heparin Lock on a Central Intravenous Catheter			
Assessment			
1. Validate the orders.			
2. Examine medication administration record (MAR) for accuracy and completeness.			
3. Review information about the medication.			

(continued)

Giving a Medication Through the Heparin Lock on a Central Intravenous Catheter *(Continued)*	Needs More Practice	Satisfactory	Comments
4. Check your unit procedure for strength of heparin.			
5. Assess patient for need for prn IV medications.			
Planning			
6. Determine needed equipment.			
7. Wash your hands.			
8. Obtain necessary supplies: **a.** Medication in syringe or small volume parenteral with 1-in needle or connector.			
b. Povidone-iodine or alcohol swab.			
c. Syringe with 2.5 mL heparinized saline.			
d. Clean gloves			
e. Optional: Saline in syringes if medication not compatible with heparin.			
Implementation			
9. Read name of medication on MAR.			
10. Check label on medication, and pick it up.			
11. Check label a second time, comparing it with MAR.			
12. Prepare the medication.			
13. Check the label with the MAR a third time.			
14. Label medication if MAR is not taken to room.			
15. Prepare and label heparinized saline.			
16. Identify the patient.			
17. Explain procedure to patient.			
18. Administer medication by IV push or piggyback set. **a.** Put on gloves.			
b. Cleanse cap by scrubbing for 1 minute with antiseptic swab.			
c. Optional steps: (1) Insert needle or connector of plain saline into cap.			
(2) Release clamp.			

(continued)

Giving a Medication Through the Heparin Lock on a Central Intravenous Catheter *(Continued)*	Needs More Practice	Satisfactory	Comments
(3) Inject 2.5 mL saline.			
(4) Reclamp line.			
(5) Remove saline syringe.			
d. Insert needle or connector for medication into cap.			
e. Release clamp.			
f. Inject medication at rate ordered, or set infusion to rate ordered.			
g. When medication completed, clamp catheter.			
h. Remove needle or connector from cap.			
i. Scrub cap again if medication is injected over more than 5 minutes.			
j. Optional Steps: Follow steps 19.c. through 19.d. again if medication not compatible with heparin: Insert needle or connector, release clamp, inject saline, reclamp line, remove syringe.			
k. Instill heparinized saline using steps 19.c.(1) through 19.c.(5) above: Insert needle or connector, release clamp, inject heparin, reclamp line, remove syringe. Optional steps: (1) Inject first 2 mL heparinized saline.			
(2) Clamp the catheter while injecting the remaining 0.5 mL of heparin and then remove syringe.			
19. Leave the patient in a comfortable position.			
20. Dispose of used equipment and gloves.			
21. Wash your hands.			
Evaluation			
22. Evaluate using the following criteria: **a.** Six rights followed.			
b. Medication given over correct time.			
c. Catheter clamp secure.			
d. Catheter not caught in clothing.			
e. Criteria established for determining medication's effectiveness used.			

(continued)

Giving Medication Through the Heparin Lock On a Central Intravenous Catheter *(Continued)*	Needs More Practice	Satisfactory	Comments
f. Side effects promptly identified			
Documentation			
23. Document medication on medication record.			
Drawing Blood Through a Central Intravenous Catheter			
Assessment			
1. Determine suitability of catheter for drawing blood.			
2. Determine which ordered laboratory tests require specimens.			
3. Consult laboratory or reference to identify amount of blood needed and type of tube to be used for sample.			
Planning			
4. Wash your hands.			
5. Gather necessary equipment. a. One empty 5-mL syringe without needle or 5 mL test tube			
b. One syringe large enough to aspirate amount of blood needed for tests or collection device with appropriate connector			
c. One syringe with 20 mL saline			
d. One syringe with 2.5 mL heparinized saline			
e. Sterile 2 × 2 gauze squares to hold cap or sterile capped needle			
f. Povidone-iodine or alcohol swab			
g. Test tubes appropriate to specimens needed			
h. Tape to retape connections			
i. Clean gloves			
j. Eye protection			
Implementation			
6. Identify patient.			
7. Explain procedure to patient.			
8. Remove protective tape holding cap in place.			

(continued)

Drawing Blood Through a Central Intravenous Catheter *(Continued)*	Needs More Practice	Satisfactory	Comments
9. Put on gloves and eye protection.			
10. Cleanse junction of catheter and cap.			
11. Open package of sterile 2 × 2 gauze squares.			
12. Check to make sure catheter is firmly clamped.			
13. Remove cap from catheter, and place cap between two sterile 2 × 2 gauze squares or place sterile capped needle on IV line.			
14. Connect empty 5-mL syringe or collection device to catheter.			
15. Release clamp on catheter.			
16. Aspirate 5 mL fluid from catheter, or engage test tube into collection device.			
17. Reclamp catheter.			
18. Remove first syringe from catheter on test tube from device and discard.			
19. Attach empty syringe on next test tube.			
20. Unclamp catheter.			
21. Aspirate desired amount of blood, or engage test tubes one at a time into collection device.			
22. Reclamp catheter after aspirating blood or between changing test tubes.			
23. Remove syringe of blood.			
24. Attach syringe with 20 mL saline.			
25. Unclamp catheter.			
26. Inject saline.			
27. Clamp catheter.			
28. Remove empty syringe.			
29. Attach syringe with heparinized saline.			
30. Unclamp catheter.			
31. Inject heparinized saline. a. Optional: Inject remaining 0.5 mL while clamping catheter.			
32. Clamp catheter.			

(continued)

Drawing Blood Through a Central Intravenous Catheter *(Continued)*	Needs More Practice	Satisfactory	Comments
33. Remove empty syringe.			
34. Replace cap or line on catheter.			
35. Inject blood into proper laboratory test tubes.			
36. Tape cap to catheter.			
37. Discard used equipment and gloves.			
38. Wash your hands.			
39. Send labeled blood to laboratory with proper forms.			
Evaluation			
40. Evaluate using the following criteria: 　a. Catheter clamp secure.			
b. Catheter not caught in clothing.			
c. Appropriate blood samples obtained.			
Documentation			
41. Record on flow sheet or on narrative record that blood was drawn and sent to laboratory.			
Accessing a Subcutaneous Catheter Port			
Assessment			
1. Check the physician's order.			
2. Identify the type and location of the port.			
Planning			
3. Wash your hands.			
4. Obtain needed equipment. 　a. Three iodine swabs			
b. Dry cotton swab			
c. Sterile gloves			
d. Mask, alcohol, and povidone-iodine swabs if facility indicates			
e. Syringe, extension tubing with clamp, and noncoring needle.			

(continued)

Accessing a Subcutaneous Catheter Port (Continued)	Needs More Practice	Satisfactory	Comments
f. One of following groups of supplies: *For temporary access:* noncoring needle, extension tubing with clamp, and syringe; other materials based on purpose			
For ongoing access: right-angle noncoring needle with extension tubing, clamp and empty syringe and IV set-up			
g. Ethyl chloride if facility indicates			
Implementation			
5. Check the patient's identification.			
6. Explain the procedure to the patient.			
7. Provide for patient privacy.			
8. Prepare a clean area for your equipment and supplies.			
9. Place the patient in a supine or semi-Fowler's position.			
10. Put on a mask, if required in your facility.			
11. Set up your equipment, and open sterile packages.			
12. Put on clean gloves.			
13. Palpate area over the port.			
14. Prepare the skin over the port. **a.** Use povidone-iodine swab in a concentric circle three times.			
b. Allow solution to remain on skin 1 full minute.			
c. Wipe off iodine solution with alcohol swab if prescribed by your facility.			
d. Dry area with sterile swab.			
e. Spray with ethyl chloride if indicated.			
15. Discard clean gloves, and put on sterile gloves.			
16. Attach noncoring needle, extension tubing with clamp, and syringe.			
17. Palpate site, and hold the edges of port firmly with nondominant hand.			

(continued)

Accessing a Subcutaneous Catheter Port (Continued)	Needs More Practice	Satisfactory	Comments
18. Insert needle firmly straight into the center of the diaphragm until you feel needle stop.			
19. Hold needle firmly in place while aspirating.			
20. After blood return, draw blood, administer medications, attach fluid set, or flush and heparinize according to performance check lists.			
21. Complete procedure: **a.** For intermittent access: remove needle after flushing and heparinizing.			
b. For ongoing access: tape connections and apply dressing according to Performance Checklist.			
Evaluation			
22. Evaluate using the following criteria: **a.** Catheter dressing and tapes intact.			
b. Site clean and free of signs of infection.			
c. Correct medication or fluids received or correct blood sample obtained.			
Documentation			
23. Document accessing of port, including time and date on flow sheet or progress notes.			
24. Document medications or heparin on medication record.			

? **Q U I Z**

Short-Answer Questions

1. What are two common reasons for the use of central intravenous (IV) catheters?

    a. _____

    b. _____

2. Name two major complications of central IV infusion catheters.

    a. _____

    b. _____

3. List four purposes for changing the dressing on a central IV catheter.

    a. _____

    b. _____

    c. _____

    d. _____

4. Why is acetone not recommended as an agent to prepare the skin when changing the dressing on a central IV catheter? _____

_____

5. What is the purpose of applying an antiseptic or antimicrobial ointment to the insertion site?

_____

6. Why should a right atrial catheter with a peripheral exit site be labeled as a central IV catheter directly on the dressing? _____

_____

7. Why might the patient be asked to perform a Valsalva maneuver when the tubing is being changed on a central IV catheter? _____

_____

8. What is the difference between the Hickman catheter and the Broviac catheter? _____

_____

9. Why is the cap removed from the Hickman line for drawing of blood? _____

_____

10. Why are the Hickman and Broviac lines always clamped when not in use? _____

_____

11. What type of needle is used to access an implanted subcutaneous central venous port such as a Port-a-cath and why? _____

_____

_____

12. What is used to prepare the skin before accessing a subcutaneous port? _____

_____

_____

MODULE

55

STARTING INTRAVENOUS INFUSIONS

MODULE CONTENTS

RATIONALE FOR THE USE OF THIS
  SKILL
NURSING DIAGNOSES
PSYCHOLOGICAL IMPLICATIONS
INDICATIONS FOR INTRAVENOUS
  FLUIDS/ACCESS
WEARING GLOVES
EQUIPMENT
SELECTING A VEIN
PROCEDURE FOR STARTING AN
  INTRAVENOUS INFUSION
  Assessment
  Planning
  Implementation

Evaluation
Documentation
PROCEDURE FOR CONVERTING AN
  INTRAVENOUS INFUSION TO AN
  INTRAVENOUS LOCK
  Assessment
  Planning
  Implementation
  Evaluation
  Documentation
LONG-TERM CARE
HOME CARE
CRITICAL THINKING EXERCISES

PREREQUISITES

Successful completion of the following modules:

VOLUME 1
Module 1 An Approach to Nursing Skills
Module 2 Basic Infection Control
Module 3 Safety
Module 5 Documentation
Module 6 Introduction to Assessment Skills

VOLUME 2
Module 33 Sterile Technique
Module 47 Administering Medications: Overview
Module 50 Giving Injections
Module 52 Preparing and Maintaining Intravenous Infusions

Review of the anatomy and physiology of the vascular system.

O V E R A L L   O B J E C T I V E

To start intravenous (IV) infusions safely and comfortably for patients, using the equipment correctly and maintaining safety for the nurse.

S P E C I F I C   L E A R N I N G   O B J E C T I V E S

Know Facts and Principles	Apply Facts and Principles	Demonstrate Ability	Evaluate Performance
1. Psychological implications			
State three reasons why patients become anxious about intravenous (IV) infusions.	Given a patient situation, assess and plan appropriate nursing intervention to decrease patient's anxiety about receiving IV infusion.	Prepare patient psychologically for IV therapy immediately before initiating. Bring equipment into room at time IV is to be started.	Evaluate own performance with instructor.
2. Indications for IV fluids			
State four indications for IV fluids.	Given a patient situation, state why patient is receiving IV fluids.	In the clinical setting, discuss reason(s) for IV therapy for assigned patient(s).	Evaluate own performance with instructor.
3. Equipment			
List three kinds of equipment generally available for starting IV infusions.	Correctly identify equipment for starting IVs.	Choose correct equipment for particular clinical situation.	Evaluate own performance with instructor.
4. Setting up an IV infusion			
List steps for setting up IV.	Given a patient situation, discuss ways basic procedure might be modified.	In the practice setting, set up IV correctly.	Check entire set-up using Performance Checklist.
5. Locating a vein			
State usual sites for adult and infant IVs, and give rationale for their use. State four methods that can be used to distend veins.	Given a patient situation, state potential IV site. Given a patient situation, discuss which method of distending veins might be used.	In the practice or clinical setting, locate potential IV sites on peers or patients. In the practice or clinical setting, demonstrate how to cause vein to distend using peer or actual patient.	Evaluate own performance with instructor.
6. Procedure for starting an IV infusion			
Describe steps in procedure.	Given a patient situation, describe how procedure might be adapted.	Start IV in practice or clinical setting.	Evaluate with instructor using Performance Checklist.
7. Documentation			
State items of information to be included when documenting insertion of IV infusion.	Given a patient situation, do sample charting for insertion of IV infusion.	In the clinical setting, correctly document insertion of IV infusion.	Evaluate with instructor.

LEARNING ACTIVITIES

1. Review the Specific Learning Objectives.
2. Read the section on administering fluids intravenously in the chapter on nutrition and fluids in Ellis and Nowlis, *Nursing: A Human Needs Approach*, or a comparable chapter in another textbook.
3. Look up the module vocabulary terms in the glossary.
4. Read through the module as though you were preparing to teach the concepts and skills to another person. Mentally practice the skills included.
5. In the practice setting, do the following:
   a. Examine the various pieces of equipment available for starting an IV. Identify each of the following:
      (1) A winged-tip or butterfly needle (these are available in various sizes)
      (2) An IV catheter over a needle (Clear-Cath, Intima)
      (3) An IV catheter inside a needle (Intracath, Venocath)
      (4) Any other available devices
   b. Read the package instructions accompanying each of the previous devices. Handle the equipment, and attempt to follow the instructions.
   c. Using a manikin or IV "arm," start an IV with a 21-gauge butterfly needle or a 22-gauge over-the-needle IV cannula. Do the complete procedure, including the explanation to the "patient," the taping, and the dressing. Review Module 52, Preparing and Maintaining Intravenous Infusions, and if time permits, set up the IV as well. When you feel you have had sufficient practice, ask your instructor to evaluate your performance.
   d. If sterile equipment is available and school policy permits, practice starting an IV on another student. Carry out the entire procedure and have the student evaluate your performance.
   e. Practice documenting, using the form used in the facility to which you are assigned, and a narrative note, SOAP, or FOCUS note.
6. In the clinical setting, do the following:
   a. Ask your instructor to arrange for you to observe an IV being started.
   b. Ask your instructor to arrange for you to start an IV under supervision in your facility, if the facility's policies permit. For your first experience, a patient with "good" veins (for example, a young male) is preferable.
   c. If your facility employs an IV nurse, ask your instructor if arrangements can be made for you to observe. If time permits, ask if you can practice locating a suitable vein, and have the nurse evaluate your choice. If policy permits, ask if you can start an IV on a patient with good veins.

VOCABULARY

antecubital space	bifurcation	laminar airflow hood	phlebitis
arm board	butterfly	patent	tortuous
bevel	infiltration	Penrose drain	tourniquet

Starting Intravenous Infusions

Rationale for the Use of This Skill

Depending on the policies of the facility, unit nurses may or may not start intravenous (IV) infusions. If it is the unit nurse's responsibility to start IV infusions, the nurse must follow the six rights and three checks and manipulate the necessary equipment skillfully, keeping the patient comfortable and safe. If specially trained IV nurses are responsible for starting IV infusions, the unit nurse must still be sufficiently familiar with the equipment and the procedure to be of assistance.[1]

▼ NURSING DIAGNOSES

Patients may require IV therapy when a wide variety of nursing diagnoses are present. The most common is Risk for Fluid Volume Deficit. Patients with this nursing diagnosis are those who are not taking oral fluids and need fluids to avoid a problem. The actual problem of Fluid Volume Deficit also may be treated by IV therapy. Those receiving IV fluids also are at Risk for Infection because normal body defenses have been breached. The various potential complications of IV therapy, such as phlebitis and infiltration, also are a concern.

PSYCHOLOGICAL IMPLICATIONS

To some patients, the knowledge that they are about to receive IV fluids is threatening. *Some patients feel the procedure implies serious illness. Others are frightened by the threat of pain, discomfort, and immobility. Still others fear contracting infections, such as acquired immunodeficiency syndrome.* Previous experience can help make the patient less apprehensive, assuming the experience was positive. For some patients, the memories of problems related to the IV make the impending experience more frightening.

Explain the procedure just a few minutes before the IV is to be started. *This prepares the patient without providing a long time for worry.* In addition, keep the equipment out of the room until you actually are going to begin. In some facilities, the policy is to use 0.1 to 0.2 mL local anesthetic intradermally before

starting an IV *to numb the skin and the vein. This make[s] it easier for the patient to cooperate and removes most [of] the pain and discomfort associated with the insertion.* However, the anesthetic sometimes makes it mor[e] difficult to identify the vein in challenging situations. Individual healthcare facilities may have specific policies governing the use of a local anesthetic before venipuncture.

INDICATIONS FOR INTRAVENOUS FLUIDS/ACCESS

IV fluids are ordered for various reasons. *They maintain the daily requirements for fluid (in the patient who i[s] NPO or who is nauseated and vomiting); they replace los[t] fluid (in the postoperative patient); they provide large amounts of fluid rapidly (for a patient who is severely dehydrated); and they are a vehicle for medications, mos[t] commonly antibiotics.*

The fluid is ordered by the physician specifically *to meet the needs of the individual patient.* Refer to Module 52, Preparing and Maintaining Intravenous Infusions, for a discussion of the variety of solutions available and of things to check before using a solution.

An IV lock or heparin lock is inserted and maintained *when there is need for IV access without need for IV fluids.* Some examples of such situations are need for IV antibiotic therapy and need for access in terms of specific prn drug therapy. Advantages of an IV lock include greater patient mobility and reduction in cost of care. Module 53, Administering Intravenous Medications, includes a discussion of IV locks.

WEARING GLOVES

Gloves protect the caregiver from the possibility of contamination by the patient's blood through skin breaks. Glove[s] do not protect from inadvertent needle sticks. Needle stick[s] present more of a risk for blood-borne infections than d[o] blood spills because the skin is penetrated. The Center[s] for Disease Control and Prevention (CDC) do no[t] specifically recommend that all individuals starting IV infusions wear gloves. The CDC recommendation is that the use of gloves be based on the individua[l] situation and the potential for blood spills. Although some healthcare facilities leave the decision o[f] whether to wear gloves to the individual, many have a policy requiring those who do any venipuncture to wear gloves *for protection from blood spills.*

Blood spills are more likely to occur with students learning the technique than with experienced nurses. There

---

[1] Note that rationale for action is emphasized throughout the module by the use of italics.

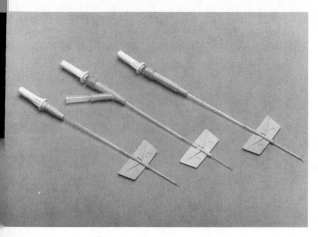

Figure 55-1. Various styles of over-the-needle IV access devices. (Courtesy Becton Dickinson, Sandy, Utah)

fore, we recommend that all students wear gloves when attempting any venipuncture. If sensitivity for palpation of a vein becomes a problem, it is possible to cut the end off of one glove index finger. This provides protection for hands that handle the needle, syringe, and tubing while allowing for sensitivity of touch.

The nurse must wash his or her hands when initiating peripheral IV access, and in most settings, clean gloves are worn. Sterile gloves must be worn when initiating a peripherally inserted central IV catheter. *The most common source of infection associated with IV devices is the IV cannula wound* (Maki, 1992). The terminology "IV cannula" refers to all types of percutaneous devices used for vascular access, including small steel needles (as found on butterfly and scalp vein devices) and plastic catheters. The IV access device provides a direct conduit between the world external to the patient and the bloodstream.

EQUIPMENT

No single type of equipment is ideal; each has advantages and disadvantages. When choosing equipment, consider the type of IV solution or medication ordered for the patient, the patient's diagnosis and history of IV therapy, the length of time the equipment will be in place, and the patient's age, mobility, and vein condition and structure. Then compare these factors to the characteristics of the equipment, and make your choice. Select the device with the shortest length and the smallest diameter that allows for appropriate administration of the fluid or other therapy prescribed.

Most facilities select a single manufacturer of IV solutions and equipment as their supplier. You will

become familiar with this equipment with time. Types of fluid containers and administration sets are discussed in Module 52, Preparing and Maintaining IV Infusions. Similar equipment is available for starting infusions.

A variety of equipment is available to initiate peripheral IV therapy. The winged-tip (*butterfly*) or scalp vein infusion set comes with plastic "wings" that are attached to the cannula hub for easier manipulation during insertion. After the vein has been entered, the wings lie flat against the skin and provide a means for securing the needle and tubing. Steel winged-tip or butterfly devices are available but are recommended only when the IV therapy is planned to last no more than a few hours.

In most other situations, a winged-tip device consisting of an over-the-needle plastic cannula with attached tubing (Angio-set/Intima IV Catheter is one brand) is preferred (Fig. 55–1). From ¾ to 1 in long, these devices are available from 16 to 24 gauge. The smaller sizes are particularly useful for infant scalp veins and for patients with small, fragile, or rolling veins.

The nurse inserts the needle and catheter. When blood returns, the needle is removed, leaving only the flexible catheter in place. Over-the-needle IV access devices also are available with protective needle shields that prevent needle stick injuries. These shields are activated after the IV cannula is in place and the nurse is ready to remove the needle (Fig. 55–2).

A through-the-needle IV cannula is threaded into the vein and is used when the IV is expected to remain in place for several days. After the needle is pulled back out of the skin, leaving the approximately 11-inch long catheter in place, a guard is secured over the needle, covering it completely. These

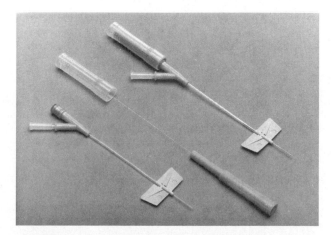

Figure 55–2. An example of an over-the-needle IV access device with needle shield. (Courtesy Becton Dickinson, Sandy, Utah)

devices have been replaced in large part by central venous catheters.

SELECTING A VEIN

For the adult patient, IV infusions are usually started in a hand. Legs are avoided *because of the danger of thrombus formation and subsequent pulmonary emboli.* Selection depends on a number of factors, including the reason for the IV, the length of time it is expected to be needed, the condition of the patient's veins, and the patient's comfort and safety.

Although it is usually easy to start an IV in the branches of either the cephalic or the basilic vein located near the antecubital space (inner aspect of the elbow), these veins are usually not a good choice. *In addition to limiting the patient's mobility in that arm, laboratory technicians often rely on these veins for blood samples. Also, these veins are the preferred site for peripheral central line access.* They should be used as a last resort and in emergency situations only.

Better sites in the adult patient are the lower branches of the basilic and the cephalic veins (Fig. 55-3).

An excellent site in infants or nonambulatory

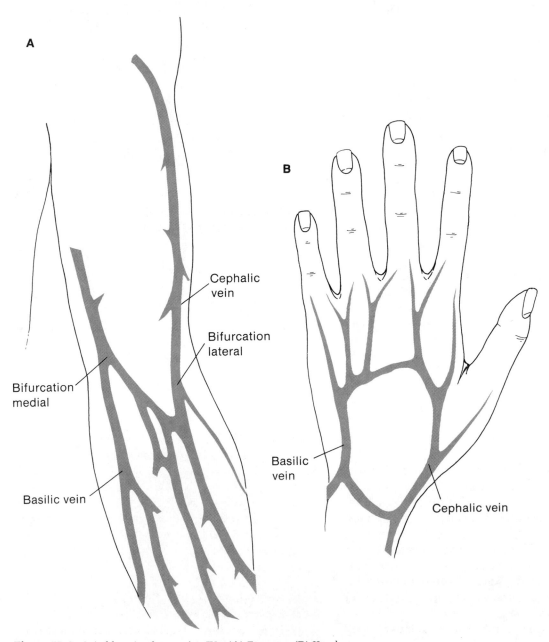

Figure 55–3. Suitable veins for starting IVs. **(A)** Forearm. **(B)** Hand.

mall children is the portion of the saphenous vein hat crosses or is anterior to the medial malleolus, ccording to researchers. When initiating IV thera-y for infants and children, avoid an infant's thumb-ucking hand, the dominant hand of an older child, or the feet of children who are ambulatory. The scalp eins also are used in infants *because there is less move-nent there and hence less chance of dislocation.* Scalp vein Vs, however, are esthetically unpleasant, and par-nts may object to their use.

It is best to start distal in the vein (in the hand or orearm). *Then, if you are unsuccessful or if the IV comes ut later, you can choose a vein proximal to or higher than he first one.* A site where there is bifurcation may be asier to enter if you can enter from below. Compare he length of the device you plan to use with the available vein. If you have a choice, it is preferable not to use the dominant hand or arm, and it is bet-ter to change sides with subsequent IVs. Your choic-es are commonly limited by the diagnosis, the con-dition of the patient's veins, or the presence of additional equipment. IVs are not started on an arm with a dialysis access nor on the side of a mastecto-my *because of concern regarding circulation on that side.*

Select the vein by looking, palpating, and at-tempting to distend any veins in the area. A clearly visible vein that can be palpated and that has a straight section for entry is most desirable. If one is not visible, look for the faint outline of a blue vein under the skin *to determine where to begin.* If not even an outline is visible, you must begin to distend the veins *to make them visible or palpable.*

To distend the veins, place a tourniquet (a length of Penrose drain will suffice if no commercial tourniquet is available) a few inches above the area where you want to start the IV, and ask the patient to "pump," opening and closing the fist. Generally, these maneuvers distend the vein, *making it easier to locate and enter.* If you still cannot locate a vein, place the arm in a dependent position for 5 to 10 minutes, or apply warm wet packs to the area (Fig. 55–4). Veins that are not visible but are palpable can be used.

Some veins can be entered without using a tour-niquet, which is advisable when a patient's veins are particularly fragile or rolling. The extra distention produced by a tourniquet can cause a vein to burst or roll even more.

If you have tried two times and have been unable to enter a vein, it is best to get assistance. *The proce-dure is uncomfortable for the patient, and it is unwise to use up all the available veins. If no member of the nursing staff can start the IV,* it may be necessary to ask the anesthesia department for assistance (depending on the policies in your facility), or the physician may

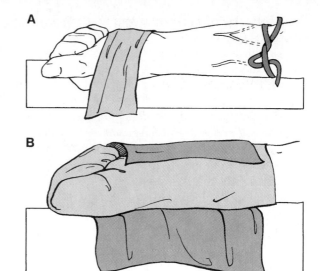

Figure 55–4. Ways to distend a vein. **(A)** Tourniquet. **(B)** Moist heat.

elect to use the jugular vein. This site often is cho-sen when other veins cannot be used and is a site for a central line.

PROCEDURE FOR STARTING AN INTRAVENOUS INFUSION

Assessment

1. Review the physician's orders. The orders include the type and amount of solution and the length of time over which the solution should run. The physician also may order additional medications to be added to the solution. Depending on the policies of the facility in which you work, you may add them yourself, or they may be added in the pharmacy under a laminar airflow hood (see Module 53, Administering Intravenous Medica-tions).

Planning

2. Wash your hands *for infection control.*
3. Choose equipment to set up the IV and to start the IV, including the following:
   a. Sterile IV solution as ordered with timing strip
   b. Administration set that contains tubing to de-liver the fluid and a means of regulating the flow rate
   c. IV pole
   d. Tourniquet
   e. Antiseptic swab
   f. Means of IV access
   g. Tape (tear four 6-in strips and place them con-veniently)

h. Antiseptic or antibiotic ointment (depending on facility policy)

i. Dressing materials

j. Armboard. Much of this equipment may be in an "IV start" package or may be kept together in a box or on a cart. This is a convenient practice *because you often will not know which device you will use until you have examined the patient.* Be sure that this box or cart is kept well stocked.

k. Clean gloves

4. Set up the IV fluid and tubing as described in Module 52, Preparing and Maintaining Intravenous Infusions.

5. Take the equipment to the bedside.

Implementation

6. Identify the patient *to be sure you are performing the procedure for the correct patient. Starting an IV infusion should be handled with the same careful checking as the administration of any medication.*

7. Prepare the patient psychologically. Just a few minutes before you plan to start the IV, tell the patient that IV fluids have been ordered and for what reason. Do not take the equipment to the bedside until you are ready to start. (See the section on Psychological Implications, and refer to Module 52, Preparing and Maintaining Intravenous Infusions.)

8. Adjust the lighting. Make sure you have adequate lighting, which is extremely important and often overlooked. If the room lights are not adequate, locate a portable lamp for temporary use.

9. Prepare the patient physically. First provide privacy. Look at the gown or pajamas the patient is wearing, and help the patient to change to more convenient clothing if necessary. *A pajama top with narrow sleeves or a long nightgown may be difficult if not impossible to remove once the IV is in place.* A patient gown with a shoulder snap opening is often the easiest and best garment for the patient to wear. Then position the patient as comfortably as possible. Place a towel under the arm *to protect the bed.* You may have to remove the patient's watch or change the position of the nameband *if either is in the way.*

10. Wash your hands, and put on clean gloves. Your hands must be clean. Gloves protect you from blood spills.

11. Position yourself. To start an IV, it is as important for you to be comfortable as it is for the patient. The position you choose does not have to be as orthodox as sitting in a chair at the bedside. Some nurses put the bed in high position

and stand. Others sit on the bed. Of course, th[e] policy in your facility may somewhat limit you[r] range of choices.

12. Locate a vein in which to start the IV. Examin[e] both hands and forearms, and select a site to be[-] gin. Place a tourniquet a few inches above th[e] area where you want to start, and ask the pa[-] tient to open and close the fist. If the vein doe[s] not distend, you may have to place the arm in [a] dependent position or apply warm, moist pack[s] to the area. Do not use a tourniquet if the vein[s] are extremely fragile or rolling *because the extr[a] distention may cause the veins to burst or roll eve[n] more.*

13. Release the tourniquet.

14. Clean the area thoroughly. Start from the point at which you want to enter, and move with a circular motion away from it, cleaning the skin thoroughly at and around the vein you have selected. If the area is especially hairy, clip or shave it before you attempt to start the IV *for aseptic reasons and to prevent the tape from pulling. Because of the risk of nicking the skin and thus increasing the potential for infection,* some facilities do not permit shaving IV sites. Clean the area after the hair has been removed. The antiseptic agent used for cleaning is usually indicated by unit or facility policy. Tincture of iodine is preferred, but 70% alcohol can be used (Centers for Disease Control, 1987). A recent study shows that site preparation with products containing chlorhexidine gluconate is associated with lower rates of inflammation or phlebitis (Larson, 1994). Try not to touch the area after it has been cleaned.

15. If it is the policy in your facility to anesthetize the area, do so now. Be sure to check first to determine if the patient is allergic to local anesthetics.

16. Reapply the tourniquet.

17. If you are using a device with a catheter, inspect it for defects.

18. Insert the needle. Using the thumb of your nondominant hand, gently retract the skin away from the site. Holding the needle at about a 15- to 30-degree angle with the bevel up, pierce the skin immediately beside the vein you have selected (Fig. 55–5). When the needle is through the skin, decrease the angle until it is almost parallel with the skin, and enter the vein. When blood comes back into the cannula hub or tubing (depending on the device you are using), insert the needle almost its full length. Advance the cannula according to package instructions and facility policy for the device you are using.

19. Holding the cannula steady with your dominant

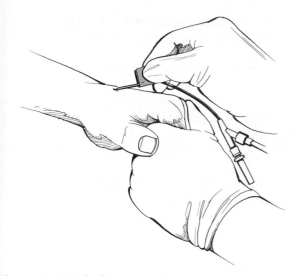

Figure 55–5. With skin retracted and needle bevel up, pinch wings on IV access device together and hold at a 15- to 30-degree angle to pierce the skin, followed by a decreased angle for entering the vein.

hand, release the tourniquet with your other hand.

20. Connect the tubing, and initiate the flow. Remove the protective cap from the IV tubing (maintaining sterile technique), connect it securely to the cannula, and open the regulator *to initiate the flow.* This should be done quickly *to prevent the patient's blood from clotting and occluding the cannula.*

21. Remove your gloves, tape the cannula securely, and dress the site. This should be done according to unit or facility procedure. If you have no procedure, use one of the three following methods:

    a. Chevron tape with gauze dressing (Fig. 55–6)
       (1) Place a sterile folded 3 × 3 or 2 × 2 gauze square under the cannula (folded side toward the cannula). *This protects the skin from the cannula hub.*
       (2) Place a small amount of antiseptic ointment at the cannula site. (Povidone-iodine ointment or a topical polyantibiotic ointment may be used.) *This decreases the incidence of infection.*
       (3) With 1/4-in adhesive tape (check for patient allergy), tape the cannula in place, using a chevron configuration *to hold the cannula securely in place.*
       (4) Place a sterile 3 × 3 or 2 × 2 gauze square open over the IV site.
       (5) Tape the cannula and tubing in place, using paper tape (if available—*it is usually*

less traumatic to the patient's skin), and make a loop of tubing near the point of entry. *This helps prevent the weight of the tubing from pulling the cannula out of place.* A commercially produced U-shaped connector is available for this purpose (Fig. 55–7).
       (6) Tape the armboard in place if necessary.
       (7) Write the date, time, type of device, catheter gauge, and your initials on the tape or label.

    b. U method of taping (Fig. 55–8)
       (1) Apply antiseptic ointment at the cannula site according to your facility's procedure.
       (2) Place the middle portion of a strip of ½-in tape, with the sticky side up, under the tubing.
       (3) Fold each end of the tape down so the sticky side is toward the skin and the tape is parallel to the cannula.
       (4) Place a piece of ½-in tape over the hub of the cannula, allowing the tape to extend out on either side over the strips parallel to the cannula.
       (5) Cover the IV site with an adhesive strip.
       (6) Make a loop in the tubing, and secure it with 1-in tape.
       (7) Write the date, time, type of device, catheter gauge, and your initials on the tape or label.
       (8) If you are using a winged IV access device, place a strip of tape over each side of the wing, parallel to the cannula. Then place a third strip of tape over the wing itself (see Fig. 55–8). Label as indicated previously.

    c. Transparent dressing (Fig. 55-9). Some facilities use transparent, moisture- and vapor-permeable adhesive dressings (OpSite, Tegaderm) rather than the traditional IV site dressings described previously. The dressing covers the IV site and seals snugly around the hub of the cannula, leaving the hub out *for ease of tubing change.* Follow specific package directions. An advantage is that this dressing does not need to be removed to assess the IV site.

22. Adjust the flow rate. The physician will have ordered a specific amount of fluid to be administered over a certain period. In some facilities, you will calculate the rate of flow yourself, based on the number of drops per milliliter administered by the equipment you are using. In others, the rate will be determined by pharma-

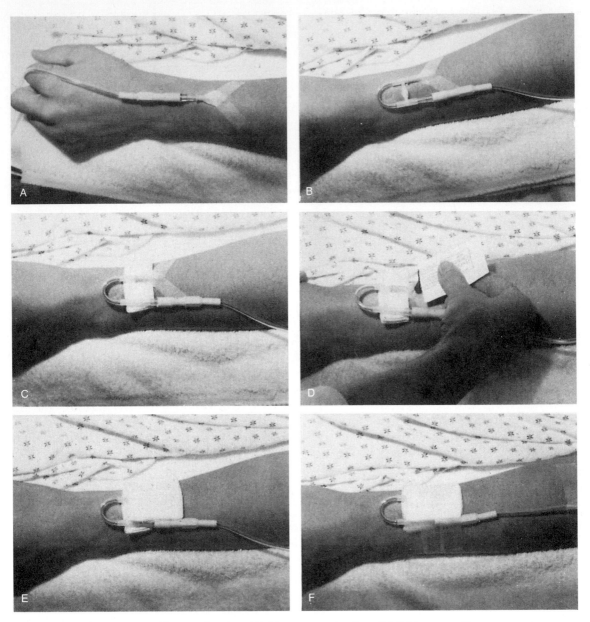

Figure 55–6. Chevron tape with gauze dressing. **(A)** Chevron tape in place. **(B)** Tubing curved by using a U-shaped connector. **(C)** Gauze square under hub to support position. **(D)** Applying antiseptic ointment on needle entry site. **(E)** 2 × 2 dressing. **(F)** Dressing and tubing taped in place. (Courtesy Ivan Ellis)

cy personnel, but you still must be able to check that rate and to calculate it again in the event the IV gets "ahead" or "behind." Many facilities stock narrow strips of paper calibrated according to the time over which the IV is to infuse (Fig. 55–10). The nurse adds the specific times appropriate for the individual IV. *These forms make it easier for the nursing staff to assess the progress of the infusion.* You also may be using a controller or pump as described in Module 52, Preparing and Maintaining Intravenous Infusions.

23. Care for the equipment appropriately.

24. Wash your hands.

Evaluation

25. Evaluate using the following criteria:

    a. The right patient received the right solution at the right time in the right amount deliv-

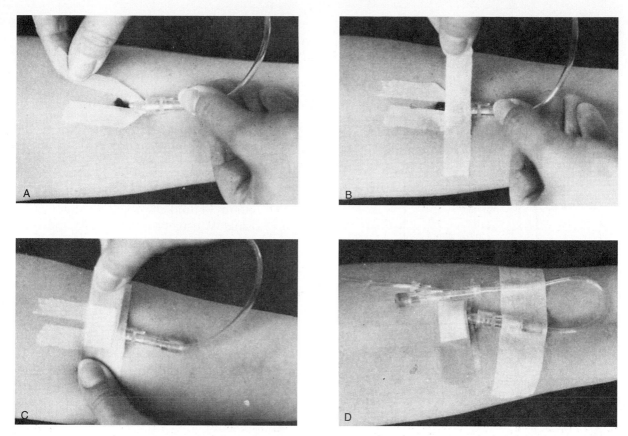

Figure 55–7. U method of taping. **(A)** Apply antibacterial ointment and U-tape. **(B)** Cross tape to secure cannula hub. **(C)** Bandage across insertion site. **(D)** Tubing looped and taped in place. (Courtesy Ivan Ellis)

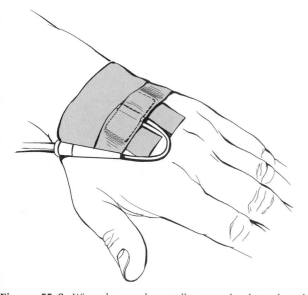

Figure 55–8. Winged over-the-needle cannula dressed and taped in place. Place a strip of tape over each side of the wing, parallel to the cannula. Place a third strip of tape over the wing itself.

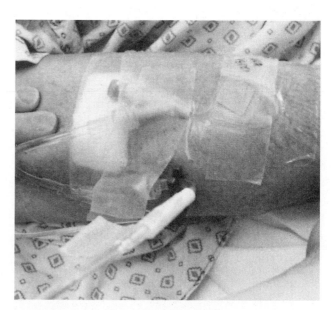

Figure 55–9. Transparent dressings are used to cover IV sites in many healthcare facilities.

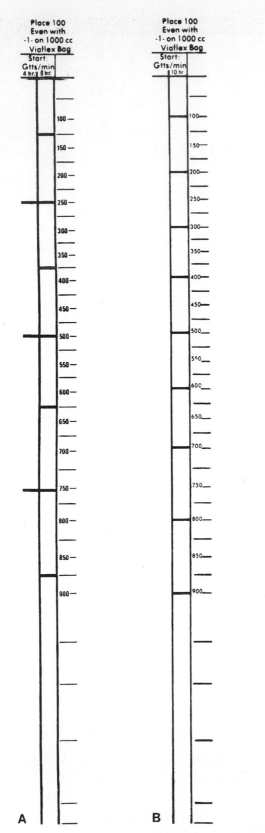

Figure 55–10. Calibration labels. **(A)** 4– or 8–hour label. **(B)** 10–hour label.

ered at the right rate, and it was correctly documented.

b. IV is secure (on arm board if positional).

c. Patient is comfortable.

Documentation

26. Document the IV insertion. Usually a special form is used for this purpose (see Module 52, Figs. 52–15 and 52–16). Include the time the IV was started, the type of fluid, any additives, where the IV was started, and by whom. When an IV is discontinued, include the time and the amount of fluid absorbed. A patient with an infusing IV usually is on intake and output as well.

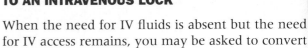

PROCEDURE FOR CONVERTING AN INTRAVENOUS INFUSION TO AN INTRAVENOUS LOCK

When the need for IV fluids is absent but the need for IV access remains, you may be asked to convert an IV infusion to an IV lock.

Assessment

1. Check the physician's orders.

2. Check the IV site for signs and symptoms of phlebitis, infiltration, and obstruction of flow.

Planning

3. Wash your hands *for infection control.*

4. Take the equipment to the bedside. You will need the IV lock adapter, heparinized or normal saline solution, dressing and taping materials, and clean gloves.

Implementation

5. Identify the patient *to be sure you are performing the procedure for the correct patient.*

6. Fill the IV lock adapter with heparinized or normal saline solution, using sterile technique, and put on clean gloves.

7. Turn off the existing IV, and disconnect it at the hub of the cannula.

8. Attach the IV lock adapter, and instill the remainder of the heparinized or normal saline solution.

9. Dress and tape according to facility policy, or refer to step 21 under Procedure for Starting an Intravenous Infusion.

10. Observe and document the amount remaining in the IV container, and dispose of the tubing and the container.

11. Dispose of your gloves, and wash your hands.

Evaluation

12. Evaluate using the following criteria:
 a. IV lock is securely in place.
 b. Patient is comfortable.

Documentation

13. Document the conversion of the IV infusion to an IV lock on the IV record or as appropriate in your facility.

LONG-TERM CARE

Because an increasing number of individuals with higher acuity levels are receiving care in long-term care facilities, there is an increasing need for IV access devices to be placed and used for fluid and medication therapy. Again, individual facilities will have chosen specific equipment and will have policies in place regarding individuals who are responsible for initiating and caring for IV infusions. The procedures remain the same.

HOME CARE

IV fluid and medication therapy are being administered to increasing numbers of individuals receiving care at home. Although clients or their caregivers are commonly successful at maintaining the prescribed therapy, skilled home care nurses are needed to assist with trouble-shooting IVs and restarting IVs that are no longer functional. Again, individual agencies choose specific equipment and have policies in place regarding who initiates and cares for those receiving IV therapy. The procedures remain the same.

CRITICAL THINKING EXERCISES

• You are to start an IV infusion for an 84-year-old female patient who has just been hospitalized for pneumonia. She had a left radical mastectomy 2 weeks ago and is dehydrated. Identify the sites commonly used for peripheral IVs, and explain which of these will you consider. Justify your choices. Tell which sites you will *not* consider and the reasons why.

• Margaret Seder will be having a minor surgical procedure this morning. You have been assigned to start an IV to provide access for IV medication administration. Given this purpose, identify what equipment you will use and what site(s) you will consider first. How will you determine if this IV is patent when a medication is ordered?

References

Centers for Disease Control (1987). Recommendations for prevention of HIV transmission in health care settings. *Morbidity and Mortality Weekly Report Supplement, 36,* 25–185.

Centers for Disease Control (1988). Update: Universal precautions for prevention of transmission of human immunodeficiency virus, hepatitis B virus, and other blood borne pathogens in health care settings. *Morbidity and Mortality Weekly Report, 37,* 1–7.

Larson, E. (1994). Does antiseptic make a difference in intravascular device-related complications? *Heart & Lung, 23*(1), 90–92.

Maki, D. (1992). Infection due to infusion therapy. In J. Bennett & P. Brachman (Eds.). *Hospital infections* (3rd ed.). Boston: Little, Brown.

✔ **PERFORMANCE CHECKLIST**

Procedure for Starting an Intravenous Infusion	Needs More Practice	Satisfactory	Comments
Assessment			
1. Review physician's orders.			
Planning			
2. Wash your hands.			
3. Choose appropriate equipment: a. Solution			
b. Administration set			
c. Intravenous (IV) pole			
d. Tourniquet			
e. Antiseptic swab			
f. Means of IV access			
g. Tape			
h. Antiseptic ointment			
i. Dressing materials			
j. Armboard			
k. Clean gloves			
4. Set up IV fluid and tubing.			
5. Take equipment to bedside.			
Implementation			
6. Identify patient.			
7. Prepare patient psychologically.			
8. Adjust lighting.			
9. Prepare patient physically.			
10. Wash your hands, and put on gloves.			
11. Select position of comfort for yourself.			
12. Locate vein. Apply tourniquet.			
13. Release tourniquet.			
14. Clean area thoroughly.			
15. If policy is to anesthetize area, do so now.			
16. Reapply the tourniquet.			

(continued)

Procedure for Starting an Intravenous Infusion *(Continued)*	Needs More Practice	Satisfactory	Comments
17. If using a device with a catheter, inspect it for defects.			
18. Insert needle and advance cannula.			
19. Release tourniquet.			
20. Connect tubing and initiate flow.			
21. Remove gloves, tape cannula, and dress site.			
22. Adjust flow rate.			
23. Care for equipment.			
24. Wash your hands.			
Evaluation			
25. Evaluate, using the following criteria: **a.** Right patient, right solution, right time, right amount, right rate, correctly documented.			
b. IV secure.			
c. Patient comfortable.			
Documentation			
26. Document IV insertion on appropriate chart form(s).			
Procedure for Converting an IV to an IV Lock			
Assessment			
1. Check physician's orders.			
2. Check IV site.			
Planning			
3. Wash your hands.			
4. Take equipment to bedside.			
Implementation			
5. Identify patient.			
6. Instill heparinized or normal saline into the IV lock adapter, and put on gloves.			
7. Turn off IV, and disconnect at cannula hub.			
8. Attach IV lock adapter, and instill remainder of heparinized or normal saline.			

(continued

Procedure for Converting an IV to an IV Lock *(Continued)*	Needs More Practice	Satisfactory	Comments
9. Dress and tape.			
10. Observe amount remaining in IV container, and dispose of tubing and container.			
11. Dispose of gloves, and wash your hands.			
Evaluation			
12. Evaluate using the following criteria: **a.** IV lock securely in place.			
b. Patient comfortable.			
Documentation			
13. Document appropriately.			

? **QUIZ**

Short-Answer Questions

1. List three reasons why patients often fear intravenous (IV) infusions.

   a. _____

   b. _____

   c. _____

2. List two reasons why a patient might be receiving IV fluids.

   a. _____

   b. _____

3. List three pieces of equipment discussed in this module that can be used to start an IV.

   a. _____

   b. _____

   c. _____

4. a. Where is an IV usually started in an infant? _____

   b. Why? _____

5. List four methods that can be used to distend a vein.

   a. _____

   b. _____

   c. _____

   d. _____

6. Name two agents that can be used to cleanse the skin before starting an IV infusion.

   a. _____

   b. _____

7. List five items of documentation to include on the tape that secures the IV dressing in place.

   a. _____

   b. _____

   c. _____

   d. _____

   e. _____

MODULE

56

ADMINISTERING BLOOD AND BLOOD PRODUCTS

MODULE CONTENTS

PREREQUISITES

Successful completion of the following modules:

OVERALL OBJECTIVE

To prepare and administer blood and blood products with comfort, safety, and maximum effectiveness for patients and to recognize common complications and intervene appropriately.

SPECIFIC LEARNING OBJECTIVES

Know Facts and Principles	Apply Facts and Principles	Demonstrate Ability	Evaluate Performance
1. *Rationale for administration of blood and blood products*			
State three reasons for administration of blood and blood products.	Given a patient situation, identify the reason for the administration of blood or a blood product.	In the clinical setting, identify the reason for the administration of blood or a blood product to a specific patient.	Verify rationale with instructor.

2. *Use of blood and blood products*
 a. Whole blood
 b. Blood products
  (1) Packed red blood cells
  (2) Platelets
  (3) Plasma
  (4) Plasma Protein fraction
  (5) Human serum albumin
  (6) Cryoprecipitate			

State rationale for the use of blood and blood products discussed. State two advantages of component therapy.	Given a patient situation, identify appropriate type(s) of blood or component therapy.	In the clinical setting, identify rationale for the use of blood or a blood product in a specific patient situation.	Verify with instructor.
3. *Typing and crossmatching*			
Name the four main blood groups in the ABO system of typing. State the major advantage of regular cross-matching over 10-minute cross-matching. State a valid reason for using a 10-minute crossmatch.	Given a patient situation, identify which type of crossmatching would be appropriate.	In the clinical setting, identify the appropriate type of crossmatching for a specific patient.	Verify with instructor.

(continued

S P E C I F I C L E A R N I N G O B J E C T I V E S (c o n t i n u e d)

Know Facts and Principles	Apply Facts and Principles	Demonstrate Ability	Evaluate Performance
4. Potential reaction to transfusion			
a. Hemolytic			
b. Febrile			
c. Allergic			
d. Transmission of disease			
e. Circulatory overload			
f. Hypothermia			
g. Hyperkalemia			
h. Hypocalcemia			
i. Air embolus			
State signs and symptoms of each type of transfusion reaction discussed.	Given a patient situation, identify type of transfusion reaction from symtoms listed.	In the clinical setting, take appropriate preventive measures as the situation allows.	Evaluate with your instructor.
State appropriate intervention for each type of transfusion reaction discussed.	Given a patient situation, identify appropriate intervention for that particular type of transfusion reaction.		
State appropriate measures to prevent various transfusion reactions.	Given a specific reaction, state appropriate preventive measures.		
7. Equipment			
Identify special equipment needed for administering blood and blood products.		In the practice or clinical setting, select the correct equipment to administer blood or a blood product.	Verify selection with instructor.
8. Procedures for administering blood and blood products (whole blood, packed red cells, platelets, albumin, cryoprecipitate)			
Describe procedure for administering whole blood, packed red cells, platelets, albumin, and cryoprecipitate.	Given a patient situation, identify whether correct procedure is being used for administering blood or blood product.	In the clinical setting, give whole blood, packed red cells, platelets, albumin, and cryoprecipitate safely.	Evaluate performance with instructor using Performance Checklist.

1996 by Lippincott-Raven Publishers

LEARNING ACTIVITIES

1. Review the Specific Learning Objectives.
2. Read the section on blood transfusion in Ellis and Nowlis, *Nursing: A Human Needs Approach,* or comparable material in another textbook.
3. Look up the module vocabulary terms in the glossary.
4. Read through the module as though you were preparing to teach the contents to another person. Mentally practice the specific procedures.
5. In the practice setting, do the following:
   a. Examine the blood administration equipment. Identify each of the following:
      (1) Y blood administration sets
      (2) Primary blood administration sets
      (3) Secondary blood administration sets
      (4) Secondary intravenous administration sets
      (5) Forms for recording blood administration
   b. Read the directions on the package regarding how to set up the blood administration equipment you will be using.
   c. Set up a blood administration set as though you were going to administer blood. Attach a secondary administration set as a normal saline line if that is the policy in your facility.
   d. Regulate the drip rate so 500 mL blood will be delivered in 4 hours. Consult the blood administration set package to identify the drops per milliliter delivered by the tubing.
   e. Demonstrate what you would do if it were necessary to stop the transfusion.
   f. Practice documenting:
      (1) The administration of a unit of whole blood is started at 1:00 PM and completed at 4:00 PM; document as appropriate to your facility.
      (2) The recipient of the blood has an allergic reaction. Simulate appropriate observation data, and indicate required nursing intervention.
6. In the clinical setting, consult with your instructor regarding an opportunity to set up and administer blood or a blood product to an adult or pediatric patient.

VOCABULARY

allergic reaction	donor	hyperkalemia	recipient
autologous transfusion	erythrocyte	hypocalcemia	salvaged blood
circulatory overload	febrile reaction	hypothermia	transfusions
citrated blood	hemodilution	packed red blood cells	serum hepatitis
compatibility	hemolytic reaction	plasma	type and crossmatch
cryoprecipitate	human serum albumin	platelets	whole blood

Administering Blood and Blood Products

Rationale for the Use of This Skill

Blood and blood products may be administered for various reasons, including restoration of circulating blood volume, replacement of clotting factors, and improvement of oxygen-carrying capacity. Whatever the situation, potential complications are involved. The nurse must be cognizant of these complications and work to prevent them and be able to intervene appropriately as necessary.[1]

NURSING DIAGNOSES

The patient's nursing diagnoses are often those that lead to the need for transfusion rather than those centered around the procedure. These may involve activity intolerance or hemorrhage, as in the following examples:

Activity Intolerance: weakness related to too few red blood cells (anemia)

Impaired Physical Mobility: fatigue related to low red blood cells (anemia)

Fluid Volume Deficit: hemorrhage related to bleeding at surgical site

Fluid Volume Excess related to increase in vascular fluid volume

Risk for Injury related to transfusion reaction

Anxiety related to the fear of pending blood transfusion

The complications or potential complications related to the transfusion procedure are referred to as collaborative problems. They are in response to the medical diagnosis rather than the nursing diagnosis. The nurse institutes action to prevent these problems if possible, identifies problems when they occur, and reports them to the physician. In addition, the nurse implements the physician's plan for treatment. One potential complication (PC) is Transfusion Reaction (specify type, such as hemolytic or allergic) related to previous transfusion reaction.

USE OF BLOOD AND BLOOD PRODUCTS

Commonly patients receive packed red blood cells or whole blood, depending on medical need. Before the various blood products are described, this chapter addresses the five methods now in use to administer blood.

Blood Donated by an Unrelated Donor

The majority of blood needed by patients is obtained from an unrelated donor. The identity of the donor is not revealed to the recipient. Through a laboratory process, the blood from each is typed, and the two samples are mixed (called crossmatching) *to make sure that the two are compatible and that a reaction will not occur.* In addition, the donor's blood is tested for a variety of blood-borne antibodies to diseases, such as hepatitis and human immunodeficiency virus (HIV). If the blood tests positive, the donor is notified, and the blood is discarded.

Blood Donated by a Related Donor

In a few states, blood may be donated by a relative of the patient. The blood is designated for use only by the family member for whom the donation is given. Statistically, these donations are no safer from disease than blood given by an unrelated donor *because of the unwillingness of family members to reveal lifestyle or medical history.* For this reason, many blood centers do not support using blood from related donors. A special charge is assessed for blood donation by a related donor because of the added tracking. The blood undergoes the same tests as blood given by an unrelated donor.

Autologous Transfusion

For patients anticipating elective surgery, the trend toward autologous transfusion is increasing. Autologous transfusions are those in which the patient is infused with his or her own blood, which was donated in advance. In some areas, 5% to 10% of all blood transfusions are now autologous.

The patient can donate at the blood center every 3 to 4 days up until 3 days before surgery to provide the blood for autologous transfusion. The blood must still pass the screening process (American Association of Blood Banks, 1994). A written referral must have previously been sent by the surgeon to the blood center. To be eligible for self-donation, the person may not have a hemoglobin value of less than 11 g/dL. The donated blood or red blood cells are labeled for the patient and stored as fresh or frozen blood until ready for use. The patient may be placed on oral iron supplements *to aid in hemoglobin regeneration.* There is a special charge to the patient for the autologous transfusion process because of

Note that rationale for action is emphasized throughout the module by the use of italics.

the added collection and tracking costs. Autologous blood that is not used is tested and may be released to another person needing blood, according to the American Association of Blood Banks, although some blood centers do not participate in this program because screening is less thorough.

This method of transfusion *eliminates the likelihood of transmission of hepatitis, HIV antibodies, and other diseases transmitted by contaminated blood.* Autologous blood donation also is acceptable to people for whom receiving blood from others is not acceptable as a religious belief. In addition, it frees up a portion of the blood supply for use by the general population, and studies have shown that people who have entered an autologous program often return to make subsequent donations for others (Drago, 1992). A disadvantage is that the patient may experience a mild anemia.

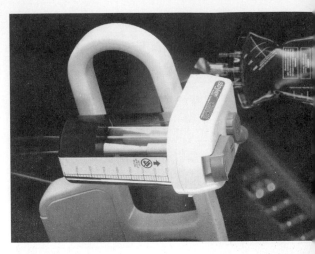

Figure 56–1. This device, the CBC II Blood Conservation System (commonly called a "cell saver") is used to recover and filter a patient's blood for reuse. (Courtesy Stryker Instruments, Kalamazoo, Michigan)

Hemodilution

As the patient is prepared for surgery, 1 to 2 U of blood may be withdrawn, and this volume replaced with an intravenous (IV) infusion of a "plasma expander" or colloidal solution *to maintain blood volume.* During the surgery, the blood that was collected immediately prior to surgery is reinfused into the patient to replace blood loss.

Salvage During and After Surgery

When there is massive blood loss during surgeries, which sometimes occurs during orthopedic, vascular, or cardiac surgeries, the blood may be recovered with a special suction device, filtered, and reinfused into the patient. The device is sometimes referred to as a "cell saver." The blood is mixed with an anticoagulant *to prevent clotting.* Some patients having major surgeries return from the operating room with a container of their own blood to reinfuse. This is a successful alternative when prior donation for autologous transfusion is not possible or when bleeding during surgery is significant.

Also used after surgery is a conservation reinfusion device. This is used when a considerable amount of blood is draining from a wound or body cavity. This autologous blood is collected into a sterile container, filtered, and then reinfused through a line into the patient (Fig. 56–1).

TYPES OF BLOOD PRODUCTS

Whole blood may be ordered as a part of patient therapy, or, because blood can be separated into its component parts, only the specific component needed in a patient's therapy may be used. Below i a discussion of indications and contraindications fo using whole blood and some of its components.

Whole Blood

Whole blood transfusion is most commonly used i instances of acute massive blood loss or for tota blood exchange in neonates. Its use should be re stricted to situations in which a need to increase th oxygen-carrying capacity and a need to increase cir culating volume of the blood are both present. A unit of blood equals approximately 500 mL (450 m of blood from a donor and 60–70 mL of preservativ or anticoagulant). Whole blood is not indicate when blood volume is normal or increased.

Blood Products

The use of blood products (or components) has in creased in recent years, making it possible to giv only the *needed* factor to the recipient. This practic also makes it possible *to serve more needs with fewer d nations and to decrease the risk of complications, such circulatory overload and blood-borne diseases, to the r cipient.*

Packed Red Blood Cells

Packed red blood cells make up the blood produ remaining after up to 80% of the plasma is remove from whole blood. *Because red blood cells provide t same oxygen-carrying capacity as whole blood but smaller volume,* they may be used when the patie is at risk for circulatory overload but needs hem lobin for its oxygen-carrying capacity. Red cells are usually infused over 2 or 3 hours and may be made ess viscous by the addition of normal saline (50–100 nL) if the patient's condition permits. A unit of red ells equals approximately 250 mL. The use of red lood cells (also called packed cells) necessitates typ- ng and crossmatching.

Platelets

latelets (thrombocytes) are used *in cases of thrombo- ytopenia caused by lack of platelet production, resulting in ncreased bleeding time.* They are indicated only *for reatment of potential life-threatening hemorrhage.* A nit of platelets consists of a large number of latelets in a small amount of plasma (50–70 mL). he usual volume for a bleeding adult with throm- ocytopenia is 6 to 10 U. Platelets should be type ompatible, but Rh antigens are not found on latelets. The risk for acquiring blood-borne diseases the same as for whole blood.

Plasma

lasma is the fluid portion of the blood remaining fter the red blood cells, platelets, and leukocytes ave been removed. Fresh frozen plasma can be ored for 12 months but must be used within 24 ours of thawing. It provides clotting factors, roteins, and fluid volume. Such IV solutions as extran and lactated Ringer's solution also are re- ommended for volume expansion. Plasma deriv- tives, such as albumin and plasma protein frac- on, are recommended for protein replacement ecause they do not expose the recipient to the risk of lood-borne diseases, as does fresh or fresh frozen lasma.

Plasma Protein Fraction

lasma protein fraction is the portion of the plasma emaining after fibrinogen and globulin have been emoved. This component is used when *the replace- ent of intravascular volume is necessary.* The risk of he- atitis is eliminated because of a pasteurizing rocess.

Human Serum Albumin

uman serum albumin *increases the colloidal osmotic ressure of the blood and is administered for shock, burns, d hypoproteinemia.* Typing and crossmatching are ot required. It is heat treated at 60°C /140°F for 10 ours *to decrease hepatitis risk and eliminate viral disease* sk.

Cryoprecipitate

Cryoprecipitate, sometimes referred to as "cryo," is prepared from fresh frozen plasma and contains large amounts of the clotting factor VIII—the factor lacking in hemophiliacs. It contains a small number of red cells, which makes crossmatching unneces- sary, but it is advisable to give ABO-compatible cry- oprecipitate if the total volume is more than 100 mL. It may be stored frozen for 12 months but must be administered within 6 hours of thawing. The remote risk for blood-borne diseases is present.

A dried, heat-treated cryoprecipitate product that has an indefinite shelf life and must be reconstitut- ed before infusing is now available. This product eliminates the possibility of transmitting blood- borne antibodies or diseases. Commonly used blood products are listed in Table 56–1.

TYPING AND CROSSMATCHING

Basic to safe administration of blood and blood com- ponents is accurate typing and crossmatching of blood. Four main blood groups are in the ABO sys- tem of blood typing: A, B, AB, and O. Blood also is classified as either Rh positive or Rh negative. In the laboratory, the recipient's blood is first tested for type. Next, blood samples from the donor and re- cipient are mixed to determine compatibility. If they are *not* compatible, antibodies in the recipient's plas- ma will agglutinate the erythrocytes from the donor's blood and cause the most serious complica- tion of blood transfusion therapy—hemolytic reac- tion (Table 56–2).

Crossmatching may be done in one of two ways. A standard crossmatch may take up to 2 hours and *includes a complete testing of compatibility, thus reducing potential for reactions.* In an urgent situation, the blood may be tested for type, and a 10-minute cross- match for blood compatibility may be done. Because the process is abbreviated, some incompatibilities may not be revealed. Therefore, the 10-minute process is reserved for emergency situations.

EQUIPMENT

A size 19 or larger needle, butterfly, or other device is used to start an IV through which blood is to be infused. If the patient is an infant or young child, a size 20 to 23 needle may be used (see Module 55, Starting Intravenous Infusions).

Whole blood, packed red blood cells, and plasma should be administered using a standard (170–
(text continues on page 623)

Table 56–1. Commonly Used Blood Products

Component	Major Indications	Special Points	Time Lapse Expected for Receipt of Blood Bank Items	Product Expiration Time After Arrival to Blood Bank	Rate of Infusion
Red blood cells	Symptomatic anemia		4–6 h (routine) 1 h (10 min type and crossmatch)	48 h	Usual rate 2–4 h For massive loss, fast as patient can tolerate
Whole blood	Symptomatic anemia with large volume deficit		4–6 h (routine) 1 h (10 min type and crossmatch)	48 h	Usual rate 4 h For massive loss, fast as patient can tolerate
Leukocyte-poor RBCs	To prevent febrile reactions from leukocyte antibodies while treating symptomatic anemia	Leukocyte-poor RBCs must be specifically prescribed by physician.	4 h	24–48 h; check expiration time on bag	Usual rate 2–4 h For massive loss, fast as patient can tolerate
Leukocyte-poor RBCs (obtained by washing)	Paroxysmal noctural hemoglobinuria and some types of immune globulin disorder	To order, physician must make special arrangement at blood center.	4 h	24 h	Should be administered stat after arrival to blood center. For massive blood loss, fast as patient can tolerate. Usual rate 2–4 h

Component	Indication	Nursing considerations	Time	Expiration	Infusion rate
Platelets	To decrease clotting times for platelet function abnormality or for decreased platelets	Do not refrigerate. Give as soon as possible after arrival. The greater the delay of administration, the less value platelets are to the patient. Platelets are probably of some value for several hours.	1½ h	Check expiration time on bag	As rapidly as possible
Granulocytes	Neutropenia and infection	Increased risk of allergic reaction. Physician must order through the blood center.	6–24 h depending on availability	Unknown—probably 24 h	Infuse over 2–4 h
Plasma (fresh frozen)	Deficit of labile plasma coagulation factors		½ h + 45 min to thaw	1 h after thaw	Approximately 10 mL/min
Cryoprecipitate	1. Hemophilia A 2. Replacement of fibrinogen 3. Replacement of factor VIII	Do not refrigerate. To minimize trauma to vessels, a new butterfly needle is inserted for each infusion and removed on completion.	1 h	1. 6 h after thawing OR 2. 4 h after pooling	10 mL diluted component per min

Swedish Hospital Medical Center Nursing Policy/Procedure Committee Revised: July 1987

Table 56–2. Reactions to Transfusions

Reaction	Cause	Assessment	Nursing Intervention

Hemolytic reaction	Incompatibility of types of red cells	Flank pain, dark urine, chest constriction, low back pain, hypotension, tachypnea, tachycardia, fever, chills, apprehension	Stop transfusion immediately and maintian IV line.
			Monitor vital signs.
			Notify physician.
			Monitor urine output.
			Collect blood and urine samples and send to laboratory.
			Prevention:
			  Careful identification of patient and blood before transfusion.
			  Careful observation of patient during first 15 min of transfusion.

Febrile reaction	Sensitivity to white cells in the blood	Fever, chills, headache, nausea, and vomiting	Mild: Slow rate of transfusion.
			       Notify physician.
			       Administer antihistamine as ordered.
			Severe: Stop transfusion, and maintain IV line.
			       Monitor vital signs.
			       Notify physician.
			       Administer aspirin or acetaminophen to reduce fever as ordered.

Allergic reaction	Antibody reaction to allergens in donor's blood	Mild: Hives, itching, flushing
		Severe: Shortness of breath, bronchospasm, wheezing
			Mild: Slow transfusion.
			       Notify physician.
			       Give antihistamine as ordered.
			Severe: Stop transfusion, and maintain IV line.
			       Notify physician.
			       Give antihistamine, epinephrine, or adrenocorticosteroid as ordered.
			Prevention: If recipient is known to be allergic, reaction may be prevented by administration of antihistamine 1 h before transfusion.

*Transmission of disease (serum hepatitis most common)**	Presence of virus in donor's blood	May appear from 6 w to 6 mo after transfusion	Prevention: Careful screening of blood donors

Circulatory overload	Excessive volume, excessive rate (infants, elderly, and those with cardiac disease especially at risk)	Dyspnea, cough, rales in bases of lungs; distended neck veins; elevated central venous pressure	Slow or stop transfusion.
			Raise patient's head, and place feet in dependent position.
			Notify physician.
			Give diuretics if ordered by the physician.
			Prevention:
			  Administer at slow rate.
			  Suggest packed cells for patients at risk.

Hypothermia	Rapid transfusion of large volume of cold blood (infants and children especially at risk)	Chills; may lead to cardiac arrhytmias, fibrillation, arrest	Slow transfusion
			Keep patient covered.
			Prevention:
			  Give blood at room temperature.
			  Suggest warming coils for rapid transfusion (microwave warmers *not* recommended, *because they cause lysis of red cells*).

(continued)

Table 56–2. Reactions to Transfusions (Continued)

Reaction	Cause	Assessment	Nursing Intervention
Hyperkalemia	Breakdown of red blood cells in stored blood—potassium released into plasma	Nausea, diarrhea, muscle weakness, slowed pulse rate, cardiac arrest	Stop transfusion. Notify physician. Prevention: Use blood of a short-storage interval.
Hypocalcemia	Rapid rate of transfusion of large quantities of blood, possibly causing calcium deficit *from ability of citrate in stored blood to combine with serum calcium.*	Tingling of fingers, circumoral tingling, muscle cramping, convulsion, laryngospasm	Stop transfusion. Notify physician. Administer IV calcium as ordered.
Air embolus	Entry of air into vein	Cyanosis, dyspnea, shock, arrhythmias, cardiac arrest	Lower patient's head, and turn patient on left side. Notify physician. Treat shock or cardiac arrest appropriately. Prevention: Cover blood filter *completely* with blood before infusing, and avoid giving blood under pressure.

Licensed antibody tests detect 97% of acquired immunodeficiency syndrome-infected donors.

micron) blood filter, which removes any particulate matter. The filter should be entirely covered with blood or blood product before blood is run through the tubing *to remove the air* (Figs. 56–2 and 56–3).

Although a standard blood filter can be used for 2 to 3 U of blood before debris accumulates and slows the rate of flow, the filter should not be left hanging for more than 6 hours *because of the hazard of bacterial contamination.*

Some facilities use a pump to infuse blood, while others do not. Check with the policy in your facility to determine this.

Platelets are administered using a component administration set with a standard 170-micron filter. A new filter should be used each time platelets are administered. Cryoprecipitate may be administered using either a primary set or a component set.

Plasma protein fraction and human serum albumin are commercially packaged. Tubing to be used for administration is enclosed in the package.

A secondary IV set (see Module 52, Preparing and Maintaining Intravenous Infusions) may be used to piggyback normal saline into the blood tubing *to maintain access to the line in case it is necessary to discontinue the blood.* Dextrose in water should not be used for this purpose because *it may hemolyze the red cells it contacts.*

In some facilities, Y blood administration sets are used, in which case one administration set is used for both the blood or blood product and the saline. The Y set is convenient for diluting some blood products, such as platelets or packed red blood cells. If the patient has a mild transfusion reaction, the blood flow can be shut off and the saline continued until an assessment can be made. If a serious reaction occurs, which is rare, stop the blood flow immediately, and place a heparin lock in the IV line to maintain access to a vein in case it is needed for treatment of the reaction. With serious reactions, even though the blood is shut off and the saline started, the small amount of blood in the tubing that would be infused ahead of the saline flow could add to the danger and inserting a heparin lock may *prevent this from occurring.*

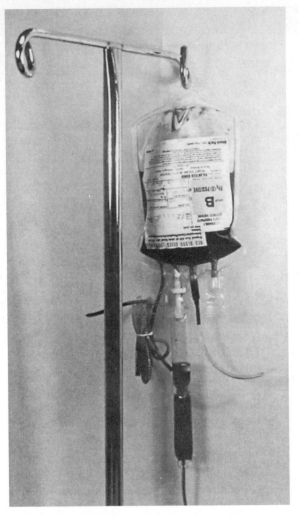

Figure 56–2. Blood administration set. (Courtesy Ivan Ellis)

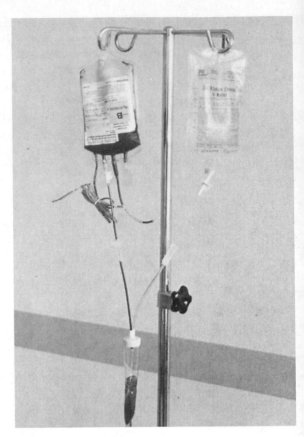

Figure 56–3. Y blood administration set used with saline. (Cour-tesy Ivan Ellis)

GENERAL PROCEDURE FOR ADMINISTERING WHOLE BLOOD AND PACKED RED CELLS

Assessment

1. Check the physician's orders. The orders include the type of blood product, the number of units, and sometimes the period over which the product is to be infused.
2. Check the existing IV infusion or heparin lock for patency and needle size, or initiate an IV infusion with a size 19 or larger needle or other means of entering the vein. A 20- to 23-gauge needle may be used for infants and other patients with small veins.

Planning

3. Wash your hands *for infection control.*
4. Gather the necessary equipment. If you will need to start an IV infusion, gather the basic equip-

ment for starting an IV infusion in addition to the following:

   a. Primary blood administration set (see Fig 56–2) or Y blood administration set (see Fig 56–3), as your facility's policy indicates

   b. 250-mL bottle or bag of normal saline with secondary administration set, if your facility policy indicates

   c. A blood pump, which may be needed *when blood volume and oxygen-carrying capacity need be increased immediately to increase flow rate*

   d. Clean gloves and tape

5. Obtain the blood product from the facility blood center immediately before using, and check it ou according to facility procedure. The transfusion should be started within 30 minutes of the time the blood is removed from refrigerated storage in the facility's blood bank. The blood should not b stored in the refrigerator on the nursing unit b *cause refrigerators used for blood storage are monitor to maintain the correct temperature.*

   In instances of massive transfusion, it may b necessary to warm the blood before transfusio *to prevent a severe temperature drop.* A blood-warn ing coil immersed in a water bath at a temperature of 37°C (98.6°F) is used for this purpose. Blood should not be warmed unless it is going to be given immediately. Blood that has been warmed may not be returned to the blood center for future use.

6. Carefully identify all blood and blood products, including autologous donations. *This prevents any possibility that a mistake has been made.* Proper identification usually includes having the hospital blood laboratory and unit personnel check the patient's name, hospital number, blood and Rh type, and blood unit identification number and sign the necessary release form before the blood is removed from the center. *Any discrepancy* must be investigated before the blood is administered. With another nurse on the unit, check the following just before infusing:

   a. Patient's name and spelling, hospital number, and physician's name on face sheet; compare these with the blood center invoice.

   b. Blood product type, Rh, and blood unit administration number on blood bag; compare these with the blood center invoice.

   c. Expiration date on the blood bag

7. You and the other nurse sign your names, titles, date, and time on the blood center invoice if all of the information is correct.

8. Prepare the equipment as follows:

   a. If blood is to be infused using a pump, obtain one. Select pump tubing, and use either a Y or a primary blood administration set as described in steps 8.b and c. Put on clean gloves.

   b. Y blood administration set

   (1) Close all control clamps on the Y set.

   (2) Insert one spike of the administration set into the blood bag according to package directions.

   (3) Open the clamp closest to the normal saline bag, and fill the drip chamber half full.

   (4) Open the lower control clamp, and flush the air from the tubing; reclamp.

   (5) Insert the other administration set spike into the normal saline bag according to package directions.

   (6) Open the clamp closest to the blood, and squeeze the filter chamber; release it until the filter is completely covered; reclamp.

   (7) Open the lower control clamp, and flush the tubing with blood.

   c. Primary blood administration set

   (1) Turn the control on the blood tubing to the off position.

   (2) Open the entry port on the blood bag.

   (3) Insert the administration set into the blood bag according to package directions.

   (4) Compress the drip chamber and release it, *allowing blood to flow into the filter chamber.* Repeat until the filter is completely covered with blood.

   (5) Clear the tubing of air, and clamp and cap it with the sterile cap provided. (In some facilities, the procedure includes the use of normal saline. Most facilities have a policy of attaching the blood tubing directly into the hub of the needle that enters the patient's vein. This method is preferable *because the red cells receive less trauma being infused directly into the patient than they do being forced through two needles, as they are when piggybacked.* It is always preferable to disconnect the existing IV tubing at the needle hub and connect the blood, but if it *is* piggybacked into the existing IV line, flush the tubing with normal saline first. The normal saline line should be *clamped* during the administration of the blood or blood product.)

Implementation

9. Identify the patient *to be sure you are performing the procedure for the correct patient.* Check the patient's identification band against the blood center invoice.

10. Explain the procedure to the patient. Your explanation should include the product to be administered, the rationale for the therapy, and approximately how long it will take. Tell the patient that transfusion reactions are uncommon but that you should be called if he or she experiences any of the following: itching, headache, tightness in the chest, shortness of breath, chills, or sudden anxiety (see Table 56–2).

11. Measure and record the patient's blood pressure, temperature, pulse, and respirations for baseline data.

12. Wearing clean gloves, hang the blood bag and normal saline, if used, on the IV stand.

13. Remove the tape securing the IV tubing.

14. Clamp the tubing on the IV infusion that is running. Medications should not be added directly to blood or a blood product. If the tubing being used to administer blood *must* be used to give medications, flush it with saline before and after.

15. Remove the tubing from the needle, and cap it with the sterile needle and cover.

16. Remove the sterile cap from the blood tubing, and connect it to the needle hub.

17. Open the clamp on the tubing, and check for patency. *Because red cells settle to the bottom, and plasma rises to the top*, gently mix whole blood before and during the transfusion. Mix packed cells by squeezing the bag gently every 20 to 30 minutes *to prevent settling of red blood cells.*
18. Clamp the saline tubing, and open the blood delivery tubing. Calculate the flow rate to run over 2 to 6 hours as indicated by the physician's order, patient condition, or policy. Blood should not be allowed to hang at room temperature longer than this time *because of the danger of bacteria proliferation and red blood cell hemolysis.* Each facility has a specific policy regarding maximum time for a blood transfusion.
19. Tape the blood tubing in place.
20. Adjust the flow rate to run at a TKO (to keep open) rate (or about half the rate you calculated) for the first 15 minutes.
21. *Because most reactions start within the first 15 minutes,* stay with the patient during this time or during the first 50 mL of the transfusion *to observe for reactions and complications.*
22. Monitor vital signs 5 and 15 minutes after the blood product is started, and compare them with baseline measurements.
23. Regulate the rate to run as calculated.
24. Check periodically (at least every 20–30 minutes) *for the rate of infusion and symptoms of reaction.*
25. If a transfusion reaction occurs, do the following:
    a. Stop the blood. Keep the IV open with normal saline or the previous IV infusion as described below.
    b. Recheck the vital signs.
    c. Notify the physician for further orders.
26. On completion of the transfusion, remove tape, put on clean gloves, and perform one of the following:
    a. If the IV is to be resumed, do the following:
       (1) Remove the tape from the blood tubing.
       (2) Clamp the blood tubing, and remove it from the needle.
       (3) Immediately connect the normal saline IV or a syringe of normal saline to flush the tubing and needle or catheter.
       (4) Clamp the normal saline tubing, and remove it from the needle.
       (5) Connect the previous IV infusion.
       (6) Release the clamp on the IV tubing; adjust the flow rate, and secure the tubing with tape.
    b. If the IV is to be discontinued (see Module 52, Preparing and Maintaining Intravenous Infusions, for detailed directions):
       (1) Clamp the blood tubing, and remove the needle or other IV device.
       (2) Check to make sure that no part of the needle has broken off and remains in the patient.
       (3) Apply pressure, and raise the patient's arm.
       (4) Apply an adhesive bandage or pressure dressing.
    c. If an IV lock is to be applied (see Module 55 Starting Intravenous Infusions, for detailed directions):
       (1) Clamp the blood tubing, and remove i from the needle.
       (2) Immediately connect the IV solution filled adapter.
       (3) Flush the lock with the remaining solution, following your facility's policy.
       (4) Secure the IV lock with tape.
27. Monitor vital signs, and compare them with baseline measurements.
28. Discard the blood administration set in the special container in the soiled utility room. *Even though all blood is tested for hepatitis B virus and HI antibodies, infectious agents could still be present.* needles have been used, remove them with gloved hands, and place them in the sharps container. Dispose of all transfusion equipment i the plastic-lined containers kept in the soile utility room and never in the wastebasket in the patient's room.
29. Discard blood bags in the same plastic-lined containers in the soiled utility room. For patient who have experienced reactions in the past, the policy of some facilities is to return the use blood bags to the facility blood center *so that th blood samples connected to the bag are available f testing in case of a delayed blood reaction.*
30. Remove gloves, and wash your hands *for infe tion control.*

Evaluation
31. Evaluate using the following criteria:
    a. Correct blood product given at correct rat
    b. TPR and blood pressure within normal limi and patient free of other signs of reaction.
    c. Patient comfortable.

Documentation
32. Document the following:
    a. Type and amount of blood product
    b. Blood unit identification number. Usually printed adhesive-backed tag is available the blood unit. This is removed and attach to the appropriate chart form.
    c. Time started and completed

d. Vital signs before, at 5 and 15 minutes after initiation of transfusion, and on completion of transfusion—or at other times as indicated by your facility's policy

e. Flow rate

f. Pertinent patient responses and clinical observations. Some facilities have a special form on which to record information about blood administration (Fig. 56–4). In others, the parenteral fluid sheet is used, along with flow sheets and nurses' notes, to record vital signs and other pertinent observations (Fig. 56-5).

Administering Platelets

To administer platelets, follow the steps of the General Procedure for Administering Whole Blood and Packed Red Cells as modified below.

Assessment

1.–2. Follow the steps of the General Procedure for Administering Whole Blood and Packed Red Cells.

Planning

3.–4. Follow the steps of the General Procedure.

5. Obtain the platelets from the facility blood center.

6. With another nurse, check the following:

a. Patient's name and spelling, hospital number, and physician's name as on the face sheet with the blood center invoice

b. Blood type of platelets with the blood type of the patient. If a discrepancy exists, look under remarks to see if the physician who ordered the platelets has accepted ABO-incompatible platelets. If the physician has accepted this risk, it is permissible to give unmatched platelets.

c. Blood type and platelet unit identification numbers listed on the platelet pack with the blood type and platelet unit identification numbers on the blood center invoice

7. and 8. Follow the steps of the General Procedure.

Implementation

9.–17. Follow the steps of the General Procedure.

18. Adjust the flow rate to administer the platelets

DATE: _7-27-99_   TIME: _0800_

Number: **MH 70530**

Group: _O_   RH: _+_

Donor: _Timothy Benson_
Whole Blood: _✓_ Packed Cells: ___
Platelets: ___ Plasma: ___
Fibrinogen: ___ Gamulin D: ___
Checked by: _P. Jones_ RN

_____ _J. Russell_ RN
Started by: _P. Jones, R.N._

Solution used: _Normal Saline_

Amount: _250 cc_

Needle size: _19_

Type: _Butterfly_
Filter: New (Yes) Changed Yes
No   No
Location: _① forearm_

Rate of flow: _25 gtts / min._

Previous Transfusion (Yes) No
Previous Reaction Yes (No)

Starting TPR: _97⁸ 64 18_ BP: _110/70_
TPR: 5" _98-66-18_ BP: _114/76_
15" _98⁴-66-18_ BP: _114/78_
TPR Completion _98⁸-66-18_ BP: _116/78_

CLINICAL SYMPTOMS OF REACTION
Low back pain Yes (No)
Chest discomfort Yes (No)
Chilling Yes (No)
Drop in BP Yes (No)
Flushing of face Yes (No)
Distended neck veins Yes (No)
Headache Yes (No)
Dizziness Yes (No)
Respiratory discomfort Yes (No)
Nausea-vomiting Yes (No)
Urticarial Eruptions Yes (No)
Urine output adequate (Yes) No

Pt. observed by: _P. Jones, R.N._
M.D. notified:

Time Completed _1100_
Amount Received: _500 cc._
D/C'd by whom: _P. Jones, RN_

Patient tolerated: _3 problems_

If reaction, was Reaction
Procedure followed? Yes No

1. Urine specimen Yes No
2. Blood samples drawn Yes No
3. Blood samples to Yes No
   Blood Bank
4. Transfusion:
   continued discontinued
5. Antihistamine antipyretic
   therapy Yes No

BALLARD COMMUNITY HOSPITAL
SEATTLE, WASHINGTON

BLOOD RECORD

Figure 56–4. The blood record documented by the nurse.

Date and Time	AMOUNT SOLUTION ADDITIVES (number consecutively)	Rate and Regulator	Added By	Needle Type Started	Size Site By:	Tubing Chng. By:	Site Care and Observations	Solu' Time	DC'd Amount Absorb.	SHIFT TOTALS Time	Total
Date: 7/27/99 Time: 0200	WB #MH70529	25 gtts/min	PJ	Vital signs: Initiation:			97^8-64-18 $^{110}/_{70}$	1100	500 cc	6-2	500
				10 Minutes:			98^4-66-18 $^{114}/_{78}$				
Date: Time:				Completion:			98^8-68-16 $^{116}/_{78}$				
				Reaction: Yes ☐ No ☒							
Date: Time:											
Date: Time:											
Date: Time:											
Date: Time:											
Date: Time:											
Date: Time:											

Identify Initials with Signature:	4.	8.
1. PJ P. Jones RN	5.	9.
2.	6.	10.
3.	7.	11.

ADDRESSOGRAPH:

Bertha Johnson F-54
537-34-1409
Dr. James Gusher

CODE: "*" = see Nurses Narrative

THE SWEDISH HOSPITAL MEDICAL CENTER
SEATTLE, WASHINGTON

N-1547 Nursing Rev. 6/80 FC/TSHMC

Figure 56–5. Documenting blood administration on a parenteral therapy record.

as rapidly as possible *because they must be administered within 4 hours of the time they were pooled together at the blood center.* Do not use pressure cuffs or pumps with platelets *because the cells are easily damaged.*

19.–30. Follow the steps of the General Procedure.

Evaluation

31. Follow the General Procedure.

Documentation

32. Follow the General Procedure.

Administering Albumin

To administer albumin, follow the steps of the General Procedure for Administering Whole Blood and Packed Red Cells as modified below.

Assessment
1.–2. Follow the steps of the General Procedure for Administering Whole Blood and Packed Red Cells.

Planning
3. Follow the General Procedure.
4. Gather the equipment. Albumin is usually available in a 50-mL glass container and is piggybacked into an existing IV infusion. If it is necessary to start an IV infusion, you will need the equipment discussed in Module 55, Starting Intravenous Infusions, in addition to the following:
 a. Albumin solution (albumin NSA)
 b. Secondary tubing
 c. Alcohol swab
 d. Tape
5. Obtain the albumin preparation from the pharmacy.
6. Check the medication administration record (MAR) to be sure this is the correct preparation.
7. Carry the albumin and the MAR or an identification card to the patient's bedside.
8. Prepare the equipment as follows:
 a. Insert the administration set into the albumin container according to the package directions.
 b. Fill the drip chamber half full.
 c. Clear the tubing of air, and clamp.

Implementation
9.–10. Follow the steps of the General Procedure.
11. Measure and record the patient's blood pressure.
12. Wearing clean gloves, hang the albumin bag on IV stand.
13. Remove the tape securing the tubing.
14. Clamp the tubing on the IV running if you are not piggybacking the albumin.
15. Remove IV tubing from the needle; cap it with the sterile needle, and cover it.
16. Remove the sterile cap from the albumin tubing, and attach it to the needle hub or piggyback; follow the policy of your facility.
17. Open the clamp on the tubing.
18. Adjust the flow rate according to the manufacturer's directions.
19. Tape the albumin tubing in place.
20. Adjust the flow rate of the primary set to slow the drip, and lower the primary bag or bottle to a point below where the albumin is hanging. Prepare the injection port closest to the patient, using an alcohol swab. Attach the albumin tubing to the injection port, using a 19-gauge or larger needle or needleless connector. Leave the clamp open on the primary tubing. It will not flow until the albumin infusion is completed.

Open the clamp on the albumin tubing. Adjust the rate of the albumin as ordered by the physician. The rate should not exceed 2 mL/min *because it can increase intravascular volume rapidly, resulting in congestive heart failure or pulmonary edema.*
21. Follow the General Procedure.
22. Monitor the patient's blood pressure.
23. Regulate the rate, not to exceed 2 mL/min.
24. Follow the General Procedure.
25. Identify any untoward reactions, and report them to the physician.
26. On completion of albumin infusion, do the following:
 a. Close the clamp on the albumin tubing.
 b. Raise the primary bag or bottle to its original position. Readjust the flow rate.
 c. Remove the albumin bottle and tubing, and discard them.
27. Monitor the patient's blood pressure, and compare it with baseline measurements.
28. Discard used equipment.
29. Place needle in sharps container.
30. Follow the General Procedure.

Evaluation
31. Evaluate using the following criteria:
 a. Albumin infused at appropriate rate.
 b. Blood pressure checked before and after albumin infusion.
 c. Patient comfortable.

Documentation
32. Document the following:
 a. Amount of albumin administered
 b. Time started and finished
 c. Patient's blood pressure before and after albumin administration
 d. Pertinent patient reactions to the procedure

Administering Cryoprecipitate

To administer cryoprecipitate, follow the steps of the General Procedure for Administering Whole Blood and Packed Red Cells as modified below.

Assessment
1.–2. Follow the steps of the General Procedure for Administering Whole Blood and Packed Red Cells.

Planning
3. Follow the General Procedure.
4. Gather the equipment. If it is necessary to start an IV infusion, you will need the equipment discussed in Module 55, Starting Intravenous Infusions, and the following:

a. Blood administration set

b. Bottle or bag of normal saline with a secondary administration set, as facility policy indicates. Normal saline is the only IV fluid that can be mixed with cryoprecipitate.

c. Tape

5. Obtain the cryoprecipitate from the facility's blood center as soon as it arrives *because it must be administered within 4 hours of the time it is thawed and pooled.*

6. With another nurse, compare the patient's name and spelling, hospital number, and physician's name on the face sheet in the chart with those on the blood center invoice. Verify the dose size by comparing the number of units ordered with the number of units listed on the cryoprecipitate bag and on the invoice.

7. You and the other nurse sign your names, titles, date, and time on the blood center invoice if all of the information is correct.

8. Prepare the equipment as follows:

a. Turn the control on the blood tubing to the off position.

b. Open the entry port on the cryoprecipitate bag.

c. Insert the administration set into the cryoprecipitate bag.

d. Squeeze the drip chamber and release it to allow cryoprecipitate to flow into the filter chamber. Repeat until the filter is completely covered.

e. Clear the tubing of air, and clamp it.

Implementation

9.–11. Follow the steps of the General Procedure.

12. Wearing clean gloves, hang the cryoprecipitate bag on the IV stand.

13.–15. Follow the steps of the General Procedure

16. Connect cryoprecipitate tubing to needle hub

17. Follow the General Procedure.

18. Adjust the flow rate. Cryoprecipitate should be administered rapidly (ie, 10–12 U [200–250 mL] can be administered in 20–30 minutes) *because it loses its effectiveness if not administered within 4 hours of the time it is thawed and pooled.*

19.–25. Follow the steps of the General Procedure

26. On completion of the cryoprecipitate, connect the normal saline or discontinue the IV infusion as ordered.

27. You do not need to monitor vital signs.

28. Discard blood administration set and cryoprecipitate bag.

29. Place needle in sharps container.

30. Follow the General Procedure.

Evaluation

31. Evaluate using the following criteria:

a. Cryoprecipitate infused at appropriate rate

b. Patient comfortable.

Documentation

32. Document the following:

a. Amount of cryoprecipitate

b. Blood center numbers, as facility policy indicates

c. Time started and completed

d. Pertinent patient responses and clinical observations

LONG-TERM CARE

Residents in long-term care facilities occasionally receive blood products. Packed red blood cells are commonly used to treat serious chronic states of anemia. Older residents with chronic leukemia may receive either red blood cells or platelets. A physician's order is needed, and an employee of the facility needs to pick up and identify the blood product. The nurse administering the blood product must be licensed and understand the policies and procedures *for safe administration.*

Elderly people have an increased risk for transfusion reactions *because their body systems are less active and more fragile than those in younger people.* Older people who require blood transfusion also may have a heightened sense of anxiety about the procedure *because they may hold the view that receiving blood is a fearful and life-saving action rather than the common treatment modality it is considered today.* Give clear, calm, and supportive explanations to allay any fear the resident may have.

HOME CARE

People who have hemophilia, including children, frequently receive factor VIII preparations or infusions of cryoprecipitate at home. This procedure may have been done by a family care provider or sometimes by the adult client. *Reactions rarely occur with the use of this product, so self-administration is considered safe.*

However, the administration of blood in the home can have serious consequences. This is presently being done experimentally under the guidelines of several central blood centers in the United States. Studies are underway *to determine whether more reactions occur at the time of transfusion in the home and whether a prompt and appropriate response can be made if a serious reaction occurs.* Blood centers strongly recommend that only specially trained and competent licensed people administer the blood. Some blood centers will not release the product unless they are assured that the person who will be administering the blood is competent to do so. Home care administration of blood products has merits *in that it would avoid having very ill and weak people who are receiving care in the home transported to and from an acute care setting for this procedure.* As more home health nurses are available for giving care, this procedure may become more common in the home setting.

CRITICAL THINKING EXERCISES

• You started an IV infusion of blood on your patient 20 minutes ago. When you check back with him after 10 minutes, he reports a feeling of apprehension and a chill. Evaluate the situation, and plan your immediate nursing actions, giving the rationale for each. Also describe your interaction with the patient.

• Your young patient with a leg fracture to be repaired requires 6 U of cryoprecipitate. Describe how you would proceed, beginning with obtaining the cryoprecipitate from the facility's blood center. Compare and contrast the steps of this procedure with those for transfusing whole blood. Explain why certain steps are different.

References

American Association of Blood Banks (1994). *Nursing guidelines for administration of blood.* US Department of Health and Human Services.

Drago, S. S. (1992). Banking on your own blood. *American Journal of Nursing, 92*(3), 61–64.

✔ PERFORMANCE CHECKLIST

General Procedure for Administering Whole Blood and Packed Red Cells	Needs More Practice	Satisfactory	Comments
Assessment			
1. Check physician's orders.			
2. Check existing intravenous (IV) for patency and needle size, or initiate IV therapy.			
Planning			
3. Wash your hands.			
4. Gather equipment. **a.** Blood administration set			
b. Normal saline			
c. Blood pump			
d. Clean gloves and tape			
5. Obtain blood product from facility blood center.			
6. With another nurse, check: **a.** Patient's name and spelling, hospital number, and physician's name on face sheet with blood center invoice			
b. Blood product type, Rh, and blood unit administration number on blood bag with blood center invoice.			
c. Expiration date on blood bag			
7. Sign blood center invoice.			
8. Prepare equipment. **a.** If used, obtain pump.			
b. Y blood administration set (1) Close all clamps on Y set.			
(2) Insert one spike of administration set into blood bag.			
(3) Open clamp closest to normal saline bag, and fill drip chamber half full.			
(4) Open lower control clamp, and flush air from tubing; reclamp.			
(5) Insert other administration set spike into normal saline bag.			

(*continued*)

General Procedure for Administering Whole Blood and Packed Red Cells (Continued)	Needs More Practice	Satisfactory	Comments
(6) Open clamp closest to blood and squeeze filter chamber, and release until filter is completely covered with blood; reclamp.			
(7) Open lower control clamp and flush the tubing with blood.			
c. Primary blood administration set (1) Turn control on blood tubing to off.			
(2) Open entry port on blood bag.			
(3) Insert administration set into blood bag.			
(4) Compress and release drip chamber to allow blood to flow into drip chamber. Repeat until filter is completely covered.			
(5) Clear tubing of air, and clamp.			
Implementation			
9. Identify patient.			
10. Explain procedure to patient, and list signs of a reaction.			
11. Measure and record vital signs.			
12. Wearing clean gloves, hang blood bag on IV stand.			
13. Remove tape securing IV tubing.			
14. Clamp tubing on IV running.			
15. Remove IV tubing from needle; cap with sterile needle and cover.			
16. Remove sterile cap from blood tubing, and connect to needle hub.			
17. Open clamp on tubing.			
18. Calculate flow rate to run over 2–6 hours.			
19. Tape blood tubing in place.			
20. Adjust flow rate to run at TKO rate for first 15 minutes.			
21. Stay with patient for first 15 minutes or for infusion of 50 mL.			
22. Recheck vital signs 5 and 15 minutes later.			

(continued)

General Procedure for Administering Whole Blood and Packed Red Cells *(Continued)*	Needs More Practice	Satisfactory	Comments
23. Regulate the rate to run as calculated.			
24. Check periodically for rate of infusion and symptoms of reaction.			
25. If transfusion reaction occurs: **a.** Stop blood, maintaining venous access.			
b. Recheck vital signs.			
c. Notify physician.			
26. On completion of transfusion: **a.** If IV is to be resumed: (1) Remove tape from blood tubing.			
(2) Put on gloves, clamp blood tubing and remove from needle.			
(3) Connect normal saline to flush tubing and needle or catheter.			
(4) Clamp normal saline tubing and remove from needle.			
(5) Connect previous IV infusion.			
(6) Release clamp on IV tubing, adjust flow rate, and secure tubing with tape.			
b. If IV is to be discontinued: (1) Put on gloves; clamp blood tubing and remove needle.			
(2) Check to make sure infusion device is intact.			
(3) Apply pressure and raise patient's arm.			
(4) Apply adhesive bandage.			
c. If IV lock is to be applied: (1) Put on gloves, and clamp blood tubing and remove from needle.			
(2) Immediately connect solution-filled lock adapter.			
(3) Flush with remaining solution or saline.			
(4) Secure with tape.			
27. Monitor vital signs, and compare with baseline measurements.			

(continued)

1996 by Lippincott-Raven Publishers

General Procedure for Administering Whole Blood and Packed Red Cells *(Continued)*	Needs More Practice	Satisfactory	Comments
28. Discard blood administration set.			
29. Place blood bag in special container or return to facility blood center.			
30. Remove gloves, and wash your hands.			
Evaluation			
31. Evaluate using the following criteria: **a.** Correct blood product at correct rate.			
b. TPR and blood pressure within normal limits and patient free of other signs of reaction.			
c. Patient comfortable.			
Documentation			
32. Document the following: **a.** Type and amount of blood product			
b. Blood unit identification number			
c. Time started and completed			
d. Vital signs before, at 5 and 15 minutes after initiation of transfusion, and on completion of transfusion			
e. Flow rate			
f. Pertinent patient responses and clinical observations			
Administering Platelets			
Assessment			
1.–2. Follow steps 1 and 2 of the Performance Checklist: General Procedure for Administering Whole Blood and Packed Red Cells: Check physician's orders, check existing IV for patency and needle size, or initiate an IV.			
Planning			
3.–4. Follow steps 3 and 4 of the General Procedure: Wash your hands and obtain necessary equipment.			
5. Obtain platelets from facility blood center.			

(continued

Administering Platelets *(Continued)*	Needs More Practice	Satisfactory	Comments
6. With another nurse check: **a.** Patient's name and spelling, hospital number, and physician's name on face sheet with blood center invoice			
b. Blood type of platelets with blood type of patient			
7.–8. Follow steps 7 and 8 of the General Procedure: Sign blood center invoice, and prepare equipment.			
Implementation			
9.–17. Follow steps 9 through 17 of the General Procedure: Identify patient, explain procedure, measure and record vital signs, put on gloves, hang platelet bag and normal saline, remove tape securing IV tubing, clamp tubing on IV running, remove tubing from needle, cap with sterile needle and cover, remove sterile cap from tubing, connect it to needle hub, and open clamp on tubing.			
18. Adjust flow rate to administer platelets as rapidly as possible. Do not use pressure cuffs or pumps.			
19.–30. Follow steps 19 through 30 of the General Procedure: Tape blood tubing in place; adjust flow rate; stay with patient for first 15 minutes; monitor vital signs 5 and 15 minutes after blood product is started; regulate the rate to run as calculated; check periodically for rate of infusion and symptoms of reaction; if transfusion reaction occurs, stop blood product, and keep IV open with normal saline; recheck vital signs; notify physician for further orders; on completion of transfusion, resume IV, discontinue IV, or apply IV lock, as ordered; monitor vital signs; discard blood administration set; place blood product bag in special container or return to facility blood center; remove gloves and wash your hands.			

(continued)

Administering Platelets *(Continued)*	Needs More Practice	Satisfactory	Comments
Evaluation			
31. Evaluate, using the following criteria: **a.** Correct blood product at correct rate.			
b. TPR and blood pressure within normal limits and patient free of other signs of reaction.			
c. Patient comfortable.			
Documentation			
32. Document the following: **a.** Type and amount of blood product			
b. Blood unit identification number			
c. Time started and completed			
d. Vital signs before, at 5 and 15 minutes after initiation of infusion, and on completion of transfusion			
e. Flow rate			
f. Pertinent patient responses and clinical observations			
Administering Albumin			
Assessment			
1.–2. Follow steps 1 and 2 of the General Procedure for Administering Whole Blood and Packed Red Cells: Check physician's orders, check existing IV for patency and needle size, or initiate an IV.			
Planning			
3. Wash your hands.			
4. Gather equipment. **a.** Albumin solution			
b. Secondary tubing			
c. Alcohol swab			
d. Tape			
5. Obtain albumin preparation from pharmacy.			
6. Check the medication administration record (MAR) to be sure this is the correct preparation.			

(continued)

Administering Albumin *(Continued)*	Needs More Practice	Satisfactory	Comments
7. Carry the albumin and the MAR record or a card to the bedside.			
8. Prepare equipment:			
a. Insert administration set into albumin container.			
b. Fill drip chamber half full.			
c. Clear tubing of air, and clamp.			
Implementation			
9.–10. Follow steps 9 and 10 of the General Procedure: Identify patient; explain procedure.			
11. Measure and record blood pressure.			
12. Wearing clean gloves, hang albumin bag on IV stand.			
13. Remove tape securing tubing.			
14. Clamp tubing on IV running if not piggybacking albumin.			
15. Remove IV tubing from needle; cap with sterile needle and cover.			
16. Remove sterile cap from albumin tubing, and attach to needle hub or piggyback, following policy.			
17. Open clamp on tubing.			
18. Adjust rate of flow according to directions from manufacturer.			
19. Tape albumin tubing in place.			
20. Adjust flow rate to TKO (to keep open) for first 15 minutes.			
21. Stay with patient for first 15 minutes.			
22. Monitor blood pressure.			
23. Regulate the rate, not to exceed 2 mL/min.			
24. Check patient periodically during infusion.			
25. Identify any untoward reactions, and report to physician.			
26. On completion of albumin infusion: **a.** Close clamp on albumin tubing.			

(continued)

Administering Albumin *(Continued)*	Needs More Practice	Satisfactory	Comments
b. Raise primary bag to original position, and readjust flow rate.			
c. Remove albumin bottle and tubing, and discard.			
27. Monitor patient's blood pressure.			
28. Discard used equipment.			
29. Place needle in sharps container.			
30. Remove gloves, and wash your hands.			
Evaluation			
31. Evaluate, using the following criteria: **a.** Albumin infused at appropriate rate.			
b. Blood pressure within normal limits.			
c. Patient comfortable.			
Documentation			
32. Document the following: **a.** Amount of albumin administered.			
b. Time started and finished.			
c. Patient's blood pressure before and after albumin administration.			
d. Other pertinent patient reactions.			
Administering Cryoprecipitate			
Assessment			
1.–2. Follow steps 1 and 2 of the General Procedure for Administering Whole Blood and Packed Red Cells: Check physician's orders, check existing IV for patency and needle size, or initiate an IV.			
Planning			
3. Wash your hands.			
4. Gather equipment. **a.** Blood administration set			
b. Normal saline with secondary set			
c. Tape			
5. Obtain cryoprecipitate from facility blood center.			

(continued)

Administering Cryoprecipitate *(Continued)*	Needs More Practice	Satisfactory	Comments
6. With another nurse, compare patient's name and spelling, hospital number, and physician's name on face sheet of chart with those on blood center invoice.			
7. Sign blood center invoice.			
8. Prepare equipment: **a.** Turn control on blood tubing to off.			
b. Open entry port on cryoprecipitate bag.			
c. Insert administration set into cryoprecipitate bag.			
d. Squeeze and release drip chamber to allow cryoprecipitate to flow into drip chamber. Repeat until filter is completely covered.			
e. Clear tubing of air and clamp.			
Implementation			
9.–11. Follow steps 9 through 11 of the General Procedure: Identify patient, explain procedure, and measure and record vital signs.			
12. Wearing clean gloves, hang cryoprecipitate bag on IV stand.			
13.–15. Follow steps 13 through 15 of the General Procedure: Remove tape securing IV tubing, clamp tubing on IV running, remove tubing from needle, and cap with sterile needle and cover.			
16. Connect cryoprecipitate tubing to needle hub.			
17. Open clamp on tubing.			
18. Adjust the flow rate to administer rapidly.			
19.–25. Follow steps 19 through 25 of the General Procedure: Tape tubing in place; adjust flow rate to run at TKO for first 15 minutes; stay with patient for first 15 minutes; recheck vital signs 5 and 15 minutes later; regulate the rate to run as calculated; check periodically for infusion rate and symptoms of reaction; if transfusion reaction occurs, stop blood product, keep IV open, recheck vital signs, and notify physician.			

(continued)

Administering Cryoprecipitate *(Continued)*	Needs More Practice	Satisfactory	Comments
26. On completion of the cryoprecipitate, connect normal saline or discontinue IV, as ordered.			
27. You do not need to monitor vital signs.			
28. Discard blood administration set and cryoprecipitate bag.			
29. Place needle in sharps container.			
30. Remove gloves and wash your hands.			
Evaluation			
31. Evaluate using the following criteria: 　**a.** Cryoprecipitate infused at appropriate rate.			
b. Patient comfortable.			
Documentation			
32. Document the following: 　**a.** Amount of cryoprecipitate			
b. Blood center numbers as facility policy indicates			
c. Time started and completed			
d. Pertinent patient responses and clinical observations			

? QUIZ

Short-Answer Questions

1. What are the five methods used in blood transfusion?

   a. _____

   b. _____

   c. _____

   d. _____

   e. _____

2. Why are more autologous transfusions now being administered?

   _____

   _____

   _____

   _____

   _____

3. What tests are done on autologous blood as compared with the tests done on nonautologous blood?

   _____

   _____

4. List three reasons for administering blood and blood products.

   a. _____

   b. _____

   c. _____

5. List two advantages of component therapy.

   a. _____

   b. _____

6. List the two indications for the administration of whole blood.

   a. _____

   b. _____

7. Name the four main blood groups in the ABO system of typing.

   a. _____

   b. _____

   c. _____

   d. _____

8. List four potential complications of transfusion.

    a. _____

    b. _____

    c. _____

    d. _____

9. List four signs and symptoms of a hemolytic reaction.

    a. _____

    b. _____

    c. _____

    d. _____

10. List three actions you would take in the event of a mild allergic reaction.

    a. _____

    b. _____

    c. _____

11. How can air embolus be prevented?

_____

12. Why is dextrose in water *not* used with blood and blood products?

_____

13. What five items should be checked before a unit of blood is administered?

    a. _____

    b. _____

    c. _____

    d. _____

    e. _____

MODULE

57

ADMINISTERING PARENTERAL NUTRITION

MODULE CONTENTS

RATIONALE FOR THE USE OF THIS
  SKILL
NURSING DIAGNOSES
TOTAL PARENTERAL NUTRITION
PARTIAL PARENTERAL NUTRITION
COMPLICATIONS OF PARENTERAL
  NUTRITION
SOLUTIONS USED FOR PARENTERAL
  NUTRITION
GENERAL PROCEDURE FOR
  ADMINISTERING PARENTERAL
  NUTRITION
Assessment
Planning
Implementation

Evaluation
Documentation
PROCEDURE FOR ADMINISTERING FAT
  EMULSIONS (LIPIDS)
Assessment
Planning
Implementation
Evaluation
Documentation
DISCONTINUING PARENTERAL
  NUTRITION
LONG-TERM CARE
HOME CARE
CRITICAL THINKING EXERCISES

PREREQUISITES

Successful completion of the following modules:

VOLUME 1

VOLUME 2

OVERALL OBJECTIVE

To safely administer parenteral nutrition through an existing intravenous line or a central venous catheter.

SPECIFIC LEARNING OBJECTIVES

Know Facts and Principles	Apply Facts and Principles	Demonstrate Ability	Evaluate Performance
1. Types of parenteral nutrition			
Know the two types of parenteral nutrition.	Given a situation, state rationale for the type of parenteral nutrition in use.	In the clinical setting, identify patients receiving the two types of parenteral nutrition.	Verify your knowledge with your instructor.
2. Equipment			
List the various items of equipment used to administer parenteral nutrition.	Given a physician's order, list the equipment needed to give parenteral nutrition.	In the clinical setting, gather the equipment needed for the ordered parenteral nutrition.	Validate your choice of equipment with your instructor.
3. Administering parenteral nutrition			
List steps in administering parenteral nutrition.	Given a specific situation, identify the steps necessary in the administration procedure.	In the clinical setting, correctly administer parenteral nutrition.	Evaluate performance with your instructor.
4. Administering lipids (fat emulsions)			
List steps in administering lipids.	Given a specific situation, identify the steps necessary in the administration of lipids.	In the clinical setting, correctly administer lipids.	Evaluate performance with your instructor.
5. Potential complications			
Name the complications that can occur with parenteral nutrition.	Given a patient situation, state appropriate assessment and preventative actions.	In the clinical setting, make appropriate assessments, and take any action needed to prevent complications.	Evaluate own performance with instructor.

LEARNING ACTIVITIES

1. Review the Specific Learning Objectives.
2. Read the section on nutrition and intravenous (IV) infusions in Ellis and Nowlis, *Nursing: A Human Needs Approach,* or comparable material in another textbook.
3. Look up the module vocabulary terms in the glossary.
4. Read through the module as though you were preparing to teach the skills to another person. Mentally practice the procedures.
5. In the practice setting, do the following:
   a. Examine the fat emulsion equipment. Identify the following:
      (1) A simulated order for fat emulsion
      (2) A practice fat emulsion bottle
      (3) An infusion pump (if one is used)
      (4) Pump or regular tubing
      (5) Pull-tapes used for connections
   b. After checking the order against the printed label on the bottle, practice setting up the fat emulsion bottle using the appropriate tubing. Insert the tubing into the pump or an existing parenteral nutrition line.
   c. Using a waste basket when practicing to catch the flow, set the flow rate and operate the pump.
   d. Practice documenting the parenteral nutrition and lipids on an IV record form.
6. In the clinical setting, examine equipment and policies and procedures for administering parenteral nutrition, including lipids. When your instructor approves your practice performance, administer both total and partial parenteral nutrition and fat emulsions (lipids) under supervision.

VOCABULARY

amino acids	finger stick	infusion pump	piggyback
cycling	hyperalimentation	lipids	positive nitrogen
dextrose	hyperglycemia	lumen	balance
fat emulsions	hypertonic	parenteral	test dose

Parenteral Nutrition

Rationale for the Use of This Skill

More individuals are receiving parenteral nutrition in the hospital, in the long-term care setting, and in the home. This has occurred because of the improvements in central venous lines, the availability of intravenous (IV) nutritional solutions, and the increasing number of people with long-term illnesses that interfere with normal nutrition. The complexity of the procedure and the potential for complications demand a high level of nursing skill.[1]

▼ NURSING DIAGNOSES

The nursing diagnosis that is most common to indicate a need for parenteral nutrition is Altered Nutrition: Less than body requirements. This nursing diagnosis follows an assessment that reveals the patient is not eating adequately and is losing weight.

Patients on parenteral nutrition have had an IV catheter inserted, disrupting skin integrity. The insertion site must be conscientiously inspected for inflammation or infection. This fact makes both Risk for Infection and Impaired Skin Integrity appropriate nursing diagnoses for the patient on parenteral nutrition.

TOTAL PARENTERAL NUTRITION

For most patients, parenteral nutrition is total in that all nutrients needed by the body are supplied by accessing a central venous catheter and infusing a specially formulated solution into the central circulation. (For details about the position of these access lines and other information, see Module 54, Caring for Central Intravenous Catheters.) The nutrients supplied by total parenteral nutrition include dextrose, protein, electrolytes, amino acids, and vitamins. These substances are mixed with sterile water into a hypertonic solution. The maximum dextrose concentration for total parenteral nutrition solutions is 35%. Several terms are used for this therapy—hyperalimentation (sometimes referred to as "hyperal" or HA) and the initials TPN, which stand for total parenteral nutrition. Some patients also receive fats or lipids in a separate solution, which is in-fused by inserting the line into the hyperalimentation line. For guidelines on this procedure, see Module 53, Administering Intravenous Medications.

Patients receiving total parenteral nutrition are usually *those who cannot eat for a long time due to major trauma, pathology of the intestinal tract, or long-term illness, such as cancer, acquired immunodeficiency syndrome, or renal failure.* Other patients who receive total parenteral nutrition are those who cannot eat normally, preventing them from taking in sufficient nutrients.

Sometimes patients are given IV fluids without additional nutrients. In most facilities, a policy states that a patient should not be sustained on peripheral IV solutions alone for more than a few (usually 3–5) days. The policy requires that after the designated time, an alternate method must be provided *for nutritional requirements.* Although peripheral IV solutions provide water, calories, and some electrolytes, it has been found that *prolonged use of fluids without additional nutrients leads to protein depletion and malnutrition.* Because of this, patients receiving peripheral IV solutions are appropriate candidates for placement of a central venous catheter and the initiation of parenteral nutrition.

PARTIAL PARENTERAL NUTRITION

Some patients who are unable to eat properly for an extended time and are nutritionally depleted may receive partial parenteral nutrition as a *temporary adjunct to their nutritional status.* These patients are able to eat some of their diet but not enough to be nutritionally healthy. In partial parenteral nutrition, the solution is infused through a peripheral IV line. This route is not recommended for any length of time *because the solution irritates the veins.* The dextrose concentration should not exceed 10%.

COMPLICATIONS OF PARENTERAL NUTRITION

There are potential complications with either total or partial parenteral nutrition. The most common complication is inflammation and sepsis of the catheter insertion site. The administration of these solutions, particularly those with lipids, does not increase the risk of developing sepsis of the central catheter. However, the nurse should carefully assess the catheter site each time parenteral nutrition is administered and report any signs of inflammation or infection.

---

[1]Note that rationale for action is emphasized throughout the module by the use of italics.

Another common complication is hyperglycemia. *The solutions contain large amounts of dextrose, which if not rapidly metabolized, may cause increased amounts of glucose in the blood.* If hyperglycemia is allowed to continue, the patient may become dehydrated and confused and experience a decreasing level of consciousness. Those receiving parenteral nutrition are assessed for the presence of hyperglycemia on a continuing basis. This is done by obtaining blood from finger sticks and using a glucose meter to measure the blood glucose level (see Module 11, Collecting Specimens and Performing Common Laboratory Tests). If hyperglycemia becomes a problem, the physician may order that a small amount of insulin be added to the solution or given subcutaneously.

During the early phases of parenteral nutrition, fluid and electrolyte imbalances also can occur. The nurse is responsible for scheduling the periodic laboratory tests, which are ordered by the physician *to detect any potential fluid or electrolyte problems.* Changes are then made in the solution *to correct any imbalance.*

Because patients on total parenteral nutrition lack adequate amounts of vitamins K and B12, bleeding tendencies and anemias can occur. These complications are prevented by adding the vitamins to the parenteral solution weekly.

SOLUTIONS USED FOR PARENTERAL NUTRITION

The solutions prepared for parenteral nutrition follow a standard for the facility with individualized adaptations for the specific needs of the patient. Figure 57–1 is a sample form listing the contents of routine parenteral nutrition solutions. The formula is ordered by the physician, who may consult with the pharmacist, nutritionist, or nurse specialist. Some nurses specialize in caring for patients receiving parenteral nutrition therapy and teach the procedure to the patient and the family when appropriate.

The solutions are prepared under sterile conditions in the facility's pharmacy. Because the dextrose and protein solution are unstable when mixed together, they are either kept separate until just before administration (Fig. 57–2) or are administered using a two-part plastic bag. The lower portion of the bag contains the dextrose solution, and the upper portion contains the protein solution. The usual ratio used is 25% dextrose solution to 5% protein solution. Standard electrolytes are added to each bag or bottle. These are allowed to mix just prior to being transported to the nursing unit. Multivitamins are added daily. Trace elements and vitamins K and B12 are added weekly.

Fat emulsions are usually referred to as "lipids" and are delivered to the nursing unit in a glass container, appearing as a white milky solution. The concentration of fatty acids contained in these solutions is ordered by the physician at either 10%, which provides 1.1 calorie/mL, or 20%, which provides 2.0 calories/mL. Only the more dilute 10% emulsion is given by the peripheral route.

GENERAL PROCEDURE FOR ADMINISTERING PARENTERAL NUTRITION

The following guidelines are for initiating parenteral nutrition to the patient for the first time.

Assessment

1. Assess the patient who is to receive parenteral nutrition. The following are essential:
   a. The patient's diagnosis. *This information may indicate whether the patient will be on long-term or short-term therapy. It also may tell you of any particular complications for which the patient may be at risk.* For example, if the patient is a diabetic, close monitoring of the glucose component of the solution may be of added importance.
   b. The patient's age and medical condition. *If the patient is an infant or a person of advanced age or in precarious health, the impact of parenteral nutrition therapy on other body systems may be much greater than if the patient is in relatively stable health.*
   c. Height and usual weight. *This information gives you baseline data so you can monitor the patient's fluid and nutritional status on an ongoing basis.*
   d. Intake and output. All patients on parenteral nutrition are placed on intake and output measurement *to assess daily nutritional and fluid status.*
   e. Allergies. A report of any previous allergies is important. Some patients have allergic reactions to tape or iodine-based solutions that are commonly used to prepare and maintain the central line insertion site. Other patients may have allergies to components of the solutions. *Reactions can typically be avoided if known allergies are reported before starting therapy.*
   f. The patient's usual vital signs. *By knowing this, you will be much more likely to detect fluctuations in vital function and complications before they become severe.* Patients receiving this therapy have their vital signs taken every 4 hours.
   g. Knowledge of procedure. *Some patients become very involved with their therapy and are helpful in*

INITIATION OF TPN — ADULT

☐ 1. STANDARD CENTRAL VENOUS FULL-STRENGTH TPN SOLUTION
   D50W 500ml (850 Calories) + Amino Acids 10% 500ml (50 Grams Protein)
   Final Concentration = Dextrose 25% & Amino Acids 5%

NaCl	30 mEq		Reg. Insulin ___0___ u.
KCl	25 mEq		Multivitamins (MVI) 1 pack (10ml) daily
KPhos	15 mEq		Multitrace Elements (MTE) 1ml daily
CaGluc	8 mEq		Vitamin C 500mg daily
MgSO4	8 mEq	(except BMT = 16 mEq)	Vitamin K 10mg weekly (Sundays)

2. RATE: TO INFUSE AT _____ ml/hr TO PROVIDE A TOTAL OF _____ liter(s)/day.

☑ 3. NON-STANDARD CENTRAL OR PERIPHERAL FORMULA   (Note: Non-standard TPN material and labor costs are higher than for the standardized solution above.)

   SPECIFY: A) solution type, strength and amount   B) additives and amounts

D10W _____ ml	Amino Acid 8.5% _____ ml	NaCl __7__ mEq	Reg Insulin __Ø__
D20W _____ ml	Amino Acid 10% _500_ ml	NaAcet _____ mEq	Multivitamins (MVI) _1_
D40W _____ ml	Hepatamine 8% _____ ml	KCl _40_ mEq	Multitrace Elements (MTE) _1_
D50W _500_ ml		KPhos _20_ mEq	Vitamin C _500_
D70W _____ ml		CaGluc _8_ mEq	Vitamin K _____
		MgSO4 _16_ mEq	Other _____

   C) FINAL Concentration Dextrose __25__ % & Amino Acids __5__ %

4. RATE: TO INFUSE AT __40__ ml/hr TO PROVIDE __1__ liter(s)/day.

☑ 5. INTRAVENOUS FAT EMULSION

   __✓__ 10% (1.1 calories/ml) __50__ ml/hr over __10__ hours (minimum 4 - 6 hours)
   _____ 20% (2.0 calories/ml) _____ ml/hr over _____ hours (minimum 8 - 10 hours)

6. Non-BMT and Non-ICU Patients: Begin fat infusion after TPN (Hyperal) Screen is drawn and before 0600.

7. Infuse initial dose slowly. 10%: begin at 60ml/hr × 30 min.; 20%: begin at 30ml/hr × 30 min.
   (Note: some patients may react adversely to subsequent exposures.)

The following orders are standard for all non-bone marrow transplant patients. Delete only if crossed out by physician.

PRE-TPN ORDERS

8. Central venous catheter placement verification: (circle one)
   ⓐ. CXR asap for placement needed
   b. Catheter tip location: _____ ; may begin TPN infusion.

9. Baseline Lab: ZINC, COPPER, TRIGLYCERIDES, TPN (Hyperal) SCREEN I (CBC w/diff, Protime, Ca, P04, Mg, GOT, Bilirubin, Lytes, BUN, Glucose, Albumin, Prealbumin)

TPN INITIATION AND MAINTENANCE ORDERS

⑩ Initiate TPN Nursing Protocol.

⑪ Nutritional Assessment – notify Unit Dietitian.

12. TPN LAB:
   Lab Draw Times: ICU Patients – draw TPN labs in AM; Non-ICU Patients – draw TPN labs in the evenings before 1900

   ✓ Daily × 1st 3 Days: lytes & glucose (already included in Monday & Thursday labs)

   ✓ Mondays: TRIGLYCERIDES, if IV fat administered.
                  TPN (Hyperal) SCREEN I (includes CBC w/diff, Protime, Ca, PO4, Mg, GOT, Bilirubin, Lytes, BUN, Glucose, Albumin, Prealbumin)

   ✓ Thursdays: TPN (Hyperal) SCREEN II (includes CBC, Lytes, Glucose, Ca, PO4, Mg)

   ✓ Chemstick: Q 8 hrs × 1st 48 hours.   Thereafter, urine fxs Q 8 hrs on fresh specimen – Chemstick for trace or greater.
   Chemstick Results: Chemstick > 240 notify MD if no sliding scale ordered
                       Chemstick > 400 notify MD & obtain stat glucose
                       Chemstick for S/S hypoglycemia: < 60 notify MD & obtain stat glucose

⑬ Daily Weight; Strict I&O

Date ___7/15/99___ MD Signature ___A. Bryant, M.D._____

SWEDISH HOSPITAL MEDICAL CENTER
Seattle, Washington

PH-390 Rev. 4/90 FC/SHMC SN-5650

Figure 57–1. The order form that is filled out by the physician.

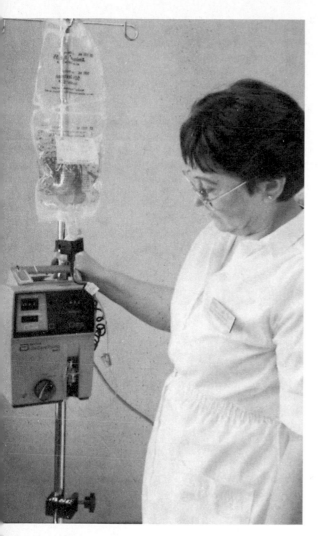

igure 57–2. The parenteral nutrition components are kept sep-
rated until just before infusing.

*the monitoring process. Other patients find it stress-
ful to become involved and choose not to participate
actively.*

h. Mental status. *The ability to understand the procedure and participate and help in its implementation may be affected* if the patient's level of
awareness is decreased or if mental status is
impaired.

, Assess the patient's unit to determine which
items of equipment are already in the room and
what needs to be obtained.

lanning

, Wash your hands *for infection control.*

, Check the physician's order, including the solution to be given and the length of infusion time
(which may be written as a part of the order or
found in the agency policy).

Remove the parenteral nutrition solution from

the refrigerator *so that it can warm to room temperature.*

6. Gather the equipment: infusion pump, filtered
tubing, an alcohol swab, tape for connections,
and clean gloves. Use an infusion pump that is
volume controlled. (See Module 52, Preparing
and Maintaining Intravenous Infusions regarding volume-controlled infusion pumps.) Parenteral nutrition is always infused by pump *to ensure that an exact amount of solution is given for a
prescribed time.* Use filtered tubing. *The filter on the
tubing prevents any particulates from entering the system.* Check the policy of your institution, and
note the time and date on either a tubing sticker
or in a space provided on the IV record *so that the
tubing will be changed if the time of infusion exceeds 24
hours.* New tubing is used with each bag of solution or changed after 24 hours *to decrease the possibility of infection.* Tubing changes are more frequent when giving parenteral nutrition than
when giving regular IV solutions *because the high
glucose content and protein component can promote
bacterial growth.*

Implementation

7. Check the bag for the date of expiration, cloudiness, or other particulate material. Compare the
written contents of the solution on the bag
against the order card *for accuracy.* Note that
multivitamins are added to one bottle or bag
every 24 hours. The solution with the multivitamins can be identified by its yellow color. Figure 57–3 is an example of an order card.

8. Depending on the type of solution bottle or bag
being used, pull off the rubber or plastic cover,
and insert the spike of the tubing into the port.

9. Flush the tubing with solution, following the directions for the specific infusion pump being
used.

10. Maintain asepsis at all times, covering the distal
end of the tubing with the sterile cap before carrying it with the pump to the bedside.

11. Hang the bag on the hook of the infusion pump
stand.

12. Identify the patient *to be sure you are carrying out
the procedure for the correct patient.*

13. Explain the procedure and rationale to the patient and family members if they are present.
Answer any questions.

14. Inspect the central or peripheral line site for
signs of inflammation or infection.

15. Administer the parenteral nutrition.
    a. *For total parenteral nutrition*: Because the tub-
ing will go directly into the central line
catheter, put on clean gloves *to protect yourself*

```
┌─────────────────────────────────────────────┐
│                 HA ORDERS                     │
│                    DATE: ___3-17-99___        │
│  Dextrose __25__ %   Amino Acids __5__ %     │
│  Rate ___1___ L/Day  _____ cc/hr            │
│  Volume _____                         │
│  ─────────────────────────────────────────    │
│  NaCl _____ mEq/ _30_  Date ord. _____  │
│  Na Acetate _____ mEq/ ____ Date ord. _____ │
│  K Cl _____ mEq/ _25_  Date ord. _____  │
│  K Phos _____ mEq/ _15_  Date ord. _____  │
│  K Acetate _____ mEq/ ____  Date ord. _____ │
│  Ca Gluc _____ mEq/ ____  Date ord. _____ │
│  Mg SO₄ _____ mEq/ _8_   Date ord. _____  │
│  _____  Date ord. _____ │
│  _____  Date ord. _____ │
│  Reg. Insulin _0_ u/ _____  Date ord. _____ │
│  MVI _____10___ ml/Day                    │
│  Trace Minerals _1_ ml/Day                    │
│  Vit. K _____10___ mg/wk   (Sun.)            │
│  Vit. C __500_____ mg/Day                    │
│  ─────────────────────────────────────────    │
│  Lipids __20__ % __500__ cc/Day               │
│  Rate: _50_ cc/hr                             │
│  ─────────────────────────────────────────    │
│  Maintenance IV rate: _____ cc/hr        │
│  Maximum IV rate: _____ cc/hr        │
└─────────────────────────────────────────────┘
```

Figure 57–3. A medication form used by the nurse to check the contents of the parenteral nutrition bag.

from contact with blood. Clamp the central line, remove the IV lock cap, and firmly attach the parenteral solution tubing. Infusing the solution directly into the catheter and not through a needle *decreases chances for infection.* Some central lines have more than one port, so verify which one is being used for parenteral nutrition.

  b. *For partial parenteral nutrition*: Put on clean gloves. Discontinue other IV fluids, or remove the IV lock device if the port is not being used. Insert the sterile parenteral nutrition tubing directly into the needle hub.

16. Place a pull-tape on the connection *for safety* (see Module 24, Applying and Maintaining Traction).

17. For the first hour of infusing every bottle or bag, give the solution at a rate not greater than 50 to 85 mL/h *to prevent fluctuations in blood glucose.* Then adjust the rate to the ordered infusion time.

  People receiving parenteral nutrition also may be "cycled." This means that for the first few days, the solution may be given over a 24-hour period, and the time is then gradually decreased to 12 hours. In this manner, the rate of administration is gradually increased until the patient is receiving the optimum calories and nutrients for each 24-hour period. This is called "cycling up." Giving the solution over fewer hours also provides for greater mobility and less restriction for the patient.

  When the parenteral nutrition is to be discontinued, a similar procedure is used in reverse. The length of time that the solution is infused is increased so that the person is getting less solution. This is called "cycling down."

  Cycling *allows the body to adjust to the rate of flow of the solutions.* Figure 57–4 is an example of a cycling form. Check the specific policy of your facility and the physician's orders.

18. Within 4 hours after beginning parenteral nutrition, check the patient's vital signs and blood glucose levels.

Evaluation

19. Evaluate using the following criteria:
  a. Equipment is functioning correctly.
  b. Patient's vital signs remain stable.
  c. No evidence of either hypoglycemia or hyperglycemia is found when testing blood.
  d. No untoward reactions, such as nausea, vomiting, or diarrhea, are present.
  e. Patient maintains desired weight over the time parenteral nutrition is administered.

Documentation

20. These fluids are usually documented as you would IV solutions. Any untoward reactions are recorded on the nursing progress notes.

PROCEDURE FOR ADMINISTERING FAT EMULSIONS (LIPIDS)

To administer fat emulsions, follow the steps of the General Procedure for Administering Parenteral Nutrition as modified below. The modified steps have been included completely, and the steps of the General Procedure that remain the same are referenced.

Assessment

1.–2. Follow the steps of the General Procedure for Administering Parenteral Nutrition.

Planning

3.–7. Follow the steps of the General Procedure.

Implementation

8. Check the order against the label on the lipid glass bottle.

9. Select macrodrip, unfiltered, vented IV, or pump tubing if a pump is used. Remove the metal band covering around the top of the bottle without

DATE	TIME	PHYSICIAN'S ORDERS	NOTED BY

TPN CYCLING ORDERS FOR NON-BMT PATIENTS

12/26/99 1000

1. CYCLE SCHEDULE

   (Final goal: **2** liters at night over **12** hours)

	DATE	START TIME	BAG #	LITERS	RATE	HOURS
DAY 1	12/26	1900	5	1	110	10
DAY 2	12/27	0500	6	1	110	10
DAY 3	12/27	1900	7	1.5	135	16
DAY 4	12/28	1900	8	1.5	155	14
DAY 5	12/29	1900	9	1.5	185	12

2. TAPERING:

   Start infusion at 50 ml/hour for ½ hour.

   End infusion at 50 ml/hour for ½ hour.

3. Infuse ___**500**___ ml intravenous Fat Emulsion (10%)/20%

   every ___**day**___ . Infuse over ___**4-6**___ hours.

   Begin when TPN started.

4. Heparin Lock catheter when TPN completed.

5. DC all sliding scale insulin coverage.

   DC previous chemstick orders.

   DC urine fractionals.

6. Obtain chemsticks each day of Cycle Schedule:

   a. 2 Hours after TPN initiated

   b. ½ hour after TPN completed

   c. Notify Dr. ___**Norman**___ if chemstick results are

   >240 or <60.

7. DC chemsticks when Cycle Schedule is completed if chemstick results are

   within normal limits.

   DATE ___**12/26**___ RPh/RN SIGNATURE ___*Nancy Alkins, R.N.*___

   PHYSICIAN SIGNATURE ___*N. Norman*___

A DRUG EQUIVALENT MAY BE DISPENSED UNLESS CHECKED ☐

SIGNATURE IS REQUIRED FOLLOWING ENTRY OF EACH ORDER

SWEDISH HOSPITAL MEDICAL CENTER
Seattle, WA

PH-122 Rev. 6/90 FC/SHMC

Figure 57–4. A "cycling" form used by the physician to prescribe the rate of flow.

touching the sterile black cap beneath. Insert the spike of the tubing into the port of the bottle.

10. Flush the tubing as you would when administering IV fluids. Replace the sterile cover over the end of the tubing *to maintain sterility*.

11. Gather an alcohol swab and a sterile needle, size 20 or 21.

12. Carry the lipids with tubing attached to the bedside.

13. Hang lipids bottle on same stand that holds the glucose–protein fluid container.

14. Put the needle on the tubing. Needleless systems are now available.

15. Choose a port *below* the infusion pump and the filter, clean with an alcohol swab, and insert the needle. The lipid solution is run below the filter *so that its viscosity will not obstruct the flow by being trapped in the filter*.

16. Secure with tape if a needle-lock device is not used.

17. Using the roller clamp, manually time the lipids that will infuse with the parenteral nutrition solution.

18. If this is the first time a patient has received lipids, give a test dose. This means starting the lipids at a very slow rate. The following examples are for equipment that delivers 15 gtt/mL:
    a. 10% solution at 1 mL/min for 15 minutes and then the remainder over 4 hours (8 drops over 15 seconds)
    b. 20% solution at 0.5 mL/min for 15 minutes and then the remainder over 8 to 10 hours (3–4 drops over 15 seconds).

Evaluation

19. Evaluate using the following criteria:
    a. Equipment is functioning correctly.
    b. No untoward reactions, such as changes in vital signs, dyspnea, dizziness, chest and eye pain, nausea and vomiting, or a metallic taste in the mouth, occur.
    c. Patient maintains desired weight.

Documentation

20. Document lipids as you would IV solutions. Record any untoward reactions on the nursing progress notes.

DISCONTINUING PARENTERAL NUTRITION

The fat emulsions may be completely infused before the parenteral nutrition solution is infused. If this occurs, discontinue the lipids as you would other "add on" or piggyback solutions. When the par-

enteral nutrition solution is completely infused, again discontinue the therapy as you would do with other IV fluids. Reinstate previous fluids using a new, sterile needle if the fluids have not expired. If no other IV fluids are ordered, replace the IV lock (see Module 52, Preparing and Maintaining Intravenous Infusions).

LONG-TERM CARE

Many long-term care facilities accept residents who are receiving parenteral nutrition. In some, the solutions are prepared and delivered by a commercial medical supply company. In others with a complete pharmacy department, the solutions may be prepared within the facility. Regardless of where the solutions are prepared, the general procedure for assessing the patient and administering and monitoring parenteral nutrition must be conscientiously followed *to ensure safety*. Your responsibility as part of the nursing staff is to be knowledgeable and competent in administering parenteral nutrition to residents.

HOME CARE

A patient may need parenteral nutrition for an extended time after discharge. The nurse teaches the procedure to the patient and caregiver(s) and gives demonstrations along with written directions. The caregiver provides the nutritional support to the patient within the hospital environment before the patient goes home. It is important that the patient and the caregiver feel comfortable and confident before the procedure is performed in the home.

The general procedure is the same as that used in the hospital or long-term care facility. In urban areas, the solutions and equipment are available from a number of commercial companies. These companies usually make deliveries to the home at least twice weekly. They also are a resource to the family *if any difficulties arise after the nurse or nutritionist makes an initial home visit*. In nonurban areas, the family may have to make special arrangements regarding where and how to obtain the solution and equipment for the procedure.

The solutions are prepared as ordered by the physician, and the caregiver is taught to add vitamins or insulin, if needed, at specific designated times.

CRITICAL THINKING EXERCISES

Evaluate each of the following situations, then describe how you would respond.

• The parenteral solution bag you are to hang has a label that says multivitamins have been added, but the solution is clear.

• The patient's central line site is slightly reddened, but the solution flow is not obstructed.

• The alarm on the pump rings several times.

• The lipid bottle arrives on the unit without pump tubing.

• After receiving the first container of parenteral nutrition, the patient has a blood glucose level of 205 mg/dL.

General Procedure for Administering Parenteral Nutrition	Needs More Practice	Satisfactory	Comments
Assessment			
1. Gather the following patient assessment information: a. Diagnosis			
b. Age and physical condition			
c. Height and usual weight			
d. Intake and output			
e. Allergies			
f. Usual vital signs			
g. Knowledge of procedure			
h. Mental status			
2. Assess the patient's unit regarding equipment needed.			
Planning			
3. Wash your hands.			
4. Check order, including solution and time for infusion.			
5. Take solution out of refrigerator to warm.			
6. Gather equipment: infusion pump, filtered pump tubing, alcohol swab, tape, and clean gloves.			
Implementation			
7. Check bag for imperfections and content orders.			
8. Pull off rubber or plastic cover, and spike bag with tubing.			
9. Flush tubing with solution.			
10. Cover distal end of tubing with sterile cap, and carry to bedside.			
11. Hang bag on stand holding pump.			
12. Identify the patient.			
13. Explain procedure and rationale to patient.			

(*continued*)

General Procedure for Administering Parenteral Nutrition *(Continued)*	Needs More Practice	Satisfactory	Comments
14. Inspect central line for signs of inflammation or infection.			
15. Administer the parenteral nutrition. **a.** *Total parenteral nutrition:* Put on clean gloves, clamp central line, remove IV lock cap, and directly attach parenteral tubing.			
b. *Partial parenteral nutrition:* Put on clean gloves, discontinue other intravenous fluids, and directly attach parenteral tubing.			
16. Place a pull-tape on connection.			
17. Infuse at 50–85 mL/h for the first hour. Follow any specific orders for "cycling."			
18. Assess blood glucose level within 4 hours (not necessary with lipid infusion).			
Evaluation			
19. Evaluate: **a.** Equipment functioning correctly.			
b. Patient's vital signs stable; no evidence of rise in temperature.			
c. No evidence of hypoglycemia or hyperglycemia.			
d. No other untoward reactions.			
e. Desired weight maintained.			
Documentation			
20. Document according to the policy of your facility.			
Procedure for Administering Fat Emulsions (Lipids)			
Assessment			
1.–2. Assess as in steps 1 and 2 of the Performance Checklist: General Procedure for Administering Parenteral Nutrition: Gather baseline information; assess unit for equipment.			

(continue

Procedure for Administering Fat Emulsions (Lipids) *(Continued)*	Needs More Practice	Satisfactory	Comments
Planning			
3.–7. Plan as in steps 3 through 7 of the General Procedure: Wash hands, check order, warm solution, gather equipment, and explain procedure to patient.			
Implementation			
8. Check the order against label on bottle.			
9. Select tubing; remove metal cover without touching sterile, black rubber cap beneath; insert tubing spike into port of bottle.			
10. Flush tubing as you would for intravenous fluids.			
11. Gather an alcohol swab and 20- or 21-gauge needle.			
12. Carry lipids and tubing to bedside.			
13. Hang lipid bottle on stand.			
14. Put needle on end of tubing.			
15. Insert needle into a port on hyperalimentation tubing, which is below infusion pump and filter.			
16. Secure with tape.			
17. Time lipids as ordered.			
18. If test dose, give as follows: **a.** 10% at 1 mL/min for 15 minutes, then over 4 hours (8 gtt/15 sec).			
b. 20% at 0.5 mL/min for 15 minutes, then over 8–10 hours (3–4 gtt/15 sec).			
Evaluation			
19. Evaluate: **a.** Equipment functioning correctly.			
b. No untoward reactions.			
c. Desired weight maintained.			
Documentation			
20. Document according to the policy of your facility.			

❓ Q U I Z

Short-Answer Questions

1. The nutrients supplied by total parenteral nutrition are _____
   _____

2. Total parenteral nutrition is appropriate for which type of patients? _____

3. Partial parenteral nutrition is appropriate for which type of patients? _____

4. An infusion pump is always used to infuse the parenteral nutrition solution because
   _____

5. The solution is given directly into the central line catheter and not through a needle to decrease
   the risk of _____

6. Peripheral parenteral nutrition is usually only given for a limited time of time because
   _____

7. A common complication of parenteral nutrition is _____

8. This complication can be detected early by performing _____
   _____

9. Lipids may be given along with parenteral nutrition to supply the patient with
   _____

10. Lipids are available in which two concentrations? _____

11. How are the test doses for giving 10% lipid solutions administered?

   a. _____

   b. _____

996 by Lippincott-Raven Publishers

MODULE
58

GIVING EPIDURAL MEDICATIONS

MODULE CONTENTS

PREREQUISITES

Successful completion of the following modules:

VOLUME 1

VOLUME 2

Review of the anatomy of the spinal cord and spinal canal.

996 by Lippincott-Raven Publishers

OVERALL OBJECTIVE

To administer analgesics through an epidural catheter, while maintaining safety for the patient.

SPECIFIC LEARNING OBJECTIVES

Know Facts and Principles	Apply Facts and Principles	Demonstrate Ability	Evaluate Performance
1. Purposes State reasons for epidural catheter is used for narcotic administration.	Given an example of a patient with an epidural catheter, identify its purpose.	In the clinical setting, identify the reason a specific patient has an epidural catheter.	Evaluate with your instructor.
2. Safety concerns State four safety concerns related to the administration of epidural narcotics.	Given an example of a patient, identify safety concerns.	In the clinical setting, plan specific actions to maintain patient safety.	Evaluate with your instructor.
3. Exit site care State usual procedure for exit site care.		In the practice setting, change an exit site dressing.	Evaluate with your instructor.
4. Administering narcotics through the epidural catheter			
List supplies needed to administer narcotics through an epidural catheter by direct injection.	Explain rationale for supplies needed.	In the practice setting, administer a narcotic through an epidural catheter by direct injection.	Evaluate with your instructor.
List supplies needed to administer narcotics through an epidural catheter by continuous infusion.	Explain rationale for supplies needed.	In the practice setting, administer a narcotic through an epidural catheter by continuous infusion.	Evaluate with your instructor.
5. Complications List the complications or adverse effects that might occur related to epidural analgesia.	Given a situation with untoward effects occurring related to epidural analgesia, identify the possible complications that might be present.	In the clinical setting, perform a comprehensive assessment of a patient receiving epidural analgesia that would reveal complications present.	Evaluate with your instructor.
6. Documentation Identify data that should be documented for the person receiving epidural analgesia.	Given a patient receiving epidural analgesia, correctly document data on appropriate forms.	In the clinical setting, document information relative to the patient receiving epidural analgesia.	Evaluate with your instructor.

LEARNING ACTIVITIES

1. Review the Specific Learning Objectives.
2. Look up the module vocabulary terms in the glossary.
3. Read through the module as though you were preparing to teach these skills to another person. Mentally practice the skills.
4. Review the policies and procedures in your facility related to caring for epidural catheters.
5. Arrange for time to practice using an epidural catheter.
6. In the practice setting, do the following:
   a. Practice the procedures outlined in the Performance Checklist.
   b. When you are ready to demonstrate these procedures, select a partner, and critique one another's performance using the Performance Checklist.
   c. Arrange for your instructor to evaluate your performance.
7. In the clinical setting, do the following:
   a. Identify patients with epidural catheters in place.
   b. Arrange for an opportunity to observe care for these patients.
   c. Ask your instructor for an opportunity to carry out the specific care needed by the patient.

VOCABULARY

analgesic
anesthetic
dura

epidural
neurotoxic
paraparesis

particulate
subdural

1996 by Lippincott-Raven Publishers

Giving Epidural Medications

Rationale for the Use of This Skill

The technology associated with providing pain relief is constantly expanding. One aspect of this technology is the administration of analgesic narcotics through an epidural catheter. To provide effective care and optimum pain relief, nurses caring for patients with epidural catheters must understand the location of the catheter, how the system works, and the specific actions of the medications instilled.[1]

▼ NURSING DIAGNOSES

Because the epidural administration of a narcotic carries hazards for patients, a narcotic antagonist, such as naloxone, should be immediately available when epidural narcotics are administered. Usually, the narcotic antagonist is kept in the patient's room with equipment for administration, but in some units it is in a central location. The physician identifies the criteria for administering the narcotic antagonist and orders the dosage.

Although one of the advantages of epidural narcotic administration is less frequent respiratory depression than with other methods of narcotic administration, Ineffective Breathing Pattern related to respiratory depression still can occur. It is more likely to occur if the patient is lying flat while an infusion is given because the medication ascends along the dura. It also may occur if there is a large absorption into the vascular system from the epidural site. When the first dose is given, pay particular attention to respiratory assessment and preparation for immediate intervention. A crash cart with a self-inflating rebreathing (Ambu) bag should be available for emergency treatment. The physician may order a narcotic antagonist for a respiratory rate of less than 8 per minute.

Other nursing diagnoses include the following:

Urinary Retention related to *disturbed innervation of the bladder caused by the narcotic's effect on spinal receptors*. Measure urinary intake and output, and palpate the bladder for distention. Catheterization may be needed.

Risk for Injury related to administering intravenous medications or solutions into an epidural catheter. *Because the epidural catheter looks exactly like an intravenous catheter*, a special safety concern is clearly identifying these two lines and not confusing them. *Medications intended for intravenous use may be neurotoxic, and the dosage of narcotic given epidurally may be life-threatening when given by direct intravenous push.* In some facilities, a brightly colored label specifying "epidural catheter" is placed on the epidural line next to the injection port. In other facilities, the policy is that two nurses verify the epidural line immediately before giving any medication. Both of these safeguards may be used. We recommend that a large, very legible label be placed on the line next to any port (if there are several ports on the line, use a label for each port). Also, as a student, you should always have a registered nurse identify the line with you. In all cases, follow the hospital policy.

Pain (in the head) related to leakage of cerebrospinal fluid from the site around the catheter. Additionally, there is Risk for Infection if cerebrospinal fluid leaks around the catheter. *This creates a pathway for microorganisms to travel into the wound and cause an infection.* The cap on the tubing is changed at regular intervals, depending on the frequency of use, *to prevent leakage from repeated puncture.* Check your facility's policy. There is no danger if air enters the catheter, as there is with an intravenous line, because the air cannot move into the circulatory system.

Impaired Skin Integrity related to a skin rash. Pruritus *that is sometimes accompanied by a rash is a fairly common adverse response to epidural narcotics.* For some individuals, it is only mildly annoying and may be alleviated by lotion on the skin. For others, it is extremely uncomfortable, necessitating administration of a narcotic antagonist. *As the narcotic antagonist relieves the pruritus, it also diminishes the pain relief.* Therefore, the narcotic antagonist may be given in small increments *to attempt relief of the pruritus without loss of pain control.* If that is unsuccessful, another drug or method of pain management is necessary.

Potential complications include the following:

Reversible paraparesis (weakness of the lower extremities). This may occur *if a medication*

---

[1]Note that rationale for action is emphasized throughout the module by the use of italics.

with a preservative or one not intended for epidural use is injected into the catheter, causing an adverse response by nervous system tissue. Fortunately, this complication is usually reversible if the medication causing the problem is discontinued and the tissue is given an opportunity to recover.

Hypotension. This may occur *because of the narcotic's action on receptor sites that control vascular responses*. Special attention to safety is necessary *because hypotension may cause dizziness*. A narcotic antagonist is ordered only if the blood pressure drop is precipitous.

Neural irritation related to particulate matter. This is identified by abnormal sensations in the lower extremities that may include tingling and numbness. A 0.22-µm filter is placed on the epidural catheter *to ensure that no particulate matter, which might cause local irritation, is injected into the catheter.*

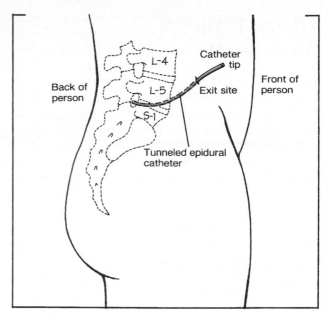

Figure 58–1. Tunneled epidural catheter for long-term use.

WHAT IS AN EPIDURAL CATHETER?

Epidural catheters are silicone rubber catheters that look like Hickman central intravenous catheters (see Module 54, Caring For Central Intravenous Catheters) and are used to administer a medication into the epidural or subarachnoid space. The catheter usually is placed in surgery by a physician (most commonly an anesthesiologist).

When the epidural catheter is used for long-term control of chronic pain, such as cancer pain, it is sutured in place and tunneled through the subcutaneous tissue to an exit site on the abdomen (Fig. 58–1).

When the catheter is intended for short-term use (such as postoperatively), it may not be sutured in place. The temporary catheter exits on the back, under the insertion site dressing. *To protect the catheter,* an extension tubing is commonly attached and secured with wide adhesive tape along the spine to the shoulder where the port at the end of the catheter is accessible.

The catheter is the same type used to administer regional anesthetic for childbirth and some types of surgery. In some instances of chronic terminal pain, a low-dose anesthetic agent (such as bupivacaine [Marcaine]) is infused continuously into an epidural catheter *to provide pain relief.* When regional anesthetic agents are used in an epidural catheter, most states require that they be administered by an anes-

thesiologist or nurse anesthetist *because of the risk of serious complications.*

This module discusses the administration of narcotic analgesics by direct injection or infusion into an epidural catheter. Although potential problems are associated with the use of narcotics in this manner, they are not as serious as those from the use of anesthetic agents. Therefore, narcotics are commonly administered by registered nurses using the epidural route. Some facilities require that nurses attend special inservice education classes and be certified in the use of epidural catheters before assuming this responsibility.

Many facilities have a special form on which the physician's orders for epidural medications and care are written. Use of these forms ensures that complete orders are clearly written. Such forms usually include medication, dose, and method of administration. Scheduled assessment may be included in the orders. Additionally, the form includes specific orders for treatment of the various complications outlined previously. In other facilities, the orders are less detailed, and there are standardized protocols in place for assessment and management of epidural catheters.

ADVANTAGES OF EPIDURAL NARCOTIC ADMINISTRATION

The major advantage of epidural administration of narcotics is that a lower total dose per day is needed to maintain adequate pain relief. Additionally, *much of this dose attaches to receptors in the spinal cord before reaching the central nervous system. This action allows the person to be more alert, more mobile, and have fewer central nervous system effects while remaining pain free.* Narcotics given epidurally also have a more prolonged effect than those administered through other routes *because they must first be absorbed and then transported to the liver for breakdown.* Respiratory depression is less common with epidural administration than with intravenous administration, as are other side effects of narcotics, such as nausea, constipation, and dizziness. Epidural medications can be given by intermittent or continuous infusion.

EPIDURAL CATHETER EXIT SITE CARE

The temporary epidural catheter is covered with a surgical dressing after insertion, and this dressing is not usually changed. If a dressing change is necessary, follow the directions for sterile dressing change. The care of the exit site for the permanent epidural catheter is usually identical to the care of the exit site of a surgically implanted central intravenous catheter. The catheter has been tunneled under the skin *to provide a barrier to infection ascending along the exterior of the catheter.* Be sure to follow the procedure outlined for your facility, or follow the general procedure for Hickman site care outlined in Module 54, Caring for Central Intravenous Catheters.

PROCEDURE FOR ADMINISTERING A MEDICATION THROUGH AN EPIDURAL CATHETER

Epidural narcotics may be injected intermittently into the epidural catheter. The medication gradually diffuses across the dura to contact opiate receptors in the spinal cord. *Because of this gradual diffusion, the injections may be made every 8 to 12 hours.* The amount used is often small, but *because it is concentrated where the receptors are located, pain relief is maintained.*

The following procedure is for the intermittent injection of narcotics into the epidural catheter. To carry out this procedure, follow the steps of the General Procedure for Administering Medications (Module 47, pages 365–366) as modified below. The modified steps are included completely, and references are made to the steps of the General Procedure that remain the same.

Assessment

1. Review the medication administration record (MAR) or the physician's order sheet *to identify the order for the epidural medication.*
2.–3. Follow steps 2 and 3 of the General Procedure for Administering Medications: Examine the MAR for accuracy and completeness, and review information about the drug to be administered, keeping in mind that preservative-free narcotics are used.
4. Check for the type of epidural catheter in place (temporary or permanent).
5. Assess the patient for baseline information:
   a. Pain level using a standard scale (ie, 1–5 or 1–10)
   b. Respiratory rate
   c. Blood pressure and pulse
   d. Ability to move lower extremities
   e. Sedation level

Planning

6.–7. Follow steps 6 and 7 of the General Procedure Determine the what equipment you will need, and wash your hands *for infection control*
8. Gather the appropriate equipment:
   a. Povidone-iodine swabs to clean the tops of the vials and to swab the injection port. *Alcohol causes pain and is toxic to nervous tissue; therefore it is not used when preparing medications for epidural administration or on the injection port of an epidural catheter.*
   b. A 10- or 12-mL syringe with a 20-gauge, 1-in needle *to administer the diluted preservative-free narcotic.* In addition, you will need a small syringe *if the narcotic comes in an undiluted form and must be drawn up and measured before dilution.*
   c. Sterile 2 × 2 gauze squares

Implementation

9. Follow step 9 of the General Procedure: Read the name of the medication on the MAR.
10. Check the label on the available medication before picking it up *for your first check.*

   Use a prediluted preservative-free narcotic solution (such as Duramorph) or a preservative-free narcotic (such as morphine, fentanyl, or hydromorphone labeled as preservative free) and preservative-free sodium chloride for diluting the narcotic.

   A large volume of fluid permits the narcotic to contact the optimum number of receptors. Preservatives used in standard multiple-dose vials may be toxic to nervous tissue. Some facilities do allow narcotics with preservatives to be used in **long-term** epidural catheters as long as they are diluted with preservative-free saline. Be sure you follow the policy in your facility.

11. Recheck the medication record, and compare it with the label on the medication after you have removed it from the drawer or shelf *for the second check*; record it on the narcotic record.
12. Prepare the medication using sterile technique according to your facility's procedure.
    a. If a prediluted narcotic is used, draw it up into the large syringe.
    b. If an undiluted narcotic is used, do the following:
       (1) Draw it up into the small syringe.
       (2) Draw up 10 mL of preservative-free saline into the large syringe, and pull back to allow enough space for the narcotic.
       (3) Cap the needle (the needle is sterile, so it is acceptable to recap it), and remove the needle from the large syringe. Hold the needle carefully while you insert the needle from the small syringe into the tip of the large syringe. Inject the narcotic into the saline in the large syringe.
       (4) Replace the needle on the large syringe or attach a needleless connector if a needleless system is in use at your facility.
       (5) Gently rotate the syringe to mix the narcotic and saline.
13. Recheck the medication record, the label on the medication container, and your syringe *for the third check*.
14.–16. Follow steps 14 through 16 of the General Procedure: Place the medication on the cart or tray; place a medication card or label with the prepared medication; and approach and identify the patient.
17. Explain the procedure to the patient, emphasizing what the patient will experience. The injection should not be painful. In some situations, you will be teaching the patient and caregivers to administer these medications at home.
18. Give the medication in the appropriate manner.
    a. Identify the epidural catheter with another nurse.
    b. Clean the injection cap on the epidural catheter with a povidone-iodine swab.
    c. Dry the injection cap with the sterile 2 × 2 gauze. *Povidone-iodine may form a sticky residue if left on the cap.*
    d. Insert the needle or needleless connector into the cap.
    e. Aspirate. *If blood is returned, the catheter may have eroded into a blood vessel. Do not give the medication; remove the syringe, and report to the physician. If more than 1 mL of clear fluid is aspi-*

rated, *the catheter may have eroded into the subarachnoid space. Do not give the medication; remove the syringe, and report to the physician.*
    f. Inject the medication. *You are injecting it into the epidural space, where it will be used gradually. It is not like an intravenous medication, which goes immediately into the circulation.* If the patient indicates discomfort, slow the injection. It may be hard to instill medication *because the catheter is small and long.* If you are unable to inject the medication, check the tubing for kinks. If you are still unable to inject, withdraw the syringe, and report to the physician.
    g. Remove the needle and syringe from the catheter. Check that the cap is secured in place *to prevent it from inadvertently coming off.* In some facilities, the cap is taped in place for extra security.
19. Follow step 19 of the General Procedure: Leave the patient in a comfortable position.
20. Dispose of the syringe and needle in the appropriate "sharps" container.
21. Follow step 20 of the General Procedure: Wash your hands *for infection control.*

Evaluation
22. Evaluate the patient's response:
    a. Level of pain relief. Use the same pain measurement scale used before giving the medication.
    b. The presence of any adverse effects (Table 58–1):
       (1) Respiratory depression
       (2) Sedation
       (3) Lightheadedness or confusion
       (4) Pain
       (5) Pruritus
       (6) Muscle weakness or lack of control
       (7) Abnormal sensation in lower extremities
       (8) Hypotension
       (9) Urinary retention

Documentation
23. Document both the medication administered and the assessment information.
    a. Include name of medication, dose, time, route, and your signature.
    b. Record assessment data at regularly scheduled intervals, such as every hour initially then gradually moving to every 2 hours and every 4 hours as pain relief and patient's response are stabilized. Include the following: pain level assessed on a consistent scale; respiratory rate, pulse, and blood pressure; as-

Table 58–1. Sample Assessment Protocol: Patients With New Epidural Catheters

Objective Data	Scale		Frequency
Pulse	Note any drop		Every 30 min × 2
Respiration	R < 10—Obtain O_2 saturation/pulse oximetry		Every 1 h × 2
Blood pressure	Notify physician R < 8—Give naloxone 0.4 mg IV stat Obtain O_2 saturation/pulse oximetry Notify physician		Every 4 h × 24, then every 8 h

Sedation	3 = Awake and responding
	2 = Sleeping but responds to normal voice
	1 = Sleeping but responds to loud voice/movement
	0 = Sedated, does not respond
	Level 1—Obtain O_2 saturation/pulse oximetry
	  Call physician
	Level 0—Give naloxone 0.4 mg IV stat
	  Obtain O_2 saturation/pulse oximetry
	  Call physician stat
	  Obtain ABGs stat		

Mental state	Light headed Confused		
Pain	5 = Severe 4 = 3 = Moderate 2 = 1 = Mild 0 = None		
Pruritus	Present Absent		
Muscle strength and Control	Note extremities checked Weak versus normal strength		

Skin sensation	*Sensation Scale*
	  N = Normal
	  T = Tingling
	  Nb = Numbness
	  A = Absent
		Anatomic Location
		  S1-5; Ankle/foot
		  L1-5; Groin/pelvis/thigh
		  T1-12–T-10; Umbilicus
		  T-4; Nipple level
		  C1-5; Hand	

Postural blood pressure	Note excessive postural drop		Every 8 hours beginning before first ambulation and continue until stable.
Urinary output	Compare with intake		Every 8 hours

sessment for potential adverse responses, such as pruritus and hypotension.

A special flow sheet may be used *to facilitate the documentation of pain management and assessment done to identify adverse effects.* See Module 53, Administering Intravenous Medications, Figure 53-3, for an example of such a flow sheet.

PROCEDURE FOR SETTING UP A CONTINUOUS EPIDURAL INFUSION

For patients with long-term pain, such as those with major trauma, a complicated recovery, or cancer, continuous infusion of an epidural narcotic may be used *for pain management.* The continuous infusion is set up using an intravenous pump that is volume controlled *to provide the precise control of the dosage that is needed.* Review Module 53, Administering Intravenous Medications, for information on setting up intravenous pumps. Follow the Procedure for Administering a Medication Through an Epidural Catheter (above) with the modifications described below.

Assessment

1. Review the MAR or the physician's order sheet *to identify the order for the epidural medication.*
2.–3. Follow steps 2 and 3 of the General Procedure for Administering Medications: Examine the MAR for accuracy and completeness, and review information about the drug to be administered, keeping in mind that preservative-free narcotics are used.
4. Check for the type of epidural catheter in place (temporary or permanent).
5. Assess the patient for baseline information:
   a. Pain level using a standard scale (ie, 1–5 or 1–10)
   b. Respiratory rate
   c. Blood pressure and pulse
   d. Ability to move lower extremities
   e. Sedation level

Planning

6.–7. Follow steps 6 and 7 of the General Procedure: Determine the equipment you will need, and wash your hands *for infection control.*
8. Gather and prepare the appropriate equipment:
   a. Volume-controlled intravenous pump. After obtaining the pump, determine how you will set the pump to deliver the correct rate of infusion. You will usually need to calculate a rate in milliliters of solution per hour that will deliver the ordered milligrams of drug per

hour. Some pharmacies print this information on the label, but others do not because it is confusing if the dosage is changed while the same bag is in use. In some facilities, policy requires that two nurses verify the dosage calculation on an epidural medication. As a student, you should always have your instructor or another registered nurse double-check your dosage calculation *for safety.*

A patient-controlled analgesia pump that has a mechanism for administering a basal rate also may be used for continuous infusion of epidural narcotics. These pumps have many safeguards in their operation that provide additional protection to the patient.
   b. Special pump tubing
   c. Appropriate in-line filter if one is not already on the epidural catheter
   d. 20-gauge, 1-in needle or needleless connector
   e. Povidone-iodine swabs
   f. Sterile 2 × 2 gauze squares
   g. Tape and labels indicating "epidural line"

Implementation

9. Read the name of the medication from the MAR, and compare it with the infusion bag label.
10. Check that the medication bag is labeled "for epidural use" and label is correct (first check).
11. Recheck the MAR and label on the infusion bag, and record use of narcotic (second check).
12. Attach the pump tubing to the medication container, set up the pump, attach the filter and needle (or connector) to the line, and attach appropriate labels.
13. Recheck the MAR and the infusion bag label (third check), and calculate the hourly rate.
14. Set up the pump on an intravenous stand.
15. Place an "epidural" label on the tubing.
16.–17. Follow steps 16 and 17 of the General Procedure: Approach and identify the patient, and explain what you are going to do.
18. Set up the infusion, and administer the medication as follows:
   a. Identify the epidural catheter by noting the written label.
   b. Clean the injection cap on the catheter with povidone-iodine *for infection control.* Do not use alcohol *because it is neurotoxic.*
   c. Dry the injection cap with a sterile 2 × 2 gauze *to prevent the formation of a sticky residue.*
   d. Attach the infusion set to the epidural catheter by inserting the needle or needleless connector into the injection cap.
   e. Tape the connection or use the built-in system connector *to secure the two lines together.*

ANALGESIA MONITORING RECORD

Date	5-22-99											
Time	1000	1200	14	16	18	20						
Resp. Rate	24	22	20	22	18	20						
Pain Scale • Appropriate box												
5–Excruciating												
4–Horrible												
3–Distressing	∗	∗										
2–Discomforting			∗	∗								
1–Mild					∗	∗						
0–None												
Sedation Scale												
SL–Sleeping/Not assessed 1–Alert 3–Rousable, drowsy frequently 2–Drowsy, occas. somnulent, hard to arouse	1	1	1	1	1	1						
Side Effects/Other Monitoring												
List if present: N–Nausea R–Respiratory Depression P–Pruris O–Other (write in) U–Urinary retention	Ø	Ø	Ø	Ø	Ø	Ø						
Numbness Level (local anesthetic/See reverse)	N/A											
Motor Function (only for local anesthetics) Y–Able to move knees U–Unable	N/A											
Analgesics and/or Local Anesthetics												
Type morphine sulfate												
Rate 1 ml/hour												
1–Cont. Infusion	✓	✓	✓	✓	✓	✓						
☐ IV ☑ Epi ☐ SQ												
New syringe/Bag hung (✓)												
Volume hung (cc)	50											
2–PCA Dose volume (ml)												
☐ IV ☐ Epi Lockout time (min)												
4 hr. limit												
3–New syringe hung (✓)												
4–Other Medications given (✓) (see M.A.R. for details)												
5–Total Narcotics infused per 8 hrs			4 mg									

Init	Signature	Init	Signature
WW	W. Wentzel RN		

Roberts, Jeffrey M. Age 67
510-02-7312
Dr. M°Carty

ADDRESSOGRAPH

Figure 58–2. Flow sheet for monitoring epidural pain management.

f. Turn on the pump, and set it according to the manufacturer's directions to deliver the prescribed dosage per hour.

19. Follow step 19 of the General Procedure: Leave the patient in a comfortable position.

20. Dispose of equipment.

21. Follow step 21 of the General Procedure: Wash your hands.

Evaluation

22. Evaluate the patient's response according to these criteria:
    a. Level of pain relief
    b. Presence of adverse effects

Documentation

23. Most facilities use flow sheets to record the data regarding medication administration and patient assessment.
    a. Document the concentration of fluid hung and the infusion rate.
    b. Record assessment data at regularly scheduled intervals, such as every hour initially then gradually moving to every 2 hours and then every 4 hours as pain relief and patient response are stabilized. Include respiratory rate, pulse, and blood pressure, and assessment for potential adverse responses (Fig. 58–2).

LONG-TERM CARE

Patients with permanent epidural catheters in place may be transferred from acute care to long-term care facilities for convalescence or terminal care. In the past, this was rare; therefore, nurses in these settings may be inexperienced in the use of epidural catheters. The acute care staff may arrange for learning materials and educational opportunities to support the long-term care nursing staff in providing quality care to the patient with an epidural catheter. This type of cooperative planning for effective care management is increasingly common. Procedures in long-term care will be the same as in acute care.

HOME CARE

Both intermittent and continuous epidural narcotics are used in the home setting to provide pain management to individuals with terminal or intractable pain. Permanent epidural catheters are usually placed while the individual is hospitalized, and response to the medications can be carefully monitored. The patient and family caregivers must be instructed in the techniques of epidural medication administration before the individual is discharged for home care. Some agencies provide excellent written and illustrated materials to support home care, including specific directions, drawings, and a place for record keeping. In addition, family caregivers will need to learn how to care for the catheter exit site. After initial teaching in the hospital, a home care nurse is needed for ongoing assessment and support for the client and family.

CRITICAL THINKING EXERCISES

• Katherine Stover has returned from surgery with a temporary epidural catheter in place. You are planning for her care. She has stated that she is not having any pain, but her back is itching, and she would like some lotion rubbed on it. As you make your plans for care, identify what assessment will be most important. Summarize the concerns you might have for her.

• Jonathan Baker has been diagnosed as being terminally ill with metastatic cancer that has spread to his spine. He was admitted for placement of an epidural catheter for pain control. He will be going home with his son. His son and daughter-in-law plan to care for him with the help of hospice nurses. Evaluate Mr. Baker's immediate and long-term care needs, and then formulate the plans you will make. Identify a variety of resources to assist this family.

PERFORMANCE CHECKLIST

Procedure for Administering a Medication Through an Epidural Catheter	Needs More Practice	Satisfactory	Comments
Assessment			
1. Review the medication administration record (MAR) or physician's order to identify the order for epidural medication.			
2.–3. Follow steps 2 and 3 of the Performance Checklist: General Procedure for Administering Medications in Module 47: Examine MAR for accuracy and completeness and review medication information.			
4. Check for type of epidural catheter (temporary or permanent).			
5. Assess the patient for baseline information a. Pain level			
b. Respiratory rate			
c. Blood pressure and pulse			
d. Ability to move lower extremities			
e. Sedation level			
Planning			
6.–7. Follow steps 6 and 7 of the General Procedure: Determine equipment needed, and wash your hands.			
8. Gather appropriate equipment. a. Povidone-iodine swabs			
b. 10–12 mL syringe with 20-gauge, 1-in needle			
c. Sterile 2 × 2 gauze sponges			
9. Read name of medication on MAR.			
10. Check label before picking up medication. Use prediluted solution or preservative-free sodium chloride for dilution.			
11. Recheck medication record and label on medication, and record use of narcotic.			
12. Prepare medication, using sterile technique. a. If prediluted, draw up into large syringe.			
b. If undiluted narcotic: (1) Draw narcotic into small syringe.			

(continued)

Procedure for Administering a Medication Through an Epidural Catheter *(Continued)*	Needs More Practice	Satisfactory	Comments
(2) Draw 10 mL of preservative-free saline into large syringe and air to equal narcotic volume.			
(3) Remove needle from large syringe, and insert needle of small syringe into large syringe tip. Inject narcotic into saline.			
(4) Replace needle on large syringe.			
(5) Gently rotate syringe to mix narcotic and saline.			
13. Recheck medication record, label on medication container, and syringe.			
Implementation			
14.–16. Follow steps 14 through 16 of the General Procedure: Place medication on cart or tray, place medication card or label on prepared medication, and approach and identify patient.			
17. Explain procedure to patient; if required, teach patient and caregivers to administer medication at home.			
18. Give the medication. a. Identify the epidural catheter by noting written label.			
b. Clean injection cap on catheter with povidone-iodine.			
c. Dry injection cap with sterile 2 × 2 gauze.			
d. Insert needle into cap.			
e. Aspirate. If blood or more than 1 mL clear fluid is returned, do not give medication.			
f. Inject medication.			
g. Remove the needle and syringe.			
19. Leave the patient in a comfortable position.			
20. Dispose of syringe and needle in sharps container.			
21. Wash your hands.			
Evaluation			
22. Evaluate patient's response: a. Pain relief			

(continued

Procedure for Administering a Medication Through an Epidural Catheter *(Continued)*	Needs More Practice	Satisfactory	Comments
b. Adverse effects			
Documentation			
23. Document on medication record of facility. Include name, dose, time, route, signature and patient's response.			
Procedure for Setting up a Continuous Epidural Infusion			
Assessment			
1. Review the MAR or physician's order to identify the order for epidural medication.			
2.–3. Follow steps 2 and 3 of the Performance Checklist: General Procedure: Examine MAR for accuracy and completeness, and review medication information.			
4. Check for type of epidural catheter (temporary or permanent).			
5. Assess the patient for baseline information. **a.** Pain level			
b. Respiratory rate			
c. Blood pressure and pulse			
d. Ability to move lower extremities			
e. Sedation level			
Planning			
6.–7. Follow steps 6 and 7 of the General Procedure: Determine equipment needed, and wash your hands.			
8. Gather appropriate equipment. **a.** Volume-controlled pump			
b. Pump tubing			
c. In-line filter			
d. 20-gauge, 1-in needle			
e. Povidone-iodine swab			
f. Sterile 2 × 2 gauze			
g. Tape and label indicating "epidural line"			

(continued)

Procedure for Setting up a Continuous Epidural Infusion *(Continued)*	Needs More Practice	Satisfactory	Comments
Implementation			
9. Read name of medication from medication record, and compare with infusion bag label.			
10. Check that medication bag is labeled "for epidural use" and label is correct.			
11. Recheck the medication record and label on the infusion bag, and record use of narcotic.			
12. Attach pump tubing to the medication bag, set up pump, and attach needle and label to line.			
13. Recheck the medication record and the infusion bag label, and calculate the hourly rate.			
14. Set up pump on IV stand.			
15. Place an "epidural" label on the tubing.			
16.–17. Follow steps 16 and 17 of the General Procedure: Approach and identify patient, and explain to patient.			
18. Set up the infusion: **a.** Identify epidural catheter.			
b. Clean injection cap with povidone-iodine swab.			
c. Dry injection cap with 2 × 2 gauze.			
d. Attach infusion set to epidural catheter.			
e. Tape the connection.			
f. Turn on and set pump.			
19. Leave the patient in a comfortable position.			
20. Dispose of equipment.			
21. Wash your hands.			
Evaluation			
22. Evaluate patient's responses: **a.** Level of pain relief			
b. Presence of adverse effects			
Documentation			
23. Record on medication record of facility. Include name of medication, dose, time, route, and patient's response.			

? Q U I Z

Short-Answer Questions

1. Give two reasons epidural narcotics may be used instead of oral narcotics.

   a. _____

   b. _____

2. Identify two safety precautions related to the administration of epidural narcotics.

   a. _____

   b. _____

3. How does the exit site care differ for a temporary and for a permanent epidural catheter?

   _____

   _____

   _____

4. List four adverse responses to epidural narcotics.

   a. _____

   b. _____

   c. _____

   d. _____

5. What action would be taken if the patient experiences respiratory depression from an epidural narcotic?

   _____

   _____

   _____

6. What action is commonly taken if the patient experiences pruritus from an epidural narcotic?

   _____

   _____

   _____

7. What assessment should the nurse make to determine whether there is any neural irritation in the patient with an epidural catheter?

   _____

8. Giving a narcotic antagonist to relieve pruritus has what effect on pain control?

   _____

GLOSSARY

abdominal breathing   Respirations in which the abdominal muscles and diaphragm are active; the abdomen moves out on inspiration and in on expiration; also called *diaphragmatic breathing.*

additive   A substance that is added to a medication or intravenous solution.

adhesive   A substance that causes two surfaces to stick to each other.

aeration   Exchanging oxygen and carbon dioxide between the blood and inspired air in the lungs.

AIDS (Acquired Immunodeficiency Syndrome)   A viral disease causing dysfunction of the immune system that can be transmitted through the blood and certain body fluids of infected persons.

air embolism   A bubble of air moving within the circulatory system.

alimental   Pertaining to nutritive material.

allergic reaction   Reaction to a blood transfusion in which the recipient experiences an antibody reaction to allergens in the donor's blood.

allergy   An abnormal body hypersensitivity to a specific antigen that is ordinarily harmless.

alveoli   Air sacs of the lungs, at the termination of a bronchiole.

ambient   Surrounding; encircling. Used to describe the normal air found in a room as ambient air.

Ambu bag   A device composed of a face mask and a large bag made of a flexible material that is used to force air into the lungs using positive pressure.

ambulatory surgery   Surgery done on a patient who has not been admitted for an overnight stay.

amino acid   An organic compound containing both an amino (nitrogen) group and a carboxylic acid (carbohydrate-related) group that is the basic component of the protein molecule.

amniotic   Fluid within the uterus that surrounds the unborn fetus.

amoeba   Any of various protozoans of the genus *Amoeba* and related genera, occurring in water, soil, and as internal animal parasites, characteristically having an indefinite, changeable form and moving by means of pseudopodia.

ampule   A small, sterile glass container that usually holds a parenteral medication.

analgesic   Any substance that relieves pain.

anastomose   To surgically connect two tubular organs.

anesthesia   (1) The total or partial loss of sensation. (2) The agents that are used to induce a loss of sensation.

anesthesiologist   A physician with special training in the science and skill of administering anesthetic agents.

anesthetist   A nonphysician who is skilled in administering anesthetic agents.

anoxia   A pathologic deficiency of oxygen.

antecubital space   A depression in the contour of the inner aspect of the elbow; also called *antecubital fossa.*

anticoagulant   Any substance that suppresses or counteracts coagulation, especially of the blood.

antiembolic stockings   Stockings that are designed to aid the venous flow of immobilized persons or persons with circulatory impairment, or to decrease peripheral venous disorders; also called *support hose* or *TEDs.*

antimicrobial   Capable of destroying or suppressing the growth of microorganisms.

antineoplastic   An agent that inhibits the growth of abnormal cell tissues or neoplasms.

antiseptic   Any substance that halts the growth of microorganisms, not necessarily by killing them.

apical pulse   The heartbeat heard through a stethoscope held over the apex of the heart.

apnea   The absence of respiration.

appliance   Any device worn by a person to facilitate the meeting of basic needs; for example, any device worn to contain drainage from an ostomy.

approximated   Wound edges that are touching.

armboard   A firm, flat padded device that is used to straighten the arm and/or hand, to keep an intravenous infusion in place.

ascitic fluid   An abnormal accumulation of serous fluid in the abdominal cavity; also called *ascites.*

aseptic   Preventing contamination by microorganisms; also see *surgical asepsis.*

asepto syringe   A medical instrument that is used to aspirate and instill a fluid. The tip is graduated in size so that it fits into tubings of various sizes; the rounded bulb is used to create suction to fill the barrel and pressure to expel the fluid.

asphyxiation   Suffocation.

aspirate   To remove gases or fluids by suction.

asymmetry   Difference in form or function on opposite sides of the body.

atelectasis   The collapse of a group of alveoli due to blockage of the bronchiole passage by secretions.

auricle   The external part of the ear; the pinna.

auscultation   Listening with a stethoscope to the sounds produced by the body.

autoclave   A device that establishes special conditions for sterilization by steam under high pressure.

autologous transfusion   A blood transfusion of the person's own blood that was donated previously or recovered and processed during a surgical procedure.

681

barrel In a syringe, the cylinder that holds the fluid.

bevel On a needle, the slanting end that contains the opening.

bifurcation The point at which a structure divides or separates into two parts or branches.

bolus A measured amount of medication delivered at one time, usually into a vein or intravenous device.

bronchi The branches of the trachea that lead directly to the lungs.

bronchial Pertaining to or affecting one or more bronchi; see *bronchi.*

bronchiole The fine, thin-walled, tubular branches of a bronchus.

Broviac catheter A single-lumen intravenous catheter with an internal diameter of 1.0 mm designed to be surgically implanted into a large central vein.

buccal Pertaining to the cheeks or oral cavity.

butterfly (1) A type of tape that is used to secure two wound edges together. (2) A device that is used to start intravenous infusions; named for its plastic "wings," which are used to secure the device in place.

button A small, round, plastic device that is used to plug a tracheostomy opening.

cannula A tube that is inserted into a bodily cavity to drain fluid or to insert medication. A tubing used to deliver oxygen to the nostrils.

canthus The corner at either side of the eye that is formed by the meeting of the upper and lower eyelids. The *inner canthus* is the corner next to the nose; the *outer canthus* is the corner to the outside of the face.

capsule A soluble gelatinous sheath that encloses a dose of oral medication.

cardiac output The amount of blood pumped by the heart in a minute. It is the volume pumped in each stroke times the number of beats per minute. In the normal resting adult it is usually 2.5–3.6 L.

catheter A slender flexible tube, of metal, rubber, or plastic, that is inserted into a body channel or cavity to distend or maintain an opening; often used to drain or to instill fluids or to provide suction.

catheterized A patient who has had a urinary catheter inserted for the purpose of draining urine from the bladder.

catheter-tip syringe Any syringe that has a smooth, funnel-type tip to allow it to fit tightly into any type of tubing.

caustic Able to burn, corrode, dissolve, or otherwise eat away by chemical action.

cauterize A technique that uses high heat to coagulate protein, thereby sealing blood vessels or cutting through tissue.

cecostomy A surgically devised opening directly from the cecum to the abdominal wall.

cephalic vein A large superficial vein of the upper arm.

cerumen A yellowish waxy secretion of the external ear; earwax.

circulatory overload A situation in which the volume of fluid circulating in the body is more than the heart can handle adequately. It can develop if a large amount of blood or fluid is infused in a short period.

citrated blood Blood that is prevented from coagulating by the presence of citrate-phosphate-dextrose or acid-citrate-dextrose.

claustrophobia A pathologic fear of confined places.

collaborative problem A patient problem that the nurse must assess for, identify when present, and report to the physician for treatment.

colostomy A surgically devised opening directly from the large intestine to the abdominal wall.

combustion Burning.

compatibility A situation in which two substances can be mixed without a reaction occurring.

compatible In agreement, harmony, or congenial combination. No reaction occurs when two agents are combined.

complete blood count (CBC) A measurement that establishes the values of a variety of components of the blood, usually including red blood count, white blood count, hemoglobin, and hematocrit.

compromised host A person with a suppressed immune system, who is therefore less capable of self-protection against pathogens.

concentration of solution The amount of a specified substance in a unit amount of another substance; may be expressed as a percentage (20% solution), or as a ratio (1:1000), or as a weight in a fluid amount (100 mg/L).

conjunctival sac The saclike inner fold of membrane on the lower eyelid.

constriction A feeling of pressure or tightness.

contaminated Having been in contact with microorganisms.

continent urinary reservoir (CUR) A surgical procedure in which a portion of the ileum is used to create a bladder-like structure for the collection of urine. A "nipple" valve on the skin surface allows intermittent self-catheterization.

cough reflex An involuntary nerve response that causes a cough.

cryoprecipitate A component of blood that contains Factor VIII—the factor hemophiliacs lack.

culture The growing of microorganisms in a nutrient medium.

cyanotic The presence of a bluish discoloration of the skin due to oxygen deficiency.

cycling Occurring in a pattern of regular repeated events. Used to refer to total parenteral nutrition or tube feeding schedules in which the daily intake is provided during a set number of hours followed by a number of hours with no feeding.

dead-air space The portion of the airway in which gas exchange does not take place.

debride To remove dead or necrotic tissue from the surface of a wound.

dehiscence The splitting or bursting open of a wound usually of the abdomen.

depilatory A substance or device that is used to remove hair.

dermatologic Pertaining to the skin.

descending colostomy A colostomy performed on a portion of the descending colon.

dextrose A simple sugar found in animal and plant tissue. Also called glucose.

diaphragm (1) A muscular membranous partition that separates the abdominal and thoracic cavities and that functions in respiration. (2) On a stethoscope, the flat, drumlike head that is used most often for listening to lung and bowel sounds.

diluent A substance that is used to dilute or dissolve.

disinfect To clean or rid of pathogenic organisms.

disinfectant An agent that disinfects by destroying, neutralizing, or inhibiting the growth of pathogenic microorganisms.

diuretic A drug that increases the production of urine.

donor One who donates blood, tissue, or an organ for use in a transfusion or transplant.

dorsal recumbent position Person lies on back with knees bent.

dose A specified quantity of a therapeutic agent, prescribed to be taken at one time or at stated intervals.

double-barrel colostomy A colostomy in which there are two openings—one that leads to the proximal colon and one that leads to the distal colon.

douche A stream of water that is applied to a part or cavity of the body for cleaning or medicinal purposes; most frequently, in relation to the vagina.

droplet nuclei Microscopic particles that, when surrounded by moisture, become airborne.

dura The outermost of the three membranes covering the spinal cord.

dyspnea Difficulty in breathing.

edema An excessive accumulation of serous fluid in the tissues. *Dependent edema* is fluid that has accumulated in the lower areas of the body due to gravity; *periorbital edema* is fluid that has accumulated in the soft tissue around the eyes; and *pretibial edema* is fluid that has accumulated over the tibia.

embolus A moving particle in the bloodstream.

emulsify To combine two solutions that do not normally mix into one liquid, resulting in a suspension of globules.

endotracheal tube A rubber or plastic tube that is placed in the trachea for purposes of ventilation.

enteral Within the gastrointestinal tract.

enteric Referring to the small intestine.

enterostomal therapist A person, often a nurse, with specialized preparation in the care of individuals with ostomies and skin management problems.

epidural Outside of the dura mater that covers the brain and spinal cord.

epithelial Related to the cellular surface of the skin or mucous membrane.

epithelialization The process by which the body creates epithelial tissue for wound healing.

erythrocyte Red blood cell.

ethmoid sinus The open cavity in the ethmoid bone that lies between the eyes and forms part of the nasal cavity.

eustachian tube A narrow opening that connects the middle ear to the pharynx that serves to equalize pressure on either side of the tympanic membrane.

evisceration Protrusion of a part through an incision after an operation.

excoriate To chafe or wear off the skin.

excoriation An abrasion or an irritated area of the skin.

expectorate To eject from the mouth; spit.

expiration Breathing out.

explosive Pertaining to a sudden, rapid, violent release of energy.

exudate Fluid drainage from cells.

fat emulsion A form of fats in which the particles are finely disbursed so as to form a smooth fluid.

febrile reaction Reaction to a blood transfusion that occurs when the recipient is sensitive to white cells in the blood being transfused and a fever develops.

fenestrated tracheostomy tube A tracheostomy tube that allows air to pass through the larynx, allowing the individual to talk while the tracheostomy tube is in place.

fibrin An insoluble protein essential to clotting of blood.

finger stick A method used to obtain a drop of blood for testing.

first-intention healing Uncomplicated wound healing that occurs when tissue is constructed between two wound surfaces that touch; also called *primary-intention healing.*

flowmeter A mechanical device that monitors the flow of oxygen or other gases or liquids.

fluid overload A situation in which there is more fluid in the circulatory system than it can handle; also called *circulatory overload.*

Foley catheter A rubber urethral catheter with an inflatable balloon at its end. When inflated, the balloon holds the catheter in place.

gag reflex A reflex action that results in gagging or vomiting when the pharynx is stimulated.

gastric sump tube (Salem) A gastric intubation tube having two lumens; one is used to apply suction and the second is used to provide an air vent to limit the level of suction that can be applied.

gatched bed A hospital bed that can be bent and raised at the knee area.

gauge A measurement of the diameter of a needle; a large number indicates a smaller diameter.

gavage Feeding by means of a tube.

Groshong catheter A central intravenous catheter that is inserted surgically and emerges from a subcutaneous tunnel on the chest. This catheter is characterized by a special tip which eliminates the need for heparin to maintain patency of the catheter.

hemodilution The dilution of blood by the presence of other fluids; done purposefully before surgery when a patient's blood is donated and then replaced with intravenous fluids. The donated blood is returned to the patient during or after the surgical procedure as replacement for the diluted blood lost during surgery.

hemolytic reaction   A reaction in which red blood cells are broken down as a result of incompatibility of the donor's red cells and the recipient's red cells.

hemophilia   A hereditary, plasma-coagulation disorder principally affecting males but transmitted by females and characterized by excessive, sometimes spontaneous bleeding.

hemophiliac   A person who suffers from hemophilia.

hemopneumothorax   The presence of blood and air in the pleural space.

hemorrhage   Bleeding; especially copious discharge of blood from the vessels.

hemothorax   The presence of blood in the pleural space.

heparin trap   A device filled with anticoagulant solution, used to provide ready access to a vein, making the presence of an infusing IV unnecessary; IV lock.

hepatitis   Inflammation of the liver, caused by infectious or toxic agents, characterized by jaundice and usually accompanied by fever and other systemic manifestations.

Hickman catheter   An intravenous catheter with an internal lumen diameter of 1.6 mm designed to be surgically implanted into a large central vein. Both single- and multiple-lumen models are available.

homeostasis   The tendency of all living tissue to restore and maintain itself in a condition of balance or equilibrium.

Homans' sign   Pain in the dorsal calf when the foot is firmly flexed; may be indicative of thrombophlebitis.

hub   On a needle, the portion that attaches to a syringe or tubing.

human serum albumin   A blood product composed of human simple proteins, which can be infused.

humidifier   An apparatus that increases the humidity of an enclosure.

hydrogen peroxide   A colorless, strongly oxidizing liquid made of hydrogen and oxygen.

hyperalimentation   Nutrition provided outside of the alimentary tract. Another term for parenteral nutrition; the introduction of nutrients into a large vein.

hypercalcemia   An excessive amount of calcium in the serum; greater than 10.5 mg/dl.

hyperglycemia   An excessive amount of glucose in the blood; greater than 120 mg/100 ml.

hyperkalemia   An excessive amount of potassium in the blood; greater than 5 mEq/L.

hypertonic   Having a higher osmotic pressure than body fluids.

hyperventilation   Abnormally fast or deep respiration in which excessive quantities of air are taken in and excessive carbon dioxide is expelled, which causes buzzing in the ears, tingling of the extremities, and sometimes fainting.

hypocalcemia   A deficit in calcium in the blood, less than 4.5 mEq/L.

hypothermia   A condition in which body temperature is lower than that necessary for body processes to function adequately.

hypoventilation   Abnormally slow or shallow respirations that result in inadequate air movement and thus inadequate oxygenation.

hypoxemia   Inadequate oxygenation of the blood.

hypoxia   An oxygen deficiency of body tissues.

ileoconduit   A surgically constructed pathway for urinary drainage in which a segment of ileum is detached from the rest of the bowel, the ureters are attached to this ileal segment, and one end of the segment is closed while the other opens onto the abdomen in a single stoma; also called *ileobladder* and *ileoloop*.

ileoloop   A surgical procedure that uses a portion of the small intestine to form a substitute or pseudobladder.

ileostomy   A surgically devised opening from the ileum to the abdominal wall, the drainage of which is liquid and contains some digestive enzymes.

incubate   To provide conditions for growth.

inferior vena cava   The large vein that returns blood to the heart from the lower body.

infiltration   Leaking of fluid from an intravenous line into the tissue surrounding the vein.

inflammation   Localized heat, redness, swelling, and pain as a result of irritation, injury, or infection.

inflatable cuff   A plastic balloonlike device, such as the one around a tracheostomy tube, that, when filled with air, expands, producing pressure on surrounding tissues.

Infus-a-port   A brand of surgically inserted subcutaneous central intravenous access port.

infusion pump   A mechanical device used to control the rate and volume of fluids administered parenterally.

infusion   The introduction of a solution into a vessel; commonly, the introduction of a solution into a vein.

inpatient   A person who has been admitted to an acute care facility.

inspiration   The act of breathing in; inhalation.

instill   To pour in drop by drop; commonly used to indicate very slow fluid introduction.

instillation   The process of pouring in drop by drop; commonly used to indicate a slow process of introducing fluid.

intensive care unit (ICU)   An area of a hospital set aside for the care of the critically ill.

intermittent   Stopping and starting at intervals.

intermittent infusion adapter   A device used to convert a regular intravenous needle into a heparin trap. (See *heparin trap*.)

intermittent infusion set   A set that delivers intravenous solutions into a vein at intermittent time periods; also called *heparin lock* or *IV lock*.

intracranial pressure   The pressure existing within the cranium.

intradermal   Injected into the skin layers.

intramuscular (IM)   Injected into the muscle tissue.

Intrasil catheter   An intravenous catheter designed to be inserted at a peripheral site on the arm and threaded through the vein until the tip rests in the right atrium.

intravenous   Placed into a vein; often used to refer to the fluid being given directly into a vein.

ntubation The placement of a tube into an organ or passage; often used to refer to placing an endotracheal tube into the trachea.

rrigate To wash out with water or a medicated solution.

solation To set apart from the environment so that organisms cannot be readily transferred from one person to another.

V lock or heparin lock A device filled with normal saline or heparized solution used to provide vascular access.

etone body A substance synthesized by the liver as a step in the metabolism of fats. May be present in abnormal amounts in situations such as uncontrolled diabetes mellitus.

aminar airflow hood A device that provides a controlled flow of microorganism-free air layers within a hood; used to create an environment for the sterile preparation of medications.

aparotomy A surgical incision into any part of the abdominal wall.

ateral Toward the side; away from the midline of the body.

ather A light foam that is formed by soap or detergent agitated in water.

avage Washing, especially of a hollow organ (stomach or lower bowel) by repeated injections of water.

esion A wound or injury in which tissue is damaged.

evin tube A slender rubber or plastic tube that is usually used for decompression or nasogastric feedings; also called *nasogastric tube.*

ingula The projection from the lower portion of the upper lobe of the left lung.

iniment A medicinal fluid that is applied to the skin by rubbing.

ipids (fats) A term used to indicate the fat emulsion given as part of total parenteral nutrition.

ter The metric equivalent of 1.0567 quarts, equal to 1000 milliliters.

obe A subdivision of the lung that is bounded by fissures and connective tissue.

ocal Of or affecting a limited part of the body; not systemic.

uer-Lok A brand name that is commonly used to refer to a type of syringe tip that fastens securely to the needle by a twisting action.

umen The inner, open space of a needle, tube, or vessel.

aceration A process in which an area of skin softens and deteriorates following prolonged contact with moisture.

eatus The opening of the urethra onto the surface of the body.

edial Toward the midline of the body.

ediastinal tube A chest drainage tube used to drain secretions from a surgical wound in the mediastinum.

ediastinum An area in the center of the chest which contains the heart, great vessels, trachea, esophagus, thymus gland, and lymph nodes.

edication administration record (MAR) A form used to identify, list, and document the medications administered to a patient.

meniscus The curved, upper surface of a liquid column.

microorganism An animal or plant of microscopic size, such as a bacterium, protozoan, fungus, or virus.

mucous Pertaining to mucus.

mucus The viscous suspension of mucin, water, cells, and inorganic salts that is secreted as a protective lubricant coating by glands in the mucous membranes.

nasal mucosa The mucous membrane lining of the nose.

nasogastric tube A long slender rubber or plastic tube that is introduced through the nose and esophagus into the stomach for purposes of feeding or aspiration.

nasopharynx The part of the pharynx immediately behind the nasal cavity and above the soft palate.

nebulizer A device that converts a liquid into a fine spray.

necrosis The death of living tissue.

neurotoxic Damaging to neural tissue.

noncoring needle A needle constructed so that it cuts a slit in a rubber stopper or diaphragm and does not cut out a cylindrical core.

normal flora Those microorganisms that are usually found at a site and that do not cause disease by their presence there.

NPO Nothing by mouth.

obturator Any device that closes the opening in a channel, such as a tracheostomy tube.

ocular Of or pertaining to the eye.

OD The right eye.

ointment One of the numerous, highly viscous or semisolid substances that are used on the skin as a cosmetic, an emollient, or a medicament; an unguent; a salve.

ophthalmic Of or pertaining to the eye or eyes; ocular.

oropharynx The part of the pharynx between the soft palate and the upper edge of the epiglottis.

OS The left eye.

ostomate A person who has an ostomy.

ostomy A surgically constructed opening from a body organ to the exterior of the body.

otic Of or pertaining to the ear.

OU Both eyes.

outpatient A patient who comes to the hospital, clinic, or dispensary for diagnosis and/or treatment but does not remain for ongoing care.

oximetry A procedure for measuring the oxygen saturation of the blood by measuring the reflectance of light transmitted by hemoglobin. Also referred to as "pulse oximetry."

oxygenation Treating, combining, or infusing with oxygen.

packed red blood cells Components of blood that make up the blood product remaining after most of the plasma is removed from whole blood.

paralytic ileus Immobilization of the intestinal wall resulting in acute obstruction and distention.

paraparesis A weakness or partial paralysis of the lower extremities.

parenteral Administered into the body in a manner other than through the digestive (enteral) tract; for example, through intramuscular or intravenous injection.

parenteral fluid Fluid given directly into tissues or blood vessels.

parietal pleura The serous membrane that lines the walls of the thoracic cavity.

Parkinson's position The patient is supine with the head tilted back hanging over the edge of the bed, and tilted to one side, to facilitate the administration of nose drops.

particulate matter Material made up of particles, often airborne or undissolved in a liquid.

patent Open.

pathogen Any agent, especially a microorganism, such as a bacterium or fungus, that causes disease.

pectoralis muscles Four muscles of the chest.

Penrose drain A flat, soft-latex tubing; short lengths are often used to provide drainage from a surgical wound, while longer lengths are sometimes used as tourniquets.

percussion (1) A process of striking a finger held against the body surface with a fingertip of the opposite hand and listening to the resulting sound as a part of assessment. (2) The striking of a hand on the chest wall to produce a vibration or shock that loosens secretions retained in the lungs.

percutaneous endoscopic gastrostomy (PEG) The insertion of a "mushroom" catheter through the abdominal wall into the stomach, using an endoscope to assure correct placement within the stomach.

perineum The portion of the body in the pelvic area that is occupied by urogenital passages and the rectum.

peristalsis Wavelike muscular contractions that propel contained matter along the alimentary canal.

pharynx The section of the digestive tract that extends from the nasal cavities to the larynx, there becoming continuous with the esophagus; functions as a passageway for both food and air.

phlebitis Inflammation of a vein.

piggyback An intravenous infusion setup in which a second container is attached to the tubing of the primary container through a short tubing.

pinna The flaring portion of the external ear that aids in the reception of sound waves. The auricle.

plasma The liquid portion of the blood after red and white blood cells and platelets are removed.

platelets Small, disk-shaped cells in the blood that adhere to any damaged surface and begin the clotting process; also called *thrombocytes*.

pleural space A potential space formed by the visceral and parietal pleura and containing only enough lubricating fluid to allow the two surfaces to slide smoothly over each other during inhalation and exhalation.

pleural tube A chest drainage tube used to drain secretions from the pleural space.

plunger In a syringe, the pistonlike rod that expels the fluid from the barrel.

pneumonitis Acute inflammation of the lung.

pneumothorax Accumulation of air or gas in the pleural cavity, occurring as a result of disease or injury or sometimes induced to collapse the lung in the treatment of tuberculosis or other lung diseases.

Port-a-cath A brand of surgically inserted subcutaneous central intravenous access port.

positive nitrogen balance A condition in which the amount of nitrogen taken into the body is greater than the amount excreted.

postanesthesia care unit (PACU) *see* postanesthesia recovery room.

postanesthesia recovery room (PARR) An area of the hospital set aside for the care of the immediate postoperative patient; also called the recovery room (RR) or postanesthesia care unit (PACU).

postural hypotension A sudden drop in blood pressure that is caused by a change in position, from lying to sitting or standing; may cause dizziness, fainting, and falling; also called *orthostatic hypotension*.

premeasured injection dose A glass container filled with a medication. The container fits into a holder in order to administer an injection.

Proetz's position The patient is supine with a pillow or other support under the shoulders, so that the head tilts straight back, to facilitate the administration of nose drops.

prongs (1) Sharp or pointed projections. (2) A device that delivers oxygen at the nares.

prophylactic Acting to defend against or to prevent something, especially disease.

pruritis Itching.

pulmonary embolus Obstruction of the pulmonary artery or one of its branches by an embolus.

purulent Containing or secreting pus.

pylorus The passage connecting the stomach and the duodenum.

recipient Person receiving blood, tissue, or an organ as a transfusion or transplant.

reconstituted A powder that has been mixed with a liquid so that it becomes a solution. Used to describe a powdered medication prepared for injection.

recovery room (RR) An area of a hospital set aside for the care of the immediate postoperative patient; also called the postanesthesia recovery room (PARR).

respirator A mechanical apparatus that administers artificial respiration; a ventilator.

right atrium The chamber on the right side of the heart that receives unoxygenated blood from the body

route In medication, a path of administration.

rubber-shod The presence of rubber tubing over the tips of hemostats or Kelly clamps to make them less traumatic.

saliva The secretion of the salivary gland, which contains mucus and digestive enzymes.

salvaged blood transfusion A transfusion using blood that is recovered and processed during a surgical procedure in order to be reinfused into the patient

anguineous Pertaining to or involving blood; containing blood.

clerose To develop scarring or connective tissue. In a blood vessel, this causes the vessel to be occluded.

econd-intention healing Healing that occurs through granulation beginning at the base of the wound; also called *secondary-intention healing.*

ecretions Substances that are exuded from cells or blood.

egment A subdivision of a lobe of the lung.

emi-Fowler's position A supine position with the head raised 12–18 inches.

ensory deprivation A lower level of sensory input than that required by an individual for optimum functioning.

epticemia An infection in which the pathogens are circulating in the bloodstream.

erosanguineous Containing both serum and blood.

erous Containing, secreting, or resembling serum.

erum hepatitis A form of hepatitis caused by a virus transmitted primarily by blood and body fluids; also called hepatitis B.

haft On a needle, the long narrow stem.

hock A syndrome characterized by insufficient blood and oxygen supply to the tissues; may be caused by hemorrhage, infection, trauma, and the like.

ilicone A flexible material used in the manufacture of tubes and prosthetic devices.

ims' position A side-lying position with the top leg flexed forward.

ingultus Hiccup.

kin barrier An agent to protect the skin from the discharge of urine or feces.

phenoid sinus The open area in the center of the sphenoid bone that lies at the base of the brain.

pore (1) An asexual, usually single-celled reproductive organism that is characteristic of nonflowering plants, such as fungi, mosses, and ferns. (2) A microorganism in a dormant or resting state that is especially resistant to destruction.

putum Expectorated matter that contains secretions from the lower respiratory tract.

tab wound A small intentional wound made with a scalpel in order to introduce a trocar, tube, or drain.

terile Free from bacteria or other microorganisms and their spores.

terile technique A method of functioning that is designed to maintain the sterility of sterile objects.

terilize To render sterile; also see *sterile.*

ternum A long flat bone that forms the midventral support of most of the ribs; the breastbone.

tethoscope An instrument that is used for listening to sounds produced in the body; also see *diaphragm.*

tock drugs Medications kept in a general supply, to be dispensed to individual patients.

toma The opening on the skin of any surgically constructed passage from a body organ to the exterior of the body.

topcock A valve that regulates a flow of liquid through a tube.

straight catheter A plain catheter without a bulb or balloon on its end.

stylet A thin metal wire or probe which fits inside a catheter or tube making it more rigid and easier to insert.

subclavian vein A vein of the upper body that lies under the clavicle.

subcutaneous (SC) Pertaining to tissue beneath the layers of the skin; sometimes called *hypodermic* (*H*), a term that can also mean "injection," and is, therefore, not recommended usage.

subcutaneous catheter port A wholly implanted device for access to a central vein consisting of a flexible rubber intravenous line and a rounded metal reservoir with a rubber diaphragm which is entered through a skin puncture with a special needle.

subcutaneous emphysema Air trapped in the subcutaneous tissue that "crackles" when palpated.

subdural Immediately under the dura mater that covers the brain and spinal cord.

sublingual Beneath the tongue.

subungual Under a fingernail or toenail.

suction Withdrawing (gas or fluids) through the use of negative pressure.

superior vena cava The large vein that returns blood to the heart from the upper body and head.

suppository A solid medication that is designed to melt in a body cavity other than the mouth.

suppurating Forming or discharging pus.

surgical asepsis The techniques that are designed to maintain the sterility of previously sterilized items and to prevent the introduction of any microorganisms into the body.

suspension A relatively coarse, noncolloidal dispersion of solid particles in a liquid.

symmetry The equal configuration of opposite sides.

syringe A medical instrument that is used to aspirate and expel fluids.

syrup A concentrated solution of sugar in water. A medicinal syrup has a drug added to the solution.

systemic Of, pertaining to, or affecting the entire body.

tablet A small flat pellet of medication that is taken orally.

TEDs A brand name that is commonly used as a synonym for antiembolic stockings; see *antiembolic stockings.*

tension pneumothorax A situation in which air gets trapped in the pleural space leading to buildup of pressure, which collapses the lung and causes mediastinal shift.

test dose A small amount of any substance that is given in order to assess for adverse reactions before regular administration is begun.

thoracentesis The insertion of a trocar into the pleural space of the chest for the removal of abnormal fluid.

thoracotomy A surgical incision of the chest wall.

three checks A safety measure that is used to ensure procuring the correct drug. The label is checked (1) before picking up the medication, (2) while holding it in the hand, and (3) after returning the container to its storage place.

thrombophlebitis   Inflammation of a vein resulting from the presence of a thrombus.

thrombus   A clot formed in a blood vessel.

thyroid gland   A two-lobed endocrine gland that is located in front of and on either side of the trachea.

tidal volume   The volume of air moved in or out during a normal breath.

tidaling   Fluctuation of the water level in the long tube in the waterseal bottle.

tolerance   In activity, the capacity to endure.

Toomey syringe   A large-barreled syringe with a graduated tip that fits into a tubing.

topical   Applied or pertaining to a local part of the body.

tortuous   Having or marked by repeated turns or bends; winding; twisting.

tourniquet   Any device that is used to stop temporarily the flow of blood through a large artery in a limb.

trachea   A thin-walled tube of cartilaginous and membranous tissue that descends from the larynx to the bronchi, carrying air to the lungs.

tracheal ring   The proximal, cartilaginous ringlike structure that surrounds the trachea.

tracheostomy   A surgically devised opening into the trachea from the surface of the neck.

transfer forceps   A sterile instrument with pincer or pronglike tips that is used to move sterile items from one sterile area to another.

transfer needle   A double-ended needle used to transfer medication from the medication container to the fluid container prior to intravenous administration.

transverse colostomy   A colostomy performed on a portion of the transverse colon.

Trendelenburg's position   Position in which the head is lower than the feet, with the body on an inclined plane.

triage   A process that prioritizes patients according to their condition so that the most expedient and appropriate treatment can be given to a large number of patients.

trocar   A sharp, pointed instrument used to enter a body cavity.

Tubex   A brand name for a system of metal or plastic syringes and prefilled medication cartridges.

tympanic membrane   The thin, semi-transparent, oval-shaped membrane that separates the middle ear from the inner ear; also called *eardrum*.

type   To determine the type of a blood sample.

type and crossmatch   A laboratory procedure used to identify whether the donor's and the recipient's blood are compatible. First, the type of blood (A, B, AB, and O and Rh factor) is determined. Then, the donor and recipient blood of the same type are mixed in order to observe for reactions.

unit dose   A system of dispensing drugs in which each dose is packaged and labeled individually.

ureterostomy   A surgically devised opening in which a ureter is brought out to drain directly through a stoma onto the abdomen.

urethra   The tubular structure leading from the bladder to the surface of the body.

uvula   The small, conical fleshy mass of tissue that is suspended from the center of the soft palate above the back of the tongue.

vagina   The passage leading from the external genital orifice to the uterus in female mammals.

vaginal   Pertaining to the vagina.

venipuncture   The puncture of a vein; for example, in drawing blood or administering intravenous fluids and medication.

vesicant   An agent which can cause blistering, necrosis, or the sloughing of tissues.

vial   A small glass container that is sealed with a rubber stopper; may be used for single or multiple doses of a parenteral medication.

vibration   A rapid, rhythmic to-and-fro motion.

visceral pleura   The serous membrane that covers the outside walls of the lungs.

viscosity   The degree of resistance to flow; thickness.

void   The emptying of urine from the bladder through the urethra; to urinate.

waterseal drainage   A chest drainage system that allows escape of air through a vent but prevents air from traveling back up the tube and into the pleural space.

wheal   A small acute swelling on the skin; may be caused by intradermal injections or by insect bites and allergies.

whole blood   Blood drawn from a living human being which contains all blood components and is prepared for use in transfusion.

xiphoid process   Bone of the sternum at the level of the seventh rib.

Z-track   A method for injecting medications that are particularly irritating or which stain the tissues; does not allow medication to track out through the needle hole.

ANSWERS TO QUIZZES

Module 32   Isolation Technique

1. **a.** To protect the patient
   b. To protect the environment
2. Strict isolation
3. Enteric isolation
4. Any three of the following: private room with running water; sign on door; stand outside door for equipment; laundry hamper inside room; wastebasket lined with plastic; thermometer and blood pressure equipment
5. No special precautions are used.
6. Thoroughly wash your hands, doing a complete scrub.
7. To protect the patient from infection
8. Sensory deprivation
9. Any three of the following: give her care first; answer her call light promptly; stop and visit often; find diversions for her
0. Disease specific: Acid-Fast Bacillus

Module 33   Sterile Technique

1. d	**6.** a, c	**11.** T
2. d	**7.** a	**12.** F
3. a	**8.** d	**13.** F
4. b	**9.** T	
5. c	**10.** F	

4. Any two of the following: heat-sensitive tape on outside of package; glass-tubing indicator inside pack; vacuum seal on bottle; intact seal on commercial package

Module 34   Surgical Asepsis: Scrubbing, Gowning, and Gloving

1. **a.** To remove microorganisms
   b. To remove dirt and oil
   c. To leave an antibacterial residue on the skin
2. Infection Control Committee
3. **a.** When serving as a scrub nurse in the operating room
   b. When serving as a scrub nurse in the delivery room
   c. When assisting with certain invasive diagnostic procedures
4. Because jewelry is a reservoir for bacteria
5. Because the wood may splinter and harbor microorganisms
6. It continues to inhibit the growth of microorganisms

7. So that the water containing dirt, oil, and microorganisms drains off the elbows, keeping the hands the cleanest part
8. It lessens the possibility of contaminating the gloves while putting them on.
9. Your back is considered potentially contaminated because you cannot see what happens to it.
10. Notify the appropriate person for assistance in changing.

Module 35   Wound Care

1. Three of the following:
   a. Protection
   b. Absorption
   c. Application of pressure
   d. Maintain a moist surface
2. **a.** To maintain sterile technique
   b. To observe and describe the wound
   c. To use appropriate dressing materials
3. **a.** Amount
   b. Color
   c. Consistency
   d. Odor
4. Any three of the following: edges approximated; smooth contour; minimal inflammation; minimal edema
5. Nonadherent
6. Paper tape
7. **a.** Breast surgery
   b. Hip surgery
   c. Perineal surgery
8. To protect the skin from the drainage
9. This action prevents spreading microorganisms from one site to another.
10. To debride the wound

Module 36   Ostomy Care

1. An opening from the ileum (small intestine)
2. The drainage is liquid and contains digestive enzymes, which increases the potential for skin breakdown.
3. Red and smooth without ulceration
4. **a.** Use a syringe without a needle to aspirate the urine.
   b. Use a tongue blade to gently remove feces from the stoma.
5. A portion of the ileum is dissected and folded back

689

on itself to form a structure for urine storage similar to the bladder. An advantage is that the patient performs self-catheterization and does not wear an appliance.
6. Seated on a toilet or commode
7. Approximately 1000 ml
8. 240 ml in each of three syringes, for a total of 720 ml
9. 3–5 inches
10. Approximately 15 minutes
11. Approximately 30 minutes after the patient gets up from the toilet
12. Because of the potential for urinary tract infection
13. Health teaching
    Referring patient and family to community resources

Module 37   Catheterization

1. Any three of the following: fear of pain; anxiety over intrusion into body; embarrassment over lack of privacy; anxiety over relationship to reproductive system
2. There was no opportunity for the patient to express concerns or ask questions.
3. It is normal to experience some frequency; often urine will be in small amounts; minimal burning; increase fluids and call the nurse to measure the output for 24 hours.

4. b	7. c	10. c
5. c	8. a	11. b
6. c	9. a	12. d

Module 38   Administering Oxygen

1. a. Oxygen tent
   b. Nasal catheter
   c. Nasal cannula
   d. Oxygen mask

2. c	5. b	8. d
3. b	6. c	9. d
4. d	7. b	10. d

Module 39   Respiratory Care Procedures

1. Because persons who are immobile tend to breathe shallowly, leaving areas of the lungs unused. These areas may collapse or accumulate secretions. Deep breathing opens and expands the areas and encourages secretions to move.
2. 1:2
3. To use gravity to facilitate the movement of secretions from the lungs to an area where they can be coughed up and expectorated
4. a. Sitting upright
   b. Leaning 45° to right
   c. Leaning 45° to left
   d. Leaning 45° forward
   e. Leaning 30°–45° backward

Module 40   Oral and Nasopharyngeal Suctioning

1. a. To allay fears
   b. To elicit cooperation
2. Because pathogens can travel down the moist, continuous respiratory tract
3. To remove amniotic fluid and mucus that accumulate in the back of the throat and interfere with breathing
4. To obtain adequate suction, or pull
5. Lateral position facing you
6. a. To promote drainage of secretions
   b. To prevent aspiration
7. 15 seconds
8. Three times
9. When the oxygen level of the patient is critical
10. When the infant is suspected of having an infection

Module 41   Tracheostomy Care and Suctioning

1. b	4. d	7. a
2. b	5. a	8. d
3. a	6. c	

Module 42   Caring for Patients with Chest Drainage

1. a. To remove air
   b. To remove fluid
   c. To restore the normal negative intrapleural pressure
2. Air in the pleural space
3. Anteriorly through the second intercostal space
4. Air rises.
5. a. Promotes drainage because of gravity
   b. Prevents backflow of bottle contents into pleural space
6. Controls amount of suction applied to the chest tube
7. a. Airtight system except for vent in waterseal bottle
   b. Vent open
   c. Waterseal in operation
8. Tension pneumothorax
9. Anxiety and pain
10. a. The lung is expanded.
    b. No air has entered the pleural space.

Module 43   Nasogastric Intubation

1. Any three of the following: feeding; instilling medications; irrigating the stomach; gastric suction
2. So as not to damage the mucosa on insertion
3. Nausea; gagging
4. c
5. b
6. c
7. c
8. b

Module 44   Preoperative Care

1. Elective surgery is planned; emergency surgery is urgent.
2. Your care must fit the specific time frame but will include the essentials of care.
3. **a.** Deep-breathing and coughing
   b. Moving in bed and getting in and out of bed
   c. Leg exercises
4. To empty the contents of the stomach, thereby preventing vomiting and possibly aspiration
5. **a.** To remove dirt, oil, and microorganisms from the skin
   b. To prevent the growth of remaining microorganisms
   c. To leave the skin undamaged and unirritated
6. Because studies have shown a reduced infection rate over earlier preoperative shaves
7. **a.** It is more comfortable for the patient.
   b. There is less chance of nicks and cuts.
8. **a.** To establish a baseline
   b. To detect whether the patient is febrile, which might indicate infection
9. **a.** Removing colored nail polish
   b. Removing makeup
   c. Removing dentures
10. **a.** To notify them in case of emergency
    b. To tell them when the surgery is completed
11. b
12. d
13. a
14. c

Module 45   Postoperative Care

1. **a.** Tissues
   b. Emesis basin
   c. Equipment for taking vital signs (thermometer, stethoscope, sphygmomanometer, blood pressure cuff)
   d. IV stand
2. Any six of the following: time of arrival on unit; responsiveness; vital signs; skin condition; dressing; presence of IV; presence of bladder catheter; presence of other drainage tubes; safety and comfort
3. **a.** Is the catheter unclamped?
   b. Is the catheter connected to the appropriate drainage container?
   c. Is the catheter freely draining?
   d. What are the amount and characteristics of the urine?
4. 2:30 PM. Received from PACU Drowsy, but answers to name call. T–97°; P–78; R–20, deep and easy; and BP–128/88. Skin warm and dry. Dressing clean, dry, and intact. P. Johnson, RN
5. Any seven of the following: operation performed; postoperative diagnosis; anesthetic agents used; estimated blood loss; blood and/or fluid replacement in surgery and PACU; type and location of drains; vital signs when patient left PACU; medications administered in PACU; output; physician's orders
6. Any three of the following: localized pain; heat and swelling in lower extremities; positive Homan's sign
7. All of the following: encourage early ambulation; encourage fluids; administer stool softeners per physician's orders
8. Any three of the following: encourage early ambulation; encourage patient's participation; keep patient and unit tidy; listen; do patient teaching
9. Place flat with legs elevated
   Report status to surgeon
   Be prepared to administer prescribed: IV fluids, blood, medications
10. Altered Patterns of Urinary Elimination:
    Urinary Retention
    Constipation
11. Decreases the incidence of postoperative complications
    Patients feel less stress.
12. Statements regarding anxiety and feelings of "nervous"
    Rapid pulse and respiration

Module 46   Irrigations: Bladder, Catheter, Ear, Eye, Nasogastric Tube, Vaginal, Wound

1. **a.** Cleaning
   b. Instilling medications
2. To instill medication
3. One of the following: eye, wound; bladder; catheter
4. One of the following: ear, nasogastric tube; vagina
5. **a.** Too high temperature
   b. Too great pressure
   c. Incorrect solution concentration
6. That the drainage or outflow tubing not be blocked or clamped while fluid is being introduced
7. When the tympanic membrane is not intact
8. The fluid will tend to drain out too quickly and not come in contact with all vaginal surfaces
9. To prevent the spread of microorganisms from one eye to the other
10. For seriously contaminated, traumatic wounds
11. Eye irrigations to remove dust particles and secretions, ear irrigations to remove buildup of ear wax, and catheter irrigations to keep catheter patent to decrease risk of infection.
12. The antiseptic powders used may cause irritation in some susceptible females.
13. When any splashing might occur.

Module 47   Administering Medications: Overview

1. **a.** Stock supply
   b. Individual patient supply
2. **a.** As it is taken off the shelf
   b. Before opening
   c. Before it is replaced

3. **a.** Right drug
   b. Right dose
   c. Right route
   d. Right patient
   e. Right time
   f. Right documentation
4. **a.** Identification band
   b. Ask to state name
5. gr 1/60
6. 30 ml
7. 15 or 16 min
8. 1 ʒ
9. 300 mg (or 325 mg)
10. 2 teaspoons
11. d
12. c
13. c
14. d
15. d

Module 48 Administering Oral Medications

1. d	5. c	9. a
2. b	6. b	10. d
3. a	7. b	11. c
4. c	8. a	12. b

Module 49 Administering Medications by Alternative Routes

1. a
2. c
3. b
4. Because of the danger of aspiration pneumonia with oil-based solutions
5. Ethmoidal and sphenoidal sinuses
6. Any three of the following: to protect, to soften, to soothe, to provide relief from itching
7. **a.** Dorsal recumbent position with knees flexed
   b. Sims' position
8. 20 minutes
9. Beyond the internal sphincter
10. To help the patient relax
11. By fully exhaling first, then inhaling when the puff is activated, and breathing in around the mouthpiece.

Module 50 Giving Injections

1. **a.** Glass or Luer-Lok
   b. Disposable plastic
   c. Prefilled
   d. Cartridge
2. There are 100 units of insulin in 1 ml.
3. Length, gauge
4. **a.** Vials
   b. Ampules
5. Vial
6. Any three of the following: almost complete absorption; more rapid absorption; gastric disturbances do not affect the medication; patient does not have to be conscious or rational
7. 25-gauge, ⅝-inch needle
8. **a.** Upper arms
   b. Anterior aspect of thighs
   c. Lower abdominal wall
9. Intramuscular route
10. 22-gauge, 1½-inch needle
11. **a.** Upper iliac crest
   b. Inner crease of the buttocks
   c. Outer lateral edge of the body
   d. Lower (inferior) gluteal fold
12. Any three of the following: no large nerves or blood vessels; cleaner; less fatty; several positions can be used; better for small children because gluteal muscle is not well developed until after a child walks
13. **a.** Small muscle, so not capable of absorbing large amounts of medication
   b. Danger of injury to the radial nerve
14. The plunger is pulled back (aspiration)
15. To see whether the needle has penetrated a blood vessel

Module 51 Administering Medications to Infants and Children

1. 25.88 mg
2. 192,000 units
3. Four or 5 years of age
4. Dosages are small, so an error that is numerically small may have profound effects.
5. To enable the parent to maintain the role of comforter and protector
6. The choice of *not* taking a medication is an unacceptable action and should not be offered to a child.
7. A tuberculin (1 ml) syringe
8. **a.** 1600 mg/24 h
   b. 400 mg/dose
9. **a.** Preference of the child
   b. Nature of the medication
   c. Taste of the medication
   d. Diet prescribed for the child
10. **a.** The infant might not take it all and you would be unable to determine dosage given.
    b. The infant might reject the bottle.

Module 52 Preparing and Maintaining Intravenous Infusions

1. Microdrip set
2. Secondary administration set
3. No contaminated air can enter the container and come in contact with the sterile fluid.
4. Obtain another container and return the cloudy one to the source.
5. **a.** Hang it so the fluid level is higher.
   b. Put the second container on an extension hanger to make it lower than the first.

6. **a.** 31 gtt/min
   b. 24 gtt/min
   c. 33 gtt/min
   d. 33 gtt/min
7. Container every 24 hours, tubing every 48–72 hours
8. Too much fluid over a short period of time will simply be excreted *or* will cause fluid overload; too little fluid may not meet the body's needs for fluid.
9. **a.** Direct pressure on the site
   b. Raising the patient's arm above the head
10. **a.** Clot over the cannula lumen
    b. Clogged filter
    c. Lumen of the needle against the vein wall
    d. Kinking or pressure on the tubing
    e. Arm position
11. **a.** Pain
    b. Redness
    c. Swelling
    d. Warmth
12. **a.** Pallor
    b. Swelling
    c. Coolness
    d. Pain
    e. Diminished IV flow
13. **a.** Review entire system.
    b. Check container.
    c. Check drip chamber.
    d. Check tubing.
    e. Check IV site.
    f. Check extremity if armboard is in use.

Module 53 Administering Intravenous Medications

1. Because ports are made of self-sealing rubber. If a needle were inserted into plastic, the system would leak.
2. Slowly (approximately 1 ml/min), because it will be less irritating
3. To prevent the patient from receiving an inaccurate dosage of a lighter or heavier additive rather than the primary solution
4. Visual and chemical
5. A drug text or the manufacturer's literature
6. To provide access to the circulatory system without having to do repeated venipuncture
7. So that the pump mechanism will deliver the drug at the desired rate
8. To keep blood from coagulating in the lock
9. 50–100, depending on the drug manufacturer's directions

Module 54 Caring for Central Intravenous Catheters

1. **a.** To permit the infusion of solutions that would be too irritating to peripheral veins
   b. When peripheral veins have been used exten-

sively or are otherwise unsuitable for intravenous lines
2. **a.** Infection
   b. Air embolism
3. **a.** To allow for assessment of the entry site
   b. To thoroughly cleanse the area and remove debris
   c. To apply antiseptic or antimicrobial ointment to decrease future growth of organisms
   d. To replace potentially contaminated dressings with sterile ones
4. Acetone increases the incidence of local skin irritation without decreasing the incidence of infection.
5. To provide a chemical and mechanical barrier to microbes
6. Because it might easily be mistaken for a peripheral IV. This could have serious consequences.
7. To prevent air embolus
8. The Hickman catheter has an internal diameter of 1.6 mm and can be used for drawing blood and administering nutrients, fluids, and medications. The Broviac catheter has an internal diameter of 1.0 mm and cannot be used for drawing blood but can be used for all infusions.
9. Repeated punctures of the cap with needles large enough to draw blood will damage the cap, leading to leakage.
10. To prevent air from entering and causing an air embolism
11. A noncoring needle (sometimes called a Huber needle)
12. Iodophor-iodine solution

Module 55 Starting Intravenous Infusions

1. **a.** May imply serious illness
   b. Pain
   c. Immobility
2. Any two of the following: to maintain daily fluid requirements; to replace past losses; to provide large amount of fluid rapidly; to provide medication
3. **a.** Butterfly
   b. Through-the-needle IV access devices
   c. Over-the-needle IV access devices
4. **a.** Scalp
   b. Less chance of dislocation because less movement in that area
5. **a.** Applying a tourniquet
   b. Hand pumping
   c. Keeping arm in dependent position
   d. Applying warm, moist heat
6. Tincture of iodine; 70% alcohol
7. Date; time; type of device; catheter gauge; initials

Module 56 Administering Blood and Blood Products

1. **a.** Blood donated by an unrelated donor.
   b. Blood donated by a related donor.

c. Blood donated by the recipient before elective surgery.

d. Blood obtained before surgery and replaced with blood expanders until blood is needed and re-infused.

e. Blood salvaged during surgery, filtered and re-infused.

2. Increasing fear of the transmission of certain diseases.

3. The same tests are performed on autologous blood and blood from an unrelated donor.

4. **a.** Restoration of circulating blood volume
   b. Replacement of clotting factors
   c. Improvement of oxygen-carrying capacity

5. **a.** Makes it possible to serve more needs with fewer donations
   b. Decreases the risk of complications

6. **a.** To increase oxygen-carrying capacity
   b. To increase circulating blood volume

7. **a.** A
   b. B
   c. AB
   d. O

8. Any four of the following: hemolytic, febrile, allergic, transmission of disease, circulatory overload, hypothermia, hyperkalemia, hypocalcemia, air embolus

9. Any four of the following: flank pain, dark urine, chest constriction, tachypnea, fever, chills, apprehension

10. **a.** Slow transfusion.
    b. Notify physician.
    c. Give antihistamine as ordered.

11. By covering the blood filter completely with blood before infusing

12. Because it may hemolyze the red cells it contacts

13. **a.** Recipient's name and spelling
    b. Recipient's hospital number as on face sheet of patient record
    c. Blood product type and Rh

d. Blood unit identification number
e. Expiration date on blood bag

Module 57 Administering Parenteral Nutrition

1. Dextrose, protein, electrolytes, amino acids, vitamins, and calories

2. Patients who cannot eat for long periods of time or those who have sustained major trauma, pathology of the intestinal tract, or long-term illness

3. Patients who only need a temporary adjunct to their nutritional status

4. The rate of infusion must be controlled accurately.

5. Infection

6. Of irritation of the veins

7. Hyperglycemia

8. Fractional urine or blood specimens

9. Fat emulsions

10. 10% and 20%

11. If 10%, 1 ml/minute for 15 minutes

12. If 20%, .5 ml/minute for 15 minutes

Module 58 Giving Epidural Medications

1. **a.** To decrease the side effects and allow the patient to be more alert
   b. To allow lower doses of narcotics to be used

2. Identification of the catheter and observation for adverse reactions

3. Permanent catheter is dressed in the same way as an indwelling central intravenous catheter. Temporary catheter has an occlusive dressing that is not changed until the catheter is removed.

4. Any four of the following: respiratory depression, urinary retention, hypotension, pruritis, reversible paraparesis

5. Administer the ordered narcotic antagonist.

6. An antihistamine is given. If that is not successful, a narcotic antagonist is given in small incremental doses

☰ INDEX

Page numbers followed by *f* indicate illustrations; *t* following a page number indicates tabular material.